50 Years of Immunization—Steps Forward

50 Years of Immunization—Steps Forward

Guest Editors

Imran Raza Mirza
Ephrem Tekle Lemango
Ann Lindstrand

MDPI

Basel • Beijing • Wuhan • Barcelona • Belgrade • Novi Sad • Cluj • Manchester

Guest Editors
Imran Raza Mirza
Program Group/Health
United Nations Children
Fund
New York, NY
USA

Ephrem Tekle Lemango
Program Group/Health
United Nations Children
Fund
New York, NY
USA

Ann Lindstrand
Essential Programme on
Immunization Unit,
Immunization Vaccines &
Biologicals Department
World Health Organization
Geneva
Switzerland

Editorial Office
MDPI AG
Grosspeteranlage 5
4052 Basel, Switzerland

This is a reprint of the Special Issue, published open access by the journal *Vaccines* (ISSN 2076-393X), freely accessible at: https://www.mdpi.com/journal/vaccines/special_issues/E78S6A5XFF.

For citation purposes, cite each article independently as indicated on the article page online and as indicated below:

Lastname, A.A.; Lastname, B.B. Article Title. *Journal Name* **Year**, *Volume Number*, Page Range.

ISBN 978-3-7258-4685-6 (Hbk)
ISBN 978-3-7258-4686-3 (PDF)
https://doi.org/10.3390/books978-3-7258-4686-3

Cover image courtesy of UNICEF/UNI503298/Al-Safadi

Contents

About the Editors

Imran Raza Mirza

Imran Mirza is a senior global public health expert and medical epidemiologist, currently serving as a Health Specialist at UNICEF headquarters in New York. He leads UNICEF's global work on COVID-19 vaccine integration into primary health care systems and the development of life course immunization platforms. With more than 20 years of experience across humanitarian, fragile, and development settings, Dr. Mirza has held strategic leadership positions at both the national and global levels.

His technical expertise spans immunization system strengthening, emergency response, maternal and child health, vaccine delivery in complex contexts, and health system integration. As a trained physician with a Master of Science in Epidemiology, he has supported governments in optimizing immunization service delivery and planning, particularly through national integration workshops developed in collaboration with the WHO, Gavi, and other global partners.

Dr. Mirza has led the development of the Global Strategy to Defeat Meningitis by 2030, global implementation guidance, eLearning platforms, and decision-making tools for immunization in emergencies and integrated service delivery. He currently serves as UNICEF's global lead for Mpox vaccination and represents the organization in several international coordination mechanisms, including the Global Task Force for Cholera Control, the International Coordinating Group for emergency vaccine stockpiles, and IA2030 working groups.

He has co-authored peer-reviewed publications on vaccine delivery, health system resilience, and immunization in the second year of life. He also served as Guest Editor for the *Vaccines* journal's Special Issue on "Challenges and Future Trends of COVID-19 Vaccination." A committed advocate for equity, Dr. Mirza champions the integration of immunization into broader primary health care strategies to reduce child and maternal mortality and advance universal health coverage.

Ephrem Tekle Lemango

Ephrem Tekle Lemango is a global public health leader currently serving as Associate Director for Immunization at the UNICEF headquarters in New York. In this capacity, he guides global strategies to strengthen immunization delivery systems and broader primary health care frameworks. With a medical degree from Addis Ababa University and a master's from the University of Leeds, he blends academic expertise with extensive practical experience across various settings. Prior to joining UNICEF, Dr. Lemango worked for the World Health Organization Regional Office for Africa as an immunization and primary health care focal. He served as the Executive Director of the International Institute for Primary Health Care under Ethiopia's Ministry of Health and led the Maternal, Child Health, and Nutrition portfolio of the country. In these roles, he was instrumental in leading the implementation of high-impact programmes that improved the access to and quality of maternal and child health services. Dr Lemango has also served as Assistant Professor of Health Management, Planning and Policy in Mekelle University.

At UNICEF, Dr. Lemango is responsible for defining global strategic directions and priorities in health and immunization programming. He represents UNICEF in high-level platforms, including Immunization Agenda 2030; Gavi, the Vaccine Alliance; and other key vaccination-focused partnerships.

Dr. Lemango has co-authored peer-reviewed articles and official UNICEF guidance on immunization system strengthening, childhood vaccination strategies, and multisectoral approaches to reaching zero-dose children. Through his technical leadership, policy influence, and scholarly engagement, Dr. Ephrem Tekle Lemango continues to shape equitable and sustainable immunization services, particularly for underserved communities in resource-constrained settings.

Ann Lindstrand

Ann Lindstrand is a Swedish pediatrician and global public health specialist who currently serves as Head of the Essential Programme on Immunization at the World Health Organization (WHO) in Geneva. Since 2018, she has led the WHO's global efforts to advance the Immunization Agenda 2030 (IA2030), providing strategic direction, policy guidance, and advocacy tools to support countries in strengthening routine immunization systems across the life course.

Dr. Lindstrand holds an MD and MPH from Harvard and a PhD from the Karolinska Institutet in Sweden. Prior to joining the WHO, she held senior positions in Sweden's national immunization programme, including National Programme Manager for Immunization, Chair of the National Immunization Technical Advisory Group, and Head of Pediatric Preventive Services in Stockholm. In these roles, she led national vaccine strategy development, enhanced child health services, and guided immunization policy.

Her extensive international field experience includes work with Médecins Sans Frontières in Mozambique, Angola, India, Guinea Conakry, and French Guiana. She has also lectured on global pediatrics with the Karolinska Institutet in countries such as Tanzania, Cuba, and India.

Dr. Lindstrand has authored numerous publications on vaccination policy, digital innovation, vaccine safety, and adult immunization. She led the development of the 2024 *Vaccine* supplement outlining IA2030's operational framework and co-authored a 2025 review on post-COVID-19 adult immunization policies. Under her leadership, the WHO has launched 16 Vaccine Value Profiles to inform evidence-based decision making.

A passionate advocate for vaccine equity, Dr. Lindstrand focuses on reaching refugees, migrants, and vulnerable populations. She actively engages in public communication to counter misinformation and promote vaccine confidence. Her leadership and commitment continue to shape global immunization policy and advance universal health coverage.

Preface

The year 2024 marks a significant milestone in global public health—the 50th anniversary of the Expanded Programme on Immunization (EPI). Launched in 1974 with the goal of ensuring equitable access to life-saving vaccines for every child, regardless of geography or socioeconomic status, EPI has since become one of the most transformative and enduring public health initiatives in history.

Over the past five decades, EPI has played a central role in expanding immunization coverage, reducing childhood mortality, and protecting communities from vaccine-preventable diseases. Reflecting its broadened scope and evolving priorities, the programme is now recognized as the *Essential Programme on Immunization*, encompassing vaccines across the life course, including those for adolescents and adults.

This *Special Issue of the journal Vaccines—"50 Years of Immunization—Steps Forward"*—brings together more than 25 contributions from global health leaders, researchers, and practitioners. The collection offers historical reflections, current analyses, and future-oriented perspectives. Articles span global reviews, regional assessments, and country-level case studies, with a strong focus on the experiences of low- and middle-income countries.

The issue also highlights the programme's catalytic role in driving innovation—across vaccine delivery systems, digital technologies, monitoring and safety frameworks, and integration with broader health systems.

As we commemorate EPI's 50-year legacy, this Special Issue serves not only as a celebration of its achievements but also as motivation to renew commitment and encourage action to strengthen immunization for all, across every stage of life.

Imran Raza Mirza, Ephrem Tekle Lemango, and Ann Lindstrand
Guest Editors

vaccines

MDPI

Editorial

Expanded Programme on Immunization (EPI): A Legacy of 50 Years and the Road Ahead

Imran Mirza [1,*], Ephrem Tekle Lemango [1] and Ann Lindstrand [2]

1 United Nations Children Fund (UNICEF) Headquarter, New York, NY 10017, USA; elemango@unicef.org
2 Essential Programme on Immunization Unit, Immunization Vaccines & Biologicals Department, World Health Organization (WHO), 1202 Geneva, Switzerland; lindstranda@who.int
* Correspondence: imirza@unicef.org; Tel.: +1-9172854670

1. A Global Health Triumph

Throughout history, disease and epidemics have shaped human survival. However, the introduction of vaccines transformed this narrative, offering powerful protection against deadly infections. After World War II, Europe faced dire living conditions that fueled the spread of diseases like tuberculosis (TB), especially among children. In response, health workers deployed the BCG vaccine widely, reaching over 11 million children by 1950 [1]. This milestone, as well as the successful smallpox eradication program, marked a turning point in public health, laying the foundation for global immunization efforts that would go on to protect millions of children from other life-threatening diseases such as measles, diphtheria, and pneumonia.

Fifty years ago, the World Health Organization (WHO) launched [2] the Expanded Programme on Immunization (EPI) to ensure that children across the world, regardless of their socioeconomic status, had access to life-saving vaccines. What began as an ambitious initiative to combat six major infectious diseases—diphtheria, pertussis, tetanus, measles, poliomyelitis, and tuberculosis—has since evolved into one of the most significant public health interventions in history [3]. A recent study [4] showed that every dollar spent on immunization during 2011–2020 produced an average return of up to USD 26 across a child's lifetime, thanks to savings on health care expenditure and lost revenues due to illness. Today, rebranded as the Essential Programme on Immunization (EPI), the initiative has expanded its reach, integrated newer vaccines, and adapted to emerging health challenges. By preventing at least 154 million deaths since 1974, the program has dramatically reshaped the trajectory of global health, contributing to infant survival, disease eradication efforts, and broader health care infrastructure development [3].

As we commemorate the 50th anniversary of EPI, it is important to take stock of the gains in public health this flagship program has accomplished (Table 1), although this global health architecture is also currently under acute financial threat. This Editorial takes an in-depth look at EPI's evolution, achievements, challenges, and the future course of immunization efforts worldwide.

Table 1. Key achievements of EPI over 50 years.

Dramatic Improvements in Child Survival Rates
• Immunization contributed to a 40% decline in global under-five mortality from 1974 to 2024. • Pneumococcal and rotavirus vaccines have significantly reduced hospitalizations due to pneumonia and diarrhea. • Countries with high routine vaccination coverage saw improved overall health indicators.
Disease Eradication and Reduction in Vaccine-Preventable Diseases
○ Smallpox was declared eradicated in 1980, proving the success of mass vaccination campaigns. ○ Measles deaths declined by 73% between 2000 and 2018 due to routine immunization and mass vaccination campaigns. ○ Polio cases dropped by over 99.9%, with wild poliovirus cornered in a few neighboring districts of two endemic countries. Neonatal tetanus has been eliminated in most countries, with 10 remaining, reducing newborn mortality significantly.
Global Immunization Reach
○ Today, over 85% of infants worldwide receive at least three doses of the DPT vaccine. Hardly any other health intervention reached as many children as possible each year, even considering a growing cohort of births, in particular in Africa. ○ Immunization programs now reach the most remote and marginalized communities, including refugee camps and conflict zones, and are now expanded to target adolescents and adults, including HPV, influenza, and COVID-19 vaccines.
Development and Deployment of New Vaccines
○ The introduction of HPV vaccines for adolescent girls has cut cervical cancer risk by over 80% in some countries. ○ The development of malaria and Ebola vaccines represents a historic milestone in immunization science. ○ Regional vaccines such as Japanese encephalitis, TCV, etc.
Key Innovations in Cold Chain Logistics
○ Vaccine Vial Monitors (VVMs): These small labels change color if a vaccine is exposed to heat for too long, reducing vaccine wastage. ○ Solar-Powered Refrigerators: A game-changer for off-grid and rural areas, ensuring continuous refrigeration without reliance on electricity. ○ Ultra-Cold Storage Solutions for mRNA Vaccines: The development of portable ultra-cold freezers has expanded mRNA vaccine distribution to low-resource settings. ○ Remote Temperature Monitoring (RTM) Systems: Digital tracking devices now send real-time alerts if vaccines are exposed to unsafe temperatures. ○ Next-Generation Cold Chain Equipment (CCE): Introduction of passive cold chain devices that can store vaccines for up to 30 days 5–7 days without electricity.

2. The Evolution of EPI: Expanding Immunization Frontiers

2.1. The Early Years (1974–1990): Laying the Foundation

The first 15 years of the Expanded Programme on Immunization focused on establishing standardized immunization schedules and ensuring access to vaccines in low-income countries through standardized vaccination programs and outreach campaigns. Vaccination coverage was alarmingly low, with only about 5% of children in low-income countries and 21% worldwide receiving basic vaccines in 1974.

The turning point came in 1980 with the certification of the global eradication of smallpox, proving that a well-coordinated vaccination campaign could wipe out a deadly disease. This success laid the groundwork for more ambitious vaccination efforts, particularly the push for polio eradication in the late 1980s.

During this phase, UNICEF, WHO, and global donors played a critical role in advocacy for immunization, funding vaccine procurement, training health care workers, and strengthening cold chain logistics to reach the most vulnerable populations.

From 1982 to 1990, coverage increased with speed globally, from around 20 to 76% of DTP3 [5], fueled by the 'Child Survival and Development Revolution' initiated by Jim Grant in UNICEF [6] and jointly supported by WHO.

However, a major challenge during this phase was the lack of robust cold chain systems that can keep vaccines potent at the last mile, especially in low-resource settings where electricity and refrigeration were unreliable.

2.2. The Growth Phase (1990–2010): Introduction of New Vaccines and Cold Chain Innovations

As global immunization coverage increased more slowly in the 1990s—reaching over 81% for diphtheria, pertussis, and tetanus (DPT3) vaccines by 2008—the EPI expanded its scope [7]. Several key milestones defined this period, such as the introduction of hepatitis B, Hemophilus influenza type b (Hib), and pneumococcal conjugate vaccines (PCV) into routine immunization schedules.

The launch of GAVI, the Vaccine Alliance, in 2000 played a transformative role in funding vaccine access for lower-income countries (LIC). Since then, the GAVI Alliance, initially formed by WHO, UNICEF, BMGF, and the World Bank and later expanding to many more partners, has helped countries to reach over 1 billion children with lifesaving vaccines and expanded the number of vaccines available for low- and middle-income countries (LMIC) from protection of 7 to 20 infectious diseases.

Innovations and an expanded use of new vaccine delivery technologies happened during the phase, such as auto-disable syringes and better cold chain storage solutions, ensuring improved vaccine safety and efficiency. Another key achievement in this phase was the introduction of vaccine vial monitors (VVMs)—a critical innovation allowing health care workers to detect heat exposure in vaccines—as well as an expansion of cold chain storage capacity, including solar-powered refrigerators, enabling better vaccine storage in rural and off-grid areas [8].

By the early 2000s, innovations in logistics, temperature monitoring, and transportation had significantly reduced vaccine wastage and improved reach to last-mile populations. By 2010, it resulted in over 100 million infants being vaccinated annually, preventing millions of deaths and hospitalizations due to vaccine-preventable diseases, and bringing global DTP3 vaccine coverage to 83% [9].

2.3. The Current Era (2010–2024): Addressing New Challenges and Expanding Immunization Technologies

Over the last decade, immunization programs have faced both remarkable achievements and unprecedented challenges—the EPI has had to navigate new obstacles such as pandemic/outbreak-related disruptions (e.g., Ebola, H1N1 influenza, Zika, COVID-19, etc.), vaccine hesitancy, and the need for advanced cold chain solutions for new-generation vaccines.

Some of the major achievements in this phase were the introduction of new vaccines such as rotavirus, HPV (human papillomavirus), and malaria vaccines [10] in many national immunization programs to significantly reduce mortality among women and child mortality due to diarrheal disease and prevent cervical cancer and the near eradication of wild poliovirus in most countries, with only a handful of endemic cases remaining. There were advances in remote temperature monitoring (RTM) technologies, allowing real-time tracking of vaccine storage conditions. A new focus became the integration of immunization into broader primary health care systems, linking vaccination to maternal and child health services. In this era, there was a significant decline in under-five mortality rates, largely due to immunization against pneumonia, diarrhea, and measles.

The COVID-19 pandemic (2020–2023) severely disrupted routine immunization services, leading to backslides in coverage, particularly in measles and polio vaccinations [11]. Reasons for this included redirection of the health workforce towards the COVID-19 response, lack of health care workers, lockdowns leading to logistical challenges, and fear of transmission in health care settings. However, despite the impact on routine immunization coverage, established immunization programs played a vital role in the COVID-19 response by providing the infrastructure, workforce, and systems needed to rapidly scale up vaccine delivery, particularly in low- and middle-income countries. Their ability to vaccinate millions, several times more than in the years before, efficiently highlights their adaptability and positions them as key tools for managing future global health emergencies such as MERS, SARS, mpox, and Ebola, reinforcing their importance in global health security. Cold chain requirements for mRNA vaccines posed a new challenge during the pandemic, requiring ultra-cold storage solutions.

Global DTP3 coverage, however, was stagnating around 85% [12], with a severe decrease during the pandemic years 2020–2023.

3. Setbacks and Emerging Challenges

Decreased acceptance or even vaccine hesitancy—driven by misinformation, distrust in institutions, and anti-vaccine movements—has become a major public health concern and, together with the coverage decrease during the pandemic, has led to the resurgence of vaccine-preventable diseases like measles and polio. The COVID-19 pandemic had a heterogeneous impact on vaccine confidence: while adult uptake of influenza, pneumococcal, and COVID-19 booster vaccines increased in several contexts [13], perceptions of childhood vaccine importance declined in multiple sub-Saharan African countries [14].

Unvaccinated and under-vaccinated children are accumulating in conflict zones, displacement crises, and areas with weak health infrastructure. Up to half of the so-called zero-dose children live in conflict and humanitarian settings where insecurities hinder vaccine delivery in fragile settings such as Afghanistan, Syria, Sudan, and Yemen [15,16].

The increasing cost of newer vaccines has raised concerns about financial sustainability and equitable access, especially in middle-income countries transitioning out of Gavi support.

When EPI started, there were six antigens included in the program, including diphtheria, tetanus, pertussis, tuberculosis, polio, and measles. EPI now handles universally recommended vaccines against 13 antigens, and there are vaccines covering more than 30 antigens and many more in the pipeline. This ever-expanding number of vaccines poses delivery challenges in countries with health care worker gaps and weak health care systems. In addition, particularly in Africa, the yearly birth cohort is expanding and requires scaling up of PHC services [17,18].

Many children remain unvaccinated because they live in areas with little or no access to primary health care—a comprehensive approach that encompasses health promotion, disease prevention, and treatment. While vaccine campaigns are effective in reaching these children, they are inherently time-bound and cannot provide consistent, ongoing services. To ensure all children are vaccinated in a reliable and sustainable way, it is crucial to integrate childhood immunization into strengthened primary health care systems.

In 2025, global health faced a major setback when key donors imposed a budget freeze, resulting in the termination of numerous health programs and tighter restrictions on those that remained [19]. This event exposed the fragility of health systems in the Global South, which remain heavily dependent on external aid. In response, low- and middle-income countries (LMICs) are being urged to reassess their financial dependencies and develop regional strategies for sustainable health financing and international collaboration. The crisis has reinforced the importance of South–South cooperation and the sharing of knowledge and best practices among LMICs. A University of Washington report [20] warned that the funding freeze could trigger a global health crisis, while the World Economic Forum emphasized [21] the urgent need for countries to invest in domestic health infrastructure, enhance local capacity, and build greater resilience and health sovereignty.

4. The Road Ahead: The Next 50 Years of Immunization

4.1. Tackling Vaccine Hesitancy and Misinformation

As immunization programs transition into a new era characterized by scientific advancement and expanded life-course vaccination platforms, one of the most enduring impediments to achieving high coverage is behavioral rather than biological. Despite significant improvements in global vaccine supply, under-vaccination—driven by both supply- and demand-side determinants, including vaccine hesitancy—remains a critical public health challenge. The pandemic underscored the profound influence of social and psychological factors on vaccine uptake. Trust, particularly in institutions and interpersonal relationships, emerged as a decisive factor. A cross-national study [22] involving 177 countries found that high levels of governmental and interpersonal trust were the only pandemic preparedness indicators consistently associated with increased COVID-19 vaccine coverage. Conversely, belief in COVID-19-related misinformation was strongly correlated with hesitancy in over 40 countries, with misinformation exposure being particularly pervasive in low- and middle-income countries (LMICs) [23].

Addressing under-vaccination requires a nuanced understanding of vaccine acceptance within the broader context of the caregiver's journey. Structural barriers—such as geographic inaccessibility, inadequate service integration, and opportunity costs associated with vaccination—often exert a greater influence on caregiver behavior than concerns related to vaccine safety or efficacy. In many cases, non-vaccination may reflect informational or logistical constraints rather than attitudinal opposition, particularly among caregivers who are unaware of where, when, or how to vaccinate. These access-related impediments disproportionately affect women [24], who frequently bear the burden of caregiving alongside structural and social constraints.

A paradigmatic shift from reactive to proactive, context-specific, and well-resourced demand generation strategies is required. Trust-building must be institutionalized as a core component of routine health systems strengthening. This includes systematic engagement with communities, the provision of equitable and high-quality health services, and the empowerment of trusted local actors. Ghana's national response to vaccine misinformation during the COVID-19 pandemic—anchored by a multisectoral task force and comprehensive training for health promotion officers in misinformation management—provides a replicable model for institutionalizing trust-building mechanisms within national health programs [25]. Effective demand strategies must also be grounded in behavioral and social insights, using, for example, the WHO-developed Behavioral Science and Demand Tool (BeSD). Routine social listening and community-level feedback mechanisms can ensure that communication efforts are contextually resonant. For example, a global cross-sectoral initiative deployed behavioral science-informed messaging to over 100 million individuals, testing variants in message content, tone, and messenger identity to optimize vaccine-related outcomes [26]. Similarly, the UNICEF-supported "Cranky Uncle Vaccine" initiative [27], a gamified mobile platform employing inoculation theory and critical thinking, has demonstrated success in improving misinformation recognition and intent to vaccinate in five countries across Africa and Asia [28].

Health care workers continue to be among the most trusted sources of vaccine information yet often lack the competencies or confidence to address caregiver concerns effectively. Evidence from six countries in Europe and Central Asia indicates that perceived vaccine safety, strong provider recommendations, and frequent health consultations are key determinants of timely childhood immunization [29]. Training programs must therefore integrate interpersonal communication (IPC) skills within broader clinical and service quality improvement efforts to maximize their impact. Community engagement, grounded in respect, co-creation, and sustained dialog, is foundational to equitable immunization coverage. In Remo North, Nigeria [30], a participatory action research approach involving community leaders, frontline providers, and local authorities led to a 30-percentage point increase in full immunization coverage among children aged over nine months. Such models enhance both the legitimacy of health interventions and the responsiveness of systems to local needs.

Looking ahead, addressing vaccine hesitancy and under-vaccination will require a systems-level transformation that integrates trust-building, real-time social and behavioral insights, digital innovation, and equity-centered community engagement. Immunization programs must move beyond top–down messaging to embrace participatory, adaptive strategies that reflect and respond to the lived realities of the populations they serve. Only through such approaches can vaccination be re-established as a shared social norm and a cornerstone of global public health.

4.2. *Investing in New Vaccine Development*

The future of immunization hinges on sustained investment in vaccine research and development (R&D) to address both longstanding and emerging infectious disease threats. The COVID-19 pandemic catalyzed a historic surge in global investment, accelerating the development and regulatory approval of new vaccine platforms—particularly mRNA-based technologies—which have since opened the door for faster, more scalable vaccine production for other diseases [31]. These shifts have not only enhanced pandemic preparedness but also unlocked new potential for combating persistent global health challenges.

Building on this momentum, the next 50 years will see an expanded pipeline targeting high-burden diseases like tuberculosis, malaria, respiratory syncytial virus (RSV), and rotavirus. Several high-priority vaccines are on the horizon. Universal influenza vaccines are under development to provide broader and longer-lasting protection against seasonal and pandemic strains. Similarly, more effective tuberculosis (TB) vaccines aim to replace or enhance the Bacillus Calmette–Guérin (BCG) vaccine, which has limited efficacy against adult pulmonary TB. With TB remaining one of the top infectious disease killers globally, novel vaccine candidates like M72/AS01E show promise in late-stage trials [32]. Furthermore, mRNA technology, validated during the COVID-19 response, is now being applied to a range of emerging and neglected diseases, including Zika, Lassa fever, HIV, and antimicrobial-resistant infections. The adaptability and scalability of mRNA platforms offer hope for more rapid, targeted vaccine responses in the future.

To expand accessibility and address delivery bottlenecks, novel vaccine formats such as mucosal vaccines (e.g., nasal sprays and oral tablets) and needle-free technologies like microneedle patches [33] are being developed. These innovations enhance immunogenicity, reduce cold chain dependencies, and facilitate administration in hard-to-reach settings.

In parallel, global efforts are strengthening local vaccine R&D and manufacturing capacity. Less than 1% of vaccines used in Africa are produced on the continent [34]—a stark inequity that the African Union seeks to remedy by targeting 60% local production by 2040. To that end, new mRNA vaccine facilities are being established across Africa, Asia, and Latin America, supported by global initiatives like the WHO mRNA Technology Transfer Hub and the Developing Countries Vaccine Manufacturers Network (DCVMN) [35]. Building on lessons from the pandemic, global partners must continue to support vaccine innovation and equitable access. Prioritizing the development of next-generation vaccines, strengthening local manufacturing, and adopting delivery innovations will be key to ensuring that every child, no matter where they live, can benefit from life-saving immunizations.

Recent breakthroughs in artificial intelligence and nanotechnology are set to transform vaccine development and delivery. AlphaFold 3, an advanced AI tool, accelerates vaccine target identification by accurately predicting molecular interactions vital for immune responses, significantly aiding research into complex diseases like malaria [36]. Simultaneously, nanotechnology innovations, including lipid nanoparticles used in mRNA COVID-19 vaccines and emerging layer-by-layer nano-delivery systems, offer precise, scalable methods for vaccine delivery and controlled antigen release [37]. Together, these technologies pave the way for faster, more adaptable, and more effective vaccines to meet evolving global health challenges.

Together, these scientific and structural investments will define the immunization agenda for decades to come—enabling broader protection, faster pandemic responses, and equitable access to life-saving vaccines for all.

4.3. *Expanding Life Course Immunization*

As we look toward the future of global immunization, transitioning from a child-centric paradigm to a life course approach will be imperative to meet the evolving health needs of populations and to realize the full potential of immunization in achieving universal health coverage (UHC), health equity, and pandemic preparedness. While childhood immunization has historically driven dramatic reductions in vaccine-preventable diseases (VPDs), the growing epidemiological burden among adolescents, adults, and older persons signals a pressing need to expand protection across all age groups.

Demographic transitions, including rapid aging in many regions, have created new challenges. By 2050, the number of people aged 60 and older will exceed 2 billion globally [38], many of whom are at heightened risk of VPDs such as influenza, pneumococcal disease, shingles, and respiratory syncytial virus (RSV). Nevertheless, few countries have established robust immunization platforms for older adults. Without integration of routine adult vaccination into primary health care, countries risk increased hospitalizations, mortality, and economic strain due to preventable disease outbreaks.

The adolescent and adult age groups have also been neglected in most national immunization schedules. HPV vaccination, which can prevent cervical cancer, remains underutilized in many low- and middle-income countries (LMICs) [39], and uptake of vaccines for tetanus, hepatitis B, and COVID-19 among adults is often inconsistent. Adolescents and adults represent both a vulnerable group and an untapped opportunity. Adolescents, for instance, are accessible through school systems, reproductive health services, and digital technologies, making them a strategic target for catch-up vaccinations and building trust in health services. Similarly, adults engaged through antenatal care, workplaces, and non-communicable disease (NCD) clinics can be reached with maternal, influenza, and COVID-19 vaccines, enhancing disease prevention and improving continuity of care [40].

Importantly, life course immunization is not only a public health imperative but also an economic and social investment. Studies have shown that expanding vaccination beyond childhood reduces productivity losses, prevents health care costs associated with preventable illnesses, and fosters healthier, longer-living populations [41]. It also enhances pandemic preparedness by maintaining immunity across the broader population, minimizing the impact of infectious disease outbreaks on health systems and economies. Adult and elderly immunization played a crucial role in reducing severe COVID-19 outcomes and helped maintain the continuity of essential services during the pandemic—an experience that underscores the value of this approach.

Operationalizing life course immunization will require structural shifts in policy, financing, and service delivery. Governments must update national immunization plans and essential benefits packages to include vaccines for all age groups. Health systems need to strengthen delivery platforms beyond childhood, integrating vaccination into maternal health, occupational health, geriatric care, and chronic disease services. Community health workers must be trained and equipped to deliver age-appropriate vaccines in outreach and home-based settings. Furthermore, digital health tools, such as electronic immunization registries, can improve tracking and targeting of populations across the lifespan, enabling better forecasting, follow-up, and impact assessment.

Equally crucial is securing sustainable financing and strong political will. Life course immunization demands long-term investment and cross-sectoral collaboration. Leveraging existing platforms—such as school health programs, social protection schemes, and mobile health campaigns—can enhance efficiency and reach. Countries should also adopt a whole-of-society approach by involving civil society, employers, and community leaders in promoting vaccine demand and countering hesitancy.

As outlined in the Immunization Agenda 2030 (IA2030), the life course approach is central to building resilient, equitable, and people-centered immunization systems. By embedding vaccination into all stages of life and across all health touchpoints, countries can transform immunization from a childhood intervention into a cornerstone of lifelong health. This transformation is not only feasible—it is essential to realizing the vision of "health for all" in an increasingly interconnected and risk-prone world. The decisions made today will determine whether future generations can live longer, healthier lives protected by the full benefits of immunization. This is not only a path to improved health outcomes but also a critical pillar of universal health coverage and pandemic preparedness.

4.4. Strengthening Health Systems and Cold Chain Infrastructure

As the world prepares for the future of immunization, the next 50 years will require transformative investments in health systems and cold chain infrastructure to ensure equitable, timely, and efficient vaccine delivery. The growing complexity of immunization programs—driven by life course vaccination platforms, new vaccine technologies, and the need for pandemic preparedness—demands a robust, resilient, and adaptive health system backbone.

At the center of this transformation is the cold chain. The cold chain ensures vaccines remain potent from manufacture to administration. However, cold chain systems in many low- and middle-income countries (LMICs) remain fragile, constrained by unreliable electricity, insufficient maintenance, and lack of real-time monitoring. Innovations are bridging these gaps. Solar direct drive (SDD) refrigeration systems now provide sustainable, off-grid cooling solutions. Since 2017, UNICEF and partners have deployed over 180,000 refrigerators, and more than half (100,000) are solar-powered, to enhance cold storage capacity in hard-to-reach settings. These systems reduce reliance on fuel-based generators and improve vaccine availability even in areas without grid power.

To further optimize vaccine potency and reduce wastage, heat-stable and Controlled Temperature Chain (CTC)-qualified vaccines are being introduced [42]. Vaccines such as MenAfriVac (meningitis A), HPV, typhoid, and cholera now tolerate controlled excursions outside the traditional 2–8 °C range, easing logistical challenges and enabling last-mile delivery to remote populations. These innovations are particularly crucial for campaigns, outreach services, and emergency response where refrigeration is limited or absent.

The WHO's PQS initiative is advancing immunization logistics by introducing Equipment Monitoring System (EMS) specifications that enable real-time monitoring of cold chain performance [43]. These standards enhance interoperability with electronic LMIS platforms, improving asset management, maintenance, and overall reliability and sustainability of vaccine delivery systems.

Active vaccine carriers [44] are enhancing immunization reach by maintaining cold temperatures during long outreach sessions, enabling safe vaccine delivery in remote areas. Simultaneously, green waste management technologies [45]—such as steam sterilization, microwave treatment, and plasma gasification—are reducing the environmental impact of vaccine waste. Together with EMS-enabled cold chain monitoring, these innovations are strengthening immunization systems to be more reliable, equitable, and sustainable globally.

New product innovations are further streamlining logistics and improving user acceptability. Microarray patches (MAPs), or microneedle patches, represent one of the most promising breakthroughs in vaccine delivery [33]. These needle-free patches deliver dry-form vaccines painlessly into the skin and offer the following multiple advantages: they are heat-stable, easy to administer by non-health professionals, and eliminate risks of needle-related injuries or contamination. For measles and rubella, MAPs are in advanced clinical development and have demonstrated strong immunogenicity and programmatic feasibility in early trials. Because they do not require reconstitution or cold-chain-intensive storage, MAPs have the potential to revolutionize outbreak response and routine immunization in resource-limited settings [33,46].

Additionally, innovations in packaging and monitoring—like vaccine vial monitors (VVMs) and threshold indicators—are empowering frontline workers to verify vaccine exposure to heat. Freeze-preventive carriers are addressing the often-overlooked threat of freezing during transport, a major cause of potency loss for freeze-sensitive vaccines.

Digital technology is another critical enabler. Electronic Logistics Management Information Systems (eLMIS), Electronic Immunization Registries (EIRs), and real-time temperature monitoring systems are revolutionizing supply chain visibility. For example, India's Electronic Vaccine Intelligence Network (eVIN) has been instrumental in reducing stockouts and improving cold chain equipment performance, resulting in higher coverage and reduced wastage [47]. In Zambia and Tanzania, EIRs have improved data accuracy, immunization tracking, and the identification of zero-dose children.

Looking ahead, future-proofing immunization will also depend on integrating cold chains and logistics within broader health systems. This means aligning with primary health care (PHC), ensuring cross-program efficiencies, and linking vaccine delivery to civil registration and vital statistics (CRVS) systems for better targeting and accountability. Moreover, embracing drone delivery, automated stock management, and regional manufacturing of cold chain equipment can ensure timely and locally relevant solutions.

The success of immunization programs heavily depends on the strength and availability of a well-trained health workforce, particularly vaccinators. A global shortage of health care personnel—especially in rural and underserved areas—hinders effective vaccine delivery. Community health workers (CHWs) play a crucial role in bridging this gap, with evidence showing they administered vaccines in 20 of 75 countries with CHW programs [48]. Despite their potential, CHWs often face challenges such as insufficient training, support, and supervision. Strengthening the health workforce is essential to enhance the reach and effectiveness of immunization programs, ultimately improving public health outcomes. In conclusion, the next 50 years of immunization hinge on building resilient, smart, and sustainable health systems that can support increasingly complex vaccine demands. This includes leveraging innovation, local capacity building, public–private partnerships, and data-driven management to create a future where no one is left behind due to cold chain failures or system inefficiencies.

4.5. Ensuring Sustainable Financing for Immunization Programs

Securing sustainable financing is one of the most critical challenges and imperatives for the future of global immunization. The estimated cost of fully vaccinating a child [49] through the second year of life, based on standard immunization schedules, is approximately USD 73.15. While investments in immunization in low- and middle-income countries (LMICs) surpassed USD 112 billion from 2000 to 2017 [50], financial inefficiencies and systemic weaknesses persist, hampering progress toward equitable coverage and long-term program resilience. These challenges have been exacerbated by the COVID-19 pandemic, which, while catalyzing additional investment—such as Gavi's cumulative support of over USD 23 billion to LMICs—also revealed the fragility of immunization systems overly reliant on external aid and unable to absorb and manage funds efficiently [51].

Across 94 low- and middle-income countries, the total projected cost of delivering 10 key vaccines from 2011 to 2030 is USD 70.8 billion under a base case scenario [52]. However, there remains a significant funding gap of USD 38.4 billion, largely driven by the cost of immunization service delivery, which accounts for 86% of the shortfall [50]. One of the main issues lies in the discrepancy between budget allocations and actual expenditures, often driven by weak public financial management (PFM) systems [53]. Underutilized budgets, procurement bottlenecks, and lack of accountability result in missed opportunities to reach children with life-saving vaccines. In many LMICs, declining tax revenues, fragmented donor assistance, and the unreliability of health insurance contributions in informal economies have placed additional pressure on already constrained health budgets. These fiscal vulnerabilities underscore the need to shift from short-term donor dependency to long-term domestic sustainability.

To chart a more resilient course, governments and partners must adopt a comprehensive strategy that blends innovation, domestic resource mobilization, and enhanced system efficiency. Innovative financing instruments such as vaccine bonds—like the USD 1 billion raised by the International Finance Facility for Immunization (IFFIm) in 2024 [54]—demonstrate the potential for rapidly converting donor pledges into immediate cash to support vaccine delivery in LICs. Meanwhile, Gavi's co-financing model has successfully encouraged countries such as India and Angola to progressively assume greater responsibility for their immunization budgets, fostering national ownership and sustainability.

Strengthening domestic financing is crucial but must be matched with improved PFM capacity. Digitalization of financial systems—including the use of integrated financial management information systems (IFMIS), real-time dashboards, and electronic procurement platforms—can enhance transparency, streamline budget execution, and improve expenditure tracking [55]. These tools help close the loop between planning, resource allocation, and delivery of immunization services, reducing delays and corruption risks.

In addition, expanding fiscal space for health can be achieved through multiple avenues: broadening the domestic tax base; earmarking "sin taxes" on tobacco, alcohol, and sugary drinks; leveraging debt relief for health investment; and exploring blended financing approaches, including insurance schemes and philanthropic contributions. Market-shaping tools such as pooled procurement (e.g., via the UNICEF Supply Division or PAHO Revolving Fund) and advanced market commitments can also lower vaccine costs and ensure supply stability [56].

However, financial sustainability cannot be achieved in isolation. It requires coordinated, whole-of-government action, where ministries of health and finance, civil society, private sector actors, and communities work together to ensure efficient and equitable use of resources. This also means aligning donor assistance with national systems, promoting flexible, predictable, and context-specific funding modalities that facilitate transition to domestic financing without compromising program continuity.

Since human resources, service delivery, supply chains, and capital costs are the primary cost drivers of immunization delivery, countries should consider integrating vaccination programs with primary health care systems to reduce overall program costs significantly [57]. Looking ahead, sustainable immunization financing must become a core pillar of resilient health systems. This will require bold political commitment, strategic investments in local capacity, and a deliberate focus on maximizing value for money. Only through such an integrated and forward-looking approach can the global community ensure that the promise of immunization—saving millions of lives each year—remains a reality for generations to come.

To ensure sustainable and equitable immunization financing, a whole-of-government approach involving health and finance ministries, civil society, and communities is essential, as it focuses on maximizing impact in resource-constrained environments.

5. Conclusions: Renewing the Global Commitment

The success of the Expanded Programme on Immunization over the past 50 years stands as one of the greatest public health triumphs in history. However, challenges such as vaccine hesitancy, pandemic-related disruptions, and equitable access remain formidable.

Looking ahead, immunization efforts must expand beyond childhood vaccination, embrace technological advancements, and strengthen health systems to ensure that every person, regardless of their circumstances, has access to life-saving vaccines.

With continued global commitment, funding, and innovation, immunization will remain a pillar of disease prevention and public health. The future of vaccination is not just about new technologies but about ensuring that every individual—regardless of where they live—has access to life-saving vaccines.

This Special Issue, called "50 Years of Immunization—Steps Forward", covers over 25 articles and offers historical perspectives as well as the state of EPI today. It includes articles with global scope, LMIC scope, regional-specific, and country-specific case studies. It covers several vaccine-specific articles, including measles, polio, HPV, cholera, dengue, influenza, zoster, hepatitis E, shigella, and pertussis.

As we celebrate the legacy of EPI, we must recommit to protecting future generations from preventable diseases since immunization is not just about vaccines or an investment in health; it is an investment in equity, humanity, and the survival of future generations, and the right to a healthier life for all.

Author Contributions: I.M. developed the outline for this editorial. The first draft of the article was jointly written by I.M., A.L., and E.T.L. All authors provided comments, edited. All authors have read and agreed to the published version of the manuscript.

Funding: This research received no external funding.

Acknowledgments: We thank all the staff from all countries that contributed to the success of EPI.

Conflicts of Interest: The authors declare no conflicts of interest.

Disclaimer: The content of this editorial is solely the responsibility of the authors and does not necessarily represent the official views of UNICEF and WHO.

Abbreviations

The following abbreviations are used in this manuscript:

BCU	big catch-up
EPI	Essential Programme on Immunization, previously called Expanded Programme on Immunization
GAVI	Global Alliance Vaccine Initiative
GPEI	Global Polio Eradication Initiative
IA2030	Immunization Agenda 2030
RI	routine immunization
ZD	zero dose
UI	under-immunized

References

1. World Health Organization. *International Work in Tuberculosis, 1949–1964*; WHO: Geneva, Switzerland, 1965; pp. 10–13.
2. World Health Assembly (27th: 1974). The Expanded Programme on Immunization: The 1974 Resolution by the World Health Assembly. *Assign. Child.* **1985**, *69–72*, 87–88.
3. Shattock, A.J.; Johnson, H.C.; Sim, S.Y.; Carter, A.; Lambach, P.; Hutubessy, R.C.W.; Thompson, K.M.; Badizadegan, K.; Lambert, B.; Ferrari, M.J.; et al. Contribution of vaccination to improved survival and health: Modelling 50 years of the Expanded Programme on Immunization. *Lancet* **2024**, *403*, 2307–2316. [CrossRef]
4. Sim, S.Y.; Watts, E.; Constenla, D.; Brenzel, L.; Patenaude, B.N. Return on Investment from Immunization Against 10 Pathogens in 94 Low- and Middle-Income Countries, 2011–2030. *Health Aff.* **2020**, *39*, 1343–1353. [CrossRef] [PubMed]
5. Burton, A.; Monasch, R.; Lautenbach, B.; Gacic-Dobo, M.; Neill, M.; Karimov, R.; Wolfson, L.; Jones, G.; Birmingham, M. WHO and UNICEF estimates of national infant immunization coverage: Methods and processes. *Bull. World Health Organ.* **2009**, *87*, 535–541. [CrossRef] [PubMed] [PubMed Central]
6. Stanfield, P. Jim Grant—UNICEF Visionary, R. Jolly (editor). Florence: UNICEF Innocenti Research Centre, 2001. 174pp. ISBN 92-806-3723-1. *Trans. R. Soc. Trop. Med. Hyg.* **2002**, *96*, 317. [CrossRef]
7. Wallace, A.S.; Ryman, T.K.; Dietz, V. Overview of global, regional, and national routine vaccination coverage trends and growth patterns from 1980 to 2009: Implications for vaccine-preventable disease eradication and elimination initiatives. *J. Infect. Dis.* **2014**, *210* (Suppl. S1), S514–S522. [CrossRef] [PubMed] [PubMed Central]
8. World Health Organization. Global programme for vaccines and immunization. In *Strategic Plan 1998–2001*; WHO/GPV/98.04; World Health Organization: Geneva, Switzerland, 1998.
9. Centers for Disease Control and Prevention (CDC). Global routine vaccination coverage, 2010. *MMWR Morb. Mortal. Wkly. Rep.* **2011**, *60*, 1520–1522. [PubMed]
10. Hyde, T.B.; Dentz, H.; Wang, S.A.; Burchett, H.E.; Mounier-Jack, S.; Mantel, C.F. New Vaccine Introduction Impact Published Literature Working Group. The impact of new vaccine introduction on immunization and health systems: A review of the published literature. *Vaccine* **2012**, *30*, 6347–6358. [CrossRef] [PubMed] [PubMed Central]
11. Shet, A.; Carr, K.; Danovaro-Holliday, M.C.; Sodha, S.V.; Prosperi, C.; Wunderlich, J.; Wonodi, C.; Reynolds, H.W.; Mirza, I.; Gacic-Dobo, M.; et al. Impact of the SARS-CoV-2 pandemic on routine immunisation services: Evidence of disruption and recovery from 170 countries and territories. *Lancet Glob. Health* **2022**, *10*, e186–e194. [CrossRef] [PubMed] [PubMed Central]
12. Muhoza, P.; Danovaro-Holliday, M.C.; Diallo, M.S.; Murphy, P.; Sodha, S.V.; Requejo, J.H.; Wallace, A.S. Routine Vaccination Coverage—Worldwide, 2020. *MMWR Morb. Mortal. Wkly. Rep.* **2021**, *70*, 1495–1500. [CrossRef]
13. Vojtek, I.; van Wouw, M.; Thomson, A. Impact of COVID-19 on vaccine confidence and uptake: A systematic literature review. *Hum. Vaccines Immunother.* **2024**, *20*, 2384180. [CrossRef] [PubMed]
14. de Figueiredo, A.; Temfack, E.; Tajudeen, R.; Larson, H.J. Declining trends in vaccine confidence across sub-Saharan Africa: A large-scale cross-sectional modeling study. *Hum. Vaccines Immunother.* **2023**, *19*, 2213117. [CrossRef] [PubMed]
15. Gavi the Vaccine Alliance. Protecting Our Future Investment Opportunity 2026–2030. Available online: https://www.gavi.org/sites/default/files/investing/funding/resource-mobilisation/Gavi-Investment-Opportunity-2026-2030.pdf (accessed on 25 April 2025).
16. UNICEF Immunization and Conflict. Children Everywhere, in Any Situation or Circumstance, Have the Right to Survive and Thrive. Available online: https://www.unicef.org/immunization/immunization-and-conflict (accessed on 25 April 2025).
17. De Maeseneer, J. Scaling up Family Medicine and Primary Health Care in Africa: Statement of the Primafamed network, Victoria Falls, Zimbabwe. *Afr. J. Prim. Health Care Fam. Med.* **2013**, *5*, 507. [CrossRef] [PubMed Central]
18. Aliyu, A.A. Family Planning Services in Africa: The Successes and Challenges [Internet]. In *Family Planning*; InTech: West Palm Beach, FL, USA, 2018. [CrossRef]

19. Sunny, M.E.; Santhosh, C. *Funding Cuts for Global Health Programs Threaten Childhood Vaccination Efforts*; Reuters: London, UK, 18 March 2025.
20. Global Health Justice (April 2025) Global Health Catastrophe from 2025, US Foreign Budget Freeze. Available online: https://depts.washington.edu/globalhealthjustice/global-health-catastrophic-from-the-2025-u-s-foreign-budget-freeze/#:~:text=By%20the%20end%20of%20March,sustainable%20and%20resilient%20healthcare%20systems (accessed on 20 April 2025).
21. Health and Healthcare Systems. Health sovereignty builds resilience in a volatile world. Here are 3 countries working towards it. Health sovereignty builds resilience in a volatile world. In Proceedings of the World Economic Forum, Davos-Klosters, Switzerland, 20–24 January 2025.
22. Bollyky, T.J.; Hulland, E.N.; Barber, R.M.; Collins, J.K.; Kiernan, S.; Moses, M.; Pigott, D.M.; Reiner, R.C., Jr.; Sorensen, R.J.D.; Abbafati, C.; et al. Pandemic preparedness and COVID-19: An exploratory analysis of infection and fatality rates, and contextual factors associated with preparedness in 177 countries, from 1 January 2020, to 30 September 2021. *Lancet* **2022**, *399*, 1489–1512. [CrossRef] [PubMed]
23. Larson, H.J.; Broniatowski, D.A. Volatility of Vaccine Confidence. *Science* **2021**, *371*, 1289. [CrossRef]
24. Feletto, M.; Sharkey, A.; Rowley, E.; Gurley, N.; Sinha, A. A Gender Lens to Advance Equity in Immunization. In *ERG Discussion Paper 05*; Equity Reference Group for Immunization: New York, NY, USA, 2018.
25. Lohiniva, A.-L.; Nurzhynska, A.; Hudi, A.-H.; Anim, B.; Aboagye, D.C. Infodemic management using digital information and knowledge cocreation to address COVID-19 vaccine hesitancy: Case study from Ghana. *JMIR Infodemiol.* **2022**, *2*, e37134. [CrossRef]
26. Winters, M.; Christie, S.; Lepage, C.; Malik, A.A.; Bokemper, S.; Abeyesekera, S.; Boye, B.; Moini, M.; Jamil, Z.; Tariq, T.; et al. Persuasive COVID-19 vaccination campaigns on Facebook and nationwide vaccination coverage in Ukraine, India, and Pakistan. *PLoS Glob. Public Health* **2023**, *3*, e0002357. [CrossRef]
27. Hopkins, K.L.; Lepage, C.; Cook, W.; Thomson, A.; Abeyesekera, S.; Knobler, S.; Boehman, N.; Thompson, B.; Waiswa, P.; Ssanyu, J.N.; et al. Co-Designing a Mobile-Based Game to Improve Misinformation Resistance and Vaccine Knowledge in Uganda, Kenya, and Rwanda. *J. Health Commun.* **2023**, *28* (Suppl. S2), 49–60. [CrossRef]
28. Cook, J.; Lepage, C.; Hopkins, K.L.; Cook, W.; Kolog, E.A.; Thomson, A.; Iddrisu, I.; Burnette, S. Co-designing and pilot testing a digital game to improve vaccine attitudes and misinformation resistance in Ghana. *Hum. Vaccines Immunother.* **2024**, *20*, 2407204. [CrossRef]
29. Jarrett, C.; Wilson, R.; O'Leary, M.; Eckersberger, E.; Larson, H.J. Strategies For Addressing Vaccine Hesitancy—A systematic review. *Vaccine* **2015**, *33*, 4185. [CrossRef]
30. Hutchings, A.; Hollywood, J.; Lamping, D.L.; Pease, C.T.; Chakravarty, K.; Silverman, B.; Choy, E.H.S.; Scott, D.G.; Hazleman, B.L.; Bourke, B.; et al. Using Participatory Action Research to Improve Immunization Utilization in Areas with Pockets of Unimmunized Children in Nigeria. *Health Res. Policy Syst.* **2021**, *19* (Suppl. S2), 803–809. [CrossRef]
31. World Health Organization. *Immunization Agenda 2030: A Global Strategy to Leave No One Behind*; WHO: Geneva, Switzerland, 2022.
32. Tait, D.R.; Hatherill, M.; Van Der Meeren, O.; Ginsberg, A.M.; Van Brakel, E.; Salaun, B.; Scriba, T.J.; Akite, E.J.; Ayles, H.M.; Bollaerts, A.; et al. Final analysis of a trial of M72/AS01E vaccine to prevent tuberculosis. *N. Engl. J. Med.* **2019**, *381*, 2429–2439. [CrossRef]
33. Peyraud, N.; Zehrung, D.; Jarrahian, C.; Frivold, C.; Orubu, T.; Giersing, B. Potential Use of Microarray Patches for Vaccine Delivery in Low- and Middle income Countries. *Vaccine* **2019**, *37*, 4427–4434. [CrossRef]
34. Scaling Up African Vaccine Manufacturing Capacity. Wellcome, January 2023. Available online: https://wellcome.org/reports/scaling-african-vaccine-manufacturing-capacity (accessed on 26 April 2025).
35. Partnerships for African Vaccine Manufacturing (PAVM) Framework for Action, P.A.V.M. March 2022. Available online: https://africacdc.org/download/partnerships-for-african-vaccine-manufacturing-pavm-framework-for-action/ (accessed on 26 April 2025).
36. Abramson, J.; Adler, J.; Dunger, J.; Evans, R.; Green, T.; Pritzel, A.; Ronneberger, O.; Willmore, L.; Ballard, A.J.; Bambrick, J.; et al. Accurate structure prediction of biomolecular interactions with AlphaFold 3. *Nature* **2024**, *630*, 493–500. [CrossRef]
37. Xu, Y.; Masuda, K.; Groso, C.; Hassan, R.; Zhou, Z.; Broderick, K.; Tsuji, M.; Tison, C. Microfluidic Synthesis of Scalable Layer-by-Layer Multiple Antigen Nano-Delivery Platform for SARS-CoV-2 Vaccines. *Vaccines* **2024**, *12*, 339. [CrossRef] [PubMed]
38. United Nations, Department of Economic and Social Affairs, Population Division. World Population Ageing 2017. ST/ESA/SER.A/408. 2017. Available online: https://www.un.org/en/development/desa/population/publications/pdf/ageing/WPA2017_Report.pdf (accessed on 12 May 2025).
39. Toh, Z.Q.; Licciardi, P.V.; Russell, F.M.; Garland, S.M.; Batmunkh, T.; Mulholland, E.K. Cervical Cancer Prevention Through HPV Vaccination in Low- and Middle-Income Countries in Asia. *Asian Pac. J. Cancer. Prev.* **2017**, *18*, 2339–2343. [CrossRef] [PubMed] [PubMed Central]

40. Wuraola, B.; Johannes, A.; Sachin, J. Considerations for Integrating COVID-19 Vaccination into Immunization Programmes and Primary Health Care for 2022 and Beyond. Document Available on WHO Website. Available online: https://www.who.int/publications/i/item/9789240064454 (accessed on 10 May 2025).
41. Nandi, A.; Shet, A. Why vaccines matter: Understanding the broader health, economic, and child development benefits of routine vaccination. *Hum. Vaccines Immunother.* **2020**, *16*, 1900–1904. [CrossRef] [PubMed] [PubMed Central]
42. World Health Organization. *Guidance on Temperature-Sensitive Vaccines and Innovations*; WHO: Geneva, Switzerland, 2021.
43. WHO. Introduction to the WHO IMD-PQS Equipment Monitoring System EMS Specification Suite. 2023. Available online: https://extranet.who.int/prequal/sites/default/files/document_files/Introduction%20to%20the%20PQS%20Equipment%20Monitoring%20System.pdf (accessed on 10 April 2025).
44. WHO. PQS Performance Specification. WHO/PQS/E003/TS01.1. 2021. Available online: https://extranet.who.int/prequal/sites/default/files/document_files/E003_TS01.1.pdf (accessed on 10 April 2025).
45. UNICEF. Children Environmental Health Collaborative Green & Safe Technologies for Health Care Waste Management: From Selection & Procurement to Implementation. 2023. Available online: https://ceh.unicef.org/events-and-resources/events/green-safe-technologies-health-care-waste-management-selection (accessed on 10 April 2025).
46. PATH; WHO; Gavi; UNICEF. Vaccine Innovation Prioritization Strategy (VIPS): Progress Report. 2022. Available online: https://www.developmentaid.org/api/frontend/cms/file/2023/10/Gavi-Progress-Report-2022.pdf (accessed on 10 May 2025).
47. UNDP. Evaluation of the eVIN System in India. 2021. Available online: https://www.undp.org/india/projects/improving-vaccination-systems-evin (accessed on 22 April 2025).
48. Gibson, E.; Zameer, M.; Alban, R.; Kouwanou, L.M. Community Health Workers as Vaccinators: A Rapid Review of the Global Landscape, 2000–2021. *Glob. Health Sci. Pract.* **2023**, *11*, e2200307. [CrossRef] [PubMed] [PubMed Central]
49. UNICEF. Costs of Vaccine and Injection Supplies. 2024. Available online: https://www.unicef.org/media/161751/file/Standard%20costs%20of%20fully%20vaccinating%20a%20child_UNICEF_2024.pdf.pdf (accessed on 22 April 2025).
50. Sriudomporn, S.; Sim, S.Y.; Mak, J.; Brenzel, L.; Patenaude, B.N. Financing and Funding Gap for 16 Vaccines Across 94 Low- and Middle-Income Countries, 2011–2030. *Health Aff.* **2023**, *42*, 94–104. [CrossRef] [PubMed]
51. The US Government and Gavi, the Vaccine Alliance. In *Fact Sheet*; KFF: San Francisco, CA, USA, 17 July 2024. Available online: https://www.kff.org/global-health-policy/fact-sheet/the-u-s-government-gavi-the-vaccine-alliance/#:~:text=In%202022,%20Gavi%20supported%2040,not%20including%20funding%20for%20COVAX) (accessed on 5 May 2025).
52. Sim, S.Y.; Watts, E.; Constenla, D.; Huang, S.; Brenzel, L.; Patenaude, B.N. Costs of Immunization Programs for 10 Vaccines in 94 Low- and Middle-Income Countries from 2011 to 2030. *Value Health* **2021**, *24*, 70–77. [CrossRef] [PubMed] [PubMed Central]
53. UNICEF. *Engaging with Public Financial Management Challenges in the Health Sector A Resource Guide for a Problem-Driven Approach for UNICEF Country Offices*; UNICEF: New York, NY, USA, 2022.
54. Wilkes, T.R. *Vaccine Bond Raises $1 Billion for Immunisations After Record Demand*; Reuters: London, UK, 24 October 2024.
55. Carlos, P.; Antonio, S. *Technological Opportunities and Recommendations for Modernizing Integrated Financial Management Information Systems in Latin America and the Caribbean*; Discussion Paper N° IDB-DP-651; Inter-American Development Bank: Washington, DC, USA, January 2019.
56. Malhame, M.; Baker, E.; Gandhi, G.; Jones, A.; Kalpaxis, P.; Iqbal, R.; Momeni, Y.; Nguyen, A. Shaping markets to benefit global health—A 15-year history and lessons learned from the pentavalent vaccine market. *Vaccine X* **2019**, *2*, 100033. [CrossRef] [PubMed] [PubMed Central]
57. Portnoy, A.; Vaughan, K.; Clarke-Deelder, E.; Suharlim, C.; Resch, S.C.; Brenzel, L.; Menzies, N.A. Producing standardized country-level immunization delivery unit cost estimates. *Pharmacoeconomics* **2020**, *38*, 995–1005. [CrossRef] [PubMed]

vaccines

Review

The Strategic Advisory Group of Experts (SAGE) on Immunization—Past, Present and Future

Melanie Marti [1,*], Hanna Nohynek [2], Philippe Duclos [3], Katherine L. O'Brien [1] and Joachim Hombach [1]

[1] Department of Immunization, Vaccines and Biologicals, World Health Organization, CH-1211 Geneva, Switzerland
[2] Finnish Institute for Health and Welfare, 00271 Helsinki, Finland
[3] Formerly Department of Immunization, Vaccines and Biologicals, World Health Organization, CH-1211 Geneva, Switzerland
* Correspondence: martim@who.int

Abstract: Background/Objectives: In November 1999, WHO established the Strategic Advisory Group of Experts (SAGE) on Immunization as a multidisciplinary group of experts to provide high-level recommendations on vaccines and immunization. Methods: This review provides an overview of SAGE's work in the past 25 years. It further outlines the processes and methods currently used by SAGE and highlights some of its major achievements. Results: SAGE's global policies have driven action toward eradication, elimination and disease control and addressed the optimization of vaccination and immunization. In total, 27 major policy positions on vaccines/vaccine-preventable diseases have guided global public health. During times of epidemics and pandemics, interim recommendations issued by SAGE have responded iteratively in real-time to provide evidence-driven response policies. SAGE is an adaptive advisory group that has modified its procedures and working approaches to meet the evolving challenges in public health and stay up-to-date with evolving scientific and guideline development standards. Conclusions: Over the last quarter century, SAGE has significantly contributed to shaping the immunization landscape. It has achieved and maintained a high level of integrity and credibility. The advisory group continues to be an authority in global public health, and its recommendations have profound implications for the health of individuals and populations across the globe.

Keywords: Strategic Advisory Group of Experts (SAGE) on Immunization; SAGE; World Health Organization advisory group; global immunization policy; immunization strategy; vaccination policy; vaccination recommendations

1. Introduction

The World Health Organization (WHO) was established with the objective of the attainment of the highest possible level of health for all people. In its constitution, the organization's function was outlined "to act as the directing and co-ordinating authority on international health work" and to "make recommendations with respect to international health matters [1]". Consequently, WHO provides leadership, including technical and normative guidance, on the control, elimination and eradication of vaccine-preventable diseases and the immunization programs to achieve those goals.

Vaccines are one of the most successful public health interventions of all time [2]. Recent modeling sought to quantify the public health impact of vaccinations globally from the inception of the Expanded Programme on Immunization 50 years ago [3]. Since 1974, the year the World Health Assembly requested WHO to provide technical advice and assistance to countries on the use of vaccines and recommended that Member States develop or maintain immunization and surveillance programs [4], vaccination against 14 diseases has averted over 154 million deaths, including 146 million among children younger than five years, of whom 101 million were infants younger than one year. During this period, vaccination has accounted for 40% of the observed decline in global infant mortality, 52% in the African region. In 2024, a vaccinated child younger than 10 years is 40% more likely to survive to their next birthday relative to a hypothetical scenario of no vaccination [3].

Many resources are devoted to the development and testing of vaccines, leading, ultimately, to their licensure and use in populations. Nevertheless, market availability of the products alone neither ensures their availability to all in need nor their appropriate use. Additional mechanisms are required to provide vaccines equitably to individuals worldwide who need them. This encompasses not only funding mechanisms to assure fair distribution and access but also strategies and policies developed to guide vaccination programs and to ensure the highest impact of vaccine utilization.

WHO established the Strategic Advisory Group of Experts (SAGE) on Immunization as a multidisciplinary group of independent experts to provide high-level guidance to WHO on vaccines and immunization. SAGE takes a population health approach with a mandate of issuing advice on vaccines of major public health importance, spanning across the life course, for programmatic use, including during health emergencies. While SAGE aims to issue global guidance targeted at regions and countries across all income strata (high-, middle- and low-income countries), its impact may be highest in low- and middle-income countries.

While SAGE is charged with the provision of guidance to WHO, SAGE also assumes, through WHO, advisory functions, inter alia, for Gavi, the Vaccine Alliance and the Global Polio Eradication Initiative (GPEI). In that function, SAGE's recommendations are also highly consequential for financial investments by technical and other partners, manufacturers and funders.

2. History of SAGE

First established in 1999 through the merging of two WHO previous advisory groups [5,6] (The Scientific Advisory Group of Experts (SAGE) of the WHO Program for Vaccine Development) and the Global Advisory Group (GAG) of the Expanded Program on Immunization.), SAGE was initially set up to advise and report to the director of the former WHO Department of Vaccines and Biologicals—the predecessor of the Department of Immunization, Vaccines and Biologicals—on the strategic objectives of WHO's immunization program.

The Global Immunization Vision and Strategy (GIVS) 2006–2015 [7], launched in 2005, was the first-ever multi-year partnership framework for realizing pre-defined immunization-related goals grouped in four strategic areas (Strategic areas: First, protecting more people in a changing world; Second, introducing new vaccines and technologies; Third, integrating immunization, other linked health interventions and surveillance in the health systems context; Fourth, immunizing in the context of global interdependence.). In parallel, SAGE underwent an adjustment of its scope and terms of reference and operating processes to ensure alignment with the guiding principles of the GIVS, outlining its tasks pertaining to the GIVS and enabling it to formulate global immunization strategies and policies. SAGE was, therefore, mandated to provide guidance on immunization priorities, advise on matters pertaining to vaccine development and research, issue immunization policies and advise on strategies extending beyond childhood immunization to all major vaccine-preventable diseases throughout all age groups. SAGE, therefore, evolved "into a body overarching global immunization" [8,9]. SAGE was asked to advise the WHO Director-General on the adequacy of progress towards the achievement of the GIVS objectives and to identify major issues and challenges.

SAGE's role was again updated in 2011 when the Global Vaccine Action Plan (GVAP) was established as the strategic framework for the new decade [10]. SAGE was asked to determine the ambitions for 2011–2020 and took on a critical role in the GVAP oversight. SAGE provided annual reviews of progress facilitated by its Decade of Vaccine Working Group. SAGE's assessment of progress on the GVAP goals fed into a subsequent review and assessment by ministers of health through WHO's Executive Board and the World Health Assembly.

The co-creation process of the current decade's vaccine and immunization strategy, Immunization Agenda 2030 (IA2030) [11,12], included a broad range of national and international stakeholders that helped shape the vision and strategy for 2021–2030 [13]. IA2030 aspires to ensure that the vision, strategic priorities and goals are strongly driven by and aligned with country needs. Once a year, SAGE provides an independent review and guidance across the IA2030 strategic priority areas, informed by a detailed analysis of annual progress as laid out by the monitoring and evaluation framework.

Notwithstanding the impact of the above-mentioned global immunization strategies on the scope of SAGE, two external evaluations have also shaped SAGE's operations. These evaluations improved the advisory group's functioning and helped to more strongly root it within the global, regional and national immunization decision-making context.

A first review looking at the overall immunization advisory architecture of WHO was conducted in 2007. It confirmed SAGE as the principal advisory committee, which makes recommendations on all aspects pertaining to vaccine and immunization policies and strategies. The evaluation stressed, though, the importance of stronger linkages between SAGE and the Regional Immunization Technical Advisory Groups (RITAGs). Further evaluations of the impact and functioning of SAGE and of WHO's immunization advisory committees took place over the years.

In 2018, the last independent external evaluation of SAGE coincided with the launch of WHO's 13th General Programme of Work as well as with the planning process for the 2021–2030 global immunization strategy [14]. It also built on a corporate evaluation of WHO's normative function, initiated in 2017 [15], and emphasized the importance of serving the needs of countries. Overall, the evaluation concluded that the immunization stakeholder community considered SAGE extremely valuable and well respected, played a critical and leadership role in global immunization and was strong in providing evidence-based recommendations. The overall SAGE modus operandi with the consensus-based decision-making, the use of Working Groups, and the robust scientific advisory structure using evidence-based methodologies were considered highly effective. At the same time, several areas for improvement were highlighted. In response to these, the SAGE terms of reference [16] were revised to more clearly reflect the primary goals and scope of SAGE. A more systematic and transparent agenda-setting process was implemented, and the interactions between SAGE, RITAGs and National Immunization Technical Advisory Groups (NITAGs) were strengthened further. Moreover, additional guidance on what constitutes a conflict of interest for SAGE members and those providing input to the SAGE reviews of evidence was put in place.

3. SAGE's Regular Proceedings

As of today, SAGE's main purpose is to provide normative and strategic guidance on the use of existing or novel vaccines within national immunization programs. SAGE is advisory to the Director General of WHO, and all major vaccine- and immunization-related topics for which WHO requires strategic and policy advice are reviewed by SAGE. For its work, SAGE also relies on technical input from other more specialized advisory groups (see below).

SAGE is engaged in communication with regions and countries via RITAGs and NITAGs. Interactions with NITAGs are facilitated through the Global NITAG Network (GNN) [17] and regional NITAG networks. RITAGs are concerned with regional immunization policies and play an important role in the adaptation of global recommendations issued by SAGE into the regional- and country-level guidance. For example, in response to SAGE's 2020 recommendation to prioritize the uses of COVID-19 vaccines in the context of limited supply, the European Technical Advisory Group of Experts on Immunization (ETAGE) adapted those recommendations based on regional epidemiology, available literature, vaccine impact modeling and published preliminary recommendations of selected

NITAGs in the region [18]. In return, national-level requests for strategic and policy advice and country experiences are considered in SAGE's work.

SAGE is composed of 15 internationally renowned experts with a strong devotion to public health, acting in their individual capacities. Candidatures are solicited through a public call for nominations. Experts are selected across a wide spectrum of academic disciplines, specialty areas and professions. Above all, SAGE members are selected based on their scientific excellence, professional experience, and seniority while ensuring diversity not only through the vast range of expertise represented on SAGE but also by appointing a geographical and gender-balanced advisory group. Members of SAGE are not remunerated for serving on SAGE and should be free of vested interests. Therefore, upon appointment and ahead of each meeting, SAGE members are asked to declare potential interests that are then assessed and managed by the WHO Secretariat and disclosed publicly ahead of each meeting [19].

SAGE meets face-to-face biannually, generally for 3 to 4 days. Meetings are scheduled years in advance and are structured into open and closed sessions. Plenary sessions, widely attended by immunization stakeholders and Members State representatives, are convened for the purpose of exchanging information and discussing policy options. Representatives of different stakeholder groups, including UN partner agencies, governmental and non-governmental organizations, funders and manufacturers via umbrella organizations, can attend the open session upon invitation, which, since the COVID pandemic, has been organized in a hybrid mode of both in-person and online. To ensure transparency and wide engagement of the immunization community, policy recommendations are made in the open session. The specific wording of the recommendations may be refined in the closed SAGE sessions, which also serve for technical briefings and managerial issues.

On special occasions, as at the onset or during public health emergencies such as Ebola and COVID-19, SAGE is convened as necessary for extraordinary sessions in order to assure that policy guidance is provided in a real-time manner commensurate as required by the public health emergency and as the evidence allows.

Topic-specific SAGE Working Groups are set up to collate and synthesize evidence and policy options for consideration by the full SAGE committee. Working Groups are established following an open call for membership and are usually time-limited. Two SAGE members ensure that liaison between SAGE and the respective Working Group [20] (see Figure 1).

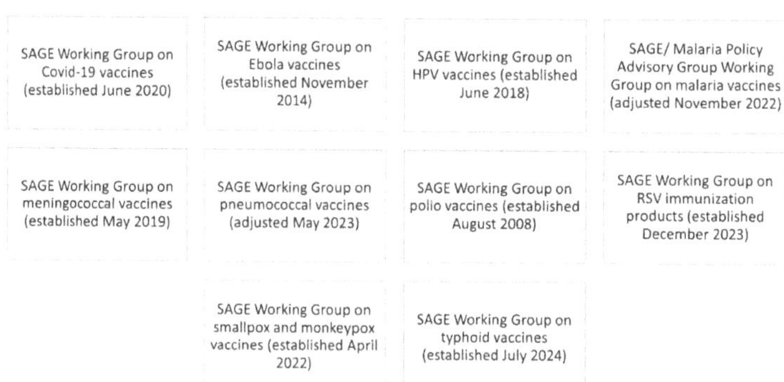
SAGE Working Group on Covid-19 vaccines (established June 2020)
SAGE Working Group on Ebola vaccines (established November 2014)
SAGE Working Group on HPV vaccines (established June 2018)
SAGE/ Malaria Policy Advisory Group Working Group on malaria vaccines (adjusted November 2022)
SAGE Working Group on meningococcal vaccines (established May 2019)
SAGE Working Group on pneumococcal vaccines (adjusted May 2023)
SAGE Working Group on polio vaccines (established August 2008)
SAGE Working Group on RSV immunization products (established December 2023)
SAGE Working Group on smallpox and monkeypox vaccines (established April 2022)
SAGE Working Group on typhoid vaccines (established July 2024)

Figure 1. Current SAGE Working Groups (November 2024).

Following each meeting, SAGE presents its policy recommendations to WHO's Director General for formal endorsement. Only thereafter can SAGE's advice be considered as official WHO guidance, most often reflected in WHO vaccine position papers. WHO publishes these vaccine position papers to provide global vaccine and immunization recommendations for diseases that have a major public health impact at a global or regional level. Vaccine position papers can be considered the flagship of global immunization guidance and are subject to a rigorous development process, which entails extensive peer-review by staff across the different levels of the organization as well as by external subject-matter experts. Over the course of the past 25 years, a total of 78 new or updated vaccine position papers (or closely related guidance) have been published on a total of 27 vaccines/vaccine-preventable diseases and two cross-cutting immunization-related topics (behavioral and social drivers of vaccine uptake and pain mitigation at the time of vaccination) (Table 1).

SAGE issues policy recommendations on vaccines against diseases of major public health importance. Policy recommendations are normally directed at a product class and indication, and product-specific considerations are only mentioned if they are public-health-relevant. Vaccines will be considered for policy if the manufacturer is regulated by a national authority of high competency (WHO-listed authority, previously termed maturity level 3 or higher). Besides the policy recommendations, WHO has a program for the prequalification of vaccines for public procurement [21]. This process is independent of the recommendation process and looks primarily at the quality, safety and efficacy of vaccines, as well as their programmatic suitability. In contrast to policy recommendations, WHO prequalification is product-specific.

Evidence-based decision-making in public health emphasizes that decisions should be informed by the best available scientific evidence as well as other criteria, such as context, equity, feasibility of implementation, affordability, sustainability and acceptability to stakeholders [22,23]. SAGE requests that all evidence on which its guidance is based be publicly available. SAGE has always recognized the necessity of providing guidance based on recent, ideally high-certainty data, assessed by internationally recognized methods, approaches and best practices. The processes, methods and approaches used by SAGE to develop evidence-based recommendations have been published as an authoritative document [24] and follow WHO's overall guidance for its core normative work.

The Grading of Recommendations, Assessment, Development and Evaluation (GRADE) approach [25] is an approach to rate the certainty of the best available evidence in developing healthcare recommendations. GRADE has been adopted by WHO and many other national and international organizations, with SAGE being an early adopter, having applied this methodology since April 2007 [26].

GRADE feeds into the Evidence-to-Decision table [27], a decision-support framework that encourages an explicit accounting of the panel's judgments based on the available evidence. These frameworks encourage the panel to consider the benefits and potential harms of an intervention but also other criteria, including resource requirements, cost-effectiveness, acceptability, feasibility and values and preferences. Documenting the assessment of each of these criteria in a systematized and transparent way allows interested parties to comprehend the thought process behind the recommendation. It further enables regional and country immunization programs to better adapt guidance to their local context.

In the context of immunization policies, SAGE follows the GRADE approach and may provide countries with strong or conditional recommendations [28]. Strong recommendations may be issued when the evidence base has been judged to be moderate to high. Strong recommendations may also be issued exceptionally based on low or very low certainty of evidence if the intervention reduces mortality in life-threatening situations or if adverse events following the intervention are deemed to be acceptable [28].

Conditional recommendations may be issued when the evidence-base has been judged to be low to very low, or when there is a close balance between the desirable and the undesirable consequences of an intervention.

All SAGE recommendations may be restrictive to a certain condition, setting, geography or population.

Table 1. New or updated vaccine position papers by year.

YEAR	1998	1999	2000	2001	2002	2003	2004	2005 ^	2006
Vaccine position paper	**Varicella vaccines *** **Japanese encephalitis vaccines ***	**Rotavirus vaccines *** **Pertussis vaccines ***	**Rubella vaccines**	**Cholera vaccines *** **Mumps virus vaccines***	**Rabies vaccines *** **Meningococcal vaccines: polysaccharide and poly-saccharide conjugate vaccines ***	Rotavirus vaccines **Pneumococcal vaccines *** **Yellow fever vaccine ***	**BCG Vaccine *** **Measles vaccines *** **Hepatitis B vaccines ***	None	**Diphtheria vaccines *** **Tetanus vaccine *** Japanese Encephalitis Vaccines **Haemophilus *influenzae* type b (Hib) conjugate vaccines ***
YEAR	**2007**	**2008**	**2009**	**2010**	**2011**	**2012**	**2013**	**2014**	**2015**
Vaccine position paper	**Mumps virus vaccines *** Rabies vaccine Pneumococcal conjugate vaccine Rotavirus vaccines Rabies vaccines	**Typhoid vaccines *** 23-valent pneumococcal poly-saccharide vaccine	**Human papillomavirus vaccines *** Measles vaccines Hepatitis B vaccines Rotavirus vaccines	Cholera vaccines **Polio vaccines and polio immunization in the pre-eradication era *** Rabies vaccines	**Vaccines against tick-borne encephalitis *** **Rubella vaccines *** Meningococcal vaccines	**Pneumococcal vaccines *** **Hepatitis A vaccines *** **Vaccines against influenza ***	Rotavirus vaccines Vaccines and vaccination against yellow fever HiB vaccination	Polio vaccines **Varicella and herpes zoster vaccines *** Human papillomavirus vaccines	Japanese Encephalitis Vaccines Meningococcal A conjugate vaccine **Hepatitis E vaccines** Pertussis vaccines **Reducing pain at the time of vaccination ***
YEAR	**2016**	**2017**	**2018**	**2019**	**2020**	**2021**	**2022**	**2023**	**2024**
Vaccine position paper	**Malaria vaccine *** Polio vaccines **Dengue vaccine ***	Tetanus vaccines Measles vaccines Human papillomavirus vaccines Hepatitis B vaccines Diphtheria vaccines Cholera vaccines	BCG vaccines Typhoid vaccines Rabies vaccines Dengue vaccines	Pneumococcal conjugate vaccines in infants and children under 5 years of age	Rubella vaccines	Pneumococcal vaccines/ their use in community outbreak settings Rotavirus vaccines	Malaria vaccine Vaccines against influenza **Understanding the behavioral and social drivers of vaccine uptake** Polio vaccines Hepatitis A vaccines Human papillomavirus vaccines	None	Meningococcal vaccines/use of multivalent meningococcal conjugate vaccines in countries of the African meningitis belt Mumps virus vaccines Dengue vaccines Malaria vaccine **Smallpox and mpox (orthopoxviruses) vaccine ***

^ SAGE took on a formal role in revising the WHO vaccine position papers as of 2005. * First position paper on a specific topic.

SAGE may issue off-label recommendations. Off-label recommendations for public health use [29] differ from the use indication on the product label provided by the manufacturer and reviewed by regulatory authorities in case there is a significant benefit from it to the target populations. The importance of SAGE's off-label recommendations is twofold: the recommendations provide global guidance to NITAGs considering going beyond the use-indication, be it in emergency situations or to optimize the efficiency and reach of the intervention at programme level. In addition, these recommendations provide a signal to manufacturers to consider seeking label extensions by national regulatory authorities. Off-label recommendations span from use in target (e.g., pregnancy) or age groups beyond those of the label, fractional doses or different routes of administration and, most commonly, alternative (often reduced) dosing schedules. Off-label recommendations are based on evidence and are the result of a benefit–risk assessment.

One highly consequential off-label recommendation resulting in great public health benefit was issued by SAGE in 2022 [30] when it was concluded that a single-dose of Human Papillomavirus (HPV) vaccine delivers comparable protection against cervical cancer as the 2-dose schedule in girls aged 9–14 years. This recommendation became a game-changer for vaccination programs, addressing serious supply constraints, easing programmatic introduction and cutting costs, thereby enabling countries to reach more girls with this life-saving vaccine. Since this recommendation, several manufacturers have initiated studies on single-dose schedules with the aim of seeking a product label variation.

The work of complementary WHO immunization-related advisory committees, with specialized remits, provides a unique resource for SAGE and plays an important role in the development of policy recommendations (Figure 2).

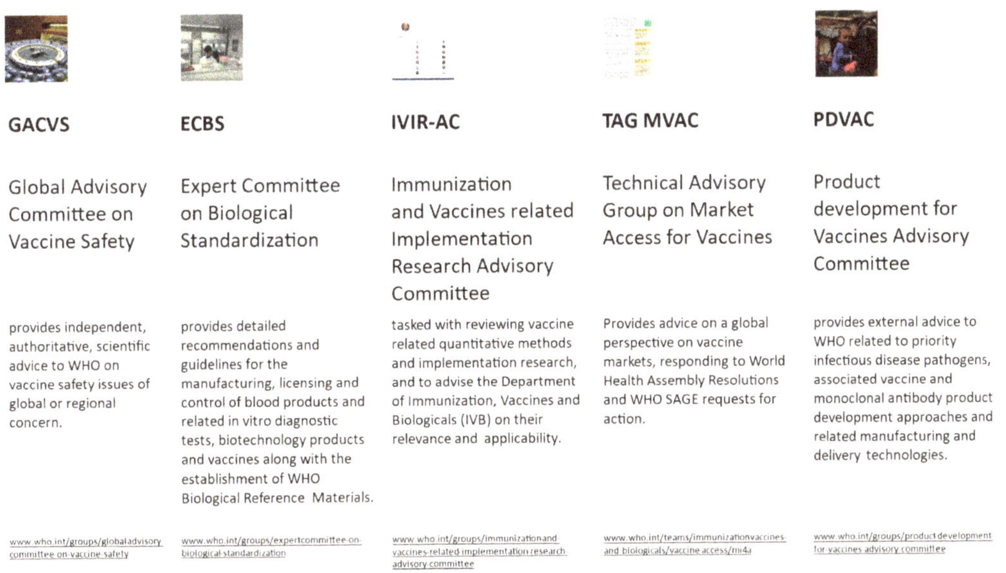

Figure 2. Other WHO advisory groups and committees relevant to immunization.

Three advisory groups are of particular relevance to SAGE:

The Product Development for Vaccines Advisory Committee (PDVAC) [31] is an advisory group of experts that provides advice to WHO on research matters related to priority infectious disease pathogens and vaccines yet under development. Early engagements with SAGE help to define key data needs for future policy development at a time when some of the questions can be integrated into late-stage vaccine development. As a result, relevant and timely data may inform SAGE policy recommendations once candidate vaccines mature to obtain regulatory approval. The Global Advisory Committee on Vaccine

Safety (GACVS) [32] is an advisory group dedicated to vaccine safety, in particular, to conduct post-introduction safety assessments. In special situations, SAGE may request a GACVS review on prelicensure vaccine safety data. The risk assessment by GACVS, as well as advice on pharmacovigilance, will be considered in SAGE's benefit–risk assessment and formulation of policy.

The Immunization- and Vaccine-related Implementation Research Advisory Committee (IVIR-AC) [33] provides an independent appraisal of and advice on questions related to vaccine implementation and, in particular, an appraisal of methods used for the quantitative effects of vaccines, such as the population impact and cost-effectiveness analysis, which are important data to shape SAGE's recommendations on policy and vaccination strategies. IVIR-ACs emphasize the suitability of methods, while the outputs of the quantitative analysis will be scrutinized by SAGE and its Working Groups.

4. SAGE Recommendations in Special and Emergency and Humanitarian Situations

SAGE's objective is to develop timely recommendations with an emphasis on equity and optimal population protection. In emergency situations, recommendations need to be issued, often on the basis of less comprehensive information, which may take the form of interim recommendations. Managing uncertainty in issuing policy recommendations requires well-balanced recommendations, maximal transparency regarding prevailing data gaps and the effective mitigation strategies of supply constraints. In all these circumstances, SAGE may issue off-label recommendations after careful assessment of the risks and benefits. In emergency situations, SAGE also advises on the use of emergency-use-authorized (or WHO emergency use listing [34]) vaccines and, in exceptional circumstances, on expanded access strategies on investigational products.

4.1. *Decision-Making in the Context of Uncertainty*

SAGE is often confronted with the task of issuing policy recommendations, while data generated during the clinical trial program used for registration are comprehensive but may be limited in terms of enrolled study populations, sample size, duration of follow-up or other elements desirable for robust policy recommendations. While this situation occurs inevitably in the context of emergency situations (see below), it also often applies to new vaccines registered for routine use. In any of these circumstances, SAGE will request additional research and more comprehensive data and adapt/complete its recommendations if needed. Without discussing the examples in detail, reference can be made to SAGE's decision-making in the context of uncertainty when advising on dengue and malaria vaccination as two examples.

4.1.1. Dengue Vaccination

In 2016, WHO issued the first WHO position paper on dengue vaccination, based on a comprehensive review of data generated from a multicentric clinical trial on a first-in-class product. Noting residual data gaps regarding the safety of the vaccine, WHO issued a conditional recommendation for limiting vaccine use in geographic areas with a high burden of disease. This was a precautionary measure against an, at that time, unproven risk of enhanced disease in vaccine recipients not previously exposed to dengue prior to vaccination. This recommendation was backed by an extensive benefit–risk analysis. Following cases of severe disease in several dengue-vaccinated children in a school-based vaccination program, a major controversy arose. While it was not possible to assess if cases occurred as a result of enhanced disease following vaccination or were cases of breakthrough disease, at WHO's request, the manufacturer conducted an additional analysis of clinical trial samples with a newly developed diagnostic procedure. SAGE rapidly reconvened in November 2017 to assess the emerging evidence from a retrospective analysis of clinical trial data. The data confirmed the previously hypothetical excess risk of severe dengue in seronegative vaccine recipients compared to seronegative non-vaccinated individuals while confirming long-term protection in seropositive individuals. While the initial positive benefit–risk assessment did not change, SAGE provided revised recommendations in April 2018 that were reflected in an updated vaccine position paper [35], providing the option of serologic pretesting of individuals prior to vaccination.

4.1.2. Malaria Vaccination

In 2015, SAGE and the Malaria Policy Advisory Committee (MPAC) (For the malaria session, SAGE was joined by the Malaria Policy Advisory Committee (MPAC) and the conclusions and recommendations concerning the malaria vaccine were those of both committees. MPAC is now called the Malaria Policy Advisory Group (MPAG). MPAG provides independent, strategic advice to WHO on all technical areas relating to malaria control and elimination.) in a joint session, assessed the evidence of a first-generation malaria vaccine, which had received a positive regulatory opinion (Using the EU-Medicines for all procedure (EU-M4all) to provide an opinion on medicines and vaccines for human use intended exclusively for markets outside of the European Union (Article 58 of the EMA Regulation (EC) No 726/2004).) by the European Medicines Agency. While the benefit–risk assessment was positive, potential safety signals had emerged from a detailed review of the phase three clinical trials program (i.e., meningitis, cerebral malaria and excess of deaths from all causes in girls compared to boys). In addition, there was uncertainty about the feasibility of implementing the vaccination schedule in a routine immunization program because it required new touchpoints. To address those uncertainties and ancillary research questions, it was recommended that additional evidence be collected through a staged pilot implementation in several countries, such as the malaria vaccine implementation program (MVIP). A framework for policy decision-making was developed for MVIP, which prospectively defined the data required for a more generalized policy recommendation. When those data became available, a second joint SAGE/MPAG[3] evidence review session was convened in October 2021, resulting in a recommendation and WHO position paper in March 2022 [36]. RTS,S was prequalified in July 2022, which then allowed for a malaria vaccine roll-out (with Gavi support) throughout *P. falciparum* malaria-endemic countries.

4.2. SAGE in the Context of Outbreaks and Pandemics

SAGE also serves as WHO's vaccine and immunization advisory body for the use of vaccines in the context of public health emergencies. Urgent strategic and policy advice by SAGE was required in the context of the H1N1 pandemic in 2009, the yellow fever outbreak in 2016, the Ebola outbreaks in 2013–2016 and 2018–2020, the COVID-19 pandemic in 2020–2023, and more recently, the mpox outbreaks in 2022–2023 and 2024, covering six of the seven Public Health Emergencies of International Concern (PHEIC) declared by WHO. Only the Zika virus PHEIC did not have a vaccination component, but the process triggered the development activities of this much-needed vaccine.

SAGE's engagement within these outbreaks varied, as described below. In each case, the aim has been to provide timely, evidence-based, pragmatic public health policy recommendations on vaccine use and prioritization in settings with incomplete and evolving evidence regarding the pathogen, epidemiology, risk factors for infection and disease and the vaccines.

4.3. Multi-Country Yellow Fever Outbreak

In 2016, large-scale yellow fever outbreaks were reported from central Africa, sharply increasing the demand for already limited yellow fever global vaccine supplies. WHO needed to swiftly respond to the rapidly depleting vaccine stockpile. In July 2016, WHO reviewed potential vaccine dose-sparing options, namely fractional doses using different modes of administration and manufacturers' reports on potency and other criteria. Given the urgent need for WHO policy guidance to its Member States and to the wider vaccine community, SAGE was asked to appraise an assessment of evidence prepared by the secretariat, which was then released as WHO guidance. This was an exceptional process, given the lack of time for the formal SAGE review of evidence and deliberation processes that usually inform and result in its recommendations [37]. A formal SAGE assessment of the available evidence, as well as the country's experience with implementing the fractional dose policy, was conducted subsequently by SAGE in October 2016. The advisory group recommended that a fractional dose could be used as part of an exceptional response [38], and these recommendations were reflected in an addendum to the WHO yellow fever position paper [39]. SAGE was also asked to provide strategic advice leading to the development of the Eliminate Yellow Fever Epidemics (EYE) strategy [40], a global effort to tackle, in a co-ordinated manner, the increased risk of yellow fever epidemics for the period 2017–2026. Since then, the research agenda advocated for by SAGE has largely been implemented, and the fractional dose strategy for yellow fever outbreaks has been recommended in other emergency situations.

4.4. The 2009 H1N1 Influenza a Pandemic

In the context of the 2009 Influenza A (H1N1) pandemic, an ad hoc Working Group on H1N1 vaccines was established. Their assessment, alongside regional perspectives, led SAGE to issue emergency recommendations on H1N1 vaccines during an extraordinary meeting on 7 July 2009. SAGE noted that "its recommendations reflected the pandemic's current estimated severity and, as the situation evolves and more evidence becomes available, the recommendations may need to be revisited" [41]. SAGE noted with great concern that in the current situation, a small number of industrialized countries would have access to most of the global vaccine supply over the next 12 months through purchase agreements, limiting vaccine availability for the rest of the world and especially in developing countries. Therefore, SAGE emphasized the importance of striving to achieve equity among countries concerning access to the vaccines developed in response to the pandemic. While H1N1's disease severity and pandemic trajectory, fortunately, did not necessitate an extended global vaccination response, the pandemic influenza preparedness (PIP) framework for the sharing of influenza viruses and access to vaccines and other benefits was developed and adopted by the Sixty-fourth World Health Assembly in 2011.

4.5. COVID-19 Pandemic

While the world was caught by surprise with the emergence of a previously unknown virus, SARS-CoV2, in late 2019 and its unprecedented spread starting in early 2020, the initial absence of vaccines provided SAGE with several months to prepare for their arrival. During this time, SAGE started proceedings under the assumption that vaccine development would be successful. In anticipation of the urgently awaited results of vaccine clinical trials, SAGE, supported by its COVID-19 Working Group set up in June 2020 [42] and several subgroups (prioritization, evidence and modeling subgroup), went beyond its usual guidance. SAGE initially developed an ethics- and value-based framework for countries on the prioritization of population groups for the anticipated initial limited vaccination supply [43].

As the COVID-19 Vaccines Global Access (COVAX) initiative, the vaccines pillar of the Access to COVID-19 Tools (ACT) Accelerator [44] was being set up—a global collaboration to accelerate the development, production and equitable access to COVID-19 tests, treatments and vaccines—and SAGE was naturally confirmed as its advisory body responsible for issuing evidence-based immunization policy recommendations.

Upon the arrival of the first vaccine doses, SAGE's functioning was pressure-tested. The committee needed to act at speed while keeping abreast of the ever-evolving evidence, often not even published in the scientific literature. Informed by a living systematic review of the evidence [45] and close exchanges with the global research community, and informed by manufacturers, SAGE, in 2021, developed a noteworthy number of 23 product-specific interim recommendations and other related COVID-19 publications, such as guidance on extended COVID-19 immunization schedules for immunocompromized individuals.

The COVID-19 Working Group met weekly over the course of the pandemic, accounting for more than 100 meetings. SAGE convened a record number of 17 times following the declaration of the COVID-19 PHEIC in 2020 to its lifting in 2023 (Figure 3).

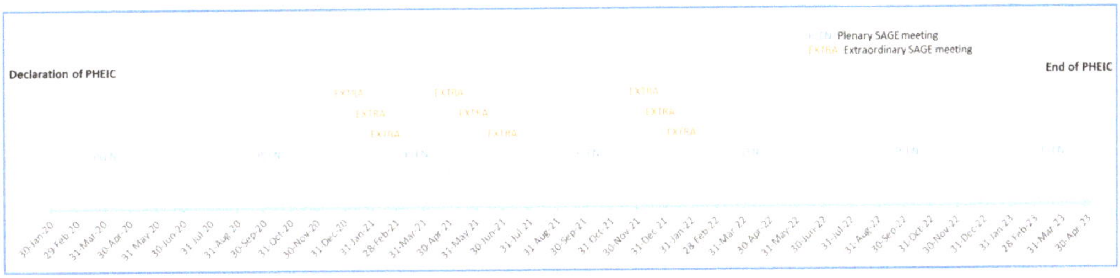

Figure 3. Occurrence of ordinary and extraordinary SAGE meetings in the period of the COVID-19 PHEIC.

The COVID-19 pandemic put exceptional strain on SAGE, the SAGE COVID-19 vaccines Working Group and on WHO staff. Meeting the needs of Member States, the global public health community, COVAX and many other stakeholders was the top priority for WHO's vaccine policy and strategy team and tremendously challenging given the evidence gaps, the need for real-time review and synthesis of newly available evidence and the soar in workload this demanded. For SAGE members, the surge in the number and scale of policy recommendations that needed to be formulated meant dedicating a huge amount of time to keep up with rapidly emerging data, revision of documents and attending multiple virtual meetings, in addition to the equally demanding surge in day-to-day activities of their regular employment.

Additionally, the necessity for SAGE to make decisions expeditiously in conditions of significant uncertainty, such as in the context of constant virus evolution and changing population immunity, was unprecedented. Unlike regular recommendations, where SAGE reviews data across a class of vaccines against a specific antigen, the COVID-19 pandemic forced SAGE to issue product-specific recommendations across the various vaccine platforms authorized by regulatory bodies using emergency procedures. This led to a massive increase in supplementary work, both for SAGE and its WHO secretariat.

The lessons learned during COVID-19 fed into updated guidance on the development of WHO vaccines and immunization policy and strategic guidance. Post-pandemic, SAGE methods and procedures were adjusted, and the type of guidance issued was more clearly defined into three categories: formal WHO recommendations issued following a comprehensive evidence review of disease epidemiology and vaccine performance compiled over an extended period; rapid advice guidance, issued within a week to three months; emergency guidance, developed within hours to days of an emergency notification, necessitating a potential vaccine response [24].

During the pandemic, many NITAGs relied on and adapted WHO's recommendations to their respective national contexts. A 2021 survey of 44 countries confirmed that SAGE recommendations concerning COVID-19 vaccines were assessed to be comprehensive and timely. Furthermore, they were seen as easy to access, understand and adapt [46].

5. Looking Ahead and Conclusions

SAGE's greatest strength emerges from those individuals serving on it. Over the years, passionate and committed experts in the field of vaccines and immunization have dedicated very significant time and energy to serve on and/or chair the panel and its Working Groups. Experts have made outstanding contributions and have genuinely committed to advancing the global immunization agenda and have left a lasting imprint. Continuing to attract the world's most distinguished vaccine and immunization experts and ensuring their engagement remains the cornerstone of SAGE's functioning.

The steadfastness of the advisory group comes from the adherence to the guiding principles of independence, transparency and scientific rigor. Mechanisms to ensure adherence to these principles have evolved over time but have always remained the key pillar of SAGE's standing.

Nevertheless, the progressive realization of these principles remains an ongoing effort. The relationship between science, policy and public opinion often remains complex, not only during exceptional circumstances, such as public health emergencies. Independence, scientific excellence, transparency and timeliness are essential qualities of credible recommendations. Beyond these attributes, effective communication is key, and SAGE aspires to make its decisions comprehensible and openly acknowledge data gaps, limitations and uncertainties. This is of particular importance during disease outbreaks where massive amounts of information (i.e., so-called infodemics), including false or misleading information by various media or individual sources, often overwhelms even knowledgeable and well-informed individuals.

Inevitably, SAGE needs to take into account novel ways of communication in a rapidly changing environment. As already remarked in the 2018 evaluation of SAGE [14], the advisory group could further improve the dissemination of its outputs. A lot of work has been performed since 2018 to facilitate access to information related to SAGE's work. A recent effort has been the development of the search tool on the WHO website, which enables the user to scan SAGE-related meetings and documents for specific search terms [47]. That said, SAGE needs to remain vigilant to the rapid developments in the field of communication while ensuring that any new strategy is tailored to the needs of its target audience.

Special emphasis should be placed on maintaining SAGE's strong linkage and relationship with RITAGs and NITAGs as well as with key actors in the immunization community, including international and non-governmental organizations, donors, manufacturers and other partners.

In the context of declining and competing financial and human resources, the capacity of countries to introduce novel vaccines into their immunization programs is increasingly saturated. The prioritization of vaccines and other public health measures in the current resource and funding environment, including dedicated cost-effectiveness analysis, is inherent to national programs and needs to be tackled at the country level. WHO and other stakeholders will continue to assist Member States with their vaccine and immunization prioritization exercises; efforts to develop respective tools are ongoing and will be reviewed by SAGE in 2025.

The ongoing mpox PHEIC has again reminded the global health community that crises necessitating a vaccination response will continue to occur, likely even at a higher frequency due to climate-change-related phenomena such as flooding, population displacements, encroachment on animal habitats, overcrowding and armed conflict. In this context, rapid, evidence-based guidance remains highly relevant and important. One of the IA2030 strategic priorities is to improve peoples' and health authorities' valuing of immunization. To reach this goal, IA2030 calls to strengthen evidence-based decision-making and points out the critical role of NITAGs. Stronger efforts are required to ensure that NITAGs and national immunization programs in low- and middle-income settings are adequately supported to take SAGE's guidance and tailor context-specific vaccination recommendations.

WHO and its partners are working to strengthen country competencies and build regional hubs and centers of excellence to that effect. Notably, the Global NITAG Network (GNN) [48] is a platform for fostering collaborations as well as sharing experiences and best practices among NITAGs. The NITAG Resource Center [49] is a unique source of information, providing national immunization programs and NITAGs with evidence, information and training to develop national immunization policies on vaccine-preventable diseases. A more systematic approach has been set up to engage NITAGs with the SAGE plenary meetings and to disseminate the outcomes and formal recommendations to the NITAG community. Through the Global NITAG Network [17], regular webinars are conducted with NITAGs across the world to debrief the community on SAGE deliberations.

Technological innovations also have a role to play: artificial intelligence (AI)-aided approaches are facilitating the work in many fields, including public health. AI will have a profound impact on how evidence-based recommendations are developed. Scientific advisory bodies, including SAGE, need to anticipate and leverage these changes. Keeping abreast of these evolutions is paramount given that resource-constrained settings, which SAGE caters specifically to, may particularly benefit from these developments. Processes are evolving at this moment and have started to provide faster and resource-sparing solutions, including AI-performed evidence syntheses. Questions remain on their validity and policy-relevant interpretation. One future scenario may be for SAGE to provide policy options that can easily be tailored to the specific context with the help of AI.

In conclusion, over the last quarter century, SAGE has significantly contributed to shaping the vaccine and immunization landscape globally. It has earned and maintained a high level of integrity and credibility. The advisory group continues to be an authority in global public health, and its recommendations have profound implications for the health of individuals and populations across the globe. SAGE's reach and impact depend on its relevance to regions and countries and for stakeholders and partners to build on SAGE's recommendations. The contextualization of recommendations to country needs, priorities, and capacities has gained major importance, and SAGE will assess strategies and tools to assist countries in prioritizing vaccines at the national level.

Against the backdrop of the plethora of crises and emerging global challenges, such as climate change, migration, armed conflict, humanitarian emergencies and aging populations, continuous critical revision and adaptation of SAGE's scope and working processes is key to ensuring the appropriateness of its guidance and relevance to the WHO Member States and partners in the decades to come.

Author Contributions: Conceptualization, M.M., K.L.O., H.N., P.D. and J.H.; writing—original draft preparation, M.M., J.H., K.L.O., H.N. and P.D.; writing—review and editing, K.L.O., P.D., J.H. and H.N.; supervision, J.H., K.L.O. and H.N. All authors have read and agreed to the published version of the manuscript. The authors alone are responsible for the views expressed in this article and they do not necessarily represent the views, decisions or policies of the institutions with which they are affiliated.

Funding: This research received no external funding.

Informed Consent Statement: Not applicable.

Data Availability Statement: Data sharing is not applicable.

Acknowledgments: We would like to acknowledge the immense contributions to SAGE of the former SAGE Chairs: Gustav Nossal, Merceline Dahl-Regis, David Salisbury, Helen Rees, Jon Abramson and Alejandro Cravioto. We would further like to express our deep gratitude to all former and current SAGE members who dedicated their time and energy to support SAGE.

Conflicts of Interest: M.M., K.L.O. and J.H are employees of the World Health Organization. K.L.O. serves as the Director of the Department of Immunization, Vaccines and Biologicals which hosts the Secretariat of SAGE, J.H. serves as Executive Secretary of SAGE and M.M. works in the SAGE Secretariat. H.N. serves as the current Chair of SAGE. P.D. previously worked for the World Health Organization and served as the Executive Secretary for SAGE.

References

1. *Constitution of the World Health Organization*; World Health Organization: Geneva, Switzerland, 1946. Available online: https://www.who.int/about/governance/constitution (accessed on 2 December 2024).
2. Greenwood, B. The contribution of vaccination to global health: Past, present and future. *Philos. Trans. R. Soc. B: Biol. Sci.* **2014**, *369*, 20130433. [CrossRef] [PubMed]
3. Shattock, A.J.; Johnson, H.C.; Sim, S.Y.; Carter, A.; Lambach, P.; Hutubessy, R.C.W.; Thompson, K.M.; Badizadegan, K.; Lambert, B.; Ferrari, M.J.; et al. Contribution of vaccination to improved survival and health: Modelling 50 years of the Expanded Programme on Immunization. *Lancet* **2024**, *403*, 2307–2316. [CrossRef] [PubMed]
4. *WHO Expanded Programme on Immunization: World Health Assembly*; World Health Organization: Geneva, Switzerland, 1947. Available online: https://iris.who.int/handle/10665/92778 (accessed on 2 December 2024).

5. *Report of the Meeting of the Scientific Advisory Group of Experts*; SAGE; World Health Organization: Geneva, Switzerland, 1998. Available online: https://www.who.int/publications/i/item/WHO-GPV-98.06 (accessed on 2 December 2024).
6. Expanded Programme on Immunization: Global Advisory Group. Geneva: World Health Organization. 1992. Available online: https://iris.who.int/handle/10665/228245 (accessed on 2 December 2024).
7. Duclos, P.; Okwo-Bele, J.-M.; Salisbury, D. Establishing global policy recommendations: The role of the Strategic Advisory Group of Experts on immunization. *Expert Rev. Vaccines* **2011**, *10*, 163–173. [CrossRef] [PubMed]
8. Meeting of the immunization Strategic Advisory Group of Experts, Geneva, 10–11 April 2006: Conclusions and recommendations. *Wkly. Epidemiol. Rec.* **2006**, *81*, 210–220.
9. Duclos, P.; Okwo-Bele, J.-M. Recommandations et politiques vaccinales mondiales: Le rôle de l'OMS. *Méd./Sci.* **2007**, *23*, 409–416. [CrossRef] [PubMed]
10. *Global Vaccine Action Plan 2011–2020*; World Health Organization: Geneva, Switzerland, 2013. Available online: https://www.who.int/publications/i/item/global-vaccine-action-plan-2011-2020 (accessed on 2 December 2024).
11. *Immunization Agenda 2030: A Global Strategy to Leave No One Behind*; World Health Organization: Geneva, Switzerland, 2020. Available online: https://www.who.int/teams/immunization-vaccines-and-biologicals/strategies/ia2030 (accessed on 2 December 2024).
12. Immunization agenda 2030: A global strategy to leave no one behind. *Vaccine* **2024**, *42*, S5–S14. [CrossRef] [PubMed]
13. O'Brien, K.L.; Lemango, E.; Nandy, R.; Lindstrand, A. The immunization Agenda 2030: A vision of global impact, reaching all, grounded in the realities of a changing world. *Vaccine* **2024**, *42*, S1–S4. [CrossRef] [PubMed]
14. *Report of the Expert Advisory Group on SAGE Evaluation. (EAGSE)*; World Health Organization: Geneva, Switzerland, 2018. Available online: https://www.who.int/publications/m/item/evaluation-of-the-strategic-advisory-group-of-experts-(sage)-on-immunization (accessed on 2 December 2024).
15. *WHO Transformation*; World Health Organization: Geneva, Switzerland, 2024. Available online: https://www.who.int/about/transformation (accessed on 2 December 2024).
16. *Terms of Reference for the Strategic Advisory Group of Experts. (SAGE) on Immunization*; World Health Organization: Geneva, Switzerland, 2022. Available online: https://www.who.int/publications/m/item/sage-terms-of-reference (accessed on 2 December 2024).
17. *Global NITAG Network*; World Health Organization: Geneva, Switzerland, 2024. Available online: https://www.nitag-resource.org/ (accessed on 2 December 2024).
18. *20th Meeting of the European Technical Advisory Group of Experts on Immunization (ETAGE)*; World Health Organization: Copenhagen, Denmark, 2020. Available online: https://iris.who.int/bitstream/handle/10665/338559/WHO-EURO-2021-1808-41559-56715-eng.pdf?sequence=1 (accessed on 2 December 2024).
19. *WHO Strategic Advisory Group of Experts (SAGE) on Immunization Meetings*; World Health Organization: Geneva, Switzerland, 2024. Available online: https://www.who.int/groups/strategic-advisory-group-of-experts-on-immunization/meetings (accessed on 2 December 2024).
20. Strategic Advisory Group of Experts (SAGE) on Immunization Working Groups. Geneva: World Health Organization. 2024. Available online: https://www.who.int/groups/strategic-advisory-group-of-experts-on-immunization/working-groups (accessed on 2 December 2024).
21. *WHO Prequalification-Vaccines*; World Health Organization: Geneva, Switzerland, 2024. Available online: https://extranet.who.int/prequal/vaccines (accessed on 2 December 2024).
22. Clark, R.; Haby, M. Chapter 7. Evidence-based policy: Why and how. In *Creating and Implementing Public Policy: Cross-Sectoral Debates*; Carey, G., Landvogt, K., Barraket, J., Eds.; Routledge: Abingdon, UK; Oxon, UK, 2015; pp. 98–112.
23. Brownson, R.C.; Fielding, J.E.; Maylahn, C.M. Evidence-Based Public Health: A Fundamental Concept for Public Health Practice. *Annu. Rev. Public Health* **2009**, *30*, 175–201. [CrossRef] [PubMed]
24. Development of WHO immunization policy and strategic guidance. In *Methods and Processes Applied by the Strategic Advisory Group of Experts on Immunization (SAGE) to Develop Evidence-Based Recommendations*; World Health Organization: Geneva, Switzerland, 2024. Available online: https://www.who.int/publications/i/item/9789240090729 (accessed on 2 December 2024).
25. Guyatt, G.H.; Oxman, A.D.; Vist, G.E.; Kunz, R.; Falck-Ytter, Y.; Alonso-Coello, P.; Schünemann, H.J. GRADE: An emerging consensus on rating quality of evidence and strength of recommendations. *BMJ* **2008**, *336*, 924. [CrossRef] [PubMed]
26. Duclos, P.; Durrheim, D.N.; Reingold, A.L.; Bhutta, Z.A.; Vannice, K.; Rees, H. Developing evidence-based immunization recommendations and GRADE. *Vaccine* **2012**, *31*, 12–19. [CrossRef] [PubMed]
27. Alonso-Coello, P.; Schünemann, H.J.; Moberg, J.; Brignardello-Petersen, R.; Akl, E.A.; Davoli, M.; Treweek, S.; Mustafa, R.A.; Rada, G.; Rosenbaum, S.; et al. GRADE Evidence to Decision (EtD) frameworks: A systematic and transparent approach to making well informed healthcare choices. 1: Introduction. *BMJ* **2016**, *353*, i2016. [CrossRef] [PubMed]
28. Andrews, J.C.; Schünemann, H.J.; Oxman, A.D.; Pottie, K.; Meerpohl, J.J.; Coello, P.A.; Rind, D.; Montori, V.M.; Brito, J.P.; Norris, S.; et al. GRADE guidelines: 15. Going from evidence to recommendation—Determinants of a recommendation's direction and strength. *J. Clin. Epidemiol.* **2013**, *66*, 726–735. [CrossRef] [PubMed]
29. Neels, P.; Southern, J.; Abramson, J.; Duclos, P.; Hombach, J.; Marti, M.; Fitzgerald-Husek, A.; Fournier-Caruana, J.; Hanquet, G. Off-label use of vaccines. *Vaccine* **2017**, *35*, 2329–2337. [CrossRef] [PubMed]
30. *Human Papillomavirus Vaccines: WHO Position Paper*; World Health Organization: Geneva, Switzerland, 2022. Available online: https://www.who.int/publications/i/item/who-wer9750-645-672 (accessed on 2 December 2024).

31. Product Development for Vaccines Advisory Committee. Geneva: World Health Organization. 2024. Available online: https://www.who.int/groups/product-development-for-vaccines-advisory-committee (accessed on 2 December 2024).
32. *WHO Global Advisory Committee on Vaccine Safety*; World Health Organization: Geneva, Switzerland, 2024. Available online: https://www.who.int/groups/global-advisory-committee-on-vaccine-safety/ (accessed on 2 December 2024).
33. *Terms of Reference for the Immunization and Vaccines Related Implementation Research Advisory Committee (IVIR-AC)*; World Health Organization: Geneva, Switzerland, 2024. Available online: https://www.who.int/publications/m/item/terms-of-reference-for-the-immunization-and-vaccines-related-implementation-research-advisory-committee-(ivir-ac) (accessed on 2 December 2024).
34. *WHO Emergency Use Listing*; World Health Organization: Geneva, Switzerland, 2024. Available online: www.who.int/teams/regulation-prequalification/eul/eul-vaccines (accessed on 2 December 2024).
35. *Dengue Vaccines: WHO Position Paper–September 2018*; World Health Organization: Geneva, Switzerland, 2018. Available online: https://www.who.int/publications/i/item/dengue-vaccines-who-position-paper-september-2018 (accessed on 2 December 2024).
36. *Malaria Vaccine: WHO Position Paper–March 2022*; World Health Organization: Geneva, Switzerland, 2022. Available online: https://www.who.int/publications/i/item/who-wer9709-61%E2%80%9380 (accessed on 2 December 2024).
37. *Fractional Dose Yellow Fever Vaccine as a Dose-Sparing Option for Outbreak Response WHO Secretariat Information Paper*; World Health Organization: Geneva, Switzerland, 2016. Available online: https://www.who.int/publications/i/item/WHO-YF-SAGE-16-1 (accessed on 2 December 2024).
38. Meeting of the Strategic Advisory Group of Experts on Immunization: Conclusions and recommendations. *Wkly. Epidemiol. Rec.* **2016**, *91*, 561–582.
39. Mondiale de la Santé, O.; World Health Organization. Yellow fever vaccine: WHO position on the use of fractional doses–June 2017. *Wkly. Epidemiol. Rec. = Relev. Épidémiologique Hebd.* **2017**, *92*, 345–350.
40. *Eliminate Yellow Fever Epidemics (EYE) Strategy 2017–2026*; World Health Organization: Geneva, Switzerland, 2016. Available online: https://www.who.int/initiatives/eye-strategy (accessed on 2 December 2024).
41. Meeting of the Strategic Advisory Group of Experts on Immunization, 7 July 2009: Extraordinary Meeting on the Influenza A (H1N1) 2009 Pandemic. Geneva: World Health Organization. 2009. Available online: https://www.who.int/publications/i/item/WER8430 (accessed on 2 December 2024).
42. SAGE Working Group on COVID-19 Vaccines. World Health Organization. Geneva, 2024. Available online: https://www.who.int/groups/strategic-advisory-group-of-experts-on-immunization/working-groups/covid-19 (accessed on 2 December 2024).
43. WHO. *WHO SAGE Values Framework for the Allocation and Prioritization of COVID-19 Vaccination*; World Health Organization: Geneva, Switzerland, 2020.
44. *ACT Accelarator and COVAX Facility*; World Health Organization: Geneva, Switzerland, 2020. Available online: https://www.who.int/initiatives/act-accelerator (accessed on 2 December 2024).
45. Graña, C.; Ghosn, L.; Evrenoglou, T.; Jarde, A.; Minozzi, S.; Bergman, H.; Buckley, B.S.; Probyn, K.; Villanueva, G.; Henschke, N.; et al. Efficacy and safety of COVID-19 vaccines. *Cochrane Database Syst. Rev.* **2022**, *2023*, CD015477. [CrossRef]
46. Kahn, A.-L.; Steffen, C.A.; Henaff, L.; MacDonald, N.E.; Morgan, C.; Faden, R.; Olayinka, F.; Desai, S. COVID-19 vaccine policy development in a sample of 44 countries- Key findings from a December 2021 survey of National Immunization Technical Advisory Groups (NITAGs). *Vaccine* **2022**, *41*, 676–683. [CrossRef] [PubMed]
47. SAGE Documentation Search Tool. Geneva: World Health Organization. 2024. Available online: https://www.who.int/groups/strategic-advisory-group-of-experts-on-immunization/sage-documentation-search-tool (accessed on 2 December 2024).
48. Adjagba, A.; MacDonald, N.E.; Ortega-Pérez, I.; Duclos, P.; Participants, G.N.N.M. Strengthening and sustainability of national immunization technical advisory groups (NITAGs) globally: Lessons and recommendations from the founding meeting of the global NITAG network. *Vaccine* **2017**, *35*, 3007–3011. [CrossRef] [PubMed]
49. Adjagba, A.; Henaff, L.; Duclos, P. The NITAG Resource Centre (NRC): One-stop shop towards a collaborative platform. *Vaccine* **2015**, *33*, 4365–4367. [CrossRef] [PubMed]

vaccines

MDPI

Article

Strengthening National Immunization Technical Advisory Groups: Twelve Years of Progress (2012–2023)

Louise Henaff [1,*], Laure Dumolard [1], Vinod Bura [2], Gerald Etapelong Sume [3], Sidy Ndiaye [4], Jennifer Sanwogou [5], Heeyoun Cho [6], Joachim Hombach [1] and Christoph A. Steffen [1]

1 World Health Organization (WHO), 1211 Geneva, Switzerland; dumolardl@who.int (L.D.), hombachj@who.int (J.H.); steffenc@who.int (C.A.S.)
2 World Health Organization (WHO) Regional Office for South-East Asia, New Delhi 110002, India; burav@who.int
3 World Health Organization (WHO) Regional Office for the Eastern Mediterranean, Cairo 11371, Egypt; sumeetapelongg@who.int
4 World Health Organization (WHO) Regional Office for Africa, Brazzaville P.O. Box 06, Congo; ndiayes@who.int
5 World Health Organization (WHO) Regional Office for the Americas, Washington, DC 20037, USA; sanwogoj@paho.org
6 World Health Organization (WHO) Regional Office for the Western Pacific, Manila 1000, Philippines; hcho@who.int
* Correspondence: henaffl@who.int

Abstract: Introduction: Well-functioning National Immunization Technical Advisory Groups (NITAGs) are valuable contributors to decision-making processes in the complex immunization policy arena. This paper describes the progress made globally on the establishment and strengthening of these key advisory groups and discusses some of their strengths, challenges, and opportunities. Methods: The data submitted annually by countries to the World Health Organization (WHO) via the WHO/UNICEF Joint Reporting Form (JRF) were analyzed, comparing the NITAG functionality criteria in 2012 and 2023. Results: In 2023 and 2012, 88% and 61% of countries, respectively, reported having a NITAG. A total of 77% of NITAGs met all six NITAG process criteria in 2023 compared to 33% in 2012. This progress was most notable in the WHO African Region, increasing from 7% (2012) to 77% (2023), and the South-East Asia Region, increasing from 45% (2012) to 91% (2023). In 2023, 84% of NITAGs issued a vaccine-policy recommendation that was adopted by decision-makers. Discussion: Marked progress has been made since 2012 on establishing and maintaining NITAGs, with a small number of countries yet to form an advisory committee. Supporting and sustaining NITAG functions remains an important means for countries to foster independent and transparent expert advice on vaccine and immunization policy. Setbacks in countries facing instability or political turmoil are a reminder of the reversibility of progress. WHO and partners play an important role in supporting countries in strengthening these advisory committees. Continuous commitment by countries to the function and involvement of NITAGs in policy recommendations is essential for enhancing the strength and resilience of immunization programs.

Keywords: National Immunization Technical Advisory Groups; NITAGs; immunization policy; WHO–UNICEF Joint Reporting Form

1. Introduction

National Immunization Technical Advisory Groups (NITAGs) are pivotal to vaccine and immunization policy processes in many countries, providing independent, transparent,

 https://doi.org/10.3390/vaccines13010080

and evidence-based advice to national immunization policymakers. Decisions to introduce new vaccines into a country's immunization program result in long-term financial and programmatic commitments and establish community expectations. Beyond advising on vaccine introductions, NITAGs also guide policymakers on optimizing existing immunization programs and addressing broader health system challenges, such as low vaccine coverage and programmatic barriers. The advice from NITAGs is also important for longer-term immunization program planning, such as that defined in the National Immunization Strategy (see the following: https://www.who.int/teams/immunization-vaccines-and-biologicals/vaccine-access/planning-and-financing/nis, accessed on 1 October 2024). Hence, through providing independent expert reviews and advice, NITAGs have become increasingly important in guiding and advising decision-makers.

The state of NITAGs at the global and regional levels in 2012 has been previously published [1]. The aim of this paper is to describe the global and regional progress on NITAG development and strengthening over the past 12 years. To this effect, this paper presents a global overview of NITAGs in 2023, comparing it to the situation in 2012 through an analysis of NITAG indicators reported via the WHO–UNICEF Joint Reporting Form on Immunization (JRF).

2. Background

The first NITAGs, established in the 1960s, included the United Kingdom's Joint Committee on Vaccination and Immunisation (JCVI) (1963); the United States' Advisory Committee on Immunization Practices (ACIP) (1964); and Canada's National Advisory Committee on Immunization (NACI) (1964). These advisory committees marked the beginning of formalized bodies providing independent, expert advice on vaccine and immunization policy.

The Agence de Médecine Préventive launched the Supporting Independent Immunization and Vaccine Advisory Committees (SIVAC) Initiative in 2008. This WHO Collaborating Center, funded by the Bill & Melinda Gates Foundation and Gavi, helped establish and strengthen more than 20 NITAGs across Africa, Asia, and Eastern Europe over a period of 10 years [2].

To better understand the progress in NITAG development globally, WHO added specific questions about their functionality to the JRF on vaccines and immunization in 2010. These additions allowed for the annual monitoring of NITAG progress and facilitated advocacy for establishing NITAGs in countries that lacked them. Data from the JRF enabled targeted capacity-building efforts and the provision of tailored technical support.

The Global Vaccine Action Plan (GVAP), endorsed by the World Health Assembly in 2012, was pivotal in advocating for the scale-up and strengthening of NITAGs globally. GVAP emphasized that every country should have access to the services of a functional NITAG and urged governments not only to establish these committees but also to equip them to support informed, independent, evidence-based decision-making regarding vaccines [3].

When the SIVAC initiative ended in 2017, WHO and technical partners swiftly transitioned the support function by assigning dedicated staff at WHO headquarters and regional offices and building regional partnerships with various institutions, such as the NITAG Support Hub (NISH), founded in 2021 and based in Cape Town, South Africa, to ensure continued support for NITAGs globally. Regional partners play a key role in assisting WHO in the training of newly formed NITAGs.

The Immunization Agenda 2030, which details the vaccination and immunization strategic priorities for 2030, reaffirms the importance of functional NITAGs for the success of immunization programs worldwide. Building on the momentum created by GVAP, the agenda identifies NITAGs as a critical component for ensuring the sustainability of immunization policies, country ownership, and the introduction of new vaccines [4].

3. Methods

Data for this paper were compiled from the 2012 and 2023 WHO–UNICEF JRFs. This standard questionnaire—sent annually to all Member States since 1998—collects data on all immunization aspects, including vaccine coverage, reported cases of vaccine-preventable diseases, immunization schedules, as well as performance indicators of the immunization program and financing. Questions relating to NITAGs in the JRF included a set of six process indicators pertaining to the characteristics and functioning of a NITAG [5]. These indicators are as follows: (i) a legislative or administrative basis for the advisory group; (ii) formal written terms of reference; (iii) a diversity of expertise among core members (referencing pediatrics, public health, infectious diseases, epidemiology, immunology, or other relevant areas of health-care expertise); (iv) the number of meetings held per year (a minimum of one meeting per year is needed to meet the requirement of this indicator); (v) circulation of the agenda and background documents at least one week prior to meetings; and (vi) the mandatory disclosure of any conflicts of interest.

In addition to these process-related indicators, WHO added in 2021 two output indicators to the JRF questionnaire: (i) did the NITAG issue one or more recommendations (during the year)?; and (ii) are one or more of the NITAG recommendations adopted by the Ministry of Health (during the year)?

More specific information on the JRF and the data collection process is published on the WHO website [6].

The results were stratified by WHO Regions, World Bank national income status categories [7], eligibility for support by Gavi [8] (which includes all countries with a gross national income of ≤USD 1810 per capita in accordance with World Bank data for the latest available year), and population size for the year 2023. Population figures used are those from the United Nations Population Division [9].

Note that all 2012 comparator figures are taken from the 2013 published analysis and are not included in the visuals of this paper.

4. Results

The 2023 status of the NITAG-related indicators at global and regional levels is presented in Table 1, while Table 2 provides an analysis of these indicators, stratified by World Bank income groups, eligibility for GAVI support, and population size.

NITAG-related JRF data were available from 193 of the 194 WHO Member States in 2023, compared with 191 Member States in 2012. With the exception of the Cook Islands, which did not report in 2023, all Member States reporting data in 2012 also reported data in 2023. Countries that did not report in 2012 but did so in 2023 include Austria, Monaco, and Serbia.

In 2023, 88% (170/193) of reporting countries, representing 98% of the global population, reported having a NITAG to guide their immunization policy decisions. By comparison, in 2012, only 61% (116/191) of reporting countries, covering 89% of the global population, reported having a NITAG (Table 1).

When examining countries that reported having a NITAG that met all six process criteria, the progress between the two periods is even more apparent. In 2023, 68% of reporting countries (131/193), representing 84% of the global population, had a NITAG meeting all six criteria. In contrast, in 2012, only 33% of countries, covering 52% of the global population, had a NITAG that met these criteria.

Table 1. Analysis of the NITAG 2024 Joint Reporting Form data for 2023, globally and by WHO Region.

Countries with NITAG Data Available/WHO Member States	Indicator	Region OVERALL N = 193/194 (99%)	AFR N = 47/47 (100%)	AMR N = 35/35 (100%)	EMR N = 21/21 (100%)	EUR N = 53/53 (100%)	SEAR N = 11/11 (100%)	WPR N = 26/27 (96%) [a]
Existence of a NITAG	Number of countries	170	41	33	21	51	11	13
	% of countries with NITAG data available	88%	87%	94%	100%	96%	100%	50%
	% of the entire population covered	98%	99%	96%	100%	99%	100%	93%
Existence of a NITAG with formal terms of reference	Number of countries	168	40	33	21	50	11	13
	% of countries reporting the existence of a NITAG	99%	98%	100%	100%	98%	100%	100%
	% of the entire population covered	97%	98%	96%	100%	94%	100%	93%
Existence of a NITAG with a legislative or administrative basis	Number of countries	168	39	33	21	51	11	13
	% of countries reporting the existence of a NITAG	99%	95%	100%	100%	100%	100%	100%
	% of the entire population covered	97%	98%	96%	100%	99%	100%	93%
Existence of a NITAG with ≥5 areas of expertise represented	Number of countries	162	40	30	19	50	10	13
	% of countries reporting the existence of a NITAG	95%	98%	91%	90%	98%	91%	100%
	% of the entire population covered	96%	99%	93%	96%	99%	99%	93%
Existence of a NITAG which met at least once in 2023	Number of countries	153	39	31	19	46	11	7
	% of countries reporting the existence of a NITAG	90%	95%	94%	90%	90%	100%	54%
	% of the entire population covered	91%	98%	83%	91%	83%	100%	83%
Existence of a NITAG for which the agenda and background documents distributed ≥1 week prior to meetings	Number of countries	153	39	31	19	46	11	7
	% of countries reporting the existence of a NITAG	90%	95%	94%	90%	90%	100%	54%
	% of the entire population covered	91%	98%	83%	91%	83%	100%	83%
Existence of a NITAG whose members are required to disclose conflicts of interest	Number of countries	168	39	31	16	45	11	12
	% of countries reporting the existence of a NITAG	99%	95%	94%	76%	88%	100%	92%
	% of the entire population covered	97%	98%	75%	87%	90%	100%	92%
Existence of a NITAG meeting all 6 criteria above	Number of countries	131	36	26	14	39	10	6
	% of reporting countries	68%	77%	74%	67%	74%	91%	23%
	% of countries reporting the existence of a NITAG	77%	88%	79%	67%	76%	91%	46%
	% of the entire population covered	84%	98%	59%	79%	73%	99%	81%

WHO Regions: AFR: African Region; AMR: Region of the Americas; EMR: Eastern Mediterranean Region; EUR: European Region; SEAR: South-East Asia Region; WPR: Western Pacific Region. [a] The only WHO Member State for which data are missing is the Cook Islands. N = total number of countries that reported in 2024 on NITAG data for 2023.

Progress varied across WHO Regions. The African Region saw an increase in countries meeting all six criteria, with 77% (36/47 countries, covering 98% of the population) in 2023 up from 7% of countries (3/46 countries representing 7% of the region's population) in 2012. Similarly, in the South-East Asia Region, 91% (10/11) of countries in 2023 had a NITAG meeting the six criteria, while only 45% (5/11) of countries had the same in 2012.

In the Region of the Americas and the European Region, the increase was also noticeable. In 2023, NITAGs that met the six criteria were reported in 74% (26/35) and 74% (39/53) of countries, respectively. In 2012 this was the case for only 37% (13/35) and 44% (22/50) of reporting countries, respectively.

Table 2. Analysis of the NITAG 2024 Joint Reporting Form data for 2023, by World Bank income status, Gavi eligibility, and population size.

	World Bank Income Status [a]			Gavi-Eligible Countries	Population Size	
	Low Income	**Middle Income**	**High Income**		**Less than 9,193,372 [b]**	**Greater than or Equal to 9,193,372**
Reporting Countries/Total (%)	26/26 (100%)	103/103 (100%)	62/62 (100%)	57/57 (100%)	96/97 (99%)	97/97 (100%)
NITAG exists/No. Reporting (%)	25/26 (96%)	87/103 (84%)	58/62 (94%)	52/57 (91%)	78/96 (81%)	92/97 (95%)
Formal terms of reference/No. Reporting (%)	25/26 (96%)	86/103 (83%)	57/62 (92%)	51/57 (89%)	77/96 (80%)	91/97 (94%)
Legislative or administrative basis for NITAG/No. Reporting (%)	25/26 (96%)	85/103 (83%)	58/62 (94%)	51/57 (89%)	76/96 (79%)	92/97 (95%)
At least 5 areas of expertise represented/No. Reporting (%)	24/26 (92%)	82/103 (80%)	56/62 (90%)	50/57 (88%)	75/96 (78%)	87/97 (90%)
Met at least once in 2023/No. Reporting (%)	23/26 (88%)	80/103 (78%)	50/62 (81%)	47/57 (82%)	71/96 (74%)	82/97 (85%)
Agenda and background documents distributed ≥1 week prior to meetings/No. Reporting (%)	23/26 (88%)	80/103 (78%)	50/62 (81%)	47/57 (82%)	71/96 (74%)	82/97 (85%)
Required to disclose conflicts of interest/No. Reporting (%)	23/26 (88%)	78/103 (76%)	53/62 (85%)	48/57 (84%)	69/96 (72%)	85/97 (88%)
Meeting all 6 criteria above/No. Reporting (%)	22/26 (85%)	66/103 (64%)	43/62 (69%)	43/57 (75%)	59/96 (61%)	72/97 (74%)

[a] The denominator is not the 194 WHO Member States but 191 countries for which the World Bank is providing the information, as of July 2024. Information on income status is missing for the Cook Islands, Niue, and Venezuela (the Bolivarian Republic of). [b] This figure was selected as being the median of the total population for the 194 WHO Member States in 2023.

In the Western Pacific Region, progress had stalled, with 50% (13/26) of countries reporting the existence of a NITAG in 2023 versus 56% (15/27) in 2012. Likewise, 23% (6/26) of NITAGs reported meeting all six process criteria in 2023, versus 26% (7/27) in 2012. This was due largely to the absence of progress in small Pacific Island countries.

In the Eastern Mediterranean Region, the proportion of countries meeting the six criteria increased slightly, rising to 67% (14/21) of countries in 2023 compared to 62% (13/21) in 2012.

The process criteria with the lowest scores in 2023 were "circulation of the agenda and background documents ahead of the meetings" and "holding at least one NITAG meeting per year". In contrast, in 2012, "mandatory disclosure of conflicts of interest" obtained the lowest achievement rate.

As shown in Table 2, the breakdown of these indicators by income class for 2023 shows that low- and high-income countries reported similar proportions of NITAG existence (94% and 96%, respectively). Middle-income countries reported a slightly lower proportion, with 84% having an established NITAG. However, when considering the proportion of NITAGs meeting all six process criteria, low-income countries led, with 84% meeting the criteria, while high- and middle-income countries reported lower scores of 69% and 64%, respectively. This is a notable shift from the pattern observed in 2012, when high-income countries consistently outperformed middle- and low-income countries in both the existence of NITAGs and meeting the six process criteria. Moreover, larger countries with populations above 10 million showed a higher proportion of reporting countries that met the six process criteria (74%) compared to smaller countries (61%).

The NITAG output indicators provide further insight into the performance of NITAGs (Figure 1). Globally, in 2023, 87% of countries with a NITAG reported issuing recommendations in the past year, with 84% having the recommendations adopted by their Ministry of Health. The regional analysis, however, reveals disparities. All countries in the South-East Asia Region reported issuing NITAG recommendations in 2023 that were adopted by their Ministry of Health, fully meeting all indicators for the NITAG. By contrast, in the Western Pacific Region, only 69% of countries issued recommendations that had been adopted in 2023. The other four WHO Regions (Africa, the Americas, Europe, and Eastern Mediterranean) displayed relatively high performance for both indicators, ranging from 78% to 94%.

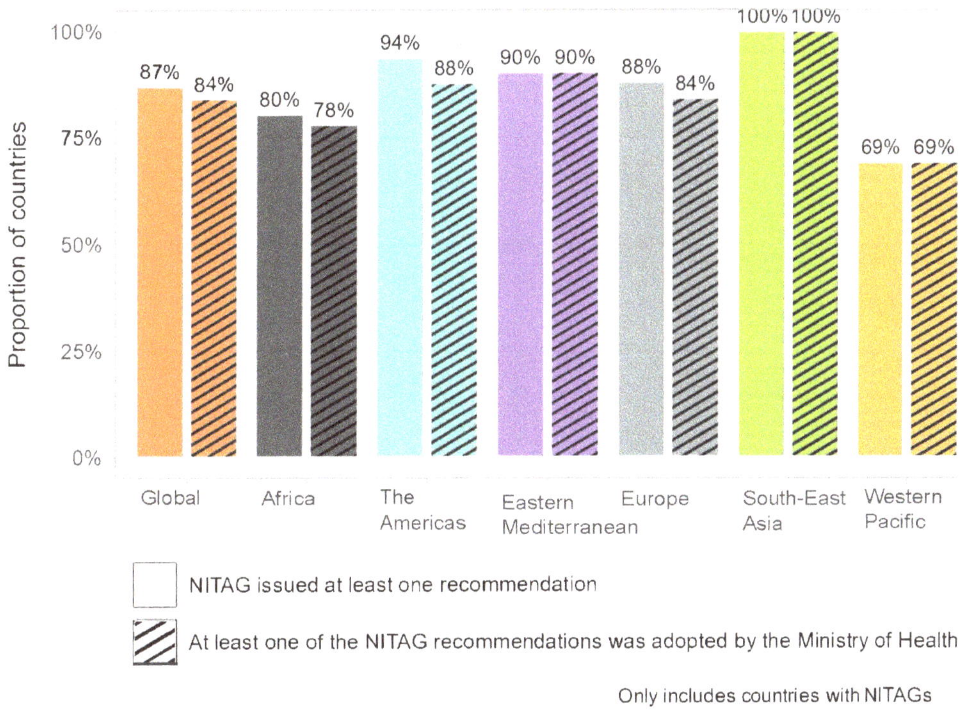

Figure 1. Proportion of countries with a NITAG that, in 2023, (i) had a NITAG issuing recommendations, and (ii) had NITAG recommendations adopted by the Ministry of Health, by WHO Region.

The ability of NITAGs to issue recommendations adopted by the Ministry of Health varied according to the functionality status of the NITAGs (Figure 2). Globally, 94% of countries with a NITAG that met the six process criteria issued at least one recommendation in 2023, compared with 64% of countries that did not meet those criteria. Likewise, 91% of countries with NITAGs meeting the six process criteria had at least one NITAG recommendation adopted by their Ministry of Health in 2023, compared with 62% of countries that did not meet those criteria.

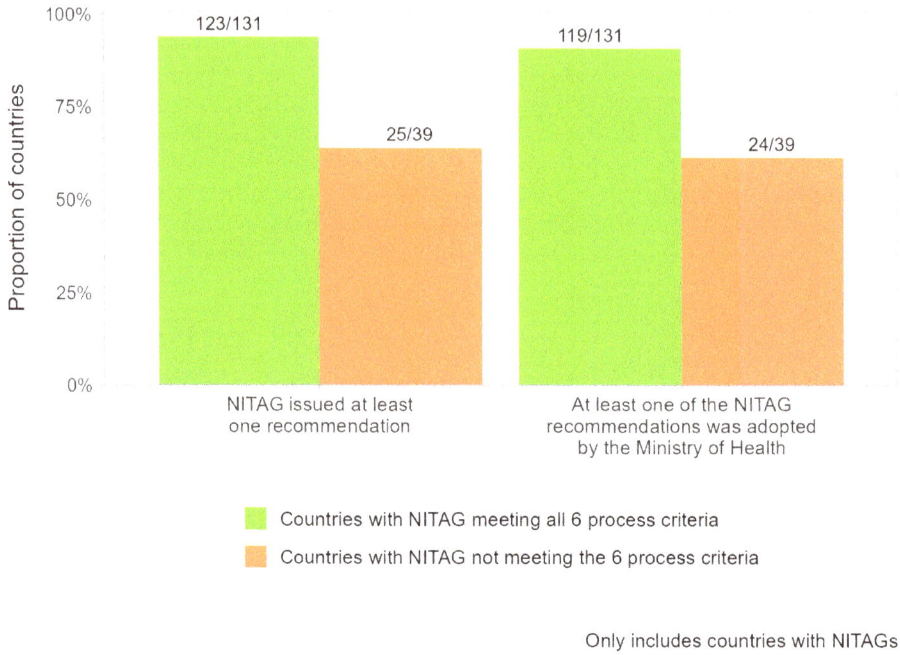

Figure 2. Proportion of countries with a NITAG that, in 2023 (i) had a NITAG issuing recommendations, and (ii) had NITAG recommendations adopted by the Ministry of Health, by their process-criteria status.

5. Discussion

The formation and functionality of NITAGs improved significantly between 2012 and 2023. During this period, global and regional stakeholders supported countries in establishing NITAGs and strengthening their capacities to carry out their important advisory role in supporting decision-makers.

Efforts have resulted in significant progress in the African Region and to a lesser degree also in the Eastern Mediterranean Region [10]. In 2023 alone, the WHO African Regional Office provided training courses for nine NITAGs on their role, responsibilities, and the evidence-to-recommendation framework, while the Eastern Mediterranean Regional Office conducted similar training for 10 countries.

In the South-East Asia Region, the progress on NITAG functionality has, likewise, been notable. The relatively small number of countries (with very large populations) facilitated more targeted support. For example, the South-East Asia Regional Office conducted independent external evaluations of NITAGs in the region during 2019–2020, enabling each NITAG to develop a clear improvement plan.

The finding that low-income countries currently have a higher proportion of NITAGs that meet all six process criteria is testament to the commitment and support these countries have mobilized, including from WHO and other partners, to strengthen their capabilities. Low-income countries also benefit from Gavi financial support, which enables the establishment of technical secretariats; the organization of meetings; the participation of NITAG members in international meetings; and NITAG-strengthening activities.

The number of NITAGs reported globally—currently in 170 of 194 countries—demonstrates how even small nations and territories have succeeded in building mechanisms to access the expertise of an advisory group. A notable example is in the Caribbean, where the first subregional Caribbean Immunization Technical Advisory Group was formed, serving 22 countries and territories. This collaborative approach highlights the creativity, adaptability, and innovation of small countries in ensuring that they are part of global immunization policy efforts [11].

The Pacific Island countries, some with populations of just tens of thousands and often scattered over wide territories, are also exploring ways to pool resources to support subregional evidence-based decision-making. The lack of a tailored solution for Pacific Island countries has contributed to the delay in forming NITAGs in the Western Pacific Region.

The fact that larger countries seem to perform somewhat better than smaller countries on the six process criteria suggests that there may be a size threshold under which it becomes increasingly difficult for small countries to have a functional committee. Pooling resources within or between countries is even more important in those settings.

The circulation of the agenda and background documents at least one week prior to meetings serves as an indicator of the ability of the NITAG secretariats to function effectively. In 2023, this was the weakest indicator, suggesting a bottleneck for many NITAGs. Indeed, without dedicated secretariat resources, the sustainability and effectiveness of NITAG operations cannot be guaranteed. Currently, there is no clear definition of "an adequately resourced technical secretariat", and the JRF does not include specific questions regarding this. However, it is increasingly evident that the absence of dedicated technical staff to manage secretariat functions leads to delays in the work of NITAGs and weakens the evidence-based recommendation process. One option to document this could be to add to the JRF an additional question regarding the existence of a dedicated technical NITAG secretariat, accompanied by a clear definition of its role and responsibilities. Reporting on this additional criterion could help programs advocate more successfully for dedicated funding and staff for the secretariat.

Over three-quarters of countries with functioning NITAGs issued at least one recommendation in 2023, most of which were adopted by their respective ministries of health. This is a relatively crude but simple way to measure the output of NITAGs annually. However, it does not allow for the drawing of granular conclusions on differences in the reported figures on those indicators. The slightly higher score on the issuance of recommendations versus the adoption by the Ministry of Health is consistent with the fact that NITAGs are advisory bodies and that other considerations come into play in the decision-making process, such as budgetary and programmatic considerations. Moreover, the finding that countries that meet the six process criteria perform better overall on these outcomes supports the approach of WHO and partners to continue strengthening NITAG secretariats.

6. Actionable Recommendations

The Global NITAG Network (GNN) has called for a detailed analysis of instances where NITAG recommendations have not been adopted by ministries of health. Understanding the delays in implementing recommendations is crucial as they may stem from various factors, including budgetary constraints, logistical challenges, competing (health) priorities, or the need for further alignment with national or subnational policies or contexts. Further investigation is needed to identify specific barriers and to support the development of strategies that facilitate faster adoption and implementation of NITAG recommendations, ensuring timely improvements in public health outcomes. Moreover, ensuring that NITAGs also consider programmatic and economic considerations in their evidence-to-recommendation process will contribute to making recommendations more fit for purpose and applicable for governments.

NITAGs operating in politically unstable contexts face unique challenges in maintaining functionality and ensuring evidence-based decision-making for immunization.

In such environments, political turmoil, conflicts, and frequent changes in government can disrupt the consistency of NITAG meetings and hinder the implementation of their recommendations—although this is not fully evident in the 2023 JRF data alone. NITAGs that had existed for several years are being dismantled by changes in government, while others, barely set up, see their work abruptly interrupted. Further analysis is needed to capture the status and challenges of NITAGs operating in these situations.

In fragile settings, often with concomitant health emergencies, NITAGs could be instrumental in addressing critical programmatic issues, such as the maintenance of cold chains, ensuring vaccination coverage in remote or conflict-affected areas, and responding to outbreaks amidst challenging conditions. Flexibility in the response is paramount, and NITAGs could play an important role in this regard. The Regional Immunization Technical Advisory Group of the Eastern Mediterranean Region called for further documentation from countries to fully capture the role of NITAGs in these volatile environments and to explore strategies that could ensure their continuity during political transitions or instability. Strengthening support mechanisms and safeguarding their operations, even amidst governmental changes, are essential for preserving the ability of NITAGs to provide informed, evidence-based decisions for national immunization programs.

The JRF questionnaire covers a wide range of immunization-related topics, limiting the opportunity to include additional questions regarding NITAGs. The current NITAG-related questions do not sufficiently capture the complexity of their functionality nor reflect the nuances of their role in national policymaking. These limitations hinder a comprehensive assessment of how well NITAGs are integrated into the broader immunization decision-making system at the country level. WHO, therefore, encourages NITAGs to regularly evaluate their committees using a standardized assessment process, which would help identify gaps and promote long-term sustainability. The NITAG Maturity Assessment Tool (NMAT) developed by the United States Centers for Disease Control and Prevention, WHO, and other partners at the request of the GNN, provides a systematic evaluation framework and offers clear recommendations for strengthening NITAG functionality. The NMAT also enables NITAGs to measure their progress over time, ensuring continuous improvement and alignment with global standards [12].

7. Conclusions

Between 2012 and 2023, NITAGs increasingly became the global standard for providing expert advice to governments on immunization policies. Functionality, as measured by the six process criteria, progressed substantially, particularly in low- and middle-income countries. With most of the world's population now covered by a NITAG, it is crucial for countries to focus on sustaining the functionality of these committees. Looking ahead, sustained support for NITAG technical secretariats and the enhanced use of assessment tools—such as the NITAG Maturity Assessment Tool—will be key to further improving their functionality and effectiveness, enabling them to provide independent, evidence-based, and transparent immunization policy guidance.

Author Contributions: Conceptualization, L.H., J.H. and C.A.S.; Methodology, L.H., L.D., J.H. and C.A.S.; Validation, L.D., V.B., G.E.S., S.N., J.S., H.C., J.H. and C.A.S.; Formal Analysis, L.D. and C.A.S.; Data Curation, L.D., V.B., G.E.S., S.N., J.S., H.C., J.H. and C.A.S.; Writing—Original Draft Preparation, L.H., L.D. and C.A.S.; Writing—Review and Editing, L.H., L.D., V.B., G.E.S., S.N., J.S., H.C., J.H. and C.A.S.; Visualization, L.D. and C.A.S.; Supervision, L.H. All authors have read and agreed to the published version of the manuscript.

Funding: This research received no external funding.

Institutional Review Board Statement: The authors are staff members of the World Health Organization. The authors alone are responsible for the views expressed in this article and they do not necessarily represent the decisions, policy, or views of the World Health Organization.

Informed Consent Statement: Not applicable.

Data Availability Statement: Data used in this analysis are officially reported by WHO Member States through the electronic Joint Reporting Form (https://www.who.int/teams/immunization-vaccines-and-biologicals/immunization-analysis-and-insights/global-monitoring/who-unicef-joint-reporting-process/, accessed 1 October 2024), and publicly available from the WHO Immunization Data Portal (https://immunizationdata.who.int/, accessed 1 October 2024).

Acknowledgments: The annual collection of country data through the Joint Reporting Form is a remarkable commitment from countries to provide up-to-date and transparent indicators on the state of their immunization system. We express our sincere appreciation to colleagues who collect and report these important indicators from their countries. We also thank colleagues in the WHO country offices, regional offices, and headquarters who provide input and contributions to produce the most accurate figures.

Conflicts of Interest: L.H., L.D., V.B., G.E.S., S.N., J.S., H.C., J.H., and C.A.S. are employees of the World Health Organization Headquarters and Regional Offices. L.H. serves as the Executive Secretary of the Global NITAG Network and coordinates all NITAG strengthening activities. L.D. coordinates the annual data collection through the JRF. The authors alone are responsible for the views expressed in this article and they do not necessarily represent the views, decisions or policies of the institutions with which they are affiliated.

References

1. Duclos, P.; Dumolard, L.; Abeysinghe, N.; Adjagba, A.; Janusz, C.B.; Mihigo, R.; Mosina, L.; Takashima, Y.; Öztürk, M.H. Progress in the establishment and strengthening of national immunization technical advisory groups: Analysis from the 2013 WHO/UNICEF joint reporting form, data for 2012. *Vaccine* **2013**, *31*, 5314–5320. [CrossRef] [PubMed]
2. Adjagba, A.; Senouci, K.; Biellik, R.; Batmunkh, N.; Faye, P.C.; Durupt, A.; Gessner, B.D.; da Silva, A. Supporting countries in establishing and strengthening NITAGs: Lessons learned from 5 years of the SIVAC initiative. *Vaccine* **2015**, *33*, 588–595. [CrossRef] [PubMed]
3. Steffen, C.A.; Henaff, L.; Durupt, A.; Omeiri, N.E.; Ndiaye, S.; Batmunkh, N.; Liyanage, J.B.L.; Hasan, Q.; Mosina, L.; Jones, I.; et al. Evidence-informed vaccination decision-making in countries: Progress, challenges and opportunities. *Vaccine* **2021**, *39*, 2146–2152. [CrossRef]
4. Immunization Agenda 2030. Available online: www.immunizationagenda2030.org (accessed on 8 December 2024).
5. WHO. National Immunization Advisory Mechanism. Available online: https://immunizationdata.who.int/global/wiise-detail-page/national-immunization-advisory-mechanism?ISO_3_CODE=&YEAR= (accessed on 8 December 2024).
6. WHO. WHO/UNICEF Joint Reporting Process. Available online: https://www.who.int/teams/immunization-vaccines-and-biologicals/immunization-analysis-and-insights/global-monitoring/who-unicef-joint-reporting-process (accessed on 8 December 2024).
7. World Bank. GNI per Capita. Available online: https://data.worldbank.org/indicator/NY.GNP.PCAP.CD?view=chart (accessed on 8 December 2024).
8. Gavi. The Vaccine Alliance. Eligibility for Gavi Support Is Determined by Countries' National Income. Available online: https://www.gavi.org/types-support/sustainability/eligibility (accessed on 8 December 2024).
9. UN Population Division Data Portal. Available online: https://population.un.org/dataportal/ (accessed on 8 December 2024).
10. Sume, G.E.; Hasan, Q.; Shefer, A.; Henaff, L.; Cavallaro, K.F.; Tencza, C.B.; Hadler, S.C.; Sidy, N.; Sardar, P.; Kagina, B.M.; et al. Region-wide assessment of National Immunization Technical Advisory Groups (NITAGs) using the NITAG Maturity Assessment Tool (NMAT)—Experience from the Eastern Mediterranean Region of the World Health Organization, 2023. *Vaccine* **2024**, *42*, 2239–2245. [CrossRef]

11. Evans-Gilbert, T.; Figueroa, J.P.; Bonvehí, P.; Melgar, M.; Stecher, D.; Kfouri, R.; Munoz, G.; Bansie, R.; Valenzuela, R.; Verne, E.; et al. Establishing priorities to strengthen National Immunization Technical Advisory Groups in Latin America and the Caribbean. *Vaccine* **2024**, *42*, 2310–2316. [CrossRef] [PubMed]
12. Dryer, E.; Shefer, A.; Desai, S.; Rodewald, L.; Bastías, M.; El Omeiri, N.; Ndiaye, S.; Cook, K.; Henaff, L.; Kennedy, E. Development of a maturity assessment tool to evaluate and strengthen National Immunization Technical Advisory Groups (NITAGs). *Vaccine* **2024**, *42*, 126005. [CrossRef] [PubMed]

vaccines

MDPI

Article

Global Status of Adult Immunization Post COVID-19 Pandemic

Alba Vilajeliu [1,*], Victor Vega [1], Randie Gibson [1], Francisco Nogareda [2], Xiaojun Wang [3], Donald J. Brooks [4], Charles Shey Wiysonge [5], Osman Niyazi Cakmak [6], Osama Mere [7], Melanie Marti [1], Phillip Lambach [1], Stephanie Shendale [1], Marcela Contreras [2], Emmanuel Njambe [8], Erin Grace Sparrow [1], Joachim Hombach [1] and Ann Lindstrand [1]

1 Department of Immunization, Vaccines and Biologicals (IVB), World Health Organization, 1211 Geneva, Switzerland; vegav@who.int (V.V.); gibsonr@who.int (R.G.); martim@who.int (M.M.); lambachp@who.int (P.L.); shendales@who.int (S.S.); sparrowe@who.int (E.G.S.); hombachj@who.int (J.H.); lindstranda@who.int (A.L.)

2 Special Program Comprehensive Immunization, Pan American Health Organization (PAHO)/World Health Organization Regional Office for the Americas, Washington, DC 20037, USA; nogaredfra@paho.org (F.N.); contrermar@paho.org (M.C.)

3 Vaccine-Preventable Diseases and Immunization Unit, Division of Programmes for Disease Control, World Health Organization, Regional Office for Western Pacific, Manila 1000, Philippines; wangxia@who.int

4 Department of Epidemic and Pandemic Threat Management, World Health Organization, 1211 Geneva, Switzerland; brooksd@who.int

5 Vaccine-Preventable Diseases Programme, World Health Organization, Regional Office for Africa, Brazzaville P.O. Box 06, Congo; sheyc@who.int

6 Vaccine-Preventable Diseases and Immunization Programme, World Health Organization, Regional Office for Europe, 2100 Copenhagen, Denmark; cakmako@who.int

7 Immunization Vaccine Preventable Disease and Polio Transition Unit, Department of Communicable Diseases and Universal Health Coverage, World Health Organization, Regional Office for the Eastern Mediterranean, Cairo 11371, Egypt; mereo@who.int

8 Immunizations and Vaccines Development, World Health Organization, Regional Office for South-East Asia, New Delhi 110002, India; emmanuelt@who.int

* Correspondence: avilajeliu@who.int

Abstract: Background/Objective: Historically, immunization programs have focused on infants, children, and women of reproductive age. COVID-19 vaccination prompted countries to vaccinate adults. The objective of this manuscript is to provide a global overview of adult immunization policies post COVID-19 pandemic. Methods: We summarized WHO Strategic Advisory Group of Experts on Immunization (SAGE) recommendations by adult group and analyzed the data reported in 2024 (2023) by WHO Member States (MS) via the WHO/UNICEF electronic Joint Reporting Form on Immunization (eJRF) on national immunization schedules, and from other sources by WHO region and income group. Results: WHO policy recommendations exist for most of the licensed vaccines targeting adults; however, the inclusion in national immunization schedules is higher in high-income (HICs) and middle-income (MICs) countries. For pregnant women, 90% of MS reported vaccination against COVID-19 (65% in low-income countries [LICs]), 63% against tetanus-containing vaccines (73% in LICs), 57% against influenza (4% in LICs), and 21% against pertussis-containing vaccines (all MICs and HICs). For health workers, 91% against COVID-19 (92% in LICs), 59% against influenza (4% in LICs), and 25% against hepatitis B (10% in LICs). For adults with chronic diseases, COVID-19 vaccination data were not available, 58% against influenza, and 23% against pneumococcal disease. For older adults, more than 90% of MS across all income groups reported COVID-19 vaccination, 59% against influenza (8% of LICs versus 89% of HICs), 17% against pneumococcal, and 7% against herpes zoster (HZ). Conclusion: The disparities in adult immunization policies across income groups highlight the need to improve access and strengthen vaccination efforts. A life course approach is essential to maximize the full potential of immunization across all ages.

Keywords: adult; immunization; health workers; pregnant women; elderly; chronic diseases

1. Introduction

Historically, national immunization programs, particularly in low- and middle-income countries (LMICs) have focused on infants, children, and women of reproductive age with the aim of preventing disease and mortality in infancy and childhood including tuberculosis, diphtheria, tetanus, pertussis, polio, and measles, among other diseases [1]. With an increasing number of vaccines becoming available for adolescents and adults, the notion of life course immunization is currently being explored by countries around the world.

The COVID-19 pandemic and associated disruptions profoundly impacted global immunization programs, and around 60% of planned mass vaccination campaigns were postponed or canceled in 57 countries as of May 2020 [2]. Global coverage for measles has not yet recovered to pre-pandemic levels [3]. The urgent need to protect other groups against COVID-19—notably older adults, those with chronic conditions, and health workers—prompted many countries to expand their focus beyond childhood immunization and catalyzed significant changes in policies, attitudes, and systems supporting adult vaccination. This has included investments in restructuring governance mechanisms to facilitate collaboration to reach new target groups (e.g., elderly care units, prison health, . . .), new vaccination sites and identification of synergies with other programs for service delivery, the expansion of the health workforce of vaccinators (e.g., pharmacists, specialists, nurses, . . .), and the embrace of technological innovations, including the use of new systems allowing for real-time monitoring of vaccination coverage and vaccine safety [4,5]. Some countries with existing seasonal influenza vaccination for adults were able to leverage those programmatic capacities and systems in service of COVID-19 vaccination [6]. By the end of 2023, more than 13.6 billion COVID-19 vaccine doses had been administered globally (mainly to adults), reaching 89% of health workers and 84% of older adults through the end of 2023 [7]. This shows the potential of programs to adapt to life course immunization.

A life course approach to immunization has been defined as a public health approach that states that persons should receive all recommended doses of vaccines through their lives to obtain maximum benefits from vaccine-preventable diseases at different ages, across generations and within their communities [8]. In addition to preventing disease and maximizing health over an individual's entire lifespan, this approach offers continuous health contact opportunities to promote synergy and integration between immunization operations and other primary health care (PHC) services [9], and contributes to shifting away from a disease-focused approach to a people-centered one [10]. It emphasizes the importance of immunization beyond childhood, addressing the evolving health risks and needs during adolescence, adulthood (including pregnancy), and older age [11]. In the context of aging populations, by 2030, almost 1 billion people will be over 65 years of age [12]; this group is already larger than the number of children younger than five across the world, so it is necessary to invest more in prevention than treatment for healthy aging [13] and to reduce healthcare costs.

In addition, vaccines play a critical role in global health security and pandemic preparedness and have been the cornerstone of the response to six of the seven Public Health Emergencies of International Concern (PHEIC) declared by the WHO to date: H1N1 influenza (2009–2010), polio (2014-ongoing), Ebola (2014–2016 and 2019–2020), COVID-19 (2020–2023) and mpox (2022–2023; 2024-ongoing). Yet, in many countries, particularly in LMICs, gaps in adult immunization platform capacity impeded efforts to achieve the vaccination targets set during the COVID-19 pandemic [14], highlighting the vulnerabilities of existing vaccination systems and reinforcing the need for routine approaches [15] to protect populations across the life course and as preparedness and readiness for future pandemics [16].

This manuscript aims to support the development of a life course approach by providing a detailed global overview of adult immunization. It summarizes current WHO recommendations for vaccines targeting adults and describes the status of adult vaccination policies by population group (pregnant women, health workers, adults with chronic conditions, and older adults), region, and country-income group. These insights contribute to the growing recognition of adult immunization as a critical component of health systems and a cornerstone of the Immunization Agenda 2030 (IA2030) vision: "a world where everyone, everywhere, at every age fully benefits from vaccines for good health and well-being" [17].

2. Materials and Methods

2.1. Study Design

This study is a review of WHO recommendations for vaccines targeting adults and national adult immunization policies in 194 WHO member states.

2.2. Data Sources

We reviewed and summarized existing WHO Strategic Advisory Group of Experts on Immunization (SAGE) [18] recommendations [19] by vaccine and by adult group (pregnant women, health workers, healthy adults not pregnant, adults with chronic conditions, and older adults). We also listed other licensed vaccines for which a WHO SAGE recommendation has not been developed.

This article considers adults to be individuals of 18 years of age and above, recognizing that pregnancy and membership in certain occupational cadres may occur before 'adulthood'. The definition of 'health worker' differs by country; in this manuscript, the term "health workers" refers to all people engaged in work actions whose primary intent is to improve health. This includes health service providers and health management and support workers, working in acute care and long-term care facilities, public health, community-based care, social care and home care, as well as other occupations in the health and social work sectors [20]. While "adults with comorbidities", "adult with chronic conditions" and "adults with underlying conditions" are all referenced in various adult vaccination recommendations, in this manuscript, we refer to them as "adults with chronic conditions". Finally, "older adults" is defined by the United Nations as a person who is over 60 years of age [21]; however, the age cut off age varies across countries.

We analyzed data collected via the WHO/UNICEF electronic Joint Reporting Form on Immunization (eJRF) [22] to assess national immunization schedules for vaccines targeting pregnant women, health workers, adults with chronic conditions, and older adults of reporting Member States (MS). We downloaded the data from https://immunizationdata.who.int/ (accessed on 9 January 2025), and analyzed them for all 194 WHO MS and regionally across the six WHO regions: Africa (AFR), 47 MS; Americas (AMR), 35 MS; Eastern Mediterranean (EMR), 21 MS; Europe (EUR), 53 MS; South East Asia (SEAR) 11 MS; and Western Pacific (WPR), 27 MS. The eJRF collects immunization data from countries on an annual basis; in 2024, 191 of 194 (~98%) of MS reported their 2023 data. For those countries for which 2023 data were not available by the time of this analysis, data from the most recent year of reporting were considered (Morocco: 2019, Israel: 2022, and Nauru: 2021).

For COVID-19 vaccination data, we used several data sources for the analysis. We downloaded data from WHO/UNICEF COVID-19 Vaccination Information Hub [23] at https://infohub.crd.co/ (accessed on 4 December 2024). COVID-19 vaccination coverage for health workers and older adults in the period 2021–2023 was used as proxy of COVID-19 vaccination policies targeting those groups. Since this source included limited information of vaccination policy of pregnant women against COVID-19, we used data from COVID-19 Maternal Immunization Tracker (COMIT) [24] (https://www.comitglobal.org/), accessed on 10 December 2024) from Berman Institute of Bioethics & Center for Immunization Research, Johns Hopkins University. This source summarizes policies on COVID-19 vaccination for pregnant and lactating women. It was last updated on 05 January 2023. For this analysis, countries with policies recommending or permitting COVID-19 vaccination for pregnant women issued by public health authorities or regulatory agencies were considered. The latest country-reported data from WHO/UNICEF COVID-19 vaccination information hub for Q1–Q2 2024 [23], regional COVID-19 vaccination dashboards [25,26], and official reports from WHO regional offices [27,28] were used to supplement and triangulate the COVID-19 vaccination results for health workers, older adults, and pregnant women. Eritrea and Democratic People's Republic of Korea were considered as not vaccinating against COVID-19 based on reports from WHO regional and country offices. Overall, data on COVID-19 vaccination were reported by 168 MS for health workers, 177 for older adults, and 186 for pregnant women at least once from January 2021 to June 2024. Data on COVID-19 vaccination policies of adults with chronic conditions were not included in the analysis due to insufficient country reporting.

For RSV, both maternal vaccines and vaccines for older adults were first licensed in 2023 and only started to be used by countries at the end that year; consequently, this was not captured in 2023 eJRF reporting. Therefore, we relied on information provided by vaccine manufacturers and available in the public domain on which countries had started to use these products.

For this analysis, we additionally used the latest World Bank income group classifications (HIC: high-income economies, UMIC: upper-middle income economies, LMIC: lower-middle-income economies, and LIC: low-income economies) as listed in November 2024 [29].

2.3. Bias

The completeness and accuracy of data from eJRF rely on the quality of reporting by countries. Additional efforts to complete missing data were conducted to reduce the risk of information bias.

2.4. Statistical Analysis

Analyses were conducted using R Studio software version 2023.03.0+386, and maps for data visualizations were developed using QGIS software version 3.40 according to WHO Operating Procedures for maps.

3. Results

3.1. Vaccines Targeting Adults

Table 1 presents a summary of recommendations for vaccines targeting adults in two categories: (1) for all immunization programs and (2) for programs with certain characteristics (i.e., funding and programmatic capacity). Table 2 presents a summary of the vaccine-preventable diseases against which an adult is recommended to be protected through vaccination (if not previously immunized) as well as vaccines recommended for some high-risk adult populations or adults in/travelling to certain regions. Where available, WHO SAGE recommendations for the different adult groups are described and referenced.

Table 1. Summary of recommendations for vaccines targeting adults.

Antigen	Pregnant Women	Health Workers (HWs) *	Healthy Adults (Not Pregnant)	Adults with Chronic Conditions	Older Adults	Considerations	Source Description
For all immunization programmes							
COVID-19 [30]	x	x	x	x	x	• One-dose primary series for those that have never received a COVID-19 vaccine and revaccination 6–12 months later for high priority-use groups and sub-populations with special considerations for COVID-19 vaccination (older adults, adults with comorbidities or severe obesity, adults with immunocompromising conditions, and health workers). • For pregnant women, a single dose is recommended in each pregnancy regardless of previous vaccination status; ideally during the second trimester or at any opportunity	WHO SAGE Roadmap for prioritizing uses of COVID-19 vaccines, 2023 Link: https://iris.who.int/handle/10665/373987 (accessed on 10 October 2024)
For programmes with certain characteristics (i.e., funding and programmatic capacity)							
Seasonal influenza [31]	x	x		x	x	• One dose, annual revaccination • WHO recommended target groups for "countries considering the initiation or expansion of seasonal influenza vaccination". • "Depending on national disease goals, capacity and resources, epidemiology, national policies and priorities, and disease burden, countries may consider additional (sub)populations for vaccination".	Vaccines against Influenza: WHO Position Paper—May 2022. Link: https://iris.who.int/handle/10665/354265 (accessed on 10 October 2024)
Herpes zoster (HZ) [32]					x	• Two doses • WHO has not provided a recommendation concerning the routine use of HZ vaccine yet (expected reco—mmendation in 2025). • "However, countries with an aging population and demographic shift towards older ages, may decide to introduce routine HZ vaccination if they have an important burden of disease and consider the programme beneficial".	Varicella and Herpes Zoster Vaccines: WHO Position Paper, June 2014. Link: https://iris.who.int/handle/10665/242227 (accessed on 10 October 2024)
Pertussis [33]	x	x	x			• "1 dose of Tdap (in the 2nd or 3rd trimester and preferably at least 15 days before the end of pregnancy) as a strategy additional to routine primary infant pertussis vaccination in countries or settings with high or increasing infant morbidity/ mortality from pertussis". • "High coverage in infants through routine immunization should be in place prior to the introduction of vaccination in adolescents and adults". • "[HWs] should be prioritized as a group to receive pertussis vaccine".	Pertussis Vaccines: WHO Position Paper—August 2015. Link: https://iris.who.int/handle/10665/242413 (accessed on 10 October 2024)

Table 1. *Cont.*

Antigen	Pregnant Women	Health Workers (HWs) *	Healthy Adults (Not Pregnant)	Adults with Chronic Conditions	Older Adults	Considerations	Source Description
Pneumococcal [34]				x	x	• "In countries that have a mature childhood pneumococcal immunization programme, decisions about initiating such a programme in adults should take into account local disease burden and cost-effectiveness considerations".	Considerations for Pneumococcal Vaccination in Older Adults, 2021 Link: https://iris.who.int/handle/10665/341722 (accessed on 10 October 2024)
Respiratory Syncytial Virus (RSV) [35]	x				x **	• One dose • "A single vaccine dose in the third trimester of pregnancy, as defined in the local context (≥28 weeks of gestation in most settings)".	Meeting of the Strategic Advisory Group of Experts on Immunization, September 2024 Link: https://iris.who.int/handle/10665/379718 (accessed on 10 October 2024)

Note: Antigens are presented in alphabetical order. * All health workers should be up-to-date with immunization as recommended in their national immunization schedule. ** Despite the availability of RSV vaccine for older adults, there is not yet a WHO SAGE recommendation for use in this group.

Table 2. Summary of vaccine-preventable diseases against which an adult is recommended to be protected through vaccination (if not previously immunized) and vaccines recommended for some high-risk adult populations or adults in/travelling to certain regions.

Antigen	Pregnant Women	Health Workers (HWs) *	Healthy Adults (Not Pregnant)	Adults with Chronic Conditions	Older Adults	Considerations	Source Description
For adults to be protected (if not previously immunized, natural or vaccination)							
BCG [36]		x				• One dose • For "unvaccinated, TST [Tuberculin Skin Test] or IGRA [Interferon gamma release assay test] -negative… adults from settings with high incidence of TB and/or high leprosy burden". • For "unvaccinated TST- or IGRA-negative… adults moving from low to high TB incidence/ leprosy burden settings". • For "unvaccinated TST- or IGRA-negative persons at risk of occupational exposure in low and high TB incidence areas (e.g., health-care workers, laboratory workers, medical students, prison workers, other individuals with occupational exposure)", travelers, and returning migrants.	BCG Vaccines: WHO Position Paper—February 2018. Link: https://iris.who.int/handle/10665/260307 (accessed on 18 December 2024)
Diphtheria [37]		x	x	x		• Three doses primary series and two subsequent booster doses.	Diphtheria Vaccines: WHO Position Paper—August 2017. Link: https://iris.who.int/handle/10665/258683 (accessed on 18 December 2024)
Hepatitis B [38]		x	x	x **		• Three doses • "Catch up of unvaccinated cohorts (if the necessary resources are available)".	Hepatitis B Vaccines: WHO Position Paper—July 2017. Link: https://iris.who.int/handle/10665/255873 (accessed on 18 December 2024)

Table 2. *Cont.*

Antigen	Pregnant Women	Health Workers (HWs) *	Healthy Adults (Not Pregnant)	Adults with Chronic Conditions	Older Adults	Considerations	Source Description
Measles [39]		x	x			• Two doses • "Vaccine should be offered to... adults likely or known to be susceptible [including travelers]".	Measles Vaccines: WHO Position Paper—April 2017. Link: https://iris.who.int/handle/10665/255705 (accessed on 18 December 2024)
Polio [40]		x	x			• "Before travelling abroad, persons residing in countries with active transmission of a wild or vaccine-derived poliovirus should complete a full course of polio vaccination in compliance with their national schedule and receive 1 dose of IPV or bOPV within 4 weeks to 12 months of travel".	Polio Vaccines: WHO Position Paper—June 2022. Link: https://iris.who.int/handle/10665/357168 (accessed on 18 December 2024)
Rubella [41]		x	x			• One dose • Women of reproductive age but contraindicated during pregnancy.	Rubella Vaccines: WHO Position Paper—July 2020. Link: https://iris.who.int/handle/10665/332952 (accessed on 18 December 2024)
Tetanus [42]	x		x			• "Vaccination history should be verified in order to determine whether a dose of TTCV [Tetanus Toxoid Containing Vaccine] is needed in the current pregnancy". • "Pregnant women and their newborn infants are protected from birth-associated tetanus if the mother received either 6 TTCV doses during childhood or 5 doses if first vaccinated during adolescence/adulthood (documented by card, immunization registry and/or history) before the time of reproductive age".	Tetanus Vaccines: WHO Position Paper—February 2017. Link: https://iris.who.int/handle/10665/254583 (accessed on 10 October 2024)
Varicella [32]		x	x	x		• Two doses • "Varicella vaccine is usually contraindicated in persons with congenital or acquired immune deficiencies. However, due to the increased severity of varicella in certain groups of immunocompromised persons, varicella vaccination may be considered in these groups. Combination MMRV [Measles-Mumps-Rubella-Varicella] vaccine has not been tested and is contraindicated in immunocompromised persons". • Contraindicated during pregnancy.	Varicella and Herpes Zoster Vaccines: WHO Position Paper, June 2014. Link: https://iris.who.int/handle/10665/242227 (accessed on 10 October 2024)

Table 2. *Cont.*

Antigen	Pregnant Women	Health Workers (HWs) *	Healthy Adults (Not Pregnant)	Adults with Chronic Condi-tions	Older Adults	Considerations	Source Description
For some high-risk adult populations or adults in/travelling to certain regions							
Cholera [43]	x	x	x	x		• Two doses • In areas at risk or where endemic cholera is present. • Pregnant and lactating women and HIV-infected individuals should be included in Oral Cholera Vaccine (OCV) campaigns. • OCV should be considered for travelers at high risk of infection. • "OCV should be considered for emergency and relief workers who are likely to be directly exposed to cholera patients or to contaminated food or water, particularly those staying in areas with poor access to health-care facilities. Other health-care workers are generally not at special risk of cholera".	Cholera Vaccines: WHO Position Paper—August 2017. Link: https://iris.who.int/handle/10665/258764 (accessed on 18 December 2024)
Dengue [44]			x	x		• Two doses • "Persons with comorbidities, [such as sickle cell anaemia, diabetes, hypertension, or underlying comorbidities that may result in bleeding tendencies (e.g., ulcerative colitis)] who live in dengue-endemic countries could be offered vaccination. Until more data on efficacy-safety profiles become available, WHO recommends the upper limit of 60 years for vaccination". • "Persons living in non-endemic countries who have previously been infected with any of the 4 dengue virus serotypes following travel to dengue-endemic countries, may benefit from vaccination to prevent a second (and hence potentially more severe) dengue infection when travelling again to an endemic country".	WHO Position Paper on Dengue Vaccines—May 2024. Link: https://iris.who.int/handle/10665/376642 (accessed on 18 December 2024)
Ebola [45]	x	x	x	x		• One dose • Countries with Ebola outbreaks: ring vaccination targeting contacts and contacts of contacts, including pregnant women. • Countries at risk of Ebola outbreaks: preventive vaccination of health workers.	Extraordinary meeting of the Strategic Advisory Group of Experts on Immunization on Ebola vaccination, May 2024: conclusions and recommendations. Link: https //iris.who.int/handle/10665/378109 (accessed on 18 December 2024)
Hepatitis A [46]			x ***	x ***		• Two doses if >40 years of age • "Groups at higher risk of hepatitis A should be vaccinated".	WHO position paper on hepatitis A vaccines—October 2022 Link: https://iris.who.int/handle/10665/363397 (accessed on 18 December 2024)
Hepatitis E [47]	x	x	x			• One dose • "The use of the vaccine to mitigate or prevent outbreaks should be considered as well to mitigate consequences in high-risk groups such as pregnant women".	Hepatitis E vaccine: WHO position paper, May 2015 Link: https://iris.who.int/handle/10665/242352 (accessed on 18 December 2024)

Table 2. *Cont.*

Antigen	Pregnant Women	Health Workers (HWs) *	Healthy Adults (Not Pregnant)	Adults with Chronic Conditions	Older Adults	Considerations	Source Description
Japanese encephalitis (JE) [48]	x		x			• "If JE risk is sufficient to warrant vaccination of pregnant women, inactivated vaccines should be used preferentially". • "For travelers to endemic areas with extensive outdoor exposure during the transmission season".	Japanese Encephalitis Vaccines: WHO Position Paper, 2015. Link: https://iris.who.int/handle/10665/242325 (accessed on 18 December 2024)
Meningococcal [49–51]		x				• One booster dose 3–5 years after the primary dose may be given to persons considered to be at continued risk of exposure.	Meningococcal Vaccines: WHO Position Paper—November 2011. Link: https://iris.who.int/handle/10665/241846 (accessed on 10 October 2024) Meningococcal A Conjugate Vaccine: Updated Guidance, February 2015. Link: https://iris.who.int/handle/10665/242320 (accessed on 10 October 2024) Meningococcal Vaccines: WHO Position Paper on the Use of Multivalent Meningococcal Conjugate Vaccines in Countries of the African Meningitis Belt, January 2024. Link: https://iris.who.int/handle/10665/375624 (accessed on 18 December 2024)
Mpox [52]	x	x	x ****	x	x	• One or two doses (depending on the vaccine product) • "Primary preventive vaccination is recommended for laboratory personnel working with orthopoxviruses and periodic revaccination should be considered". • "For persons at high risk of exposure to mpox during an outbreak".**** • During pregnancy, where consideration is given to vaccination, non-replicating vaccine ... should be used.	Smallpox and Mpox (Orthopoxviruses): WHO Position Paper, August 2024. Link: https://iris.who.int/handle/10665/378526 (accessed on 10 October 2024)
Rabies pre-exposure prophylaxis (PrEP) [53]			x			• Two doses • "Sub-populations in highly endemic settings with limited access to timely and adequate PEP [Post Exposure Prophylaxis], individuals at occupational risk, and travelers who may be at risk of exposure". • "PrEP may be considered for medical professionals who regularly provide care to persons with rabies".	Rabies Vaccines: WHO Position Paper—April 2018. Link: https://iris.who.int/handle/10665/272372 (accessed on 18 December 2024)
Tick-borne encephalitis [54]	x		x		x	• Three doses followed by additional booster doses for those who will continue to be at risk • "The vaccine should be used in pregnant women who live in areas where the incidence of the disease is high (>5 cases/100,000 population per year)". • "People travelling from nonendemic areas to endemic areas should be offered vaccination if their visits will include extensive outdoor activities".	Vaccines against Tick-Borne Encephalitis: WHO Position Paper—2011. Link: https://iris.who.int/handle/10665/241769 (accessed on 18 December 2024)

Table 2. *Cont.*

Antigen	Pregnant Women	Health Workers (HWs) *	Healthy Adults (Not Pregnant)	Adults with Chronic Conditions	Older Adults	Considerations	Source Description
Typhoid [55]			x			• One or more doses depending on the product • "Catch-up vaccination with TCV [Typhoid Conjugate Vaccine] up to 15 years of age is recommended when feasible and supported by epidemiologic data". • "Travelers from non-endemic to endemic areas". • "In typhoid-endemic areas, professional food handlers can be vaccinated against typhoid". • "Clinical microbiology laboratory staff with a recognized risk of occupational exposure to S. Typhi should be offered vaccination against typhoid".	Typhoid Vaccines: WHO Position Paper—March 2018. Link: https://iris.who.int/handle/10665/272273 (accessed on 18 December 2024)
Yellow fever [56]			x			• One dose • Individuals in endemic countries and travelers to these countries. • There is currently no recommendation regarding HWs.	Vaccines and Vaccination against Yellow Fever: WHO Position Paper—June 2013. Link: https://iris.who.int/handle/10665/242089 (accessed on 18 December 2024)

Note: Antigens are presented in alphabetical order. * All health workers should be up-to-date with immunization as recommended in their national immunization schedule. ** Hepatitis B: Adults with chronic definition includes "patients who frequently require blood or blood products, dialysis patients, diabetes patients, recipients of solid organ transplantation, person with chronic liver disease including those with Hepatitis C, person with HIV infection, men who have sex with men, persons with multiple sexual partners, as well as health workers and others who may be exposed to blood, blood products or other potentially infectious body fluids during their work". *** Hepatitis A: High risk groups include "[travelers] from low-endemic countries to areas of intermediate or high endemicity, men who have sex with men, at-risk occupational groups (such as sewage workers or laboratory personnel handling hepatitis A virus specimens), people who inject drugs, people who experience homelessness, migrants, refugees, incarcerated persons; and patients with chronic liver disease or people living with HIV, particularly in countries with low and very low endemicity". **** Mpox: in the context of an mpox outbreak, vaccination is recommended for persons at high risk of exposure. Populations to consider for vaccination may include: "based on local epidemiology, members of a defined area or community (e.g., village), with a documented high risk of exposure to persons with mpox; sex workers; gay, bisexual or other men who have sex with men (MSM) with multiple sexual partners; or other individuals with multiple casual sexual partners; health workers at risk of repeated exposure; clinical laboratory and health-care personnel performing diagnostic testing for mpox or providing care; and outbreak response team members (as designated by national public health authorities); contacts of persons with mpox, ideally within 4 days of first exposure".

3.2. Status of Immunization Policies for Pregnant Women

The WHO provides guidance for the vaccination of pregnant women where there is specific interest to protect the mother or the newborn. As reflected in Table 1, vaccines against COVID-19, seasonal influenza, pertussis, and RSV are recommended for pregnant women. Tetanus vaccination is also recommended if the mother did not receive either six TTCV doses during childhood or five doses if first vaccinated during adolescence/adulthood before the time of reproductive age. Other vaccines can be also recommended to pregnant women at high risk of exposure as summarized in Table 2.

Based on 2023 data, 90% of 194 WHO MS were identified as recommending vaccinating pregnant women against COVID-19, 57% against seasonal influenza, 63% with tetanus-containing vaccine, and 21% with pertussis-containing vaccine (Table 3). Figure 1 shows the geographical distribution of countries reporting vaccination with these four vaccines.

Table 3. Status of immunization policies for pregnant women by WHO region and income group.

		Number of Member States (MS)	COVID-19 Vaccine (%)	Seasonal Influenza Vaccine (%)	Tetanus-Containing Vaccine ** (%)	Pertussis-Containing Vaccine (Tdap/aP) (%)
Number of reporting countries		194	186 (96%)	116 (60%)	194 (100%)	194 (100%)
WHO Region	Africa	47	35 (74%)	4 (9%)	37 (79%)	1 (2%)
	Americas	35	35 (100%)	31 (89%)	30 (86%)	16 (46%)
	Eastern Mediterranean	21	17 (81%)	14 (67%)	12 (57%)	2 (10%)
	Europe	53	52 (98%)	48 (91%)	17 (32%)	17 (32%)
	South East Asia	11	10 (91%)	4 (36%)	9 (82%)	0
	Western Pacific	27	25 (93%)	9 (33%)	17 (63%)	4 (15%)
Country-income group	HIC	63	62 (100%)	54 (87%)	37 (60%)	28 (45%)
	UMIC	53	49 (92%)	42 (79%)	24 (45%)	10 (19%)
	LMIC	50	43 (86%)	12 (24%)	40 (80%)	1 (2%)
	LIC	25	17 (65%)	1 (4%)	19 (73%)	0
	Not classified *	3	3	1	2	1
All regions		194	174 (90%)	110 (57%)	122 (63%)	40 (21%)

* Not included in the WB income classification: Niue and Cook Islands. Not classified by WB due to unavailability of data: Venezuela. ** Includes Td, TT, Td-IPV, Tdap, and Tdap-IPV.

As mentioned above, countries did not report RSV in the 2023 eJRF. However, as of end of 2024 some countries had started to use RSV maternal immunization in their national programs, including seven countries in Europe and three in the Americas, Communication from Pfizer, January 2025.

3.3. Status of Immunization Policies for Health Workers

The WHO recommends an annual revaccination of health workers against two antigens: COVID-19 and seasonal influenza. Also, following WHO guidance [57], health workers should be vaccinated against nine additional antigens if not previously immunized: Bacillus Calmette–Guérin (BCG), diphtheria, hepatitis B, measles, meningococcal, pertussis, polio, rubella, and varicella. In addition, in appropriate high-incidence settings (including emergencies), other vaccines should also be considered for health workers as described in Table 2.

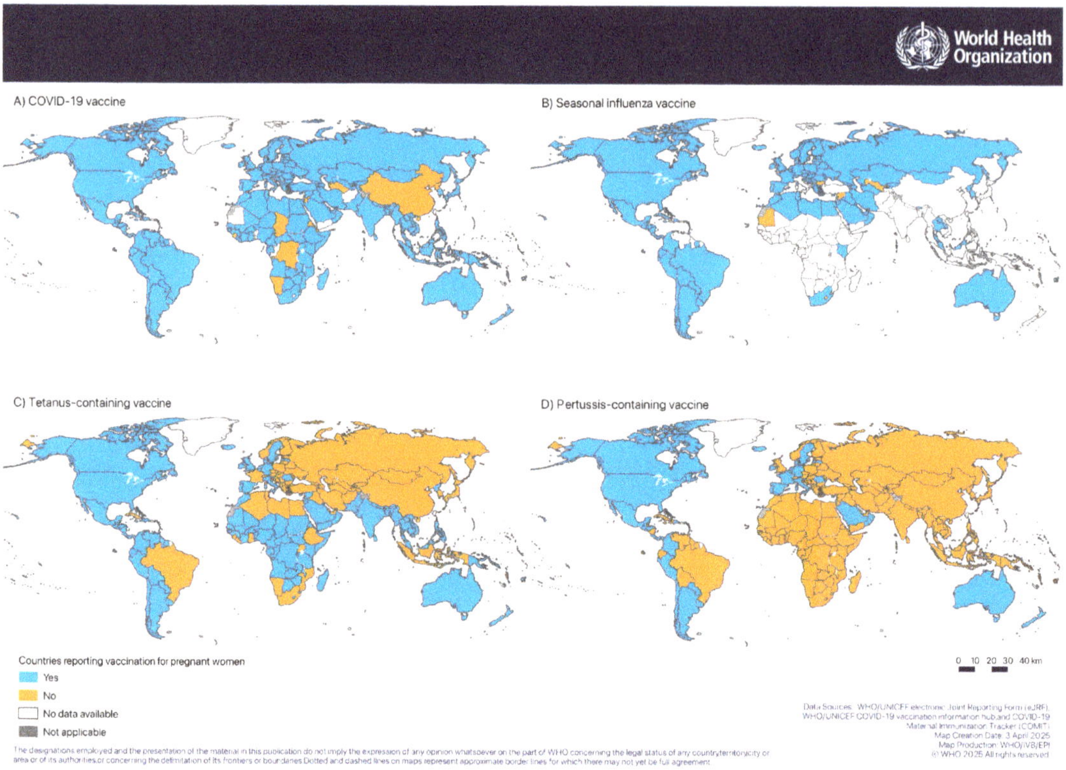

Figure 1. Geographical distribution of countries that reported vaccination for pregnant women with (**A**) COVID-19 vaccine, (**B**) seasonal influenza vaccine, (**C**) tetanus-containing vaccine, and (**D**) pertussis-containing vaccine.

Based on 2023 data, 91% of 194 MS reported vaccinating health workers against COVID-19, 59% against seasonal influenza, 24% against hepatitis B, 6% against measles-rubella, and 5% against varicella (Table 4). Other vaccines that were reported by fewer number of countries included those against polio, meningococcal disease, mpox, pneumococcal disease, hepatitis A, BCG, tetanus, diphtheria and pertussis.

3.4. *Status of Immunization Policies for Adults with Chronic Conditions*

The WHO recommends annual revaccination against COVID-19 and seasonal influenza for adults with chronic conditions. Additional vaccines, such as those against pneumococcal disease and hepatitis B, may be advised based on individual health risks, as described in Table 2.

Limited information is reported in the eJRF regarding vaccination of people with chronic conditions. The two main vaccines reported by countries for this group were seasonal influenza and pneumococcal vaccine (Table 5). Overall, 113 countries (58% of MS) report vaccination against seasonal influenza for high-risk groups. Among them, 105 countries report "vaccination for adults with chronic conditions", 94 report vaccination for "people living in long-term care facilities", and 69 report vaccination for "other groups".

Table 4. Status of immunization policies for health workers by WHO region and country income- group.

		Number of Member States (MS)	COVID-19 Vaccine (%)	Seasonal Influenza Vaccine (%)	Hepatitis B Vaccine (%)	Measles-Rubella Containing Vaccines (%)	Varicella Vaccine (%)
Number of reporting countries		194	178 (92%)	119 (61%)	194 (100%)	194 (100%)	194 (100%)
WHO Region	Africa	47	46 (98%)	5 (11%)	2 (4%)	0 (0%)	0 (0%)
	Americas	35	35 (100%)	32 (91%)	21 (60%)	3 (9%)	4 (11%)
	Eastern Mediterranean	21	13 (62%)	14 (67%)	5 (24%)	1 (5%)	2 (10%)
	Europe	53	45 (85%)	51 (96%)	17 (32%)	5 (9%)	3 (6%)
	South East Asia	11	10 (91%)	4 (36%)	1 (9%)	1 (9%)	0 (0%)
	Western Pacific	27	27 (100%)	9 (33%)	2 (7%)	1 (4%)	0 (0%)
Country-income group	HIC	63	52 (84%)	55 (89%)	23 (37%)	5 (8%)	6 (10%)
	UMIC	53	51 (96%)	42 (79%)	19 (36%)	4 (8%)	3 (6%)
	LMIC	50	46 (92%)	15 (30%)	5 (10%)	1 (2%)	0 (0%)
	LIC	25	24 (92%)	1 (4%)	0 (0%)	0 (0%)	0 (0%)
	Not classified *	3	3	2	1	1	0
	All regions	194	176 (91%)	115 (59%)	48 (25%)	11 (6%)	9 (5%)

* Not included in the WB income classification: Niue and Cook Islands. Not classified by WB due to unavailability of data: Venezuela.

Table 5. Status of immunization policies for adults with chronic conditions and older adults by WHO Region and country income group.

		Number of Member States (MS)	COVID-19 Vaccine (%)	Seasonal Influenza Vaccine (%)		Pneumococcal Vaccine ** (%)		HZ Vaccine (%)
			Older Adults	Older Adults	Adults with Chronic Conditions	Older Adults	Adults with Chronic Conditions	Older Adults
Number of reporting countries		194	184 (95%)	118 (61%)	116 (60%)	194 (100%)	194 (100%)	194 (100%)
WHO Region	Africa	47	46 (98%)	5 (11%)	4 (9%)	0	0	0
	Americas	35	35 (100%)	32 (91%)	32 (91%)	12 (34%)	13 (37%)	2 (6%)
	Eastern Mediterranean	21	15 (71%)	15 (71%)	15 (71%)	1 (5%)	7 (33%)	2 (10%)
	Europe	53	50 (94%)	49 (92%)	50 (94%)	16 (30%)	22 (42%)	7 (13%)
	South East Asia	11	9 (82%)	4 (36%)	4 (36%)	0	0	0
	Western Pacific	27	27 (100%)	9 (33%)	8 (30%)	4 (15%)	3 (11%)	2 (7%)
Country-income group	HIC	63	58 (94%)	55 (89%)	55 (89%)	25 (40%)	32 (52%)	13 (21%)
	UMIC	53	51 (96%)	40 (75%)	41 (77%)	7 (13%)	12 (23%)	0
	LMIC	50	46 (92%)	15 (30%)	13 (26%)	1 (2%)	1 (2%)	0
	LIC	25	24 (92%)	2 (8%)	2 (8%)	0	0	0
	Not classified *	3	3	2	2	0	0	0
	All regions	194	182 (94%)	114 (59%)	113 (58%)	33 (17%)	45 (23%)	13 (7%)

Notes: * Not included in the WB classification: Niue and Cook Islands. Not classified by WB due to unavailability of data: Venezuela. ** Includes those countries reporting use of PCV13, PCV15, PCV20, and/or PPV23.

Concerning vaccination against pneumococcal disease, 45 countries (23% of MS) reported vaccination for high-risk groups. Among them, 32 countries reported "high-risk groups" (generic term), eight reported "chronic conditions" (generic term), 10 reported specific conditions (for example, asplenia), 5 reported "immunocompromised individuals" (generic term), and 3 target "people living in long-term care facilities".

3.5. Status of Immunization Policies for Older Adults

The WHO recommends annual revaccination against COVID-19 and seasonal influenza for older adults. Pneumococcal vaccination for older adults can also be considered. Additional vaccines, such as HZ (expected update of WHO recommendation in 2025) and RSV, are also available (Table 1).

Based on 2023 data, 94% of 194 WHO MS reported vaccinating against COVID-19, 59% against seasonal influenza, 17% against pneumococcal disease (mainly in the Americas and Europe), and 7% against HZ (Table 5). Figure 2 shows the geographical distribution of countries reporting vaccination with these four vaccines.

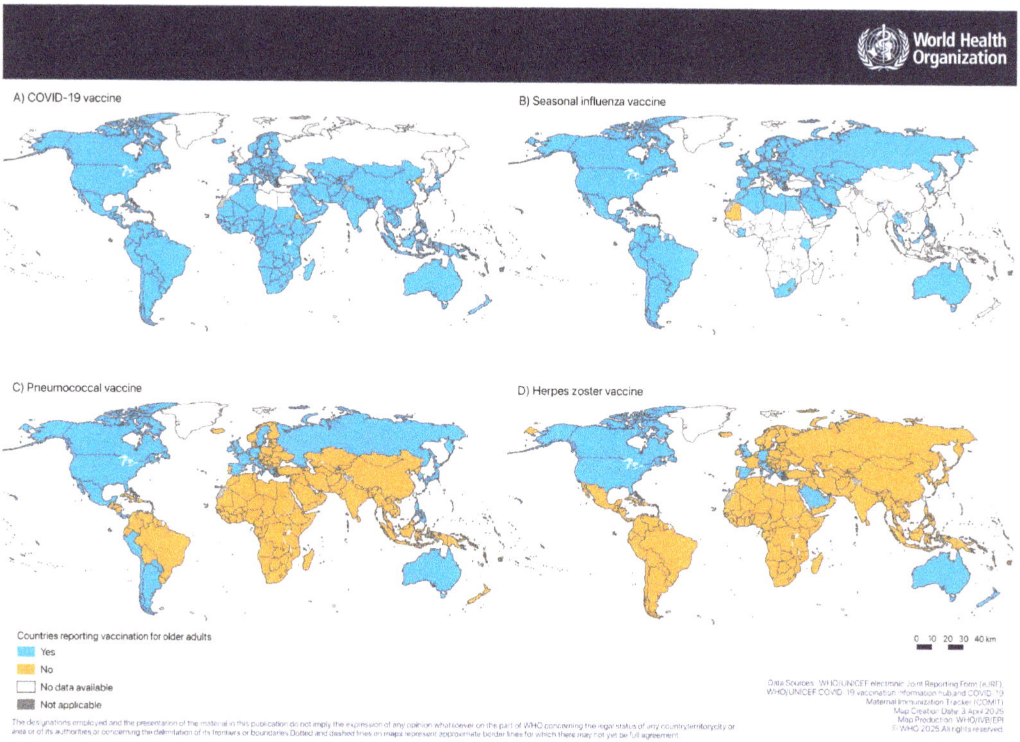

Figure 2. Geographical distribution of countries that reported vaccination for older adults with (**A**) COVID-19 vaccine, (**B**) seasonal influenza vaccine, (**C**) pneumococcal vaccine, and (**D**) HZ vaccine.

In 2024, no information about other recently licensed vaccines was reported in eJRF by countries. However, by the end of 2024, five European countries, one from the Western Pacific, and two from the Americas (all HICs) had introduced the RSV vaccine for older adults. (Communication from Pfizer and GSK, January 2025).

4. Discussion

Adult immunization policy recommendations exist for most available vaccines; however, inclusion in national immunization schedules has predominantly been reported in HICs and MICs. The global COVID-19 vaccination effort, which saw 99% of countries introduce the vaccine, brought adult immunization to the forefront of national immunization programmes. The COVID-19 experience can have lasting effects on how countries, particularly LMICs, approach immunization programs, encouraging a shift from the traditional childhood-centric focus to a life course approach to immunization [58].

The maternal immunization approach had been used for many years across geographies and income groups prior to the COVID-19 pandemic across a wide range of countries. This is a main component of the WHO's maternal and neonatal tetanus elimination (MNTE) strategy [59]. To date, 80% of LMICs and 73% of LICs are offering tetanus-containing vaccines to pregnant women. During the pandemic, 90% of countries (65% of LICs) targeted pregnant women with vaccines against COVID-19. Looking to other antigens, 57% of the countries (only 4% of LICs) report vaccinating against seasonal influenza, and only 21% (mainly HICs) are using tetanus-pertussis-containing vaccines to protect infants against emerging pertussis cases. Looking forward, a number of vaccines targeting pregnant women are expected to be available and accessible in the coming years for other pathogens causing high burden, notably RSV (claims the lives of more than 45,000 young infants worldwide each year) [60], and group B streptococcus (GBS), the leading cause of neonatal/infant sepsis and meningitis globally (around 91,000 infant deaths and 46,000 stillbirths per year) [61]. Gavi, the Vaccine Alliance (Gavi) has already committed to an in-principle investment for maternal RSV and GBS vaccine introduction in Gavi-eligible countries in the near future [62]. These new and existing vaccines further represent an opportunity to strengthen maternal immunization as a platform for improved quality of care during antenatal care visits.

Despite 91% of countries reporting vaccinating health workers against COVID-19, fewer countries report having policies for this group for other antigens. Fifty-nine percent of countries report vaccinating health workers against seasonal influenza, though only 4% of LICs reported as such, compared with 89% of HICs. More than 85% of countries in the European and Americas regions include seasonal influenza vaccination for health workers in their national schedules. Vaccination of health workers against other antigens such as hepatitis B, measles and rubella or varicella is mainly reported by HICs. Vaccines targeting health workers play a critical role in safeguarding the health workforce while also reducing the likelihood of transmission to patients. In addition, health workers play a key role in recommending vaccines to other key groups. Given this, targeted strategies to effectively engage, protect, and empower this group on communicating the benefits of adult immunization must be prioritized [63].

Similarly, while more than 90% of MS across all income groups vaccinated older adults against COVID-19, the situation for other vaccines targeting this population groups is heterogeneous, with important differences observed between regions and income groups. For seasonal influenza, for instance, 59% of reporting MS indicate vaccinating this group (8% of LICs and 30% of LMICs compared with 89% of HICs). Pneumococcal and HZ vaccination for older adults is reported to be part of national immunization schedules by even fewer countries, 17% and 7%, respectively, with inclusion limited to the Americas, Eastern Mediterranean, European and Western Pacific regions. While each of these vaccines has the potential to reduce the burden of preventable diseases among older adults, their inclusion in national programs remains inconsistent. As older adults constitute increasingly large proportions of national populations, vaccination efforts targeting this group will be a key strategy for improving long-term health while reducing burden on health systems [64]. To unlock the full potential of vaccines for this group, further study is required to understand the unique immunological, socio-behavioral, programmatic adaptations, and full economic value that influence vaccination efforts in these groups [63].

In 2024, the WHO, UNICEF, Gavi, and the Gates Foundation launched a global advocacy campaign alongside World Immunization Week: "Humanly Possible". This campaign aims to celebrate the 50th anniversary [65] of the Expanded Programme on Immunization (EPI) and inform the vision for the future of immunization. In the coming years, it is expected that a number of new vaccines targeting groups beyond childhood will become available, such as next generation of tuberculosis vaccines, group B streptococcus vaccines, cytomegalovirus vaccine and combination vaccines for respiratory viruses, among others. With the emergence of new platform technologies, such as mRNA, vaccine candidates can advance into clinical testing at a much faster rate, shortening development timelines. Mechanisms to facilitate access to existing and new products in LMICs will be required as well as t, strong adult immunization platforms. [66]. New innovations in vaccine delivery such as heat-stable micro-array patches and digital health tools like mobile phone reminders could facilitate vaccine uptake. However, these new vaccines and delivery innovations will need to be affordable and cost-effective to countries. An analysis of lessons learned from countries with successful adult vaccination programs could identify which innovations have proven to be the most successful and cost-effective, but would need to be applicable to LMIC contexts. National Immunization Technical Advisory Groups (NITAGs) or equivalent bodies will need to broaden their expertise to assess new products for potential inclusion in immunization schedules across all age groups, considering national priorities and the capacity of health systems. At the same time, governments will need to prioritize, where relevant, vaccines targeting adults as part of their National Immunization Strategy processes, while ensuring alignment with broader public health goals.

In preparation for these anticipated advancements in life course vaccines, we need to ensure there is a solid foundation upon which to build. A proactive approach to designing immunization schedules and investing in programs that include adults more comprehensively is needed, considering specific adult metrics to estimate public health impact, economic impact (at both the individual- and society-levels), and impact on health systems. While data from high and upper middle-income countries highlight the socio-economic value of adult immunization programs based on the use of four vaccines (seasonal influenza, respiratory syncytial virus (RSV), herpes zoster and pneumococcal diseases), which can return up to 19 times their initial investment to society [67], additional data, especially from LMICs, is crucial to fully assess the potential and impact of these programs.

It will be also important to establish tailored adult delivery strategies as part of the PHC services (e.g., antenatal care, adult/older adult care) and leveraging EPI structure through which vaccines are offered regularly by knowledgeable health workers and where the adult population can seek to be vaccinated. Additionally, in the current environment, and considering the stagnation of global childhood immunization coverage, addressing misinformation—particularly in the wake of the COVID-19 pandemic and the rise of anti-vaccine movements—will be crucial to sustaining public trust in vaccines and generating demand among adult populations. Engaging community leaders and healthcare professional networks will be essential for developing tailored communication for adult populations. Finally, these strategies will need to be accompanied by indicators and electronic systems (such as leveraging COVID-19 vaccine innovations), adapted to track adult immunization progress as part of the life course immunization approach and that are interoperable with other registries. Without adequate coverage, the effectiveness and impact of these programs will be compromised.

Our analysis is based on country reports to WHO and other sources and has some limitations. While the reporting in the national immunization schedules section of the eJRF follows a standardized format for all target groups, the use of open text fields for vaccines recommended for high-risk groups introduces ambiguity. This format, intended to reduce the reporting burden on MS, may lead to overlapping information between children and adult groups, making it difficult to analyze data by specific subcategories of risk groups. Furthermore, while the data reported in the schedule for all vaccines, except for seasonal influenza, are prepopulated each reporting year—requiring countries to update or add new information annually—the data on seasonal influenza target groups are not prepopulated. As a result, countries must enter this information annually, which may introduce inconsistencies or gaps in the data. While nearly all MS reported data for 2023 through the eJRF (191 of a total of 194 WHO MS), COVID-19 vaccination data were not yet being collected through this system, and the number of countries that reported COVID-19-related data during the 2021 to 2023 was fewer. At the same time, the numbers of countries currently vaccinating adult groups against COVID-19 might be already lower than the 2023 reported data. In addition, given the evolving epidemiology and the need for adapted vaccines targeting current circulating variants [68], the sunset of Gavi COVID-19 program at the end of 2025 [69], and the decreased demand of COVID-19 vaccines, the mid-to-long term sustainability of COVID-19 vaccination particularly in LMICs is uncertain. Another limitation is that the analysis primarily relies on stratification by income group, as the reported data do not allow for assessing a broad range of factors such as country-specific policy priorities, cultural norms, or infrastructure limitations, which likely influence decisions to adopt vaccine policies for adult populations.

5. Conclusions

The use of existing adult-targeted vaccines, coupled with the COVID-19 vaccination experience, has created an opportunity to advance adult immunization. With more vaccines expected for adults in the coming decade, and as evidence to understand their full value continues to grow, the concept of life course immunization is set to become a social norm. Improving access and integrating adult vaccination into national immunization strategies and primary health care promises to unlock the full potential of immunization across all ages and regions.

Author Contributions: Conceptualization, A.V. and A.L.; design of the work, F.N., X.W., C.S.W., O.N.C., O.M., M.M., P.L., S.S., E.N., E.G.S. and J.H.; methodology, A.V., V.V., R.G., D.J.B. and M.C., formal analysis, A.V., V.V., R.G. and D.J.B.; writing—original draft preparation, A.V., V.V. and A.L.; writing—review and editing, R.G., F.N., X.W., D.J.B., C.S.W., O.N.C., O.M., M.M., P.L., S.S., M.C., E.N., E.G.S., J.H. and A.L.; visualization, V.V., R.G. and A.V. All authors have read and agreed to the published version of the manuscript.

Funding: This research received no external funding.

Institutional Review Board Statement: Not applicable.

Informed Consent Statement: Not applicable.

Data Availability Statement: The original data presented in the study are openly available in WHO Immunization Data portal at https://immunizationdata.who.int/ (accessed on 9 January 2025), WHO/UNICEF COVID-19 vaccination information hub at https://infohub.crd.co/ (accessed on 4 December 2024), and COVID-19 Maternal Immunization Tracker (COMIT) from the Berman Institute of Bioethics & Center for Immunization Research, Johns Hopkins University at https://www.comitglobal.org/about/data (accessed on 10 December 2024).

Conflicts of Interest: The authors declare no conflicts of interest. The authors are staff members of the World Health Organization. The authors alone are responsible for the views expressed in this article and they do not necessarily represent the decisions, policy or views of the World Health Organization.

References

1. Wallace, A.S.; Ryman, T.K.; Privor-Dumm, L.; Morgan, C.; Fields, R.; Garcia, C.; Sodha, S.V.; Lindstrand, A.; Lochlainn, L.M.N. Leaving No One behind: Defining and Implementing an Integrated Life Course Approach to Vaccination across the next Decade as Part of the Immunization Agenda 2030. *Vaccine* **2024**, *42*, S54–S63. [CrossRef] [PubMed]
2. Ho, L.L.; Gurung, S.; Mirza, I.; Nicolas, H.D.; Steulet, C.; Burman, A.L.; Danovaro-Holliday, M.C.; Sodha, S.V.; Kretsinger, K. Impact of the SARS-CoV-2 Pandemic on Vaccine-Preventable Disease Campaigns. *Int. J. Infect. Dis.* **2022**, *119*, 201–209. [CrossRef] [PubMed]
3. World Health Organization. Progress and Challenges with Achieving Universal Immunization Coverage—2023 WHO/UNICEF Estimates of National Immunization Coverage (WUENIC). Available online: https://www.who.int/publications/m/item/progress-and-challenges (accessed on 7 April 2025).
4. Doherty, T.M.; Pasquale, A.D.; Finnegan, G.; Lele, J.; Philip, R.K. Sustaining the Momentum for Adult Vaccination Post-COVID-19 to Leverage the Global Uptake of Life-Course Immunisation: A Scoping Review and Call to Action. *Int. J. Infect. Dis.* **2024**, *142*, 106963. [CrossRef] [PubMed]
5. Brooks, D.J.; Kim, C.I.; Mboussou, F.F.; Danovaro-Holliday, M.C. Developing National Information Systems to Monitor COVID-19 Vaccination: A Global Observational Study. *JMIR Public Health Surveill.* **2024**, *10*, e62657. [CrossRef]
6. McCarron, M. Lessons Learned from Leveraging Seasonal Influenza Vaccination Infrastructure in COVID-19 Vaccination. In Proceedings of the The Global Exchange Forum on Integrated Immunization Programs and Enhanced Pandemic Preparedness, London, UK, 18–19 October 2023.
7. World Health Organization. COVID-19 Vaccination Insights Report—4 March 2024. Available online: https://www.who.int/publications/m/item/covid-19-vaccination-insights-report-4-march-2024 (accessed on 18 December 2024).
8. Pan American Health Organization. Immunization Across the Life Course—Resource Center. Available online: https://www.paho.org/en/topics/immunization/immunization-across-life-course-resource-center (accessed on 19 December 2024).
9. World Health Organization. Working Together: An Integration Resource Guide for Planning and Strengthening Immunization Services Throughout the Life Course. Available online: https://www.who.int/publications/i/item/9789241514736 (accessed on 19 December 2024).
10. World Health Organization. Life Course. Available online: https://www.who.int/our-work/life-course (accessed on 19 December 2024).
11. Pan American Health Organization. *Building Better Immunity: A Life Course Approach to Healthy Longevity*; PAHO: Washington, DC, USA, 2023; ISBN 9789275127445.
12. United Nations. World Population Prospects 2024. Available online: https://population.un.org/wpp (accessed on 9 October 2024).
13. Philip, R.K.; Attwell, K.; Breuer, T.; Pasquale, A.D.; Lopalco, P.L. Life-Course Immunization as a Gateway to Health. *Expert Rev. Vaccines* **2018**, *17*, 851–864. [CrossRef]
14. Nabia, S.; Wonodi, C.B.; Vilajeliu, A.; Sussman, S.; Olson, K.; Cooke, R.; Udayakumar, K.; Twose, C.; Ezeanya, N.; Adefarrell, A.A.; et al. Experiences, Enablers, and Challenges in Service Delivery and Integration of COVID-19 Vaccines: A Rapid Systematic Review. *Vaccines* **2023**, *11*, 974. [CrossRef]
15. World Health Organization. Considerations for Integrating COVID-19 Vaccination into Immunization Programmes and Primary Health Care for 2022 and Beyond. Available online: https://www.who.int/publications/i/item/9789240064454 (accessed on 19 December 2024).
16. Privor-Dumm, L.A.; Poland, G.A.; Barratt, J.; Durrheim, D.N.; Deloria Knoll, M.; Vasudevan, P.; Jit, M.; Bonvehí, P.E.; Bonanni, P. A Global Agenda for Older Adult Immunization in the COVID-19 Era: A Roadmap for Action. *Vaccine* **2021**, *39*, 5240–5250. [CrossRef] [PubMed]
17. World Health Organization. 50th Anniversary of the Expanded Programme on Immunization (EPI). Available online: https://www.who.int/news-room/events/detail/2024/01/01/default-calendar/50th-anniversary-of-the-expanded-programme-on-immunization-(epi) (accessed on 20 November 2024).
18. Marti, M.; Nohynek, H.; Duclos, P.; O'Brien, K.L.; Hombach, J. The Strategic Advisory Group of Experts (SAGE) on Immunization—Past, Present and Future. *Vaccines* **2024**, *12*, 1402. [CrossRef]
19. World Health Organization. WHO Vaccine Position Papers. Available online: https://www.who.int/teams/immunization-vaccines-and-biologicals/policies/position-papers (accessed on 19 October 2024).
20. United Nations. International Standard Industrial Classification of All Economic Activities (ISIC) Rev. 4. Available online: https://unstats.un.org/unsd/classifications/isic/revision (accessed on 9 December 2024).
21. United Nations High Commissioner for Refugees. Older Persons | UNHCR. Available online: https://emergency.unhcr.org/protection/persons-risk/older-persons (accessed on 17 December 2024).

22. World Health Organization. WHO/UNICEF Joint Reporting Form Process. Available online: https://www.who.int/teams/immunization-vaccines-and-biologicals/immunization-analysis-and-insights/global-monitoring/who-unicef-joint-reporting-process (accessed on 9 January 2025).
23. World Health Organization; UNICEF. COVID-19 Vaccination Information Hub. Available online: https://infohub.crd.co/ (accessed on 3 December 2024).
24. Berman Institute of Bioethics & Center for Immunization Research Johns Hopkins University. COVID-19 Maternal Immunization Tracker (COMIT). Available online: www.comitglobal.org (accessed on 9 December 2024).
25. Regional Office for South-East Asia World Health Organization. WHO SEA Region COVID-19 Vaccination Dashboard. Available online: https://www.who.int/southeastasia/health-topics/immunization/covid-19-vaccination (accessed on 18 December 2024).
26. Regional Office for Africa World Health Organization. Africa COVID-19 Vaccination Dashboard—COVID-19 Vaccination Policies. Available online: https://www.afro.who.int/health-topics/coronavirus-covid-19/vaccines (accessed on 17 December 2024).
27. Doshi, R.H.; Nsasiirwe, S.; Dahlke, M.; Atagbaza, A.; Aluta, O.E.; Tatsinkou, A.B.; Dauda, E.; Vilajeliu, A.; Gurung, S.; Tusiime, J.; et al. COVID-19 Vaccination Coverage—World Health Organization African Region, 2021–2023. *MMWR. Morb. Mortal. Wkly. Rep.* **2024**, *73*, 307–311. [CrossRef]
28. Nogareda, F.; Ghiselli, M.; Velandia-González, M.; de Mucio, B.; Jara, J.; Couto, P.; Rodriguez, A.; Rondy, M.; Vicari, A.; Ozturk, M.H.; et al. Seasonal Influenza Vaccination Programs in the Americas: A Platform for Sustainable Life-Course Immunization and Its Role for Pandemic Preparedness and Response. *Vaccines* **2024**, *12*, 1415. [CrossRef]
29. The World Bank. World Bank Country and Lending Groups. Available online: https://datahelpdesk.worldbank.org/knowledgebase/topics/19280-country-classification (accessed on 15 December 2024).
30. World Health Organization. WHO Roadmap on Uses of COVID-19 Vaccines in the Context of Omicron and High Population Immunity. Available online: https://www.who.int/publications/i/item/WHO-2019-nCoV-Vaccines-SAGE-Prioritization-2023.1 (accessed on 9 October 2024).
31. World Health Organization. Vaccines Against Influenza: WHO Position Paper—May 2022. *Wkly. Epidemiol. Rec.* **2012**, *97*, 185–208.
32. World Health Organization. Varicella and Herpes Zoster Vaccines: WHO Position Paper, June 2014. *Wkly. Epidemiol Rec.* **2014**, *89*, 265–288.
33. World Health Organization. Pertussis Vaccines: WHO Position Paper—August 2015. *Wkly. Epidemiol. Rec.* **2015**, *90*, 433–460.
34. World Health Organization. Considerations for Pneumococcal Vaccination in Older Adults. *Wkly. Epidemiol. Rec.* **2021**, *23*, 217–228.
35. World Health Organization. Meeting of the Strategic Advisory Group of Experts on Immunization, September 2024: Conclusions and Recommendations. *Wkly Epidemiol. Rec.* **2024**, *99*, 719–740.
36. World Health Organization. BCG Vaccines: WHO Position Paper—February 2018. *Wkly. Epidemiol. Rec.* **2018**, *93*, 73–96.
37. World Health Organization. Diphtheria Vaccines: WHO Position Paper—August 2017. *Wkly. Epidemiol. Rec.* **2017**, *92*, 417–435.
38. World Health Organization. Hepatitis B Vaccines: WHO Position Paper—July 2017. *Wkly. Epidemiol. Rec.* **2017**, *92*, 369–392.
39. World Health Organization. Measles Vaccines: WHO Position Paper—April 2017. *Wkly. Epidemiol. Rec.* **2017**, *92*, 205–227.
40. World Health Organization. Polio Vaccines: WHO Position Paper—June 2022. *Wkly. Epidemiol. Rec.* **2022**, *92*, 277–300.
41. World Health Organization. Rubella Vaccines: WHO Position Paper—July 2020. *Wkly. Epidemiol. Rec.* **2020**, *95*, 306–324.
42. World Health Organization. Tetanus Vaccines: WHO Position Paper—February 2017. *Wkly. Epidemiol Rec.* **2017**, *92*, 53–76.
43. World Health Organization. Cholera Vaccines: WHO Position Paper—August 2017. *Wkly. Epidemiol. Rec.* **2017**, *92*, 477–498.
44. World Health Organization. WHO Position Paper on Dengue Vaccines—May 2024. *Wkly. Epidemiol. Rec.* **2024**, *99*, 203–224.
45. World Health Organization. Extraordinary Meeting of the Strategic Advisory Group of Experts on Immunization on Ebola Vaccination, May 2024: Conclusions and Recommendation. *Wkly. Epidemiol. Rec* **2024**, *99*, 355–362.
46. World Health Organization. WHO Position Paper on Hepatitis A Vaccines—October 2022. *Wkly. Epidemiol. Rec.* **2022**, *97*, 493–512.
47. World Health Organization. Hepatitis E Vaccine: WHO Position Paper, May 2015. *Wkly. Epidemiol. Rec.* **2015**, *90*, 185–200.
48. World Health Organization. Japanese Encephalitis Vaccines: WHO Position Paper. *Wkly. Epidemiol. Rec.* **2015**, *90*, 69–88.
49. World Health Organization. Meningococcal Vaccines: WHO Position Paper—November 2011. *Wkly. Epidemiol. Rec.* **2011**, *86*, 521–540.
50. World Health Organization. Meningococcal A Conjugate Vaccine: Updated Guidance, February 2015. *Wkly. Epidemiol. Rec.* **2015**, *8*, 57–68.
51. World Health Organization. Meningococcal Vaccines: WHO Position Paper on the Use of Multivalent Meningococcal Conjugate Vaccines in Countries of the African Meningitis Belt, January 2024. *Wkly. Epidemiol. Rec.* **2024**, *99*, 1–10.
52. World Health Organization. Smallpox and Mpox (Orthopoxviruses): WHO Position Paper, August 2024. *Wkly. Epidemiol. Rec.* **2024**, *99*, 429–456.
53. World Health Organization. Rabies Vaccines: WHO Position Paper—April 2018. *Wkly. Epidemiol. Rec.* **2018**, *93*, 201–219.

54. World Health Organization. Vaccines against Tick-Borne Encephalitis: WHO Position Paper—2011. *Wkly. Epidemiol. Rec.* **2011**, *86*, 241–256.
55. World Health Organization. Typhoid Vaccines: WHO Position Paper—March 2018. *Wkly. Epidemiol. Rec.* **2018**, *93*, 153–172.
56. World Health Organization. Vaccines and Vaccination against Yellow Fever: WHO Position Paper—June 2013. *Wkly. Epidemiol. Rec.* **2013**, *88*, 269–283.
57. World Health Organization. Implementation Guide for Vaccination of Health Workers. Available online: https://www.who.int/publications/i/item/9789240052154 (accessed on 19 December 2024).
58. Bak, J.; Hasan, Q.; Kissa, J.; Mere, M.O.; Samhouri, D.; Gillespie, A.; Aynsley, T.R.; Abubakar, A.; Hajjeh, R.; Hutin, Y.J. Deployment of COVID-19 Vaccine in the WHO Eastern Mediterranean Region 2021–2023: How Do We Switch to a Life Course Approach? *Vaccine* **2024**, *42*, 3744–3750. [CrossRef]
59. World Health Organization. Protecting All Against Tetanus Guide to Sustaining Maternal and Neonatal Tetanus Elimination (MNTE) and Broadening Tetanus Protection for All Populations. Available online: https://www.who.int/publications/i/item/protecting-all-against-tetanus (accessed on 13 January 2025).
60. Li, Y.; Wang, X.; Blau, D.M.; Caballero, M.T.; Feikin, D.R.; Gill, C.J.; Madhi, S.A.; Omer, S.B.; Simões, E.A.F.; Campbell, H.; et al. Global, Regional, and National Disease Burden Estimates of Acute Lower Respiratory Infections Due to Respiratory Syncytial Virus in Children Younger than 5 Years in 2019: A Systematic Analysis. *Lancet* **2022**, *399*, 2047–2064. [CrossRef]
61. Trotter, C.L.; Alderson, M.; Dangor, Z.; Ip, M.; Le Doare, K.; Nakabembe, E.; Procter, S.R.; Sekikubo, M.; Lambach, P. Vaccine Value Profile for Group B Streptococcus. *Vaccine* **2023**, *41*, S41–S52. [CrossRef]
62. Gavi the Vaccine Alliance. Vaccine Investment Strategy 2024. Available online: https://www.gavi.org/our-alliance/strategy/vaccine-investment-strategy-2024 (accessed on 12 December 2024).
63. Bloom, D.E.; Pecetta, S.; Scorza, F.B.; Carfi, A.; Carleton, B.; Cipriano, M.; Edwards, K.; Gasperini, G.; Malley, R.; Nandi, A.; et al. Vaccination for Healthy Aging. *Sci. Transl. Med.* **2024**, *16*, eadm9183. [CrossRef]
64. Stancu, A.; Khan, A.; Barratt, J. Driving the Life Course Approach to Vaccination through the Lens of Key Global Agendas. *Front. Aging* **2023**, *4*, 1200397. [CrossRef] [PubMed]
65. World Health Organization. Humanly Possible Campaign. Available online: https://www.who.int/campaigns/world-immunization-week/2024 (accessed on 10 December 2024).
66. World Health Organization. An Investment Case for New Tuberculosis Vaccines. Available online: https://www.who.int/publications/i/item/9789240064690 (accessed on 18 October 2024).
67. El Banhawi, H.; Chowdhury, S.; Neri, M.; Radu, P.; Besley, S.; Bell, E.; Brassel, S.; Steuten, L. The Socioeconomic Value of Adult Immunisation Programmes OHE Contract Research Report: Office of Health Economics. Available online: https://www.ohe.org/publications/the-socio-economic-value-of-adult-immunisation-programmes/ (accessed on 18 December 2024).
68. Plans-Rubió, P. What COVID-19 Vaccination Strategy Should Be Implemented and Which Vaccines Should Be Used in the Post-Pandemic Era? *Vaccines* **2024**, *12*, 1180. [CrossRef] [PubMed]
69. Gavi The Vaccine Alliance. Gavi Board Approves next Five Year Strategy; Outlines Plans to Support Access to New Vaccines, Global Health Security, and Sustainability. Available online: https://www.gavi.org/news/media-room/gavi-board-approves-2030-strategy-new-vaccines-key-decisions-vaccine-sovereignty (accessed on 21 December 2024).

vaccines

MDPI

Opinion

Polio Epidemiology: Strategies and Challenges for Polio Eradication Post the COVID-19 Pandemic

Lucia F. Bricks [1,*], Denis Macina [2] and Juan C. Vargas-Zambrano [2]

1 Sanofi Vaccines Medical, Av Nações Unidas, São Paulo 14401, Brazil
2 Sanofi Vaccines Medical, 14 Espace Henri Vallee, 69007 Lyon, France; denis.macina@sanofi.com (D.M.); juan.vargas@sanofi.com (J.C.V.-Z.)
* Correspondence: lucia.bricks@sanofi.com

Abstract: The Global Polio Eradication Initiative (GPEI), launched in 1988, has successfully reduced wild poliovirus (WPV) cases by over 99.9%, with WPV type 2 and WPV3 declared eradicated in 2015 and 2019, respectively. However, as of 2024, WPV1 remains endemic in Afghanistan and Pakistan. Since 2000, outbreaks of circulating virus derived of polio vaccines (cVDPVs) have emerged in multiple regions, primary driven by low vaccine coverage rates (VCRs). The COVID-19 pandemic disrupted routine immunization, resulting in millions of unvaccinated children, and leaving many countries vulnerable to both WPV1 and cVDPVs outbreaks. This paper reviews the epidemiological landscape of poliomyelitis post the COVID-19 pandemic, and the strategies and challenges to achieve the global polio eradication.

Keywords: poliomyelitis; epidemiology; vaccine coverage; surveillance; polio eradication

1. Introduction

Poliomyelitis presenting as acute flaccid paralysis (AFP) can be caused by three WPV types: 1, 2, and 3. Two of these WPVs were globally eradicated: WPV2 since 2012, and WPV3 since 2019 [1]. In 2024, only WPV1 persists in two endemic countries, but outbreaks caused by circulating vaccine-derived poliovirus (cVDPVs) have been reported since 2000, the year initially proposed for global polio eradication [1–9].

The success in reducing by more than 99.9% the number of AFP cases caused by WPV involved massive vaccination campaigns with the trivalent oral polio vaccine (tOPV), which is composed of live attenuated polio strains—Sabin 1, 2, and 3 [1,3,8]. In 1994, the American region was declared free of WPV by the WHO [1], but in 2000 the first outbreak caused by cVDPV1 was detected in this region [1,8,10].

Before 2000, few countries had adopted the inactivated polio vaccine (IPV) in their routine immunization (RI) schedules. The majority were European countries [8,9,11], where rare cases of AFP caused by polio were recorded, mainly in unvaccinated or inadequately vaccinated individuals, and WPV1 was the most frequent strain [8,9]. Most countries adopted tOPV on the basis of its ease of administration, its low cost, its robust immunogenicity, and its capacity to induce intestinal mucosal immunity (IMI), which helps reduce poliovirus shedding in breakthrough infections [9]. Sabin vaccine is considered one of the safer vaccines, but Sabin live virus strains are genetically unstable, and in rare occasions they can mutate and reacquire neurovirulence. As a result, OPV can cause vaccine-associated paralytic poliomyelitis (VAPP) in recipients or contacts of recipients. The risk is higher after the first dose, in communities with low vaccine coverage rates (VCRs), and among immunocompromised individuals. These revertant strains named vaccine-derived polioviruses (VDPVs) can cause paralysis, with indistinguishable clinical signs and severity from those caused by WPV [8].

VDPVs are classified in three categories: cVDPVs (circulating), when there is evidence of transmission (more than one case), iVPVD, when the infections are confirmed in immunocompromised individuals, and aVDPV (ambiguous) that can represent the initial isolates from cVDPV outbreaks, samples isolated from individuals without documented immunodeficiencies or that are environmental samples, with no evidence of community circulation [8]. Low VCRs are the most important factor associated with the emergence and circulation of these new pathogenic strains [1,3,8,9].

At the onset of the 21st century, Canada and the USA replaced tOPV by IPV, considering that the number of VAPP cases outnumbered those caused by WPV, and these countries changed tOPV to IPV. The IPV vaccine is highly immunogenic, safer, and more effective than OPV to prevent polio, but it induces low IMI. After 2000, as outbreaks caused by cVDPVs emerged in all WHO regions [3,8–10], high-income countries (HICs), where high VCRs were achieved with three doses of tOPV [6,7], progressively included IPV in their national immunization programs (NIPs) [8,9,11].

Initially, IPV was included in NIPs concomitantly with DPT-based whole-cell or acellular pertussis vaccine (DTPw or DTPa). As the acellular pertussis vaccine quickly proved amendable to be combined with IPV, DTPa combination vaccines including IPV and other antigens were developed and introduced into RI. HICs adopted acellular pertussis vaccines in combination with IPV earlier, while low-income countries (LICs) and middle-income countries (MICs) continued using OPV and combination vaccines with DTPw [8,9,11]. Nowadays, HICs use pentavalent or hexavalent combination vaccines formulated with IPV and aP, while most LICs and MICs still rely on pentavalent vaccines containing whole cell pertussis vaccines and the separate administration of at least one dose of IPV and more than two OPV doses [11,12].

The GPEI strategy recommended for global polio eradication focused on tOPV until 2016. The amazing success in eradicating WPV2 and WPV3 in four of the six WHO regions—the Americas (1994), the Western Pacific (2000), Europe (2002), and Southeast Asia (2014), associated with the fact that OPV induces IMI and the rare occurrence of VAPP cases before 2015, were the main reasons invoked to maintain the use of tOPV in RI. Between 2004 and 2009, monovalent oral polio vaccines (mOPV) were also used during specific outbreaks [1,3,8,13,14].

Despite this success, even in areas declared polio-free, many AFP cases were associated with the continued use of OPV [2]. This was especially the case in areas with low VCR, where cVDPV2 caused the majority of outbreaks [2,3,8–11].

Polioviruses are highly infectious [8] and the WHO recommends a minimum of 90% of VCR with three doses of OPV in the first year of life to achieve global polio eradication [1]. In 2018, the global VCR was 84%, but with large variations between different countries and regions of the same country [6,7]. In addition, the COVID-19 pandemic caused a reduction in the global VCR for all vaccines, resulting in millions of children remaining unprotected against polio and other serious diseases [3,6].

Since 2017, the number of AFP cases caused by VDPVs has surpassed those caused by WPV1 [2–5] (Figure 1).

Poliovirus transmission, whether WPV and cVDPV, has been declared by the WHO as a Public Health Emergency of International Concern (PHEIC) since 2014, and is still a PHEIC in 2024 [3].

The objective of this article is to review the polio epidemiology after the COVID-19 pandemic, the strategies and challenges to achieve global polio eradication, and the plans for the post-eradication era.

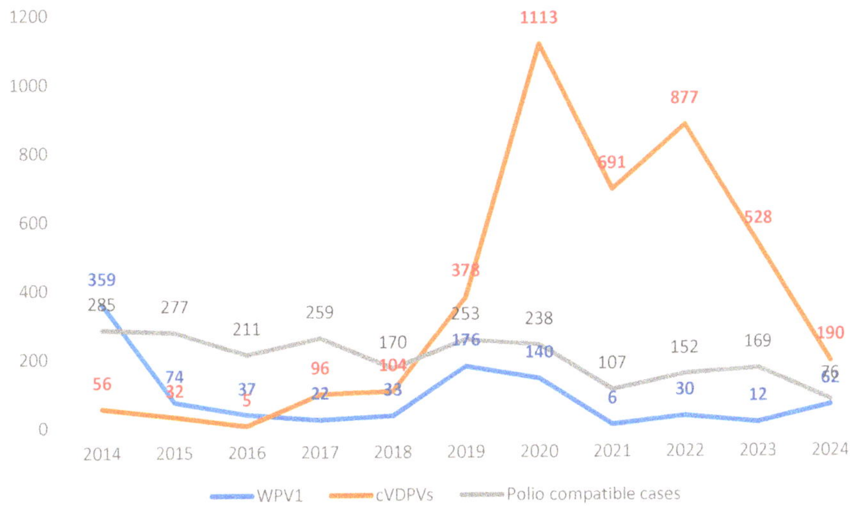

Figure 1. AFP cases caused by WPV, cVDPVs (1,2,3), and polio-compatible cases notified to the WHO from 2014 until 2024 [2]. * Data as of 24 October 2024 [2].

2. Polio Epidemiology After the COVID-19 Pandemic

Since 2019, WPV1 is the only WPV still in circulation, but the number of AFP cases and outbreaks caused by VDPVs is a cause of concern [4]. The minimum number of AFP cases caused by WPV1 before the onset of the COVID-19 pandemic was 22, in 2017. In 2019 and 2020, an increase in AFP cases caused by WPV1 was observed, with 176 and 140 cases, respectively. Most of these cases were notified in Afghanistan and Pakistan, but nine children and adolescents outside these endemic countries developed AFP caused by WPV1 in 2021 and 2022: one in Malawi (November 2021) and eight in Mozambique (2022) [5]. Extensive national and subnational campaigns of immunization were conducted in these countries and in neighboring countries (Tanzania, Zambia, and Zimbabwe) to avoid WPV1 spreading in the region. No new AFP or detection of WPV1 through environmental surveillance (ES) was registered in these countries after 2022, and they were not considered as endemic countries [12].

In 2024, the WHO considers only Pakistan and Afghanistan as endemic countries, i.e., countries where the transmission of indigenous wild poliovirus never stopped. Thanks to the work of the WHO and many partners (UNICEF, Rotary International, the US Centers for Disease Control and Prevention, the Bill and Melinda Gates Foundation, and Gavi, the Vaccine Alliance) to increase VCR in endemic and recent outbreak countries, including numerous and extensive campaigns of immunization, the number of APF cases caused by WPV1 was reduced to only six, in 2021. Yet this is no reason to let the guard down, as in 2024, this number is more than five times higher, with 62 AFP cases caused by WPV1 confirmed in Afghanistan (23) and Pakistan (39) as of 22 October 2024 compared with 12 AFP cases in 2023 (full year) [4].

Despite the success of maintaining a geographically limited circulation of WPV, the number of countries that previously stopped indigenous WPV but are experiencing either the importation of WPV or VDPVs from other countries or the local emergence of cVDPVs has grown since 2016.

In 2016, there were 37 AFP cases caused by WPV1 and five caused by cVDPVs. In 2017, the number of AFP cases caused by cVDPV2 (96) surpassed the number of AFP cases caused by WPV1 (22), reaching a peak in 2020 (1082), affecting 24 countries (Table 1).

Table 1. Number of WPV1 and cVPDVs APF cases from 2020 to 2024 [4,5].

AFP	2020 Cases (No. Countries)	2021 Cases (No. Countries)	2022 Cases (No. Countries)	2023 Cases (No. Countries)	2024 Cases (No. Countries) *
WPV1	140 (2)	6 (3)	30 (3)	12 (2)	62 (2)
cVDPV1	35 (4)	14 (2)	192 (5)	134 (3)	8 (2)
cVDPV2	1082 (24)	629 (22)	367 (20)	383 (23)	182 (16)
cVDPV3	0 (0)	0 (0)	1 (1)	0 (0)	0 (0)

* Partial data. Cases reported to the WHO as of 22 October 2024.

There was a reduction in the number of AFP cases caused by cVDPV2 over the last 4 years, but new countries have been infected, reaching a total of 51 countries with detection of cVDPV2. In 2024, cVDPV2 strains were detected only through environmental surveillance in 13 countries (Figure 2) [2–5,13,14].

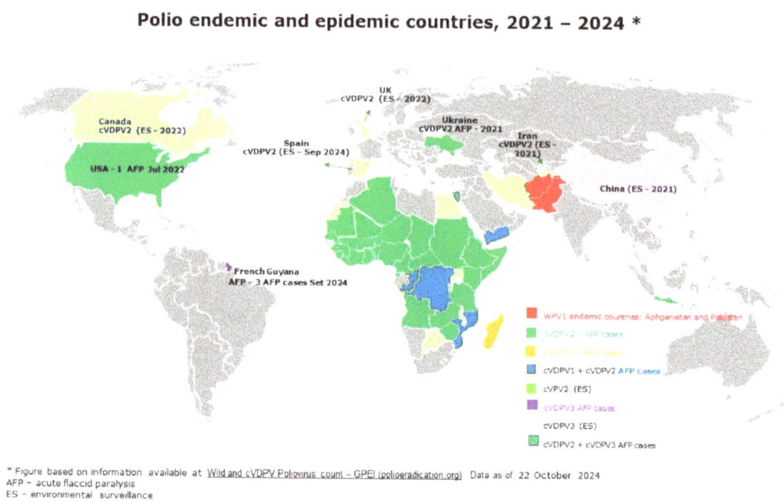

Figure 2. WPV1 polio endemic countries and cVDPVs epidemic countries in the last years (2021 to 2024 as of 22 October 2024).

In 2023, the WHO reported 12 AFP cases caused by WPV1 and 527 AFP cases caused by cVDPVs. From 1 January to 22 October 2024, 62 AFP cases caused by WPV1 were confirmed and cVDPV2 persists as the predominant strain detected through AFP surveillance and having caused paralysis in 182 individuals from 16 countries, including one case in Gaza confirmed on 25 July 2024 [3] (Table 1).

In the last four years, outbreaks caused by cVDPV1 were registered in six countries: Congo, the Democratic Republic of the Congo, Madagascar, Malawi, and Mozambique. Despite the substantial reduction in these numbers, as recently as 25 September 2024, cVDPV1 was still circulating in the Democratic Republic of the Congo (five AFP cases) and Mozambique (one APF case); additionally, one AFP case caused by cVDPV3 was confirmed in Israel in 2022 [2,5].

3. Strategies Recommended by the WHO for Polio Eradication

The GPEI strategies to achieve polio eradication changed many times over the years. From 1988 to 2005, the WHO recommended the exclusive use of tOPV in routine and immunization campaigns. Monovalent OPV vaccines (mOPV) became the vaccines of choice for supplemental immunization campaigns between 2005 and 2009 in polio-endemic or polio-epidemic countries. Indeed, the single-strain vaccine can help avoid the issue of the immunological interference between the three Sabin strains, especially with Sabin-2, the most immunogenic [8]. The massive use of mOPV1 (mOPV) resulted in the virtual elimination of WPV1 in India. Bivalent OPV containing Sabin strains 1 and 3 (bOPV1,3) has superior immunogenicity against polio 1 and 3 as compared with tOPV, without loss of immunogenicity as compared with mOPV1 and mOPV3, and was also largely used after WPV2 global eradication [8].

In 2012, with the dramatic reduction in WPV and eradication of WPV2, the WHO started to recommend the introduction of one dose of IPV to prepare for the post-eradication era. In that year, an IPV based on Sabin strains (sIPV) started to be used in Asia (Japan in 2012 and China in 2015) [9]. The WHO considers that these vaccines are as immunogenic and safe as IPV manufactured from WPV. HICs adopted a full IPV schedule before 2015, preferentially in combination with other vaccines, but most of the MIC and LIC persisted using tOPV and mOPVs until 2016. That year, with the declaration of the eradication of WPV2, the WHO recommended the substitution of tOPV by bOPV1,3 and one IPV dose [8,9,13,14]. The limitation in the supply of IPV, and a delay in the introduction of this vaccine in the poorest countries, resulted in a substantial gap of protection against polio 2, the most likely cause of the emergence of several cVDPV2 outbreaks in more than 40 countries. To overcome the short supply of IPV, the WHO recommended the use of one-fifth of an IPV dose (fractional IPV—fIPV), a strategy that was adopted by a limited number of LICs and MICs [8,9,11,13,14].

The last Polio Eradication Strategy 2022–2026 has two main goals: (1) permanently interrupting WPV1 transmission in endemic countries and (2) stopping cVDPV transmission and preventing outbreaks in non-endemic countries, both by the end of 2023, with the aim of reaching eradication by 2026 [1,3,13,14]. However, in 2024, these two goals were not achieved [1–5].

One dose of IPV or two fIPV are not sufficient to protect against polio 2 or guarantee durable protection [9].

The challenges encountered in the substitution of tOPV for bOPV1,3 resulted in a higher number of cVDPV2 outbreaks and countries affected by them [1,3,13,14]. The attempt to control cVDPV2 outbreaks with large immunization campaigns with mOPV2 was not successful. Between 1 January 2016 and 22 October 2024, 518 AFP cases caused by WPV1 were confirmed and 3983 AFP cases were caused by cVDPVs 1, 2, or 3, especially cVDPV2 [2]. The delay in the implementation of immunization campaigns and the incapacity to achieve high VCRs contributed to the emergence of new cVDPV2 cases, that spread to new areas and neighboring countries. The low VCR for bOPV1,3 in RI was responsible for the emergence of cVDPV1 outbreaks and one AFP case caused by cVDPV3 in the last 4 years. The absent or weak environmental surveillance in many countries also contributed to the late detection of VDPV emergences and late response to control its dissemination [13,14].

In 2020, the WHO recommended the introduction of a second IPV dose for all countries, considering that there was a sufficient supply of IPV, fIPV and sIPV [1,3].

In 2021, one novel OPV vaccine (nOPV2), formulated with Sabin 2 strains genetically attenuated to reduce the risks to revert to the neurovirulence observed with mOPV2, was introduced under an emergency list [15–18]. More than one billion doses of nOPV2 were used in 35 epidemic countries, including almost 500 million doses in Nigeria [15], but new countries have been infected by cVDPV between 2021 and 2024 (eight in 2023 and two in 2024) [5]. On 16 March 2024, the WHO informed that the GPEI received notification of the detection of cVDPV2 in Burundi and the Democratic Republic of the Congo (DRC) linked with the nOPV2. The viruses were isolated from the stool samples of seven children with acute flaccid paralysis—six in the DRC and one in Burundi, and from five environmental samples collected in Burundi [16]. Between January 2023 and June 2024, a total of 74 cVDPV outbreaks were detected in 39 countries, with 672 confirmed AFP cases identified in 27 of the

39 countries. Most outbreaks (70) were caused by cVDPV2, and 29 (comprising 19 VDPV2 emergencies) were linked to nOPV2 use in 19 countries [17].

On 19 July 2024, the WHO informed that a variant type 2 of poliovirus was isolated from sewage samples in Gaza [18], and one AFP case caused by cVDPV2 was confirmed in Gaza on 25 July 2024 [5]. On 13 August 2024, the WHO reported that a total of 16 new nOPV2-derived cVDPV2 emergences had been detected in the African Region, which now exclusively uses nOPV2 for outbreak response, and one had been identified in Egypt, in the Eastern Mediterranean Region. The AFP case caused by cVDPV2 confirmed in Gaza is genetically related to the lineage identified in Egypt [19].

4. Discussion

Many factors can be associated with the delay in global polio eradication, and for this paper we will focus our discussion on four: (1) vaccine coverage rates; (2) polio surveillance; (3) the benefits and risks associated with live and inactivated vaccines; (4) plannings for the final polio eradication and post-global eradication era.

4.1. Vaccine Coverage Rates

The best way to reduce polio infections is to maintain strong population immunity levels through high VCRs. This has proven difficult, especially in the poorest countries and conflict areas, since before 2019, and more so during the COVID-19 pandemic, when lockdowns and the reduction in basic health services reduced even more the VCRs in most countries. Even in high-income countries, vaccine hesitancy and loss of confidence in immunization increased because of fake news in the media [1,3,8,9,13,14]. Despite the alerts about the risks of polio resurgence, in 2023, three-dose polio VCRs (considering both OPV and IPV vaccines) were <90% in 89 out of 195 countries, including in Afghanistan and Pakistan, and countries from different WHO regions reported three-dose polio VCRs $\leq$ 60%, leaving millions of children unprotected [6,7]. Countries with outbreaks caused by cVDPV1 and cVPDV2, like the DRC, have three-dose polio VCR rates that are close to 50% [5].

The surprise was not the emergence of polio outbreaks in countries with low VCRs, but the absence of polio in some of the countries where VCRs are extremely low, such as Ecuador, Haiti, and Vietnam. In 2023, all countries had introduced the first IPV dose (IPV-1), but more than 60% did not achieve VCR $\geq$ 90% for the IPV-1, and from 85 countries that reported VCR for IPV-2, only 57.6% achieved IPV-2 VCR $\geq$ 90% [6,7].

In 2021, two cases of AFP caused by cVDPV2 were confirmed in Ukraine (the last on 24 December 2021) [5]. The three-dose polio VCR rate in Ukraine in 2021 was 78%, and it dropped to 69% in 2022 because of the war [6,7]. With the persistence of the conflict, the risk of polio resurgence is remarkably high in this country.

The risk of polio resurgence does not exist only in countries with low VCRs. In 2022, one AFP case caused by cVDPV2 was confirmed in the USA and one, caused by cVDPV3, in Israel. In 2023, Israel also reported one AFP case caused by cVDPV2. These two countries have high VCRs and good infrastructure to investigate and organize catch-up immunization in at-risk areas, impairing the spread of VDPVs [5]. In the UK and Canada, cVDPV2 was detected in 2022 through ES without causing paralysis, and the strains detected in the USA, the UK, and Canada were genetically related. In these three countries, only IPV vaccines were used to carry out catch-up vaccination, with no new AFP case or detection of VDPVs in sewage water in 2023 and 2024. In Israel, despite the use of IPV and OPV to control the emergence of cVDPVs, on 19 July 2024, the WHO alerted of the detection of cVDPV2 in six environmental samples in Gaza collected on 23 June 2024 from two different collection sites in two sub-regions [18], and one AFP case caused by cVDPV2 was confirmed on 25 July 2024 [5]. The three-dose polio routine VCR in the occupied Palestinian territory was 99% in 2022 but has declined to 89% after the onset of the conflict, and there is great concern that it will decrease even more as the war drags on [18].

Both OPV and IPV cannot eliminate the risk of polio resurgence in areas with low VCRs.

4.2. Polio Surveillance

The other major challenge for polio eradication is surveillance to detect polio infections. Less than 1% of poliovirus infections result in symptomatic disease.

According to the WHO, the strategies for detecting the poliovirus involve AFP surveillance: active surveillance among at least 1/100,000 individuals younger than 15 years of age in non-endemic countries, and passive surveillance with investigation of notified AFP cases with 80% adequate stool collection, supplemented by the environmental surveillance of sewage samples to detect early indicators of silent transmission in a population (i.e., non-paralytic cases) [3,4].

From 2020 to 2024, the number of AFP cases caused by cVDVPs and polio-compatible cases (those for which it is not possible to confirm or exclude polio) were higher than those caused by WPV1 (Figure 1). Additionally, in 2024, there were 11,127 polio-pending cases as of 24 October 2024 (AFP without lab test confirmation) [2].

From 2019 to 2024, according to the WHO, the incidence rate of non-polio AFP cases ranged from 3.83 to 6.53 per 100,000, but the surveillance for AFP is not uniform, and in many regions and countries the AFP surveillance rates are lower than 1/100,000 [2]. Failures in surveillance of AFP cases, the time necessary to confirm the etiology of AFP reported cases, and difficulties to perform laboratory investigations in cases and contacts are important challenges to the timely identification of VDPV circulation and outbreaks, and thus to the timely implementation of control measures, especially in areas with low VCRs and weak surveillance systems [14,20].

In Latin America, for example, no cVDPV cases have been reported [2], but several countries have identified VAPP cases and VDPVs. In the few countries where ES samples were collected, Sabin strains with mutations associated with neurovirulence have been identified [20,21] and rare cases of iVPDV has also been confirmed [20–22]. Mexico was the first MIC to introduce an acellular pertussis combination vaccine containing IPV in 2007, after the detection of 2 VAPP cases in healthy infants, but persisted in using OPV for boosters until 2020. Other MICs adopted IPV in RI (standalone or in combination with other antigens) but persisted in using OPV for boosters or during national immunization campaigns. More recently, a greater number of MICs are using only IPV, like Argentina, Chile, Uruguay, and Mexico.

Independently of the rarity of AFP cases caused by VDPV strains, VAPP cases have been confirmed in different countries, in addition to some iVDPV cases and some ambiguous AFP cases [2,10,20–22]. Many countries of this region reported exceptionally low three-dose polio VCRs after the COVID-19 pandemic. In Venezuela, five polio-compatible cases were registered in 2020, and six in 2022. It is impossible to know if they were caused by poliovirus, but considering the extremely low three-dose polio VCR (51%) and the political situation in this country, the probability that some are cVDPVs is high [2].

In regions where the population is seriously under-immunized, and a high number of susceptible children are immunized with OPV, Sabin strains can circulate for a prolonged period, which increases the probability to mutate and, over the course of 12–18 months, to reacquire neurovirulence [1,8,9]. On 27 December 2022, one AFP case was reported in Peru in a non-immunized healthy infant. Only in March 2023, three months thereafter, the genetic characterization of the strain was classified as VDPV type 1, and a regional alert was issued by the PAHO in April (4 months after case detection) [23]. In Peru and Venezuela there is no ES, and in Guatemala, where one VDPV case was reported, a retrospective trial showed that more than 30% of AFP cases were not reported through the AFP surveillance system [24].

Polio cases can be missed by AFP cases surveillance alone, emphasizing the importance of ES. In China, a total of 624 sewage samples were collected from domestic sewage in Guangzhou City, from 2009 to 2021. Poliovirus was identified in 66.67%. After inoculation and replication in three cell lines, 3370 viruses were isolated during a 13-year surveillance period. Among these, 1086 isolates were identified as polioviruses: type 1 PV (21.36%), type 2 PV (29.19%), and type 3 PV (49.48%). Based on VP1 capsid protein genome sequences,

1057 strains were identified as Sabin-like, 21 strains were high-mutant vaccines, and eight strains were classified as VDPVs. The numbers and serotypes of poliovirus isolates in sewage were influenced by the vaccine switch strategy. After 2016, no Sabin-2 was isolated from sewage and type 3 PV isolates increased significantly and became the dominant serotype [25]. The risk for cVDPV3 outbreak reemergence did not disappear from China, where on 25 January 2023 one cVDPV3 was detected through ES [5].

China introduced sIPV in its RI in 2015, and reports an extremely high VCR for three-dose polio vaccination [6,7]. The origin of this cVDPV3 strain is unknown.

The time for the detection of wild polio virus and VDPVs detected in AFP cases or through ES is key to the implementation of immunization campaigns. As an example, in Israel, cVDPV3 strains were detected through ES in 2021, and the AFP case caused by this strain was confirmed in 2022 [5].

Between 2004 and 2019, in a total of 74 outbreaks caused by cVDPVs registered in 24 countries, the median time from seeding until outbreak detection for serotype 1 was 572 days (95% CI 279–2016), in 10 outbreaks; for serotype 2 (in 59 outbreaks), it was 276 days (95% CI 172–765), and for serotype 3 (in 5 outbreaks), was 472 days (95% CI 392–603) [10].

The same problem related to a delay in the identification of polio strains was noted with WPV1. In the recently isolated WPV1 in Malawi, extensive nucleotide changes were detected, indicating that WPV1 had been circulating in southeastern Africa for approximately 2 years before the detection of these strains [12].

Recently, the time for detection of VDPVs seems to have been reduced, as observed in the USA, when one case of AFP was confirmed in 2022, and the genetic analysis of the cVDPV2 isolated from this case was related to strains identified through ES in the UK only a few months before [3]. In Yemen, cVDPV2 was isolated from 227 AFP cases and from 83% (39/47) of environmental samples with an average of 7 months' delay from sample collection [26]. Regardless of this reduction in detection time, this was insufficient to implement the campaigns of immunization to control cVDPV2 outbreaks in African countries [27]. Additionally, a review of VAPP cases proved the strong correlation with immunodeficiencies and also that clinical manifestations can develop 2 months to 4 years after the last OPV dose [28]. Immunocompromised people can excrete the virus for years and infect close contacts that can also shed the virus, maintaining silent circulation and transmission in the community [28].

The most recent alert from the WHO about the emergence of the cVDPV2 strain in Gaza reported that the genomic sequencing of the six cVDPV2 isolates had close genetic links with each other and are also closely related to the poliovirus variant that was circulating in Egypt during the second half of 2023. In Israel, the last detection of cVDPV2 was in December 2023, and it was estimated that cVDPV2 was introduced in Gaza as early as September 2023. These strains have probably been circulating for 10 months before their detection through ES in Gaza [18]. The isolates have limited divergence from the parental nOPV2 vaccine strain in the VP1 capsid protein coding area (6 to 16 nucleotide substitutions), indicating that surveillance detected emergence early after vaccination [18].

ES is recommended by the WHO to facilitate the identification of VDPVs, contributing to organizing a fast response to outbreaks, but in many outbreak countries, the ES was only introduced after the confirmation of AFP cases. Similarly to VCRs, ES is not uniform. As an example, the DRC, where 75% of cVDPV1 AFP cases confirmed in 2021 and 2022 were reported, had no VDPV1 identified by ES, and Madagascar, where 12% of cVDPV1 were reported, reported more cVDPV1 by ES from 2021 to 2024 [5].

4.3. Benefits and Risks Associated with Live and Inactivated Vaccines Recommended by the WHO

The WHO estimates that the large use of oral polio vaccines prevented more than 6.5 million children from developing polio caused by WPV in the last decade [1], but despite the success of the tOPV vaccine in eradicating WPV2 and WPV3 and the huge reduction of countries infected by WPV1, the emergence of VDPVs is now a difficult-to-control public health emergency.

To reduce the risk of polio, in many countries where VCRs are low, the strategy is to start the RI with bOPV followed by IPV, because IPV can boost the serologic and mucosal immunity in infants previously immunized with OPV. Many low-income countries also include a dose of OPV to newborns in an attempt to improve the VCRs. Even though the OPV and nOPV2 vaccines are considered safe for newborns, most immunodeficiencies are not diagnosed in the first months of life, and many times, AFP is the first alert to investigate immunodeficiency [22]. Recently, in China, one 7 month-old immunocompromised child developed AFP and infected his father, who shed the virus without any symptom [29]. In China, the genetic evolution of iVDPV3 showed the recombination of different Sabin strains [30].

The lower seroconversion of OPV observed in many developing countries was considered responsible for AFP cases in children who received five or more doses of OPV. This problem was detected especially in areas where there is a high circulation of other enteroviruses, low hygiene, and malnutrition, exactly those where it was more difficult to eliminate WPV and cVDPVs [8,9]. In addition, when tOPV was substituted for bOPV1,3, there was a substantial reduction in immunity against polio 2 that was even more reduced after the COVID-19 pandemic. The results of a study in 51 African countries showed that type 2 OPV immunity among children under 5 years declined from a median of 87% in January–June 2016 to 14% in January–June 2020 [27]. The probability of cVDPV2 poliomyelitis among children under 5 years was negatively correlated with OPV-induced and IPV-induced immunity. Campaigns with mOPV2 in response to cVDPV2 outbreaks covered only 11% of children under 5 years who are predicted to be at risk within the first 6 months and only 56% within the first 12 months, resulting in a failure to protect against cVDPV2 spreading [27].

In 2013–2014, Israel experienced an outbreak of wild poliovirus type 1 (WPV1), detected through the environmental surveillance of the sewage system. No cases of AFP were reported, and the epidemic subsided after a bivalent oral polio vaccination campaign. However, Brower et al. [31] estimated that 59% (95% CI 9–77%) of susceptible individuals (primarily children under 10 years old) had been infected with WPV1 over a little more than six months, mostly before the vaccination campaign's onset, and that the vaccination campaign had averted 10% (95% CI 1–24%) of WPV1 infections.

Many mathematical models have estimated the risks of the emergence of new VDPV strains, especially cVDPV2 and cVDPV1 in areas with extremely low VCR [32–34]. Recent publications showed that the introduction of at least one dose of IPV in addition to mOPV or bOPVs can contribute substantially to protect against polio [19,35–38]. Despite the low impact on intestinal immunity, IPV is highly immunogenic in higher-, middle-, and lower-income countries [8,9]. IPV contributes to boost the serologic response to all strains and/or to offer protection in naïve children and children that did not seroconvert after OPV [36–38].

IPV is the safest vaccine against polio because it cannot cause VAPP or VDPVs emergence and according to many experts, in polio-free regions, ethical reasons support the exclusive adoption of the IPV vaccination [38,39]. Children immunized with IPV can be infected by WPV or VDPVs without developing symptoms; these strains can multiply in the gastrointestinal tract and the silent circulation will put at risk people with incomplete protection, whether they live in high-, middle-, or low-income countries. The same can occur when OPV is used in areas where OPV has low VCRs or have demonstrated low efficacy because of the interference of other enteroviruses [8,9].

Devaux et al. (2024) affirmed that the intestinal microbiota can contribute to increasing poliovirus infection, replication, recombination, and transmission. There is evidence that the exposure to bacteria, and especially to lipopolysaccharides, is a potent enhancer of poliovirus infectivity. They also suggested that some bacterial strains increase co-infections by different polioviruses, promoting genetic recombination between different viruses. In LICs, these new aspects related to infection can make the use of IPV more favorable [39].

The viral shedding after the first OPV dose is high, peaking 2 weeks after vaccination, and is null after IPV. In areas with low VCRs, the use of OPV has been responsible for VPDV emergence and cVDPVs outbreaks. Inactivated strains cannot replicate and never cause VAPP or give origin to VDPVs.

Connor et al. (2002), in a review of mucosal immunity against poliovirus, showed that intestinal immunity after oral polio vaccines wanes over time to undetectable levels 1 to 4 years after the primary schedule with OPV. It is not observed also in adolescents and adults, probably because of an age-related defect in enteric mucosal immunity to poliovirus. Older children, adolescents, and adults immunized with OPV more than 1 year before can shed live polio strains for more than 2 months upon challenge. This new knowledge can impact the strategies proposed for the final phase of polio eradication [35].

To solve the problems associated with low seroconversion after immunization with Sabin vaccines, new genetically attenuated live vaccines have been developed over the last decade. The nOPV2 was used since 2021 in epidemic countries, and it was expected that it could reduce the risks of VAPP and VDPV emergences. In fact, it was proven that nOPV2 was 80% less likely to seed new-variant polio outbreaks. However, a lower risk for mutation is different from zero risk, and recently it was confirmed that nOPV2 can also cause paralysis [15–17]. Additionally, it also induces lower seroconversion and showed low effectiveness in Nigeria and Libera [40,41], as was seen with classic Sabin OPV vaccines [8,9].

In Liberia, a study including 371 children who had received two doses of nOPV2, showed that only 38.3% had antibodies against type 2 poliovirus, demonstrating that nOPV2 can be poorly immunogenic in some developing countries. In this trial, the seroprevalence against polioviruses type 1 (59.6%) and type 3 (53.0%) was also extremely low, despite the large use of bOPV(1,3) [40].

A recent case-control study performed in Nigeria showed that nOPV2 had low effectiveness to protect against cVDPV2, even after two doses. On the contrary, the IPV demonstrated higher effectiveness and efficacy [41]. Despite the large use of nOPV2 in Nigeria, and the reduction of AFP cases caused by cVDPV2 from 2021 to 2024, >40% of cVDPV2 AFP cases confirmed in 2024 (49 of 117) were from this country [19].

A new cause for concern about nOPV2 was the detection of strains derived from this vaccine in countries that never used it. In South Sudan, a new emergence of cVDPV2 strains was detected with whole-genome sequencing (WGS), indicating that the origin of the virus was the novel OPV2, although the vaccine has never been used in the country [12]. In the Russian Federation, VDPV2 strains detected in migrant children from Tajikistan [42] and in Gaza, cVDPV2 detected through ES were both genetically related to nOPV2 vaccine strains used in Egypt [18].

The other relevant point to discuss is the duration of protection offered by OPVs and IPVs. In the past, the circulation of wild poliovirus could provide a natural booster, but large outbreaks involving adolescents and adults demonstrated that it is not possible to guarantee this natural protection [8,9]. Gao et al. (2022), in a meta-analysis about the duration of protection after vaccines, reported only eight papers discussing polio duration of protection post-OPV or -IPV, and the majority were focused on combined vaccines containing IPV. The studies with available prevaccination records suggested that the geometric medium titers and geometric medium concentration of antibodies (GMT/GMC) remained around three times higher than prevaccination levels for all three poliovirus types at 5–6 years postvaccination, but only one article reporting results for 10 years postvaccination was included in this meta-analysis. There were no data about the duration of protection offered by OPV in LICs/MICs in the absence of poliovirus circulation and campaigns with OPV [43]. A study performed in Italy showed a long duration of protection with both OPV and IPV, but Italy is a HIC, where OPV has higher immunogenicity as compared with MICs/LICs [44].

A cross-sectional study for poliovirus seroprevalence performed in Guangdong, China, carried out in 2014 (before the change in the polio vaccine in 2015), including 6339 people, showed that the seropositivities for PV1, PV2, and PV3 were 95.2%, 94.9%, and 88.7%, and the respective GMTs were 82.9, 55.8, and 26.3, respectively. The highest seropositivity and GMT were observed in the 1–9-year-old age group. However, similarly to other seroprevalence studies, lower immunogenicity was observed for PV3 [45]. Another study conducted in Chongqing, China tested 636 people for poliovirus neutralizing antibodies. The overall seroprevalence rates for PV1, PV2, and PV3 were 93.40%, 96.38%, and 91.82%, and GMTs were 61.14, 66.78, and 21.47, respectively. GMTs were negatively associated with age in the geographic districts with poor economic conditions, which will increase the risk of the emergence of VDPVs after a polio vaccine switch. More than one dose of IPV should be introduced into the polio vaccine schedule, and the supplementary immunization of polio should still be annually carried out after the polio vaccine switch, especially among older children and adults [46].

In the DRC, an outbreak was caused by WPV1 in 2010, affecting 16% of adults. It is now one of the countries with the largest number of AFP cases caused by cVDPV1 and cVDPV2. A study assessing poliovirus seroprevalence in 5526 adults aged 15–59 years was performed in this country in 2013–2014. The results showed that 74%, 72%, and 57% of adults were seropositive for neutralizing antibodies for poliovirus types 1, 2, and 3, respectively. These results show that adults can be at risk also for cVDPVs [47]. Two doses of full-dose IPV can elicit more than 90% protection against polio, but HICs adopted three or more doses to ensure long-lasting protection, and all trials that estimated the duration of protection included a preschool IPV dose [9]. IPV can boost the immunity to polio 1 and 3 after bOPV1,3, but two IPV doses can be insufficient to ensure a long duration of protection against polio I 2. In countries that use fIPV, despite the good seroconversion after two doses, the antibody titers are lower as compared with full IPV, and there is no study confirming the long-term protection offered by this vaccine [9]. India recently adopted three fIPV doses (the last one at 9 months concomitantly with measles) [3,11].

4.4. Plannings for the End of the Game and Post-Eradication Era

In the last decade we learned that we should consider not only the advantages and disadvantages of each type of vaccine, but also other factors, like logistics, acceptance, supply, regulatory challenges involving clinical trials and time for approval, and the industrial capacity to supply the new vaccines to LMICs [19,48–52].

Considering that WPV1 and cVDPVs were not eradicated until the middle of 2024, a new plan for polio eradication will be proposed by the GPEI, and the best strategies for this phase are debated [39,48–51]. The strategy proposed by the GPEI to eradicate polio assumes that the route of transmission of WPV and cVDPVs is feco-oral, but this hypothesis remains controversial, and recent evidence based on the transmission of cVDPVs showed that there is a higher possibility that the route is mostly respiratory rather than only feco-oral, which is one more factor to support the exclusive use of IPV [51].

There is no doubt that only IPV can eradicate both WPV and cVDPVs [1]. Combination vaccines containing IPV and three (DPT) or more antigens (Hib, HepB) have been extensively used in HICs, and in some MICs, showing an excellent safety profile, improving timely vaccination, and leading to higher VCRs for many serious diseases. China and Japan adopted an IPV based on Sabin strains, approved since 2012, and a few LMICs adopted an fIPV, which cannot be combined with other antigens. The biggest challenge persists in the poorest countries, exactly where VCRs are low, OPVs induce lower seroconversion, intestinal infections are frequent, and there is recurrent civil unrest, conflicts, and natural disasters that have dramatic impacts on public services [52–55]. The lack of access to medical services, combined with the destruction of the already weak infrastructure (water, sewage, distribution of food and medicines), have been responsible for population displacements. The great number of migrants from regions where oral vaccines are still used and the travelers to these countries, including military, healthcare professionals, and volunteers, can contribute to the importation of polioviruses into areas considered polio-free [8,9,12,14,17–19,39,43,44,49–54].

The WHO considers that there is a sufficient supply of IPV (including fIPV and Sabin IPV), but the estimation was made for only two doses. If a transition to the exclusive use of an IPV or at least more than two doses of an IPV is expected, close coordination with manufacturers should be engaged to account for the time required to ramp up production and deliver sufficient capacity. Additionally, it is fundamental to consider that many people older than 5 years were not protected, and catching up will be necessary for non-immunized children, adolescents, and adults, increasing the need for an IPV supply [56].

There are some new vaccines in development proposed to finish polio eradication. Among the candidates, those produced with live strains (including nOPV1, nOPV3, and nOPV1,3) can pose the same challenges as recently discovered with nOPV2 (transmission, a low but confirmed risk of mutation, and the possibility to cause paralysis). The S19-IPV vaccine, now on phase I of clinical development, is formulated with the S19 virus—a hyper-attenuated, genetically stabilized strain that cannot replicate at human body temperature and has been highly restricted in its potential to revert to a neurovirulent form during the manufacturing process. It is impossible to know if this strain could recombine with other Sabin strains or enterovirus in the case of an escape from manufacturing sites [50].

The VLP vaccine is also a promise, not a reality. There are substantial regulatory challenges for its approval. It will not be possible to demonstrate its efficacy/effectiveness against WPV and VDPVs. It will be difficult to prove if it will induce intestinal immunity and if it can be combined with other antigens. The clinical development plan to have pentavalent or hexavalent combinations with new vaccines requires time and funding that could be better invested in combination vaccines containing IPV that are already available and have confirmed efficacy/effectiveness against polio and other diseases, like diphtheria, pertussis, tetanus, Hib, and Hepatitis B, for which the burden and case fatality rates are higher in the poorest countries.

5. Conclusions

The lessons learned from recent years show that the plannings to substitute tOPV for bOPV, IPV, and nOPVs did not precisely consider the low VCRs and the necessity of a large global supply of vaccines, resulting in a substantial number of outbreaks.

VCRs are not uniform, and the difficulties in implementing environmental surveillance lead to the frequent underestimation of the occurrence of gaps in immunity, as well as of the silent circulation of polioviruses, before and after global polio eradication.

The recommendation for two doses of IPV makes the routine immunization more complex, but IPV can be combined with other antigens to simplify vaccination schedules.

The duration of protection offered by polio vaccines is not known, but considering the evidence of waning antibody titers, it is considered that more than three IPV doses are necessary to guarantee a long duration of protection.

Despite the success of oral vaccines and the hopes that nOPV2 will control cVDPV2 outbreaks, the risks of VAPP and VDPV emergences cannot be acceptable anymore for ethical reasons and social equity.

All countries should make efforts to achieve high and uniform VCRs to minimize the risk of a poliomyelitis outbreak and improve the surveillance of AFP and ES. It will also be necessary to guarantee a sufficient supply and have plans to identify VDPVs and offer a fast response to outbreaks.

Finally, it is key to remember that polio can affect people of all ages, and besides guaranteeing high VCRs in primary series, it is fundamental to guarantee that children, adolescents, and adults (especially healthcare professionals and travelers to risk areas) who were unvaccinated or incompletely vaccinated against polio can also be immunized with IPV.

Author Contributions: L.F.B. conceived the study and prepared the first draft. D.M. and J.C.V.-Z. critically reviewed the first draft and added new references. All authors contributed to the interpretation of the data, discussion, and conclusions. All authors have read and agreed to the published version of the manuscript before submission.

Funding: This research received no external funding.

Institutional Review Board Statement: This study did not require ethical approval.

Informed Consent Statement: Not applicable.

Data Availability Statement: All data were based in the references mentioned in the paper.

Conflicts of Interest: L.F.B., D.M., and J.C.V.Z. are employees of Sanofi and may hold shares and/or stock options in the company.

Acronyms and Abbreviations

aVDPV	ambiguous vaccine derived poliovirus
AFP	acute flaccid paralysis
bOPV	bivalent OPV
cVDPV	circulating virus derived of polio vaccine
DRC	Democratic Republic of the Congo
DTP	diphtheria tetanus and poliomyelitis vaccine
DTPa	DPT based acellular pertussis vaccine
DTPw	DPT based whole-cell vaccine
ES	environmental surveillance
fIPV	fractional IPV
GMT	geometric medium titers of antibody
GMC	geometric medium concentration of antibody titers
GPEI	Global Polio Eradication Initiative
HIC	high-income countries
IMI	intestinal mucosal immunity
LIC	low-income countries
MIC	medium-income countries
mOPV	monovalent OPV
nOPV	novel OPV
IPV	inactivated polio vaccine
iVDPV	vaccine derived poliovirus in immunocompromised individuals
NIP	national immunization program
OPV	oral polio vaccine
PHEIC	Public Health Emergency of International Concern
RI	routine immunization
sIPV	IPV based on Sabin strains
tOPV	trivalent oral polio vaccine
USA	United States of America
UK	United Kingdom
VAPP	vaccine associated paralytic poliomyelitis
VCR	vaccine coverage rate
VLPs	virus-like particles
WPV	wild poliovirus
WGS	whole genome sequencing
WHO	World Health Organization

References

1. Poliomyelitis. Available online: https://www.who.int/news-room/fact-sheets/detail/poliomyelitis (accessed on 25 July 2024).
2. AFP/Polio Data. Available online: https://extranet.who.int/polis/public/CaseCount.aspx (accessed on 24 October 2024).
3. Cavestany, R.L.; Eisenhawer, M.; Diop, O.M.; Verma, H.; Quddus, A.; Mach, O. The Last Mile in Polio Eradication: Program Challenges and Perseverance. *Pathogens* **2024**, *13*, 323. [CrossRef] [PubMed]
4. Polioeradication. Global wild AFP and Environmental Samples, 2018–2024. p. 1. Available online: https://polioeradication.org/wild-poliovirus-count/ (accessed on 24 October 2024).
5. Polioeradication. Global Circulation Vaccine Derived (cVDPV) AFP and Environmental Samples, 2021–2024. p. 2. Available online: https://polioeradication.org/wild-poliovirus-count/ (accessed on 21 October 2024).
6. Vaccination and Immunization Statistics—UNICEF DATA. Available online: https://data.unicef.org/resources/immunization-coverage-estimates-data-visualization/ (accessed on 4 September 2024).

7. Polio (Pol3) Immunization Coverage Among 1-Year-Olds (%). Available online: https://www.who.int/data/gho/data/indicators/indicator-details/GHO/polio-(pol3)-immunization-coverage-among-1-year-olds-(-) (accessed on 24 July 2024).
8. Sutter, R.W.; Kew, O.M.; Cochi, S.L.; Aylward, R.B. Poliovirus vaccine live. In *Plotkin's Vaccines*, 7th ed.; Plotkin, S., Orenstein, W.A., Offit, P., Eds.; Elsevier: Philadelhia, PA, USA, 2018; pp. 866–917.
9. Vidor, E. Poliovirus vaccine inactivated. In *Plotkin's Vaccines*, 7th ed.; Plotkin, S., Orenstein, W.A., Offit, P., Eds.; Elsevier: Amsterdam, The Netherlands, 2018; pp. 841–865.
10. Muslin, C.; Mac Kain, A.; Bessaud, M.; Blondel, B.; Delpeyroux, F. Recombination in Enteroviruses, a Multi-Step Modular Evolutionary Process. *Viruses* **2019**, *11*, 859. [CrossRef] [PubMed]
11. Vaccination Schedule for Poliomyelitis. Available online: https://immunizationdata.who.int/global/wiise-detail-page/vaccination-schedule-for-poliomyelitis (accessed on 29 July 2024).
12. Update on Wild Poliovirus Type 1 Outbreak—Southeastern Africa, 2021–2022 MMWR. Available online: https://www.cdc.gov/mmwr/volumes/72/wr/mm7215a3.htm (accessed on 26 July 2024).
13. Geiger, K.; Stehling-Ariza, T.; Bigouette, J.P.; Bennett, S.D.; Burns, C.C.; Quddus, A.; Wassilak, S.G.; Bolu, O. Progress Toward Poliomyelitis Eradication—Worldwide, January 2022–December 2023. *MMWR Morb. Mortal. Wkly. Rep.* **2024**, *73*, 441–446. [CrossRef] [PubMed]
14. Statement Following the Thirty-Eighth Meeting of the IHR Emergency Committee for Polio. 8 April 2024. Available online: https://www.who.int/news/item/08-04-2024-statement-following-the-thirty-eighth-meeting-of-the-ihr-emergency-committee-for-polio (accessed on 24 July 2024).
15. GPEI Press Release on nOPV2 Prequalification—GPEI. Available online: https://polioeradication.org/news/gpei-press-release-on-nopv2-prequalification/ (accessed on 25 July 2024).
16. GPEI Statement on cVDPV2 detections in Burundi and Democratic Republic of the Congo. Available online: https://polioeradication.org/news-post/gpei-statement-on-cvdpv2-detections-in-burundi-and-democratic-republic-of-the-congo (accessed on 27 July 2024).
17. Namageyo-Funa, A.; Greene, S.A.; Henderson, E.; Traoré, M.A.; Shaukat, S.; Bigouette, J.P.; Jorba, J.; Wiesen, E.; Bolu, O.; Diop, O.M.; et al. Update on Vaccine-Derived Poliovirus Outbreaks—Worldwide, January 2023–June 2024. *MMWR Morb. Mortal. Wkly. Rep.* **2024**, *73*, 909–916. [CrossRef] [PubMed]
18. Variant Type 2 Poliovirus Isolated from Sewage Samples in Gaza—GPEI. Available online: https://polioeradication.org/news/variant-type-2-poliovirus-isolated-from-sewage-samples-in-gaza/ (accessed on 24 July 2024).
19. Statement of the Thirty-Ninth Meeting of the Polio IHR Emergency Committee. 13 August 2024. Available online: https://www.who.int/news/item/13-08-2024-statement-of-the-thirty-ninth-meeting-of-the-polio-ihr-emergency-committee (accessed on 11 September 2024).
20. Falleiros-Arlant, L.H.; Ayala, S.E.G.; Domingues, C.; Brea, J.; De Colsa-Ranero, A. Estado actual de la poliomielitis en Latinoamérica. *Rev. Chil. Infectologia* **2020**, *37*, 701–709. (In English, Spanish) [CrossRef]
21. Alfaro-Murillo, J.A.; Ávila-Agüero, M.L.; Fitzpatrick, M.C.; Crystal, C.J.; Falleiros-Arlant, L.-H.; Galvani, A.P. The case for replacing live oral polio vaccine with inactivated vaccine in the Americas. *Lancet* **2020**, *395*, 1163–1166. [CrossRef]
22. Macklin, G.; Diop, O.M.; Humayun, A.; Shahmahmoodi, S.; El-Sayed, Z.A.; Triki, H.; Rey, G.; Avagyan, T.; Grabovac, V.; Jorba, J.; et al. Update on Immunodeficiency-Associated Vaccine-Derived Polioviruses—Worldwide, July 2018–December 2019. *MMWR Morb. Mortal. Wkly. Rep.* **2020**, *69*, 913–917. [CrossRef]
23. Pan American Health Organization; World Health Organization. *Epidemiological Update: Poliomyelitis in the Region of the Americas*; PAHO/WHO: Washington, DC, USA, 2023. Available online: https://www.paho.org/en/documents/epidemiological-update-poliomyelitis-region-americas-23-march-2023 (accessed on 26 September 2024).
24. Rodríguez, R.; Juárez, E.; Estívariz, C.F.; Cajas, C.; Rey-Benito, G.; Amézquita, M.O.B.; Miles, S.J.; Orantes, O.; Freire, M.C.; Chévez, A.-E.; et al. Response to Vaccine-Derived Polioviruses Detected through Environmental Surveillance, Guatemala, 2019. *Emerg. Infect. Dis.* **2023**, *29*, 1524–1530. [CrossRef]
25. Chen, M.; Zhang, Y.; Zhang, W.; Huang, S.; Zhu, S.; Li, C.; Guo, X.; Zeng, H.; Fang, L.; Ke, B.; et al. Dynamic changes in polioviruses identified by environmental surveillance in Guangzhou, 2009–2021. *J. Med Virol.* **2023**, *95*, e28668. [CrossRef]
26. Al-Qassimi, M.A.; Al Amad, M.; Al-Dar, A.; Al Sakaf, E.; Al Hadad, A.; Raja'a, Y.A. Circulating vaccine derived polio virus type 2 outbreak and response in Yemen, 2021–2022, a retrospective descriptive analysis. *BMC Infect. Dis.* **2024**, *24*, 321. [CrossRef]
27. Cooper, L.V.; Bandyopadhyay, A.S.; Gumede, N.; Mach, O.; Mkanda, P.; Ndoutabé, M.; Okiror, S.O.; Ramirez-Gonzalez, A.; Touray, K.; Wanyoike, S.; et al. Risk factors for the spread of vaccine-derived type 2 polioviruses after global withdrawal of trivalent oral poliovirus vaccine and the effects of outbreak responses with monovalent vaccine: A retrospective analysis of surveillance data for 51 countries in Africa. *Lancet Infect. Dis.* **2022**, *22*, 284–294, Erratum in *Lancet Infect. Dis.* **2022**, *22*, e41. [CrossRef] [PubMed]
28. Suares, J.E.; Khan, S.; Aadrika, A.; Poojari, P.G.; Rashid, M.; Thunga, G. Vaccine-associated paralytic poliomyelitis in oral polio vaccine recipients: Disproportionality analysis using VAERS and systematic review. *Expert Opin. Drug Saf.* **2024**, *23*, 855–867. [CrossRef] [PubMed]
29. Mohanty, M.C.; Govindaraj, G.; Ahmad, M.; Varose, S.Y.; Tatkare, M.; Shete, A.; Yadav, S.; Joshi, Y.; Yadav, P.; Sharma, D.; et al. Immunodeficiency-Related Vaccine-Derived Poliovirus (iVDPV) Excretion in an Infant with Severe Combined Immune Deficiency with Spillover to a Parent. *Vaccines* **2024**, *12*, 759. [CrossRef] [PubMed]

30. Guo, Q.; Zhu, S.; Wang, D.; Li, X.; Zhu, H.; Song, Y.; Liu, X.; Xiao, F.; Zhao, H.; Lu, H.; et al. Genetic characterization and molecular evolution of type 3 vaccine-derived polioviruses from an immunodeficient patient in China. *Virus Res.* **2023**, *334*, 199177. [CrossRef] [PubMed]
31. Brouwer, A.F.; Eisenberg, J.N.S.; Pomeroy, C.D.; Shulman, L.M.; Hindiyeh, M.; Manor, Y.; Grotto, I.; Koopman, J.S.; Eisenberg, M.C. Epidemiology of the silent polio outbreak in Rahat, Israel, based on modeling of environmental surveillance data. *Proc. Natl. Acad. Sci. USA* **2018**, *115*, E10625–E10633. [CrossRef]
32. Kalkowska, D.A.; Wassilak, S.G.; Pallansch, M.A.; Burns, C.C.; Wiesen, E.; Durry, E.; Badizadegan, K.; Thompson, K.M. Outbreak response strategies with type 2-containing oral poliovirus vaccines. *Vaccine* **2023**, *41*, A142–A152. [CrossRef]
33. Kalkowska, D.A.; Badizadegan, K.; Thompson, K.M. Outbreak management strategies for cocirculation of multiple poliovirus types. *Vaccine* **2023**, *41*, 3718–3727. [CrossRef]
34. Kalkowska, D.A.; Wassilak, S.G.F.; Wiesen, E.; Burns, C.C.; Pallansch, M.A.; Badizadegan, K.; Thompson, K.M. Coordinated global cessation of oral poliovirus vaccine use: Options and potential consequences. *Risk Anal.* **2024**, *44*, 366–378. [CrossRef]
35. Connor, R.I.; Brickley, E.B.; Wieland-Alter, W.F.; Ackerman, M.E.; Weiner, J.A.; Modlin, J.F.; Bandyopadhyay, A.S.; Wright, P.F. Mucosal immunity to poliovirus. *Mucosal Immunol.* **2021**, *15*, 1–9. [CrossRef]
36. Saleem, A.F.; Kazi, Z.U.; Zehra, S.M.; Parkar, S.; Macklin, G.; Sifontes, G.; A Mainou, B.; Alam, M.; Cavestany, R.L.; Mach, O. Mucosal Immunity to Poliovirus in Children 0–15 Years of Age: A Community-Based Study in Karachi, Pakistan in 2019. *J. Infect. Dis.* **2024**, *230*, 736–740. [CrossRef]
37. Habib, M.A.; Soofi, S.B.; Hussain, I.; Ahmed, I.; Hussain, Z.; Tahir, R.; Anwar, S.; Cousens, S.; Bhutta, Z.A. Does IPV Boost Intestinal Immunity among Children under Five Years of Age? An Experience from Pakistan. *Vaccines* **2023**, *11*, 1444. [CrossRef] [PubMed]
38. Bandyopadhyay, A.S.; Cavestany, R.L.; Blake, I.M.; Macklin, G.; Cooper, L.; Grassly, N.; Nery, A.L.M.d.S.; Mach, O. Use of inactivated poliovirus vaccine for poliovirus outbreak response. *Lancet Infect. Dis.* **2023**, *24*, e328–e342; Erratum in *Lancet Infect. Dis.* **2024**, *24*, e83. [CrossRef] [PubMed]
39. Devaux, C.A.; Pontarotti, P.; Levasseur, A.; Colson, P.; Raoult, D. Is it time to switch to a formulation other than the live attenuated poliovirus vaccine to prevent poliomyelitis? *Front. Public Health* **2024**, *11*, 1284337. [CrossRef] [PubMed]
40. Kennedy, S.B.; Macklin, G.R.; Ross, G.M.; Cavestany, R.L.; A Moukom, R.; Jones, K.A.V.; A Mainou, B.; Massaquoi, M.B.F.; Kieh, M.W.S.; Mach, O. Poliovirus antibodies following two rounds of campaigns with a type 2 novel oral poliovirus vaccine in Liberia: A clustered, population-based seroprevalence survey. *Lancet Glob. Health* **2023**, *11*, e917–e923. [CrossRef] [PubMed]
41. Cooper, L.V.; Erbeto, T.B.; A Danzomo, A.; Abdullahi, H.W.; Boateng, K.; Adamu, U.S.; Shuaib, F.; Modjirom, N.; Gray, E.J.; Bandyopadhyay, A.S.; et al. Effectiveness of poliovirus vaccines against circulating vaccine-derived type 2 poliomyelitis in Nigeria between 2017 and 2022: A case-control study. *Lancet Infect. Dis.* **2024**, *24*, 427–436. [CrossRef]
42. Ivanova, O.E.; Eremeeva, T.P.; Baykova, O.Y.; Krasota, A.Y.; Yakovchuk, E.V.; Shustova, E.Y.; Malyshkina, L.P.; Mustafina, A.N.-I.; Mikhailova, Y.M.; Chirova, A.V.; et al. Detection of Polioviruses Type 2 among Migrant Children Arriving to the Russian Federation from a Country with a Registered Poliomyelitis Outbreak. *Vaccines* **2024**, *12*, 718. [CrossRef]
43. Gao, H.; Lau, E.H.Y.; Cowling, B.J. Waning Immunity After Receipt of Pertussis, Diphtheria, Tetanus, and Polio-Related Vaccines: A Systematic Review and Meta-analysis. *J. Infect. Dis.* **2021**, *225*, 557–566. [CrossRef]
44. Larocca, A.M.V.; Bianchi, F.P.; Bozzi, A.; Tafuri, S.; Stefanizzi, P.; Germinario, C.A. Long-Term Immunogenicity of Inactivated and Oral Polio Vaccines: An Italian Retrospective Cohort Study. *Vaccines* **2022**, *10*, 1329. [CrossRef]
45. Tan, Q.; Zhu, Q.; Zheng, H.; Zhang, B.; Wu, C.; Guo, X.; Li, H.; Liu, L.; Liu, Y.; Rutherford, S.; et al. Epidemiological serosurvey of poliovirus in Guangdong, China: A cross-sectional study. *Hum. Vaccines Immunother.* **2018**, *14*, 2644–2648. [CrossRef]
46. Xu, J.; Kuang, S.; Rong, R.; Zhang, Y.; Tang, W.; Wang, Q. Sero-survey of polio antibodies and quality of acute flaccid paralysis surveillance in Chongqing, China: A cross-sectional study. *Medicine* **2020**, *99*, e21298. [CrossRef]
47. Alfonso, V.H.; Voorman, A.; Hoff, N.A.; Weldon, W.C.; Gerber, S.; Gadoth, A.; Halbrook, M.; Goldsmith, A.; Mukadi, P.; Doshi, R.H.; et al. Poliovirus immunity among adults in the Democratic Republic of the Congo: A cross-sectional serosurvey. *BMC Infect. Dis.* **2022**, *22*, 30. [CrossRef] [PubMed]
48. John, T.J.; Dharmapalan, D.; Steinglass, R.; Hirschhorn, N. Novel OPV is Still not the Right Tool for Polio Eradication. *Indian Pediatr.* **2024**, *61*, 387. [CrossRef] [PubMed]
49. Fine, P.E.M. Population Immunity and Polio Eradication. *Pathogens* **2024**, *13*, 183. [CrossRef] [PubMed]
50. Sutter, R.W.; Eisenhawer, M.; Molodecky, N.A.; Verma, H.; Okayasu, H. Inactivated Poliovirus Vaccine: Recent Developments and the Tortuous Path to Global Acceptance. *Pathogens* **2024**, *13*, 224. [CrossRef] [PubMed]
51. John, T.J.; Dharmapalan, D.; Steinglass, R.; Hirschhorn, N. The respiratory route of transmission of virulent polioviruses. *Infect. Dis.* **2024**, *56*, 918–924. [CrossRef]
52. Wahid, B.; Kumari, B.; Saifullah, K.M.; Idrees, M. The History and Current Killings of Polio Vaccinators in Pakistan: A Need for Targeted Surveillance Strategy. *Asia Pac. J. Public Health* **2023**, *35*, 183–188. [CrossRef]
53. Abbasi, F.H.; Shaikh, A.A.; Mehraj, J.; Raza, S.M.; Rasool, S.; Bullo, U.F.; Mehraj, S.; Phul, Z.A.; Sahitia, S.; Zardari, A.A.; et al. Vaccine Hesitancy and Perceptions of the Community about Polio in High-Risk Areas of Karachi, Sindh, Pakistan. *Vaccines* **2022**, *11*, 70. [CrossRef]

54. Gebremedhin, S.; Shiferie, F.; Tsegaye, D.A.; Alemayehu, W.A.; Wondie, T.; Donofrio, J.; DelPizzo, F.; Belete, K.; Biks, G.A. Oral and Inactivated Polio Vaccine Coverage and Determinants of Coverage Inequality Among the Most At-Risk Populations in Ethiopia. *Am. J. Trop. Med. Hyg.* **2023**, *109*, 1148–1156. [CrossRef]
55. Jacobson, A.; Spitzer, S.; Gorelik, Y.; Edelstein, M. Barriers and enablers to vaccination in the ultra-orthodox Jewish population: A systematic review. *Front. Public Health* **2023**, *11*, 1244368. [CrossRef]
56. Kidd, S.; Clark, T.; Routh, J.; Cineas, S.; Bahta, L.; Brooks, O. Use of Inactivated Polio Vaccine Among U.S. Adults: Updated Recommendations of the Advisory Committee on Immunization Practices—United States, 2023. *MMWR Morb. Mortal. Wkly. Rep.* **2023**, *72*, 1327–1330. [CrossRef]

vaccines

MDPI

Article

Securing the Future: Strategies for Global Polio Vaccine Security Amid Eradication Efforts

Vachagan Harutyunyan [1,*], Ann Ottosen [2], Rachel M. Burke [3], Derek Ehrhardt [1], Meredith Shirey [4], Rissa Durham [3] and David Woods [1]

[1] World Health Organization, 1211 Geneva, Switzerland
[2] UNICEF, 2150 Copenhagen, Denmark
[3] Gates Foundation, Seattle, WA 98109, USA
[4] Independent Researcher
* Correspondence: harutyunyanv@who.int

Abstract: Background/Objectives: As we commemorate 50 years of the Expanded Programme on Immunization (EPI), the global mission to eradicate polio stands at a critical juncture. While remarkable progress has been made over the past decades, ensuring a steady supply of polio vaccines remains a significant challenge that could undermine these achievements. This manuscript aims to address the complexities of polio vaccine security within the context of the Immunization Agenda 2030 (IA2030) and the Global Polio Eradication Strategy 2022–2029, proposing actionable strategies to strengthen the vaccine supply. **Methods:** This manuscript analyzes obstacles to vaccine security, including supply disruptions and market uncertainties. It presents the Polio Vaccine Security Framework as a key strategy for addressing these challenges. Data were gathered from Global Polio Eradication Initiative (GPEI) reports, consultations with key stakeholders, and analyses of past vaccine shortages. **Results:** The findings indicate that the primary risks to vaccine security include the lack of a coherent long-term policy framework on polio vaccination, the absence of a clear polio vaccine development roadmap, and insufficient long-term, predictable forecasting. Additionally, stronger coordination is needed between stakeholders involved in vaccine supply, polio containment, and research, as well as addressing challenges related to financing and access to resources. **Conclusions:** A robust, adaptable, and sustainable approach to vaccine security, proposed in the Polio Vaccine Security Framework, is critical to achieving and sustaining polio eradication. Collaboration among policymakers, manufacturers, and stakeholders to implement it is essential to ensure the uninterrupted supply of polio vaccines, protecting the progress made over the past half century, and preventing a resurgence of poliovirus in the future.

Keywords: polio eradication; vaccine security; global OPV stockpile; immunization policy; inactivated poliovirus vaccine (IPV); oral poliovirus vaccine (OPV); vaccine production and distribution; global health security; poliovirus containment

1. Introduction

The year 2024 marks the 50th anniversary of the Expanded Programme on Immunization (EPI), a monumental public health initiative that has been instrumental in reducing childhood mortality and combatting infectious diseases globally. Since its inception in 1974, the EPI has expanded access to life-saving vaccines, preventing millions of deaths and substantially lowering the global burden of vaccine-preventable diseases [1].

Building on the successes of the EPI, the Immunization Agenda 2030 (IA2030) sets forth a visionary framework for the next decade, focusing on universal access to vaccines and achieving equitable immunization coverage worldwide. Central to the IA2030 are the key pillars of supply and sustainability, and research and innovation. By highlighting the need for a reliable and uninterrupted supply of vaccines, the IA2030 aims to prevent shortages and uphold the gains achieved through disease control initiatives. This involves strengthening supply chains, enhancing production capabilities, and fostering international collaboration to maintain vaccine security [2]. Furthermore, the agenda emphasizes the importance of research and innovation to address emerging health challenges and improve vaccine efficacy and delivery methods [1].

Among the EPI's many achievements, the global effort against polio stands out as one of the most significant public health victories. Thanks to the widespread use of polio vaccines, global wild polio cases have been reduced by more than 99% since 1988, from over 350,000 cases annually to just a handful of cases today, confined to oneregion. This success has brought the world to the brink of eradicating a disease that once caused widespread paralysis and death, particularly among children [3,4].

Polio eradication, however, cannot be viewed as a singular achievement, but rather as an ongoing commitment to sustaining progress. Central to this commitment is the concept of polio vaccine security, which aims to ensure the timely, sustained, and uninterrupted supply of appropriate types of affordable, quality-assured vaccines. As the world approaches polio eradication, ensuring an uninterrupted supply of polio vaccines remains critical—not only for achieving the final goal of global eradication but also for preventing a resurgence of the virus in a post-eradication world [5–7]. This is particularly important as countries face evolving epidemiological risks requiring the continued use of the OPV, while, at the same time, the global health community transitions away from OPV use toward the Inactivated Poliovirus Vaccine (IPV) to mitigate the risk of vaccine-associated paralytic poliomyelitis (VAPP) and vaccine-derived poliovirus outbreaks. The withdrawal of the trivalent oral polio vaccine (tOPV) in 2016 marked a significant step in this transition [8].

Maintaining polio vaccine security is thus pivotal to sustaining the successes achieved to date and protecting future generations from poliovirus. The cessation of certain polio vaccines, such as the trivalent OPV (tOPV) in 2016 and the Sabin monovalent OPV type 2 (mOPV2) between 2020 and 2023, along with upcoming transitions like the expected bOPV cessation, presents challenges. Addressing these challenges requires a strong, coordinated effort from national and international stakeholders to ensure an adequate global supply of vaccines for both routine immunizations and outbreak responses [6,7,9,10]. Past experiences with vaccine shortages, such as the IPV shortage in the aftermath of the global switch from the tOPV to the bivalent OPV (bOPV) in 2016, underscore the critical importance of having a reliable supply chain, adaptable production systems, and effective international cooperation [4,7,11].

In this context, polio vaccine security becomes not only a matter of achieving and maintaining the gains of polio eradication but also an important element of the broader framework of global health security. By ensuring that suitable polio vaccines of assured quality are always available, the global community can prevent any potential resurgence and safeguard the hard-won progress achieved through decades of effort. As we reflect on the 50-year journey of the EPI, the ongoing challenges and achievements in polio eradication remind us that vaccines are a powerful and critical tool in the fight against infectious diseases.

2. Background

The landscape of polio vaccines is highly complex, as evidenced in Figure 1, which illustrates the various vaccine types in use and under development, their timelines, and the potential transitions between them. Over the past decades, it has undergone multiple transitions, including the shift from the trivalent oral polio vaccine (tOPV) to the bivalent OPV (bOPV), the introduction of the Sabin monovalent OPV2 (mOPV2) followed by the novel OPV2 (nOPV2), and the rollout of hexavalent IPV-containing vaccines. Each transition, driven by evolving epidemiological needs and public health strategies, has created opportunities while also posing challenges to maintaining a consistent vaccine supply.

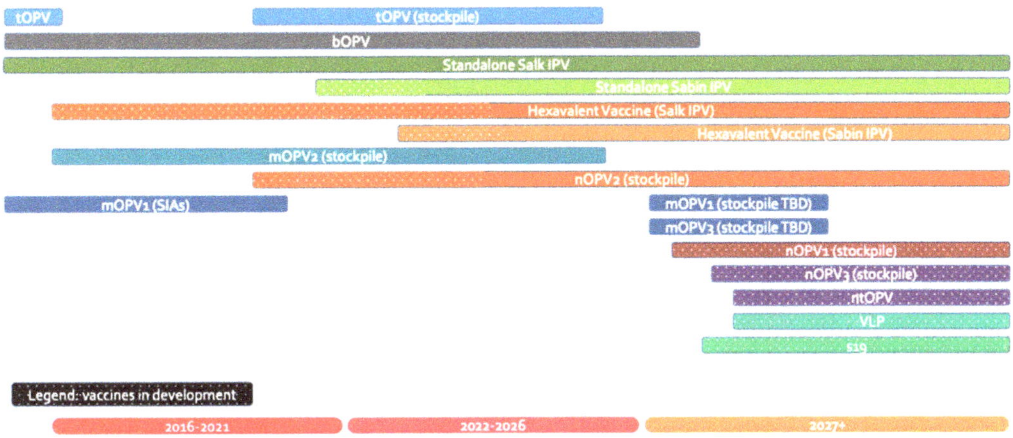

Figure 1. Current and future polio vaccines.

A notable example is the IPV shortage following the global switch from the tOPV to the bOPV in 2016 [4,7,11]. The introduction of at least one dose of IPV was recommended to protect children from type 2 poliovirus-induced paralysis. However, global IPV production could not ramp up quickly enough to meet the sudden surge in demand, resulting in 28% of countries experiencing stockouts or delays in introducing the IPV [4]. Similarly, the Global OPV Stockpile, designed as an emergency reserve to combat Circulating Vaccine-Derived Poliovirus Type 2 (cVDPV2) after the switch, faced significant challenges in meeting demand. Initially, the rapid expansion of cVDPV2 outbreaks outpaced the capabilities of traditional consumption-based forecasting methods, leading to shortages. Later, following the introduction of the nOPV2 in 2020, reliance on a single supplier, coupled with production issues, resulted in prolonged periods of vaccine scarcity. These disruptions delayed responses, allowing the virus to spread unchecked in some cases [4,12–14]. These examples highlight the critical need for a more resilient vaccine supply system, capable of adapting to unforeseen production challenges to sustain eradication efforts.

Pricing is a critical factor, especially in low-resource settings, where affordability can impact access to essential immunization. Vaccine costs are shaped by substantial investments in research and development, production scale-up, and compliance with stringent manufacturing standards [1,6,11].

A major component of these production processes is the adherence to biosafety and biosecurity measures. Strict containment practices are required during vaccine manufacturing to prevent the accidental or intentional release of live poliovirus strains, which could threaten global eradication efforts. Investments in biosecurity infrastructure, high-containment laboratories, and training are crucial to meet these standards [9,15], thereby contributing to the overall cost of vaccine production.

Further complicating decision making is the fact that the slim profit margins on the OPV offer manufacturers less incentive to produce it compared to more profitable vaccines. The heavy reliance on a small number of manufacturers for the production of critical components, such as Sabin bulk types 1 and 3 and novel oral polio vaccines (nOPVs), heightens the risk of supply chain disruptions. This dependence results in a delicate supply network, susceptible to significant impacts from unforeseen production or regulatory challenges, as demonstrated by the shortages experienced with the Inactivated Poliovirus Vaccine (IPV) and nOPV2 [4,10,15,16].

Longstanding uncertainties surrounding polio eradication timelines have led to ever-evolving polio vaccination policies, resulting in a complex and unpredictable market for polio vaccines. To address this problem, it is essential to develop a well-defined, consolidated long-term vaccination policy framework and a polio vaccines roadmap. This framework should clearly specify the necessary vaccines, their characteristics, timelines for introduction and withdrawal, and conditions for use. Providing such clarity would enable manufacturers to make informed decisions, facilitating effective long-term planning within the vaccine industry.

Addressing these multifaceted challenges requires close coordination among the following three critical operational areas: vaccine supply, research and product development, and poliovirus containment. Synchronizing efforts across policy and normative work, communication, and access to resources within these domains is essential to ensure that vaccine production aligns with public health needs, that innovative vaccines are developed and brought to market efficiently, and that containment measures are effectively implemented to prevent virus resurgence. This collaboration is vital not only for sustaining a healthy vaccine market but also for achieving the ultimate goal of global polio eradication [1,2,6,9,14,15].

Origins and Development of the Polio Vaccine Security Framework

The development of the Polio Vaccine Security Framework was initiated in response to the growing need for a long-term, strategic approach to securing a reliable and uninterrupted supply of polio vaccines. This process began following recommendations from key advisory groups to the Global Polio Eradication Initiative (GPEI), including those from the Global Certification Commission (GCC) and the Containment Advisory Group (CAG), which were issued during the Sixth Meeting of the Poliovirus Containment Advisory Group (CAG6). Additionally, the Independent Monitoring Board (IMB) reflected its recommendations in its 22nd report [17]. These groups emphasized the critical importance of a coherent vaccine strategy (Figure 2) [17,18] aligning the vaccine supply, containment, and research efforts to ensure polio vaccine security during the eradication process and beyond.

RECOMMENDATIONS FROM THE CHAIRS OF THE ADVISORY GROUPS

1. CAG recommends the development of an inclusive strategy for new polio vaccines including research-safe and cost-effective production technologies- and containment. Whenever possible, CAG recommends the development of new vaccines that would require less stringent containment requirements to provide incentives to newer developments. This should involve WHO Containment (CNT) programme, WHO Polio Research (PRD) programme and the GPEI Vaccine Supply Group (VSG).

2. CAG recommends the development of an inclusive blueprint for polio research, if not already available with approaches for accelerating research in new polio products (polio vaccine, diagnostics and treatment) and other initiatives, expedited regulatory pathways such as using the WHO Emergency Use Assessment and Listing Procedure (EUAL), containment consideration, where applicable and other approaches modelled after the WHO R&D Blueprint for Action to Prevent Epidemics for research on epidemic-prone emerging pathogens.

Figure 2. Recommendations for the chairs of the advisory groups, as outlined in the Report from the Sixth Meeting of the Poliovirus Containment Advisory Group (CAG6).

The framework's development was overseen by a dedicated steering team consisting of representatives from the GPEI's Vaccine Supply Group (VSG), the Polio Research and Analytics Group (PRAG), and the Containment Management Group (CMG). This multidisciplinary team worked collaboratively to integrate insights from various operational areas, ensuring that the framework addresses the challenges posed by shifting vaccine needs and the requirement to meet poliovirus containment standards.

Shaping the framework were insights gathered during the Twenty Second Annual Consultation between the GPEI, vaccine manufacturers, National Authorities for Containment (NACs), and National Regulatory Authorities (NRAs). This consultation provided an important platform for dialogue, where key stakeholders emphasized the need for robust demand forecasting, a clear regulatory and normative framework, sustainable financial mechanisms, and support in implementing containment strategies.

Following this, additional consultations were carried out within the GPEI, as well as WHO and UNICEF regional offices, to incorporate both global and regional perspectives. Through this consultative approach, the framework was shaped to address the evolving challenges in vaccine supply, research, and containment, ensuring long-term security and readiness.

3. Introducing Polio Vaccine Security Framework

As highlighted in the previous sections, achieving global polio eradication demands a secure, sustained, and uninterrupted supply of vaccines. The Polio Vaccine Security Framework was developed by the GPEI to address the complex challenges associated with the vaccine supply and to ensure long-term security. This framework seeks to secure the availability of affordable, quality-assured vaccines both for poliovirus eradication and to protect the gains of the global eradication efforts in the post-certification period.

The Polio Vaccine Security Framework is built on the following five key principles that form the foundation for achieving its objectives:

1. Interdependence of Operational Areas: The framework emphasizes the interconnected nature of the vaccine supply, research and development, and poliovirus containment. These elements influence one another, and their coordination is crucial for overall success. The alignment of activities in these areas ensures the availability of suitable vaccines and the safe and secure handling of polioviruses.
2. Long-Term Strategic Planning: The framework shifts the focus from reactive, short-term approaches to long-term strategic planning. A comprehensive vaccine policy and roadmap, supported by clear demand forecasts and product transitions, to be developed within the scope of the framework, will provide essential visibility for stakeholders, ensuring that production and supply can be aligned with global eradication goals.
3. Building on Existing Frameworks: The Polio Vaccine Security Framework complements and enhances existing policies and strategies (Figure 3), including the Immunization Agenda 2030 (IA2030), the Polio Eradication Strategy 2022–2026, and the Global Poliovirus Containment Strategy (Figure 2). By aligning with these frameworks, the initiative aims to foster a unified, effective approach to maintaining a polio-free world.
4. Sustainable Market for Polio Vaccines: Ensuring a sustainable market for polio vaccines is essential. This involves incentivizing manufacturers to continue production, particularly during transition periods or market uncertainty. Risk-sharing mechanisms, financial support for product development, and transparent communication of long-term demand are critical to maintaining engagement from manufacturers and ensuring a healthy, competitive market.
5. Ongoing Monitoring and Adaptation: Given the evolving nature of polio eradication and the vaccine landscape, the framework stresses the importance of continuous monitoring and adaptation. Regular updates and revisions will be necessary to respond to new challenges, ensuring the framework remains effective in securing the vaccine supply.

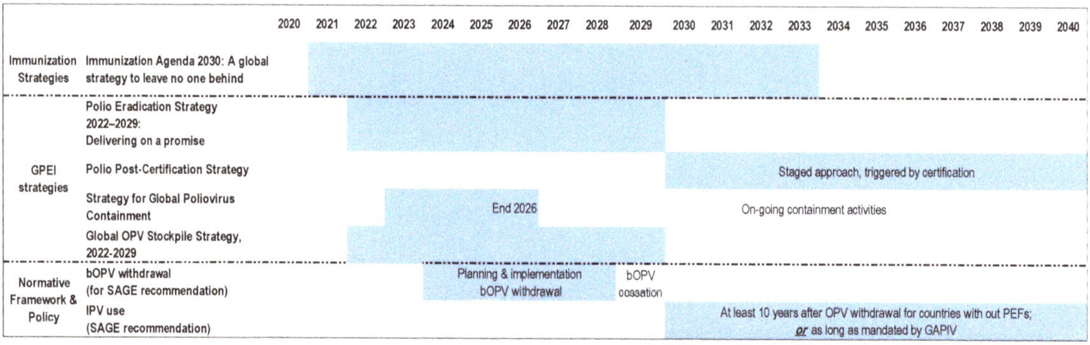

Figure 3. Mapping of strategies and policies related to Polio Vaccine Security (note: timelines presented as applicable at the time of drafting this framework; some timelines are under revision and will be noted in future versions).

3.1. Goal and Objectives

The goal of the Polio Vaccine Security Framework is to ensure the timely, sustained, and uninterrupted supply of affordable, quality-assured polio vaccines. Achieving this goal is critical to the success of global polio eradication efforts and to preventing the re-emergence of poliovirus in the future.

3.1.1. The Framework Outlines Three Primary Objectives

1. Strengthened Communication, Coordination, and Advocacy: Foster enhanced communication and coordination between global health stakeholders, manufacturers, and policymakers to ensure that vaccine security challenges are addressed comprehensively and strategically.
2. Development of a Coherent Normative and Policy Framework: Establish a unified policy framework that supports the long-term use of polio vaccines. This includes aligning vaccine supply and development efforts with containment and research requirements, ensuring that global standards and guidelines are adhered to across all areas from research to production and distribution.
3. Improved Financing and Access to Resources: Identify and mitigate financial risks by securing sustainable resources for vaccine production and distribution. This includes ensuring access to financing across key areas such as supply, containment, research, and development to support uninterrupted vaccine availability.

By integrating these objectives, the Polio Vaccine Security Framework creates a comprehensive strategy that strengthens the global capacity to prevent vaccine shortages, supports manufacturers' efforts, and ensures that the infrastructure required for polio eradication remains robust and adaptable.

3.1.2. Elements of the Polio Vaccine Security Framework

The Polio Vaccine Security Framework is organized around six key elements, designed to ensure a holistic, sustainable approach to maintaining the supply of polio vaccines. These elements include three operational workstreams—vaccine supply, research and product development, and poliovirus containment—along with the following three cross-cutting themes: normative work and policy development, communication and advocacy, and financing and access to resources (Figure 4). Together, they form an interconnected structure that supports the long-term success of global polio eradication efforts.

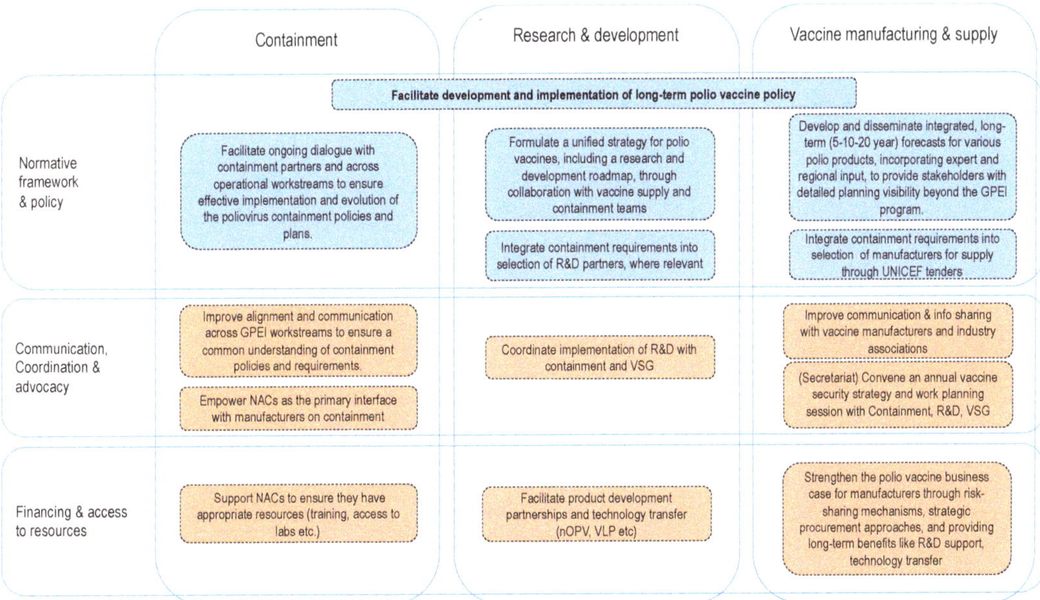

Figure 4. Key elements of the Polio Vaccine Security Framework.

Operational Workstreams

1. Vaccine Supply: Ensuring a continuous supply of vaccines is fundamental to the polio eradication effort. This involves robust forecasting, efficient production, procurement strategies, and stockpiling. It also means strengthening the supply chain to avoid disruptions. The Vaccine Supply Group (VSG) is tasked with overseeing this process, working closely with manufacturers and stakeholders to secure both OPVs and IPVs, which are critical for sustaining immunization efforts during and after eradication.
2. Research and Product Development: As we progress towards and beyond polio eradication, new products and innovations will be required to meet the evolving public health needs. This operational area focuses on the development of new and improved polio vaccines and other products to address emerging challenges and ensure long-term vaccine security; these include next-generation OPVs (nOPV1, nOPV3, and trivalent nOPV), the Sabin-based IPV (sIPV), the attenuated Sabin strain 19 (S19) vaccine, virus-like particles (VLPs), lower-cost hexavalent vaccines (Figure 1), and therapeutic options for the iVDPV. The GPEI partners coordinate closely in this domain to ensure alignment with long-term vaccine security goals, while also adapting to scientific and technological advancements.
3. Poliovirus Containment: Poliovirus containment is critical to minimize the risk of a facility-associated release of poliovirus, such as manufacturers and laboratories. The unintentional or intentional release of poliovirus could result in the re-establishment of poliovirus transmission, particularly in the post-OPV phase. This involves stringent safe and secure measures in laboratories, vaccine production sites, and other facilities that retain polioviruses. It involves implementing biorisk management policies and standards, as outlined the WHO Global Action Plan for Containment, 4th edition 2022 (GAPIV) [9]. It also includes a globally harmonized and rigorous conformity assessment process for facilities retaining poliovirus.

Cross-Cutting Themes

1. Normative Work and Policy Development: A clear and adaptable policy environment is crucial for guiding the strategic direction of all three operational areas. This includes

establishing a long-term polio vaccination policy framework that outlines the types of vaccines needed, timelines for introduction and withdrawal, and how these decisions align with evolving research and development, containment requirements, and global eradication goals. There is a need for greater clarity and collaboration on several key aspects, including the bOPV cessation strategy, regulatory pathways for novel vaccines, long-term IPV strategies, and the application of containment standards in vaccine development and production. This clarity is essential for enabling manufacturers to make informed decisions about production capacity, investments in new technologies, and engagement in the polio vaccine market, ultimately contributing to a more secure and sustainable vaccine supply.
2. Communication and Advocacy: Coordinated communication among global stakeholders, governments, and vaccine manufacturers is vital for maintaining vaccine security. This includes fostering dialog between GPEI workstreams, vaccine manufacturers, national regulatory authorities, and other relevant organizations to ensure aligned priorities, consistent messaging, and efficient resource allocation. The existing communication platforms, such as the annual GPEI consultation with manufacturers and the UNICEF Vaccine Industry Consultation, provide valuable platforms for this collaboration. However, there is a need to enhance these platforms and expand communication efforts to ensure greater transparency, share long-term demand forecasts, and provide manufacturers with clear insights into the evolving policy landscape, fostering trust and enabling them to make informed decisions about their engagement in the polio vaccine market.
3. Financing and Access to Resources: This area of work emphasizes the need for predictable financing to mitigate risks to the polio vaccine industry and strengthen the business case for vaccine production. Key to this approach are risk-sharing mechanisms that help manufacturers maintain production during periods of uncertainty, such as the withdrawal of the bivalent oral polio vaccine (bOPV). These mechanisms reduce the financial burden on manufacturers, ensuring that production continues even when future demand is unclear.

Additional mechanisms such as financial support for product development and technology transfer will remain important to keep the polio vaccine pipeline dynamic and absorb the vaccine R&D costs. Long-term demand forecasting, offering visibility over 5 to 20 years, is another essential tool for ensuring that manufacturers can plan for sustained production. By creating a more predictable market environment and providing financial stability, the framework encourages continued investment in polio vaccine production, safeguarding the supply in the post-eradication era.

These six elements are not only complementary but highly interdependent. The effectiveness of each operational workstream is bolstered by the cross-cutting themes, creating a comprehensive strategy that ensures long-term polio vaccine security.

4. Discussion

As the global health community stands on the cusp of eradicating polio, ensuring polio vaccine security is even more critical than before. The sustained availability of necessary types of affordable, quality-assured vaccines is not only essential to achieving global eradication but also to maintaining a polio-free world in the post-eradication era [19]. The Polio Vaccine Security Framework aims to address both the present and future needs of the vaccine supply chain. The framework provides an umbrella strategy to mitigate the challenges to the polio vaccine security through fostering closer engagement among the vaccine supply, research and product development, and poliovirus containment.

4.1. Present and Future Challenges

Several significant challenges persist in the ongoing fight against poliovirus. The fragmented approaches and short-term planning within the GPEI and among stakeholders jeopardize long-term vaccine security. For example, product-specific and short-term forecasting, often linked to procurement cycles, restricts manufacturers' visibility and hampers their capacity planning efforts. Uncertainties within the normative and policy framework, especially concerning the timeline for bOPV cessation and the future role of nOPVs post-bOPV, complicate manufacturers' long-term investment decisions. Financial risks for manufacturers abound due to uncertain future demand and potential supply chain disruptions.

As a result, the vaccine market remains susceptible to supply disruptions driven by evolving timelines and fluctuating demand for various vaccine types like OPVs and IPVs. Against this background, there is hesitance on the part of vaccine manufacturers to commit to long-term production investments without a clear business case. Relying on a limited number of manufacturers for critical vaccine components further weakens the supply chain, creating vulnerabilities should market fluctuations or production bottlenecks occur.

The requirement to achieve safe and secure poliovirus containment is a necessary part of polio eradication and the post-eradication period. However, there is a current need for a stronger collaboration on the implementation of containment measures while effectively conducting supply and research activities. The intricate task of balancing global supply with containment requirements, especially in laboratories and production environments, highlights the need for coordinated strategies [15].

4.2. *Opportunities Through the Polio Vaccine Security Framework*

The Polio Vaccine Security Framework offers a strategic opportunity to address these challenges and secure a sustainable, long-term supply of vaccines. The framework's focus on a coordinated vaccine supply, research and development, and poliovirus containment ensures that these operational areas work in tandem, mitigating the risks of supply shortages while fostering innovation in vaccine development.

There is broad recognition that a reliable and appropriate vaccine supply is a critical factor for the success of the eradication program. Without a steady and dependable supply of vaccines, efforts to control and eventually eradicate poliovirus will be jeopardized, potentially threatening the substantial progress made thus far.

Another significant opportunity lies in the recognition that securing the polio vaccine supply is not a task that can be achieved by supply or procurement agencies alone. It requires multi-sectoral coordination guided by a coherent normative and policy framework. This collaborative approach ensures that all facets of vaccine security are addressed, from product development and scale-up, and production and distribution to regulatory compliance and public health policies.

Another opportunity lies in leveraging existing platforms and structures that are already in place to address polio vaccine supply issues. For instance, the GPEI has well-established structures and processes that can be utilized to enhance the coordination and implementation of the polio vaccine supply.

Additionally, the Annual Consultation platform, which brings together GPEI stakeholders, the vaccine industry, and national regulatory and containment authorities, presents a valuable opportunity for fostering collaboration and alignment. By building on these existing mechanisms, the Polio Vaccine Security Framework can enhance its effectiveness and efficiency, ultimately contributing to a more robust and resilient vaccine supply system.

4.3. *Implementation and Adaptability*

The success of the Polio Vaccine Security Framework hinges on several of the following factors:

First, it needs to be effectively implemented and managed, with clear lines of responsibility and accountability. The GPEI Vaccine Supply Group (VSG) will play a critical role in coordinating these efforts, ensuring alignment between the framework's objectives and the work of other GPEI workstreams and partners.

Second, the successful implementation of the Polio Vaccine Security Framework relies on its ability to remain adaptable to the changing landscape of polio eradication. As new scientific advancements are made and epidemiological risks evolve, the framework must respond dynamically, offering clear direction to both the polio vaccine industry and the GPEI partnership. Continuous monitoring and regular updates to the framework will ensure that it remains responsive to emerging challenges, such as new vaccine technologies, containment protocols, and changing demand patterns.

Furthermore, the framework's integration of regional and global perspectives, through ongoing consultations with WHO and UNICEF regional offices, ensures that it addresses the specific needs of different regions. The coordinated efforts of these stakeholders, supported by clear communication channels and transparent decision-making processes, will be critical in aligning global vaccine supply with eradication goals.

5. Conclusions

As the global health community approaches polio eradication, ensuring a consistent and uninterrupted supply of polio vaccines is critical to achieving and maintaining a polio-free world. The Polio Vaccine Security Framework is a robust strategy that aligns with the broader goals of the Immunization Agenda 2030 (IA2030) and the Polio Eradication Strategy 2022–2026 (2029). These global strategies emphasize the need for strong, resilient vaccine supply systems that are responsive to evolving epidemiological challenges.

The Polio Vaccine Security Framework thus plays a key role in safeguarding the progress made through decades of immunization efforts under the EPI. By addressing the complexities of vaccine supply, containment, and research, the framework helps ensure that future generations are protected from poliovirus re-emergence. Its integration with the IA2030 goals of equity, sustainability, and innovation in immunization provides a broader context for ensuring that the lessons learned from polio eradication contribute to strengthening global vaccine security for all vaccine-preventable diseases.

As we move into the post-eradication phase, the continued implementation of this framework, in coordination with the IA2030 and the GPEI partnership, will be vital to preventing any resurgence of polio and to maintaining global health security. The long-term planning, financing, and adaptability embedded in the Polio Vaccine Security Framework will not only support polio eradication, but also provide a model for securing vaccines for other global immunization efforts, marking a significant step toward a healthier, more resilient world.

Author Contributions: Conceptualization, V.H.; writing—original draft preparation, V.H.; writing—review and editing, A.O., R.M.B., D.E., M.S., R.D. and D.W.; research and development contributions, R.M.B.; vaccine supply and market contributions, A.O.; poliovirus containment contributions, D.E. All authors were involved in the development of the Polio Vaccine Security Framework that informed this article. All authors have read and agreed to the published version of the manuscript.

Funding: This research received no external funding.

Institutional Review Board Statement: Not applicable. This study does not involve human or animal subjects.

Informed Consent Statement: Not applicable. This study does not involve human subjects.

Data Availability Statement: The data presented in this study are available within the article.

Acknowledgments: The authors would like to express their sincere gratitude to the Global Polio Eradication Initiative (GPEI) partners for their invaluable support throughout the development of the Polio Vaccine Security Framework. We extend our appreciation to the vaccine industry for their technical expertise and continued collaboration in addressing the challenges related to vaccine production and supply. Special thanks go to the representatives of the member states involved in vaccine regulation and poliovirus containment, whose guidance and insights were instrumental in shaping the policy recommendations and strategic directions discussed in this article.

Conflicts of Interest: The authors declare no conflicts of interest. The funders had no role in the design of the study; in the collection, analyses, or interpretation of data; in the writing of the manuscript; or in the decision to publish the results.

References

1. World Health Organization. *Immunization Agenda 2030*; WHO: Geneva, Switzerland, 2021.
2. Rey-Jurado, E.; Tapia, F.; Muñoz-Durango, N.; Lay, M.K.; Carreño, L.J.; Riedel, C.A.; Bueno, S.M.; Genzel, Y.; Kalergis, A.M. Assessing the importance of domestic vaccine manufacturing centers: An overview of immunization programs, vaccine manufacture, and distribution. *Front. Immunol.* **2018**, *9*, 26. [CrossRef] [PubMed]
3. Poliomyelitis WHO 2023. Available online: https://www.who.int/news-room/fact-sheets/detail/poliomyelitis (accessed on 10 October 2024).
4. Sutter, R.W.; Cochi, S.L. Inactivated poliovirus vaccine supply shortage: Is there light at the end of the tunnel? *J. Infect. Dis.* **2019**, *220*, 1545–1546. [CrossRef] [PubMed]
5. Tebbens, R.J.D.; Thompson, K.M. Poliovirus vaccination during the endgame: Insights from integrated modeling. *Expert Rev. Vaccines* **2017**, *16*, 577–586. [CrossRef] [PubMed]
6. Batson, A.; Glassman, A.; Federgruen, A.; Diment, J.; Ganguly, N.K.; Makoni, S.; Plotkin, S. The world needs to prepare now to prevent polio resurgence post eradication. *BMJ Glob. Health* **2022**, *7*, e011485. [CrossRef] [PubMed]
7. Rubin, J.; Ottosen, A.; Ghazieh, A.; Fournier-Caruana, J.; Ntow, A.K.; Gonzalez, A.R. Managing the planned cessation of a global supply market: Lessons learned from the global cessation of the trivalent oral poliovirus vaccine market. *J. Infect. Dis.* **2017**, *216* (Suppl. 1), S40–S45. [CrossRef] [PubMed]
8. Tebbens, R.J.D.; Hampton, L.M.; Wassilak, S.G.; Pallansch, M.A.; Cochi, S.L.; Thompson, K.M. Maintenance and intensification of bivalent oral poliovirus vaccine use prior to its coordinated global cessation. *J. Vaccines Vaccin.* **2016**, *7*, 340. [CrossRef] [PubMed]
9. World Health Organization. *WHO Global Action Plan for Poliovirus Containment GAPIV*; WHO: Geneva, Switzerland, 2023.
10. Batson, A.; Federgruen, A.; Ganguly, N.K.; Glassman, A.; Makoni, S.; Plotkin, S. Polio eradication vaccine investment: How do we ensure polio vaccines are available to keep the world polio-free after transmission of wild poliovirus (wPV) has been interrupted? *BMJ Glob. Health* **2021**, *6*, e006447. [CrossRef] [PubMed]
11. Lewis, I.; Ottosen, A.; Rubin, J.; Blanc, D.C.; Zipursky, S.; Wootton, E. A supply and demand management perspective on the accelerated global introductions of inactivated poliovirus vaccine in a constrained supply market. *J. Infect. Dis.* **2017**, *216* (Suppl. S1), S33–S39. [CrossRef] [PubMed]
12. Thompson, K.M.; Kalkowska, D.A. Reflections on modeling poliovirus transmission and the polio eradication endgame. *Risk Anal.* **2021**, *41*, 229–247. [CrossRef] [PubMed]
13. Thompson, K.M.; Badizadegan, K. Review of Poliovirus Transmission and Economic Modeling to Support Global Polio Eradication: 2020–2024. *Pathogens* **2024**, *13*, 435. [CrossRef]
14. Geiger, K.; Stehling-Ariza, T.; Bigouette, J.P.; Bennett, S.D.; Burns, C.C.; Quddus, A.; Wassilak, S.G.V.; Bolu, O. Progress Toward Poliomyelitis Eradication—Worldwide, January 2022–December 2023. *MMWR Morb. Mortal. Wkly. Rep.* **2024**, *73*, 441–446. [CrossRef] [PubMed]
15. World Health Organization. *Global Polio Eradication Initiative. Polio Eradication Strategy 2022–2026: Delivering on a Promise*; WHO: Geneva, Switzerland, 2021.
16. Thompson, K.M.; Kalkowska, D.A. Potential future use, costs, and value of poliovirus vaccines. *Risk Anal.* **2021**, *41*, 349–363. [CrossRef] [PubMed]
17. Independent Monitoring Board of the Global Polio Eradication Initiative. *Closing in on Zero: Adapting to Complexity and Risk on the Path to End Polio*; WHO: Geneva, Switzerland, 2023.
18. World Health Organization. *Sixth Meeting of the Poliovirus Containment Advisory Group (CA6) 23–25 January 2023: Report*; WHO Global Polio Eradication Initiative: Geneva, Switzerland, 2023. Available online: https://www.archive.polioeradication.org/wp-content/uploads/2023/05/CAG6-Jan-2023-Report-EN-FINAL.pdf (accessed on 10 October 2024).
19. Lopez Cavestany, R.; Eisenhawer, M.; Diop, O.M.; Verma, H.; Quddus, A.; Mach, O. The Last Mile in Polio Eradication: Program Challenges and Perseverance. *Pathogens* **2024**, *13*, 323. [CrossRef]

vaccines

MDPI

Commentary

Missed Measles Immunisations Places Individuals and Communities at Risk: The Equity Argument for Including Measles in Under-Immunised Definitions

Stefanie Vaccher [1,*], Moses Laman [2], Margie Danchin [3,4,5], Fiona Angrisano [1] and Christopher Morgan [1,6,7]

1 Burnet Institute, 85 Commercial Rd, Melbourne, VIC 3004, Australia
2 Papua New Guinea Institute of Medical Research, Boroko, National Capital District 111, Goroka P.O. Box 60, Papua New Guinea
3 Vaccine Uptake Group, Murdoch Children's Research Institute, Royal Children's Hospital, 50 Flemington Road, Parkville, VIC 3052, Australia
4 Department of Paediatrics, Faculty of Medicine, Dentistry and Health Sciences, University of Melbourne, 161 Barry St, Carlton, VIC 3010, Australia
5 Department of General Medicine, Royal Children's Hospital, 50 Flemington Road, Parkville, VIC 3052, Australia
6 Jhpiego, The Johns Hopkins University Affiliate, 1615 Thames Street, Baltimore, MD 21231, USA
7 Melbourne School of Population and Global Health, 207 Bouverie Street, Carlton, VIC 3053, Australia
* Correspondence: stefanie.vaccher@burnet.edu.au

Abstract: Background: Measles is consistently one of the leading causes of death from vaccine-preventable diseases in children, and cases and deaths have increased globally since 2019. While measles often serves as a 'canary in the coalmine' for health system weaknesses, global definitions of zero-dose and under-immunised children continue to centre on those who have missed diphtheria-tetanus-pertussis (DTP) containing vaccine. We propose that lack of receipt of measles vaccine is included in global definitions of 'under-immunised' children. Methods: We used publicly available WHO/UNICEF estimates of national immunization coverage (WUENIC) data to determine the number and proportion of children missing out on routine immunisations in each country globally in 2019 and 2022. We stratified countries by income status to further investigate inequalities in vaccine coverage between different countries. Results: In 2022, 50% more children missed out on their first dose measles-containing vaccine compared to DTP1, and 96% of these children resided in low-middle income countries (LMICs), highlighting the compounding inequities in measles immunisations globally. Furthermore, countries with the largest number of children missing out on DTP1 were not reflective of countries with the lowest measles immunisation coverage rates, suggesting targeted programs are needed to reach children who are missing out on measles vaccination. Recommendations: Given the high transmissibility and inequitable burden measles outbreaks pose to both at-risk individuals and communities, especially in LMICs, measles immunisation coverage should be included as a key metric when reporting and estimating the number of under-immunised children globally.

Keywords: measles; vaccination; under-immunized; zero-dose; vaccine inequity

1. Introduction

Globally in 2019, there were an estimated 1.5 million deaths in children under five years of age attributed to vaccine-preventable diseases [1]. Measles is consistently one of the leading causes of death from vaccine-preventable diseases in children. It is highly transmissible and as such, requires 95% vaccination coverage across the population to reach herd immunity levels, compared to 90% for most other vaccines [2].

Although measles deaths declined by approximately 80% between 2000 and 2016, representing over 21 million deaths averted [1], in 2019 there were over 207,500 deaths from measles, an increase of almost 50% since 2016 [3].

Measles cases and deaths have continued to increase globally since 2019 [2]. This has been exacerbated by declines in routine immunisation coverage during the COVID-19 pandemic, especially in low- and middle-income countries (LMICs). As well as reductions in outreach services, clinic closures, and healthcare worker shortages [4], the politicisation of vaccination and growing vaccine misinformation have led to reduced trust in and uptake of routine childhood immunisations, which may have substantial ongoing future implications [5,6].

Only 83% of children globally received their first dose of measles-containing vaccine (MCV1) in 2022 [2]. Although this is an improvement from the low of 81% in 2021, prior to the COVID-19 pandemic, global MCV1 coverage had been stable around 85–86% since 2015. This represents an additional 2.7 million children globally who missed out on MCV1 in 2022 compared with 2019 [7].

The infectiousness of measles means it often serves as a canary in the coalmine for health system weaknesses, gaps in immunisation programs, and health inequities [8]. There is a dual risk for people who are not vaccinated against measles—both the lack of individual protection, but also the immunity gaps created in under-vaccinated communities that can lead to disruptive outbreaks.

Recent modelling from the World Health Organization (WHO) has shown that of the 154 million lives saved by immunisation since 1974, measles vaccination has accounted for over 60% of these [9]. Additionally, measles vaccination was shown to be the most substantial contributor to reductions in preventable mortality and morbidity.

The importance of achieving high coverage with two doses of measles vaccine has been recognised in the Sustainable Development Goals [10]. The Immunisation Agenda 2030 notes that "high coverage with measles vaccine is an indicator of a strong immunization programme, which may signal a solid foundation for primary health care services" [11]. It is also a key prevention indicator in the WHO Immunisation Joint External Evaluation (JEE) tool, which aims to understand the degree to which countries measure measles vaccination coverage to inform supplementary immunisation activities [12].

Gavi, the Vaccine Alliance, defines "zero-dose" as children who have not received their first dose of DTP (DTP1). Similarly, children are considered "under-immunised" if they have not received their third dose of diphtheria-tetanus-pertussis containing vaccine (DTP3) [13]. While these definitions are important in highlighting priority groups or settings that need to be targeted to ensure vaccine equity, further work is needed to understand if children who have not received DTP1 are representative of all children missing out on routine immunisations, including measles vaccination.

This analysis aims to compare the number of zero-dose and under-immunised children globally, based on the Gavi definitions, with the number and proportion of children who have missed out on measles immunisations in each country worldwide to estimate the additional burden of missed measles vaccination. In addition, equity issues with current immunisation program gaps will be highlighted to argue for the inclusion of measles immunisation coverage as part of the global definitions of 'under-immunised'.

2. Methods

We used the publicly available 2022 WHO/UNICEF estimates of national immunization coverage (WUENIC) data to assess immunisation coverage for DTP1, DTP3, and MCV1 in each country globally in 2019 and 2022 [7]. These data were combined with the under-1 and under-2-year populations in each country in 2019 and 2022, which were extracted from the United Nations Population Estimates for children under five years [14].

Publicly available data were downloaded as comma-separated files and imported into Stata (v18, StataCorp, College Station, TX, USA) for analysis.

Country income status (low, lower-middle, upper-middle, and high income) was determined using the 2022 World Bank country classifications by income level [15].

The number of children missing each of DTP1, DTP3, and MCV1 in each country in 2019 and 2022 was calculated by multiplying the inverse of immunisation coverage with the number of children in the 12–23-month cohort in each country. This age cohort was chosen as there is no clear consensus on the age at which children should be considered 'zero-dose', but to ensure sufficient time had passed in which they could have been vaccinated, and to account for the differing ages at which children receive MCV1 globally [16].

Dropout is the difference in the proportion of children receiving one vaccine who do not go on to receive a second, later vaccine. For this analysis, dropout was calculated by country for three different indicators in 2022: the percentage of children receiving DTP1 minus the percentage of children receiving MCV1, the percentage of children receiving MCV1 minus the percentage of children receiving MCV2, and the percentage of children receiving DTP1 minus the percentage of children receiving DTP3. Change in coverage was calculated as 2022 coverage minus 2019 coverage for DTP1, DTP3, and MCV1.

Countries were also ranked on the number and proportion of children between 12 and 23 months who had not received DTP1 and MCV1. Ranks were calculated for each country based on DTP1 and MCV1 coverage, in ascending order, and number of children not vaccinated for DTP1 and MCV1, in descending order. If two countries shared a rank position for coverage, the higher number was assigned to both countries, and marked with an equal ("=") sign. For example, if three countries (rank 14, 15, and 16) all reported 56% coverage for MCV1, they all received the rank of =16.

Wilcoxon signed-rank tests were used to compare the number of children who missed immunisations between different groups (e.g., by World Bank income strata).

3. Results

Globally in 2022, 14 million children missed out on their first dose of DTP vaccine, and 21 million children missed out on their first dose of MCV (Figure 1). This equates to 50% more children globally not receiving MCV1, compared to those missing out on DTP1. Almost all (96%) of these children resided in LMICs, highlighting the disproportionate burden resource-limited settings face in both preventing and responding to infectious disease threats.

The number of children missing MCV1 in 2022 was significantly higher than the number of children missing DTP1 or DTP3 ($p < 0.001$ for both, Wilcoxon signed-rank test). The number of children missing out on each of these three vaccines has also increased since 2019 (Figure 2).

Countries with the largest number of children aged 12–23 months who had missed immunisations are relatively consistent across DTP1, DTP3, and MCV1. In both 2019 and 2022, these were (in alphabetical order): Afghanistan, Angola, the Democratic Republic of Congo, Ethiopia, India, Indonesia, Nigeria, Pakistan, the Philippines, and Somalia. This is perhaps unsurprising given these countries are some of the most populous globally. The median coverage for DTP1 and MCV1 in these 10 countries was 76% and 64%, respectively.

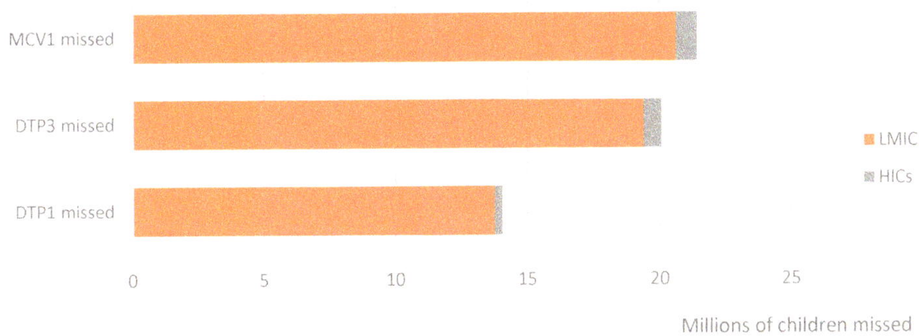

Figure 1. Number of children globally missing out on diphtheria-tetanus-pertussis (DTP) and measles-containing (MCV) vaccines in 2022, by World Bank strata. LMICs, low- and middle-income countries; HICs, high-income countries.

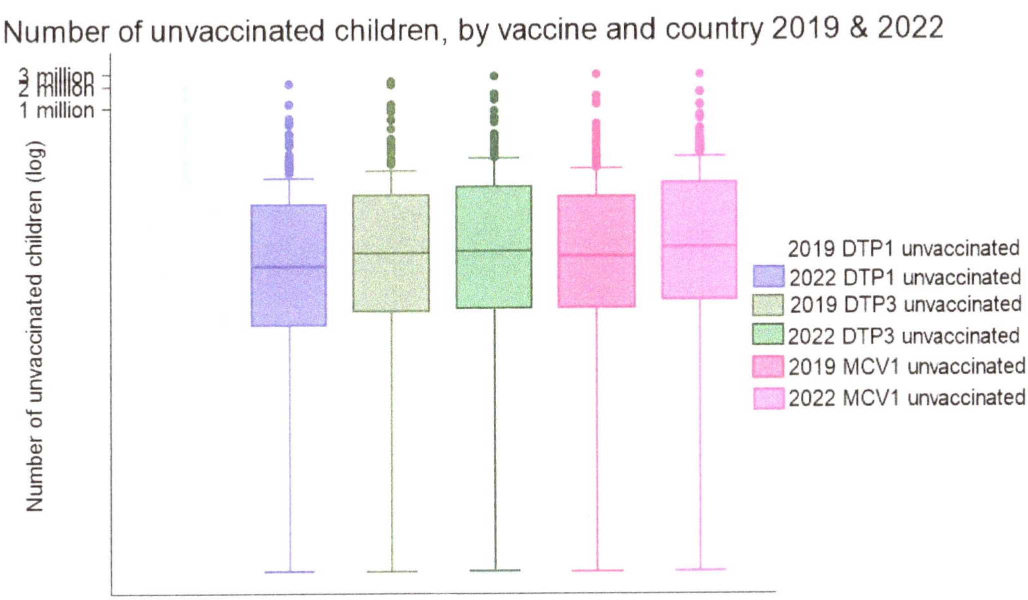

Figure 2. Median (IQR) number of children aged 12–23 months missing immunisations by country (N = 195) and vaccine, 2019 and 2022. DTP, diphtheria-tetanus-pertussis vaccine; MCV, measles-containing vaccine. Note: Data are log-transformed to aid visual interpretation.

Median MCV1 coverage globally (90%) was significantly lower than DTP1 (95%) or DTP3 (91%) coverage in 2022 (Table 1), and below the 95% coverage threshold required for herd immunity. When high-income countries were excluded from the analysis, median MCV1 coverage declined to 83%. Coverage of MCV1 also reduced more during the COVID-19 pandemic than coverage of DTP1 ($p < 0.001$, Wilcoxon signed-rank test).

Dropout is another way of measuring knowledge of vaccine schedules, accessibility, and service continuity and acceptability. Generally, immunisation coverage declines with subsequent doses as children age [17,18]. This is a particular concern for measles vaccination, where the second dose is not given until a child is 15–18 months of age or older.

Table 1. Median (interquartile range) immunisation coverage and change in coverage 2019–2022.

Outcome of Interest	All Countries	Low-Middle Income Countries Only [a]
MCV1 coverage 2022	90% (76–96%)	83% (71–93%)
DTP1 coverage 2022	95% (87–98%)	92% (82–97%)
DTP3 coverage 2022	91% (78–97%)	85% (75–94%)
Change in MCV1 coverage between 2019 and 2022	−2% (−7–0%)	−3% (−9–0%)
Change in DTP1 coverage between 2019 and 2022	0% (−3–0%)	−0.5% (−5–0%)

[a] Country income status according to the World Bank 2022 country classifications [15]. DTP, diphtheria-tetanus-pertussis vaccine; MCV, measles-containing vaccine.

Median DTP1 to MCV1 dropout in 2022 was 2 percentage points (interquartile range: 1–5%) in high-income countries (HICs), but 6 percentage points in LMICs (Table 2). There was further sustained dropout between MCV1 and MCV2 vaccination receipt in 2022. This highlights the additional challenge of continuing to engage with and reach children who have had some contact with the health system and previously received at least one vaccine in resource-limited settings. Further work is needed to identify and address barriers specific to this cohort.

Table 2. Median (interquartile range) immunisation coverage–dropout in percentage points.

Outcome of Interest	All Countries	Low-Middle Income Countries Only [a]
MCV1–MCV2 dropout 2022	5% (1–14%)	8% (1–17%)
DTP1–MCV1 dropout 2022	4% (1–11%)	6% (2–12%)
DTP1–DTP3 dropout 2022	3% (1–7%)	5% (2–10%)

[a] Country income status according to the World Bank 2022 country classifications [15]. DTP, diphtheria-tetanus-pertussis vaccine; MCV, measles-containing vaccine.

Global efforts often focus on the number of zero-dose children [13,19]. This risks leaving behind smaller countries with higher proportions of un-immunised children, and increases the likelihood of future vaccine-preventable disease outbreaks.

When examining the top 20 countries ranked by the number of children who have not received DTP1 or MCV1, and by the percentage of children who have not received DTP1 or MCV1 (Table 3) some interesting differences emerge between countries. For instance, the United States appears to have the 19th-highest population of children who have not received MCV1 globally but is not featured in any of the other top 20 rankings.

Countries with the highest proportion of children missing DTP1 and MCV1 are not always aligned with countries with the highest number of children missing these vaccinations. This is especially the case in fragile or small island developing states, or countries with more rural and remote populations.

For instance, in 2022, 55% of children in Papua New Guinea missed out on DTP1 vaccination and 56% missed out on MCV1 [7]. Papua New Guinea is the largest country in the Pacific region by an order of magnitude, yet the number of children estimated to have missed out on DTP1 and MCV1 in 2022 was 134,812 and 137,263, respectively.

This compares to nearby Philippines, another lower-middle income country, which is generally recognised as having a high number of un-vaccinated children. The birth cohort is almost 10-fold larger than Papua New Guinea, so despite MCV1 coverage rates being 34% higher, the number of children who have not been vaccinated against measles is over five times larger, at almost 752,000.

Table 3. Top 20 countries ranked by number and percentage of children who have not received DTP1 or MCV1, and by income status.

Rank	Number of Children Without DTP1	Percentage of Children Without DTP1	Number of Children Without MCV1	Percentage of Children Without MCV1
1	Nigeria	Democratic People's Republic of Korea	Nigeria	Democratic People's Republic of Korea
2	Ethiopia	Papua New Guinea	Ethiopia	Montenegro
3	India	Somalia	Democratic Republic of the Congo	Angola
4	Democratic Republic of the Congo	Angola	India	Syrian Arab Republic (=5)
5	Philippines	Central African Republic	Pakistan	Central African Republic (=5)
6	Angola	Guinea	Angola	Madagascar (=7)
7	Indonesia	Syrian Arab Republic	Philippines	Papua New Guinea (=7)
8	Brazil	Gabon	Indonesia	Somalia
9	Pakistan	Madagascar	Brazil	Guinea
10	Mozambique	Mozambique	Madagascar	Djibouti
11	Somalia	Nigeria (=13)	Afghanistan	Gabon
12	Afghanistan	Ethiopia (=13)	Niger	Equatorial Guinea
13	Madagascar	Djibouti (=13)	Somalia	Paraguay
14	Cameroon	Venezuela *	Democratic People's Republic of Korea	Ethiopia (=16)
15	Democratic People's Republic of Korea	Philippines (=18)	Cameroon	Democratic Republic of the Congo (=16)
16	United Republic of Tanzania	Chad (=18)	United Republic of Tanzania	Chad (=16)
17	Chad	Ecuador (=18)	Cote d'Ivoire	Bosnia and Herzegovina
18	Myanmar	Libya (=18)	Chad	Nigeria
19	Guinea	Cameroon	United States	Cook Islands
20	South Africa	Haiti	Sudan	Cameroon

Key: White = low income; light blue = lower middle income; dark grey = upper middle income; black = high income, based on World Bank 2022 country classifications [15]; * no recent income data. DTP, diphtheria-tetanus-pertussis vaccine; MCV, measles-containing vaccine.

Using DTP1 coverage as a proxy for MCV1 coverage underestimates countries most at risk of measles outbreaks as coverage across the two vaccines is not always closely aligned. Out of the top 50 countries globally with the lowest MCV1 coverage in 2022, 20% (10 countries) did not appear on the list of the top 50 countries with the lowest DTP1 coverage (Figure 3). That means that one in five countries with the lowest MCV1 coverage is globally missed when we focus zero-dose efforts only on children who have not received DTP1.

Most critically, Montenegro was reported to have the second-lowest MCV1 coverage globally in 2022, but was not in the top 50 lowest DTP1 countries. This emphasises the need to measure and address measles-specific drivers and barriers to immunisation coverage. Notably, among the top 10 countries with the lowest coverage for MCV1 in 2022, the maximum coverage was 50%, with an average coverage across the 10 countries of 38%. For DTP1, average coverage among these 10 countries was 57% and maximum coverage reached 67%.

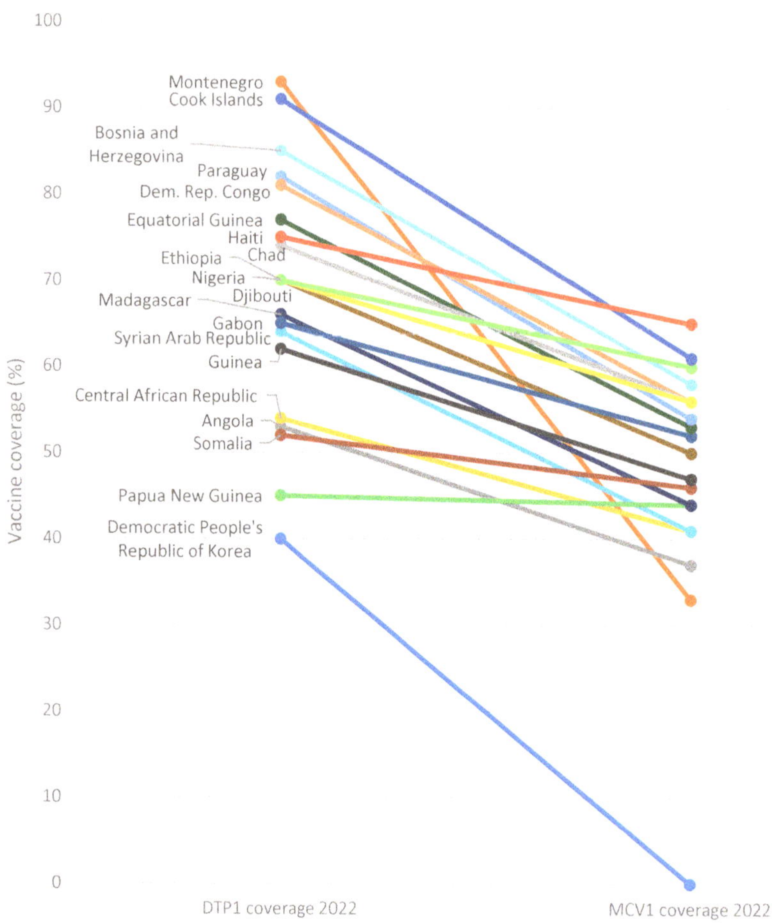

Figure 3. Difference in diphtheria-tetanus-pertussis (DTP) and measles-containing vaccine (MCV) coverage in 20 countries with lowest MCV1 coverage, 2022.

Of the 10 countries shown in Table 3 with the largest number of missed children, only two of these, Angola and Madagascar, appear in the list of the top 10 countries with the highest proportion of children who have not received MCV1. Although this analysis uses population-level data, and thus direct individual comparisons between children are not possible, examining trends at the country level can highlight areas of structural and systemic inequities within country immunisation programs.

There are many disparities in immunisation coverage within and between populations, and assessing just one vaccine cannot adequately represent the challenges with immunisation programmes. Thus, incorporating measles vaccine coverage into global definitions of under-immunised children can help to elucidate which populations are most at risk of future measles outbreaks and of being left behind in global efforts to increase vaccine coverage when the focus remains on receipt of DTP-containing vaccine.

4. Discussion

Globally, almost all children who have missed out on measles immunisation reside in LMICs, highlighting the inequities in measles immunisation coverage. Dropout between

DTP1 and MCV1 was also three times higher in LMICs than HICs and was exacerbated during the COVID-19 pandemic.

Given the huge healthcare, social, and economic burden posed by measles outbreaks, combined with high transmissibility of measles and lower MCV1 coverage compared to DTP3 globally, we propose that the absence of a first dose of measles-containing vaccine is considered in global definitions of under-immunised children. This is important as coverage across DTP and measles vaccines is not always closely aligned, as shown in this study.

In countries with large populations, even with relatively high vaccine coverage, there can be large pockets of un- and under-immunised individuals. Reducing the risk of outbreaks by reducing clusters of susceptible individuals is critical, even in less populous settings [20]. The risk of an outbreak increases with a higher relative proportion of people who are unimmunised, especially for highly infectious diseases like measles.

Measles elimination remains a priority for the WHO and is a key indicator in the JEE, with all regions committing to eliminating measles but none yet achieving sustained elimination [2]. Given the differences identified in this analysis about where children live who have not been vaccinated with MCV1 compared to DTP1, routine data collection on the number and proportion of children at a national and sub-national level who have not been vaccinated with MCV1 is critical as a standalone indicator of immunisation program performance, progress towards elimination, and to assess the potential risk of future measles outbreaks.

In terms of equity, the enduring impacts of measles infection and outbreaks do not affect all individuals and populations equally. For instance, Papua New Guinea has reported a high incidence of subacute sclerosing panencephalitis (SSPE) following measles outbreaks, with increases in SSPE cases tracking closely with prior measles outbreaks [21]. In an under-resourced healthcare system, the double burden of vaccine-preventable disease outbreaks leading to extended morbidity and mortality is even more pronounced. This was also supported by recent WHO modelling highlighting that of the 9.0 billion life-years and 10.2 billion years of full health gained globally through vaccination since 1974, 5.7 and 5.8 billion years, respectively, are directly attributable to measles vaccination, more than all other vaccines combined [9].

Although receipt of DTP1 is important as it represents early contact with the healthcare system, previous research has shown that among children who have only received one vaccine, polio was the most likely vaccine to have been administered in low and lower-middle-income countries, and BCG in upper-middle income countries [22]. MCV was the least likely vaccine to have been received, and there were substantial disparities in DTP1 to MCV1 dropout by wealth quintile, highlighting further equity issues with MCV receipt.

Gavi uses DTP3 coverage as a proxy for overall health system performance and the ability to reach children with immunisations [13]. However, as this is administered to children around 3–4 months of age, it represents less sustained engagement with the healthcare system than measles vaccination, which is usually in the second year of life [23]. Thus, measles vaccination serves as a good proxy for 'full immunisation', ensuring that a child has received all critical age-appropriate vaccines and has ongoing access to healthcare.

Incorporating missed measles immunisations into global definitions and calculations of missed immunisations can also provide insights into the reasons behind low immunisation coverage. Utazi and colleagues [24] have identified that in areas with high DTP1 coverage but low DTP3 or MCV coverage, challenges are likely to be systematic. This includes inadequate follow-up, missed opportunities for immunisation, poor previous experience with health facilities, and low knowledge of immunisation schedules. Conversely, when both DTP1 and MCV coverage are low, structural challenges such as conflict, vaccine unavailability, and difficult terrain are likely contributing to poor immunisation rates.

This nuance exemplifies why consideration of measles vaccination coverage alongside currently used DTP indicators is useful to assess overall health system status, including in high-income settings. The inclusion of the United States on the list of countries with the highest number of un-vaccinated children for measles (Table 3) highlights that, while it has the third largest population of any country globally, there are issues specific to measles vaccination, or broader constraints around ongoing access and utilization of the health system that warrant further attention.

Attention to vaccine-specific barriers in resource-limited settings is also needed, as acceptance and willingness for uptake can differ between vaccines. This is especially the case for MCV, where previous research has identified fear of autism as an enduring piece of misinformation which can lead to hesitancy, despite being comprehensively rebuked [25]. Tools such as the WHO Behavioral and Social Drivers of Vaccination [26] or UNICEF's Journey to Immunisation [27], which aim to understand the complex interplay of both access and acceptance barriers, can also be adapted for this purpose.

Focusing zero-dose efforts on countries with the largest number of un-immunised children may underestimate the risks of outbreaks in countries that have smaller populations but higher proportions of un- or under-vaccinated children. Additional immunisation challenges may also be present in conflict and fragile settings, or countries with greater gender disparities [13,28]. With increasing global mobility, outbreak risks are further exacerbated in more fragile health systems.

This analysis is limited by the lack of sub-national and demographic data publicly available in the WUENIC dataset. Additionally, as individual-level vaccination data were not available, some nuance may be lost during analysis. Further exploration of individual-level factors, particularly among under-immunised children, is warranted to better understand why some children are only partially immunized. The availability of high-quality data to provide evidence for gaps in MCV coverage at the local level is necessary to inform decision-making and enable corrective action. Routine immunisation data are already collected through the WHO/UNICEF Joint Reporting Form, but further utilisation of this data, including using MCV1 coverage as a key indicator for health equity and immunisation coverage can lead to renewed advocacy efforts to remove inequities around measles vaccination, at the same time as reducing the risk of future measles outbreaks.

Strategies that can lead to more equitable measles vaccination coverage globally may include transition from 10-dose to 5-dose vaccine vials, to reduce healthcare worker reluctance to open new vials for a few vaccines, or in coming years, implementation of measles microarray patches, which may reduce the need for cold chain and enable trained community members to administer vaccines.

Going forward, global health organisations and policymakers should emphasise the importance of measuring, reporting on, and advocating for the inclusion of measles immunisation coverage as a key metric when estimating numbers of un- and under-immunised children. This will be essential to create awareness of the need to increase measles vaccine coverage globally and reduce the number of children who currently miss out on life-saving immunisations each year. Re-focusing efforts on children who have missed out on measles immunisation will provide an opportunity to reach those who may have missed out on other childhood vaccinations or routine health checks and ensure the most vulnerable members of our communities can receive essential healthcare services.

Author Contributions: Conceptualization, S.V., F.A. and C.M.; Methodology, S.V. and C.M.; Data curation, S.V.; Formal Analysis, S.V.; Writing—Original Draft Preparation, S.V.; Writing—Review and Editing, S.V., M.L., M.D., F.A. and C.M.; Validation, M.L.; Visualization, S.V.; Supervision, M.D., C.M. All authors have read and agreed to the published version of the manuscript.

Funding: This research received no external funding. S.V. is supported by a fellowship from the Baker Foundation.

Institutional Review Board Statement: All data were publicly available, so ethical approval was not required for this research.

Informed Consent Statement: Not applicable.

Data Availability Statement: Immunization data are publicly available from the WHO/UNICEF estimates of the national immunization coverage portal (https://worldhealthorg.shinyapps.io/wuenic-trends/, accessed 21 November 2023) and population data are publicly available from United Nations Population Estimates (https://population.un.org/wpp/Download/Standard/Population/, accessed 29 November 2023).

Acknowledgments: Thank you to Leanne Robinson and Caroline Homer who reviewed an early draft of the manuscript and provided support during its development.

Conflicts of Interest: The authors declare no conflicts of interest.

References

1. UNICEF. Ending Preventable Child Deaths: How Britain Can Lead the Way. 2020. United Kingdom. Available online: https://www.unicef.org.uk/wp-content/uploads/2020/01/Unicef-UK-Ending-Preventable-Child-Deaths_Report-2020.pdf (accessed on 20 August 2024).
2. Minta, A.A. Progress Toward Measles Elimination—Worldwide, 2000–2022. *MMWR. Morb. Mortal. Wkly. Rep.* **2023**, *72*, 1262–1268. [CrossRef] [PubMed]
3. WHO. Worldwide Measles Deaths Climb 50% from 2016 to 2019 Claiming Over 207 500 Lives in 2019. Available online: https://www.who.int/news/item/12-11-2020-worldwide-measles-deaths-climb-50-from-2016-to-2019-claiming-over-207-500-lives-in-2019 (accessed on 17 July 2024).
4. Dalton, M.; Sanderson, B.; Robinson, L.J.; Homer, C.S.E.; Pomat, W.; Danchin, M.; Vaccher, S. Impact of COVID-19 on routine childhood immunisations in low- and middle-income countries: A scoping review. *PLOS Glob. Public Health* **2023**, *3*, e0002268. [CrossRef] [PubMed]
5. Pandey, A.; Galvani, A.P. Exacerbation of measles mortality by vaccine hesitancy worldwide. *Lancet Glob. Health* **2023**, *11*, e478–e479. [CrossRef] [PubMed]
6. Kaufman, J.; Hoq, M.; Rhodes, A.L.; Measey, M.; Danchin, M.H. Misperceptions about routine childhood vaccination among parents in Australia, before and after the COVID-19 pandemic: A cross-sectional survey study. *Med. J. Aust.* **2024**, *220*, 530–532. [CrossRef] [PubMed]
7. WHO and UNICEF. WHO and UNICEF Estimates of Immunization Coverage. 2022. Available online: https://immunizationdata.who.int/ (accessed on 21 November 2023).
8. WHO. *Measles and Rubella Strategic Framework 2021–2030*; World Health Organization: Geneva, Switzerland, 2020. Available online: https://iris.who.int/bitstream/handle/10665/339801/9789240015616-eng.pdf?sequence=1 (accessed on 20 August 2024).
9. Shattock, A.J.; Johnson, H.C.; Sim, S.Y.; Carter, A.; Lambach, P.; Hutubessy, R.C.; Thompson, K.M.; Badizadegan, K.; Lambert, B.; Ferrari, M.J.; et al. Contribution of vaccination to improved survival and health: Modelling 50 years of the Expanded Programme on Immunization. *Lancet* **2024**, *403*, 2307–2316. [CrossRef] [PubMed]
10. United Nations Department of Economic and Social Affairs. The Sustainable Development Goals Report 2023: Special Edition-July 2023. New York, NY, USA, 2023. Available online: https://unstats.un.org/sdgs/report/2023/ (accessed on 17 July 2024).
11. WHO. Immunization Agenda 2030: A Global Strategy to Leave No One Behind. 2020. Available online: https://www.who.int/publications/m/item/immunization-agenda-2030-a-global-strategy-to-leave-no-one-behind (accessed on 19 June 2024).
12. WHO. *Joint External Evaluation Tool: International Health Regulations (2005)*, 3rd ed.; WHO: Geneva, Switzerland, 2022. Available online: https://www.who.int/publications/i/item/9789240051980 (accessed on 20 August 2024).
13. Gavi. Reaching Zero-Dose Children. 2021. Available online: https://www.gavi.org/our-alliance/strategy/phase-5-2021-2025/equity-goal/zero-dose-children-missed-communities (accessed on 13 December 2023).

14. United Nations. *World Population Prospects 2022, Online Edition*; Department of Economic and Social Affairs: New York, NY, USA, 2022. Available online: https://population.un.org/wpp/Download/Standard/Population/ (accessed on 29 November 2023).
15. Hamadeh, N.; Van Rompaey, C.; Metreau, E.; Eapen, S.G. *New World Bank Country Classifications by Income Level: 2022–2023*; World Bank: Washington, DC, USA, 2022. Available online: https://blogs.worldbank.org/en/opendata/new-world-bank-country-classifications-income-level-2022-2023 (accessed on 21 November 2023).
16. Corrêa, G.C.; Uddin, J.; Wahed, T.; Oliveras, E.; Morgan, C.; Kamya, M.R.; Kabatangare, P.; Namugaya, F.; Leab, D.; Adjakidje, D.; et al. Measuring Zero-Dose Children: Reflections on Age Cohort Flexibilities for Targeted Immunization Surveys at the Local Level. *Vaccines* **2024**, *12*, 195. [CrossRef] [PubMed]
17. Mmanga, K.; Mwenyenkulu, T.E.; Nkoka, O.; Ntenda, P.A. Tracking immunization coverage, dropout and equity gaps among children ages 12–23 months in Malawi—Bottleneck analysis of the Malawi Demographic and Health Survey. *Int. Health* **2021**, *14*, 250–259. [CrossRef] [PubMed]
18. Hull, B.; Hendry, A.; Dey, A.; Brotherton, J.; Macartney, K.; Beard, F. *Annual Immunisation Coverage Report 2022*; NCIRS: Sydney, Australia, 2023. Available online: https://ncirs.org.au/sites/default/files/2024-01/NCIRS%20Annual%20immunisation%20coverage%20report%202022.pdf (accessed on 7 July 2024).
19. WHO; UNICEF; Gavi. *The Big Catch-Up: An Essential Immunization Recovery Plan for 2023 and Beyond*; WHO: New York, NY, USA, 2023. Available online: https://iris.who.int/bitstream/handle/10665/371801/9789240075511-eng.pdf?sequence=1 (accessed on 2 February 2024).
20. Truelove, S.A.; Graham, M.; Moss, W.J.; Metcalf, C.J.E.; Ferrari, M.J.; Lessler, J. Characterizing the impact of spatial clustering of susceptibility for measles elimination. *Vaccine* **2019**, *37*, 732–741. [CrossRef] [PubMed]
21. Manning, L.; Laman, M.; Edoni, H.; Mueller, I.; Karunajeewa, H.A.; Smith, D.; Hwaiwhanje, I.; Siba, P.M.; Davis, T.M.E. Subacute Sclerosing Panencephalitis in Papua New Guinean Children: The Cost of Continuing Inadequate Measles Vaccine Coverage. *PLOS Neglected Trop. Dis.* **2011**, *5*, e932. [CrossRef] [PubMed]
22. Cata-Preta, B.O.; Santos, T.M.; Mengistu, T.; Hogan, D.R.; Barros, A.J.; Victora, C.G. Zero-dose children and the immunisation cascade: Understanding immunisation pathways in low and middle-income countries. *Vaccine* **2021**, *39*, 4564–4570. [CrossRef] [PubMed]
23. WHO. Table 2: Summary of WHO Position Papers—Recommended Routine Immunizations for Children. 2023. Available online: https://www.who.int/publications/m/item/table-2-summary-of-who-position-papers-recommended-routine-immunizations-for-children (accessed on 24 May 2024).
24. Utazi, C.E.; Thorley, J.; Alegana, V.A.; Ferrari, M.J.; Takahashi, S.; Metcalf, C.J.E.; Lessler, J.; Cutts, F.T.; Tatem, A.J. Mapping vaccination coverage to explore the effects of delivery mechanisms and inform vaccination strategies. *Nat. Commun.* **2019**, *10*, 1633. [CrossRef] [PubMed]
25. Novilla, M.L.B.; Goates, M.C.; Redelfs, A.H.; Quenzer, M.; Novilla, L.K.B.; Leffler, T.; Holt, C.A.; Doria, R.B.; Dang, M.T.; Hewitt, M.; et al. Why Parents Say No to Having Their Children Vaccinated against Measles: A Systematic Review of the Social Determinants of Parental Perceptions on MMR Vaccine Hesitancy. *Vaccines* **2023**, *11*, 926. [CrossRef] [PubMed]
26. WHO. *Behavioural and Social Drivers of Vaccination: Tools and Practical Guidance for Achieving High Uptake*; WHO: Geneva, Switzerland, 2022. Available online: https://apps.who.int/iris/handle/10665/354459 (accessed on 28 February 2023).
27. UNICEF. *Journey to Health and Immunization*; UNICEF: New York, NY, USA, 2018. Available online: https://www.hcd4health.org/resources (accessed on 22 March 2023).
28. Fuertes, C.V.; Johns, N.E.; Goodman, T.S.; Heidari, S.; Munro, J.; Hosseinpoor, A.R. The Association between Childhood Immunization and Gender Inequality: A Multi-Country Ecological Analysis of Zero-Dose DTP Prevalence and DTP3 Immunization Coverage. *Vaccines* **2022**, *10*, 1032. [CrossRef] [PubMed]

vaccines

MDPI

Systematic Review

Immunization Coverage, Equity, and Access for Children with Disabilities: A Scoping Review of Challenges, Strategies, and Lessons Learned to Reduce the Number of Zero-Dose Children

Godfrey Musuka [1], Diego F. Cuadros [2], F. DeWolfe Miller [3], Zindoga Mukandavire [4], Tapiwa Dhliwayo [5], Patrick Gad Iradukunda [6], Oscar Mano [7] and Tafadzwa Dzinamarira [8,9,*]

1 International Initiative for Impact Evaluation, Harare P.O. Box 0002, Zimbabwe
2 Digital Epidemiology Laboratory, Digital Futures, University of Cincinnati, Cincinnati, OH 45221, USA
3 Department of Tropical Medicine and Medical Microbiology and Pharmacology, University of Hawaii at Manoa, Honolulu, HI 96822, USA
4 Institute of Applied Research and Technology, Emirates Aviation University, Dubai P.O. Box 53044, United Arab Emirates
5 Department of Community Medicine, Midlands State University, Gweru P.O. Box 9055, Zimbabwe; dhliwayot@staff.msu.ac.zw
6 Rwanda Food and Drug Authority, Kigali P.O. Box 3243, Rwanda; gadpatrickiradukunda@gmail.com
7 Department of Public Health, University of the Western Cape, Robert Sobukwe Road, Bellville 7535, South Africa
8 School of Health Systems and Public Health, University of Pretoria, Pretoria 0002, South Africa
9 ICAP in Zimbabwe, Harare P.O. Box 263, Zimbabwe
* Correspondence: td2581@cumc.columbia.edu

Abstract: Background: Children with disabilities, particularly in low- and middle-income countries (LMICs), face heightened risks of vaccine-preventable diseases due to a range of systemic and social barriers. Although immunization is a fundamental human right and a proven public health intervention, this vulnerable group is often overlooked in policy and practice. Understanding the factors compromising vaccine equity for these children is critical to reducing zero-dose prevalence and improving health outcomes. **Methods**: This scoping review examined peer-reviewed, gray literature from 2010 to 2024. Searches were conducted in PubMed, Google Scholar, and relevant organizational reports (WHO, UNICEF). Studies addressing children with disabilities and focusing on immunization barriers, interventions, or lessons learned were selected. English-language publications were screened in title/abstract and full-text stages. Key data extracted included population, barriers, and immunization outcomes. Since this review focused on articles in English, this is a key limitation. Results were synthesized thematically to identify recurring patterns and to guide improved interventions and policies. **Results**: Twelve articles met the inclusion criteria. Key barriers identified were inadequate healthcare infrastructure, insufficient provider training, limited follow-up services in rural regions, societal stigma, and pervasive misconceptions around both disability and vaccines. Factors such as maternal education, logistical support for caregivers, and using low-sensory, inclusive vaccination settings were consistently linked with better outcomes. Effective strategies included mobile vaccination units, tailored interventions (e.g., distraction or sedation techniques), school-based immunization programs, and robust community engagement to address stigma. Lessons learned underscored the importance of flexible, individualized care plans and empowering families through transparent communication. **Conclusions**: Children with disabilities continue to experience significant gaps in immunization coverage, driven by intersecting barriers at the individual, health system, and societal levels. Scaling tailored interventions, inclusive policies, strengthened infrastructure, and ongoing research can help ensure these children receive equitable access to life-saving vaccinations.

 https://doi.org/10.3390/vaccines13040377

Keywords: immunization equity; children with disabilities; low- and middle-income countries; vaccine barriers; vaccination strategies; inclusive healthcare

1. Introduction

Immunization is widely recognized as one of the most effective public health interventions to prevent infectious diseases, particularly among children [1]. Vaccines have been critical in reducing mortality and morbidity from vaccine-preventable diseases, significantly improving global health outcomes. However, achieving high immunization coverage remains a challenge, especially in low- and middle-income countries (LMICs) [2], where barriers such as geographical remoteness, poverty, limited healthcare infrastructure, and resource constraints hinder access to life-saving vaccines [3]. Within these populations, certain groups face even more significant obstacles, including children with disabilities, who are often excluded from mainstream health services due to systemic gaps and societal stigma [4–6].

Children with disabilities face significant barriers to accessing healthcare, including immunization, due to physical, environmental, and cultural challenges. In LMICs, these children are less likely to receive timely vaccinations, partly because of inadequate healthcare facilities, a lack of disability-inclusive services, logistics, and societal discrimination. For example, Thota et al. revealed that research on improving access to healthcare for children with disabilities in LMICs is lacking in several critical areas, including the provision of general health services and the accessibility of healthcare settings [7]. Their evidence and gap mapping highlighted the need for more effective interventions in areas such as non-discrimination, tackling harmful stereotypes, and ensuring access to essential services like water, sanitation, and hygiene [7]. The study also identified gaps in policies and programs that promote inclusion and participation, which are essential for ensuring that children with disabilities can fully enjoy their rights, including the right to health, as outlined in international frameworks like the Convention on the Rights of the Child (CRC). Immunization, as a fundamental human right, must be accessible to all children, including those with disabilities, to protect them from preventable diseases and reduce their disproportionate health risks.

Numerous studies reveal significant gaps in immunization coverage between children with disabilities and their non-disabled peers, even in countries with robust health systems and strong immunization programs. For example, in the UK, Emerson et al. found that children with intellectual disabilities were less likely to be fully vaccinated compared to their peers without disabilities [8]. The study, which analyzed data from the Millennium Cohort Study, showed that vaccination rates for children with intellectual disabilities were lower at the ages of nine months and three years, with these children being more than twice as likely to be non-vaccinated compared to non-disabled children [8]. This disparity persisted despite adjustments for socioeconomic factors. Similarly, O'Neill et al.'s review highlighted that 78% of studies across various countries, including the USA and the UK, found lower immunization uptake in children with disabilities [6]. The review emphasized that these vulnerabilities were often linked to various factors, including inadequate access to healthcare services, logistical barriers, and the broad and inconsistent definitions of disability used in different studies. For example, while some studies from the USA suggested no significant difference in vaccine uptake among children with special healthcare needs, other studies found that specific populations, such as children with spina bifida or autism, had notably lower vaccination rates [6]. These disparities, occurring even in high-income countries with established immunization programs, underscore the urgency of addressing this challenge, specifically in LMICs, where healthcare access and systems may be even more constrained.

This scoping review examined the factors contributing to disparities in immunization coverage for children with disabilities. We also aimed to identify effective strategies for designing and prioritizing immunization interventions to ensure that children with disabilities are included, aiming to reduce zero-dose children and reach underserved communities in LMICs. Additionally, the review assessed key lessons learned from past initiatives in delivering immunization programs to children with disabilities in LMICs.

2. Methods

2.1. Study Design

A scoping review of the available literature was conducted. The review was guided by the Preferred Reporting Items for Systematic Reviews and Meta-Analysis Protocols (PRISMA-P) guidelines [9] and aligned with the Centre for Reviews and Dissemination (CRD) guidance for undertaking systematic reviews in healthcare [10].

2.2. Research Question and Study Eligibility

The population–concept–context (PCC) framework (Table 1) was used to set the eligibility criteria for the review question following recommendations from the Joanna Briggs Institute [11].

Table 1. Population–concept–context framework for this scoping review.

Criteria	Operational Definition
Population	Children with disabilities - Defined in line with the WHO's International Classification of Functioning, Disability, and Health (ICF), encompassing physical, sensory, intellectual, or developmental impairments. - Includes individuals under 18 who experience functional limitations or activity restrictions due to these impairments.
Concept	Immunization coverage and equity - Refers to the availability, accessibility, acceptability, and quality of routine vaccinations. - Encompasses the overall coverage rates (e.g., fully immunized vs. zero-dose) and equity aspects (e.g., disparities by disability type, socioeconomic status, or geography). - Examines barriers, facilitators, interventions, and outcomes related to immunization uptake.
Context	- Healthcare Systems: The context includes healthcare infrastructure and systems, examining how these systems either support or hinder immunization efforts for children with disabilities. - Global Health and Disability Policy: The review takes place within the context of global health frameworks and disability inclusion policies. This includes the United Nations' Sustainable Development Goals (particularly Goal 3: Good Health and Well-Being, and Goal 10: Reduced Inequalities). - Barriers in Low-Resource Settings: The review may also consider the challenges in low- and middle-income countries (LMICs), where children with disabilities face compounded barriers to accessing healthcare and immunization services. - Public Health and Immunization Campaigns: The broader public health context of immunization programs and campaigns aimed at increasing vaccination rates, particularly in vulnerable groups.

This review addresses the two research questions outlined below.

1. What are the key barriers and systemic factors contributing to inequities in immunization coverage for children with disabilities globally?

2. What strategies have been identified or implemented to ensure children with disabilities are not left out by immunization programs?

2.3. Literature Sources

A search was conducted on the PubMed and Google Scholar electronic databases. Additional sources, such as grey literature and reports from WHO, UNICEF, and other relevant international organizations, were also consulted for relevant publications reporting routine immunization service delivery among children with disabilities.

2.4. Inclusion Criteria

This review included peer-reviewed publications on immunization access for children with disabilities published between 2010 and 2024. To be eligible, articles were required to focus on either barriers to immunization or strategies for improving access for children with disabilities. Only articles published in English were considered eligible. Studies were excluded if they did not address children with disabilities or did not relate to immunization access.

To address the varying definitions of disability across studies, this scoping review adopted the World Health Organization's International Classification of Functioning, Disability, and Health (ICF) as its conceptual framework [12,13]. The ICF defines disability as an umbrella term encompassing impairments, activity limitations, and participation restrictions, where a health condition interacts with personal and environmental factors. In line with this holistic view, we included studies focusing on a broad range of physical, sensory, intellectual, and developmental disabilities. This approach is intended to capture the diverse experiences and needs of children who may face barriers to immunization due to their functional limitations or social/environmental constraints.

2.4.1. Operational Criteria

Physical disabilities: Conditions significantly limiting mobility or motor functions (e.g., cerebral palsy).

Sensory disabilities: Vision or hearing impairments that require specific accommodations (e.g., Braille materials, sign language interpretation).

Intellectual disabilities: Diagnosed conditions affecting cognitive functioning, such as Down syndrome or global developmental delay.

Developmental disabilities: Neurodevelopmental conditions like autism spectrum disorder (ASD), attention deficit hyperactivity disorder (ADHD), or other pervasive developmental delays.

2.4.2. Handling Varied Definitions During Screening

Inclusive Screening: We used broad search terms (e.g., "children with disabilities", "special healthcare needs", "neurodevelopmental disorders", "physical impairment") to capture studies even if they employed alternative or narrower definitions of disability.

Cross-Checking Against ICF: In cases where authors used non-standardized definitions (e.g., "children with learning difficulties" or "children with special needs"), we compared these descriptions against the ICF framework to verify whether the study population fit our overall criteria of functional impairment and potential participation restrictions.

Contextual Judgement: When an article's definition of disability was ambiguous, we reviewed the detailed methods and population characteristics to determine alignment with the ICF perspective. If the study population overlapped substantially with the recognized categories of disability outlined above, the article was retained.

2.4.3. Rationale

By grounding our inclusion criteria in the ICF, we aimed to avoid overly restrictive or overly broad definitions of disability, thus maximizing relevance and comparability among included studies. This ensures we capture the multifaceted nature of disability (biological, psychological, social) and retain studies that reflect the diverse obstacles and facilitators to immunization.

This clear operationalization allows for a consistent interpretation of "children with disabilities" and mitigates the risk of excluding relevant subgroups who might not neatly fit a single diagnostic label. It also promotes transparency in how we approached articles that used differing or less-formalized disability definitions.

2.5. Search Strategy

The search strategy was co-developed and pilot-tested with the assistance of a senior health science librarian and pediatrician. The search strategy accounted for the number of terms used to describe disability, incorporating broad descriptors and specific diagnoses to ensure a comprehensive search of disability literature. The search terms included a combination of keywords and medical subject headings (MeSH), such as "children with disabilities", "immunization", "health equity", "vaccination access", and "zero-dose children". The strategy was tailored to each database to ensure comprehensive retrieval of relevant studies. The search dates included 2010 to 2024.

2.6. Title, Abstract, and Full-Text Screening

Two independent reviewers screened titles, abstracts, and full-text articles for eligibility. Studies identified through database searches were exported to EndNote [14]. Duplicate articles were removed. Studies were then exported from EndNote to the Covidence systematic review management platform [15]. This desk review followed the PRISMA-P guidelines.

2.7. Data Abstraction and Analysis

A customized data extraction form was developed to systematically collect information from each eligible study. Extracted data points included author(s), publication year, study design, study location, population characteristics, barriers identified, strategies implemented, key findings, and conclusions. The extracted data were analyzed thematically to identify common patterns and recurring themes related to immunization coverage and access for children with disabilities. These themes were then categorized under the PCC framework to better understand the interplay between systemic barriers, strategies for improvement, and the context of immunization programs. The analysis also considered lessons learned from past initiatives, focusing on actionable insights that can inform future interventions to improve immunization equity for children with disabilities.

2.8. Justification of Exclusion Criteria

The exclusion of 102 articles during the screening process was based on rigorous criteria to ensure relevance and quality. At the abstract level, studies were excluded if they did not specifically address immunization for children with disabilities or if the focus was unrelated to barriers, strategies, or lessons learned in improving vaccine access. For example, articles discussing general healthcare systems without mentioning vaccination programs or disability-inclusive practices were excluded. At the full-text level, studies were excluded if they lacked primary data, provided only anecdotal evidence, or did not meet quality appraisal benchmarks, such as unclear methodologies or small, unrepresentative sample sizes. For instance, a study focusing on adult vaccination programs with a brief mention of childhood immunization was excluded due to insufficient relevance. These exclusion criteria were applied consistently to maintain the integrity and focus of the review.

3. Results

3.1. Characteristics of Included Studies

Our search retrieved 109 articles. After removing duplicates, 82 articles remained. Upon screening, 49 articles were removed at the title screening stage, 13 at the abstract screening stage, and another eight at the full-text screening stage, leaving 12 articles for inclusion in this scoping review [16–27] (Figure 1). Table 2 provides more details on the characteristics of the included articles. The data were synthesized into three themes, and Table 3 provides more details.

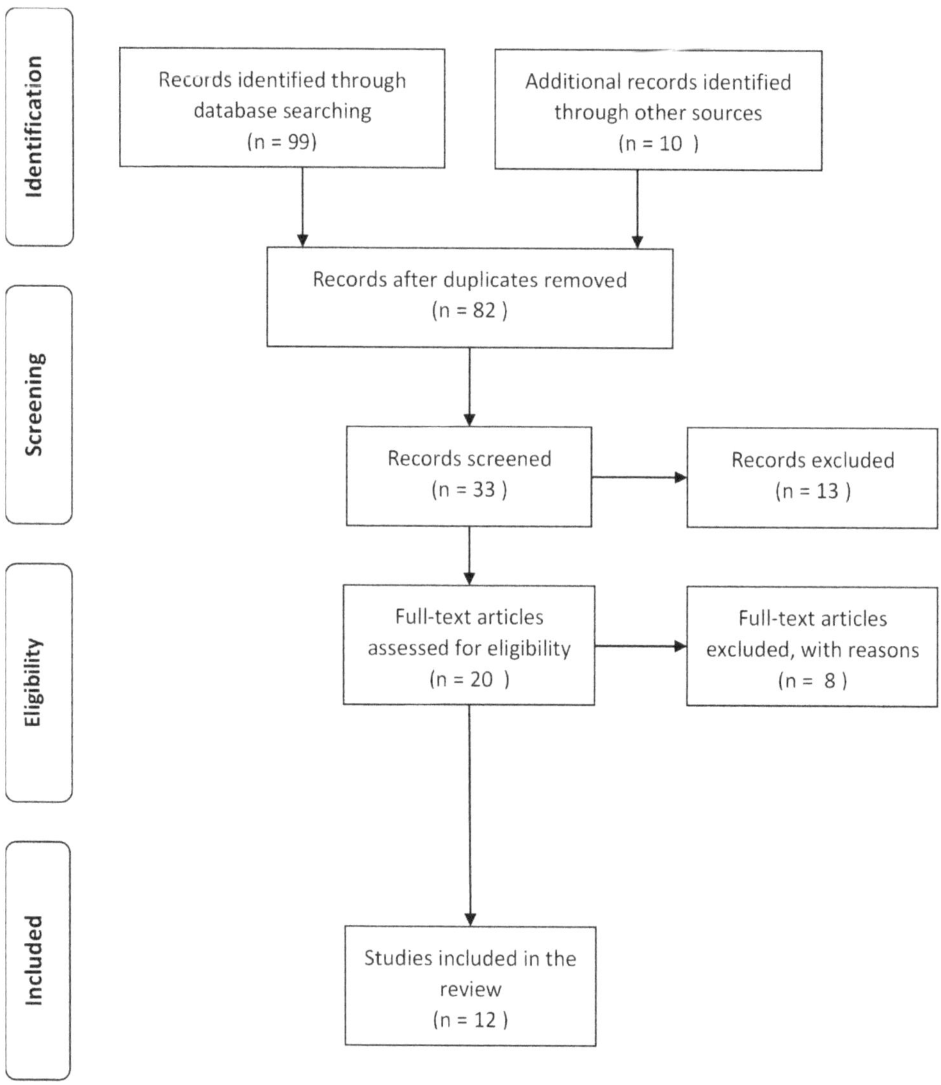

Figure 1. PRISMA flow chart of the selection of studies included in the analysis.

Table 2. Characteristics of studies included in the analysis.

Study Authors	Country/Region	Economic Setting	Method	Study Period	Total Sample	Population	Participants	Themes
Lin et al. (2010) [16]	Taiwan	HICs	Cross-sectional	NA	495	Primary caregivers of children and adolescents with ID	3–24 years	Theme 3
Tuckerman et al. (2024) [17]	Australia	HIC	Qualitative cross-sectional study	June and September 2022	32	Stakeholders linked to adolescents with disability in specialist schools in Victoria, Australia	Principal/Vice Principal, $n = 6$ Other school staff, $n = 7$ Council staff, $n = 10$ Parent, $n = 7$ Adolescent, $n = 2$	Themes 1, 2, and 3
Ong et al. (2023) [18]	Australia	HIC	Qualitative cross-sectional study	September 2017 to February 2020	36	Children with intellectual and developmental disability and needle fear	Persons who took the children to vaccination	Themes 1, 2, and 3
Rosenberg et al. (2013) [19]	US	HIC	Not specified	January 14 to October 15 2009	10,000 diagnosed with ASD and 20,000 direct family members	Autism spectrum disorder (ASD)	Consented affected participants between 4 and 18 years who had completed primary history questionnaires and their consented younger siblings aged above 4.5 years and born after family concern about index development ($n = 486$ families)	Theme 1
Fong et al. (2024) [20]	Canada	HIC	Cross-sectional survey	November 2022–April 2023	109	Children diagnosed with Autism spectrum disorder (ASD), intellectual disorder (ID), and/or global developmental delay (GDD) aged 6–17 years, seen through outpatient clinics at the Ron Joyce Children's Health Centre of McMaster Children's hospital in Hamilton	Families with children aged 6–17 years	Themes 1 and 2
Bray (2022) [21]	General	All settings	Information from expert	Not applicable	Not applicable	Children with special needs Healthy	Not applicable	Themes 1, 2, and 3
Okoro et al. (2015) [22]	Nigeria	HIC	Cross-sectional	NA	168	children with neurological disorders	6 months to 5 years	Themes 1, 2, and 3
Mactaggart et al. (2016) [24]	Cameroon and India	LMIC	Case–control study	February–April 2014	1548	People with disabilities	India: 508 cases and 337 controls Cameroon: 429 cases and 274 controls	Theme 1
UNICEF and Leonard Cheshire Disability (2020) [25]	Not applicable	Not applicable	Not applicable	Not applicable	Not applicable	People with disabilities	Not applicable	Themes 2 and 3
UNICEF (2024) [26]	Not applicable	Not applicable	Not applicable	Not applicable	Not applicable	Children with disabilities	Not applicable	Themes 1, 2, and 3
UNICEF (2013) [27]	Not applicable	Not applicable	Not applicable	Not applicable	Not applicable	Children with disabilities	Not applicable	Themes 2 and 3
UNICEF (2023) [28]	Indonesia	UMIC	Mixed-method	2022	68	Key policymakers and implementers	Government: 55 OPD: 11 Civil Society: 1 Academic Institution: 1	Themes 1, 2, and 3

Theme 1: Barriers and systemic factors that contribute to inequities in immunization coverage for children with disabilities. Theme 2: Strategies that have been identified or implemented to ensure children with disabilities are reached by immunization programs. Theme 3: Lessons learned in ensuring equitable access for children with disabilities. Abbreviations: HIC: High-income country; LMIC: Low- and middle-income country.

Table 3. Barriers and systemic factors that contribute to inequities in immunization coverage for children with disabilities.

S/N	Subthemes	Authors	Findings
1.1	Barriers related to healthcare systems and social factors	Tuckerman et al. (2024) [17]	Some children do not deliver consent paperwork to their parents, failing to obtain parental or guardian consent for vaccinating. Furthermore, some parents do not trust school workers to deliver immunizations, complicating the process and not providing consent. Schools may also have insufficient resources to assist vaccination efforts, which adds logistical challenges successfully. The level of comfort with disability and assistance received during immunizations significantly impact the vaccination outcome. Meeting the individualized needs of children with disabilities can be difficult, especially when staff have little expertise managing children's anxiety and disruptive behavior during immunization. Furthermore, the lack of a defined follow-up protocol and parents' inadequate information regarding sedation choices create further impediments. Inappropriate follow-up settings that are not parent-friendly impede good communication and care, making it difficult to guarantee a smooth and supportive immunization procedure for these children.
		Fong et al. (2024) [20]	Vaccine administration failure due to children's behavior.
		Okoro et al. (2015) [22]	The type of chronic neurological disorder also significantly affects the immunization coverage of children.
		Mactaggart et al. (2016) [24]	Most individuals who seek care at healthcare facilities present with illness, leading to failure to accommodate the special needs of children with disabilities. This is exacerbated by the geographical and financial constraints. which limit the families' access to essential services like immunization.
		UNICEF (2024) [26]	Humanitarian efforts predominantly fail to make provisions for the special needs of children with disabilities, preventing them from accessing essential services like vaccination campaigns that are generally held in schools or child-friendly venues.
		UNICEF (2023) [28]	Essential health services, such as immunization, are not reaching rural areas and do not take into consideration the unique needs of children with disabilities when accessing them, despite the progress that has been made in healthcare in general.
1.2	The influence of education, stigma, and misconceptions	Tuckerman et al. (2024) [17]	Concerns regarding potential HPV vaccine reactions, as well as preferences for some vaccines over others, impact vaccination follow-up and completion rates, and this is more evident among caregivers with high education status.
		Rosenberg et al. (2013) [19]	Vaccination may be delayed due to the misconceptions about vaccines causing autism.
		Mactaggart et al. (2016) [24]	There was a low level of knowledge about rehabilitation services, which impacted the access to those services.
		Fong et al. (2024) [20]	Parent's perspective about the influence of the children's behavior on vaccination success.
		Bray (2022) [21]	Parents may be hesitant to vaccinate children with special needs with a history of antimicrobial allergies.
		Okoro et al. (2015) [22]	The mother's educational attainment and father's occupation were observed to significantly affect the immunization coverage of children with chronic neurological disorders. Children with obvious neurological deficits whose mothers have low educational attainment are at risk of low immunization coverage. Furthermore, stigma also plays a role in lowering the immunization coverage.
		UNICEF (2023) [28]	The belief in a relationship between the vaccination and autism influenced the decision of the mothers, leading to delaying or omitting some vaccinations that were supposed to be taken in early childhood.

3.2. Barriers and Systemic Factors That Contribute to Inequities in Immunization Coverage for Children with Disabilities

The findings from the studies on immunization coverage inequities for children with disabilities were categorized into two primary themes: barriers related to healthcare systems and social factors, and the influence of education, stigma, and misconceptions. These themes reflect the multifaceted nature of inequities in vaccination access for children with disabilities and highlight systemic and societal challenges that contribute to lower immunization rates. Both themes highlight the intersectionality of healthcare accessibility and societal attitudes, which contribute to the inequities faced by children with disabilities in accessing immunization services. Our review revealed that barriers and systemic factors contributing to inequities in immunization coverage for children with disabilities include healthcare system challenges and social factors, such as the failure to obtain parental consent, logistical issues in schools with limited resources, and a lack of staff expertise in managing children's anxiety and disruptive behavior during immunization. The absence of follow-up protocols and insufficient communication with parents further complicate the process. Additionally, geographical and financial constraints limit access to immunization services, particularly in rural or underserved areas, while humanitarian efforts often overlook the special needs of children with disabilities. Education-related factors also play a significant role, as misconceptions, such as the belief that vaccines cause autism, can lead to delayed or missed vaccinations. Stigma surrounding disabilities and the low educational attainment of caregivers, especially mothers, contribute to lower vaccination rates, as does the lack of awareness about available rehabilitation services. These systemic challenges combine to create significant barriers to equitable vaccination for children with disabilities.

A. Barriers related to healthcare systems and social factors

The first theme, barriers related to healthcare systems and social factors, is deeply rooted in the accessibility and responsiveness of health services. One key issue is the lack of resources and preparation in health facilities, which often fails to accommodate the specific needs of children with disabilities. Studies by Ong et al. (2024) [18] and Tuckerman (2024) [17] identify inadequate staff training and lack of preparation techniques as significant obstacles, particularly in LMICs with limited healthcare infrastructure. For instance, children with needle phobia, common in those with autism and ADHD, experience heightened anxiety and unsuccessful vaccination attempts, which further discourage participation in immunization programs. Additionally, the inconsistency in follow-up services, especially in rural areas, creates a barrier to maintaining vaccination schedules. Ong et al. (2024) also point out the absence of specialized services tailored for children with disabilities, which exacerbates the challenge of ensuring equitable access to immunization [18]. This systemic neglect can lead to physical and psychological barriers, such as failed vaccination attempts and the resultant avoidance of vaccination by parents and children. Furthermore, such problems as the miscategorization of symptoms, particularly in children with severe disabilities like cerebral palsy or epilepsy, contribute to lower vaccination uptake, as documented in Okoro's study [22]. These healthcare-system-related inadequate healthcare resources and the lack of stable, accessible services in many LMICs compound barriers.

B. The influence of education, stigma, and misconceptions

The included studies underscored how societal attitudes and knowledge gaps exacerbate inequities in immunization coverage. Okoro et al. [22] highlighted that maternal education levels strongly correlate with higher vaccination rates, suggesting that a lack of knowledge about the benefits and safety of vaccines is a key driver of inequity. In many cases, parents' limited understanding, compounded by misinformation or myths about vaccines, particularly those related to intellectual disabilities, leads to delayed or omitted vaccinations. Rosenberg (2013) discusses how parents of children with autism spectrum disorder (ASD) may delay vaccinations due to misconceptions about vaccines causing autism [19]. This mistrust is more prevalent among highly educated mothers, who may be more susceptible to misinformation. Similarly, Tuckerman (2024) identifies that parents from culturally and linguistically diverse (CALD) backgrounds may face difficulties navigating vaccination systems, resulting in a lower immunization uptake for their children with disabilities [17]. Stigma also plays a significant role, as children with more visible disabilities, such as cerebral palsy, often face social exclusion and discrimination, leading to lower vaccination rates. In comparison, children with less-visible disabilities tend to have higher vaccination rates [22]. This stigma can affect both the willingness of parents to seek vaccinations for their children and the attitude of healthcare providers toward these children.

3.3. Strategies That Have Been Identified or Implemented to Ensure Children with Disabilities Are Reached by Immunization Programs, and How These Can Be Scaled or Improved

The strategies identified in the studies to improve immunization coverage for children with disabilities and reduce the number of zero-dose children were categorized into three primary themes: enhancing healthcare accessibility and service delivery, implementing tailored interventions for children with disabilities, and addressing societal factors like stigma and education (Table 4). Each theme had sub-themes that could be scaled and improved to ensure more children with disabilities are reached by immunization programs. Figure 2 illustrates a flowchart describing the tailored immunization pathways for children with disabilities.

Table 4. Strategies that have been identified or implemented to ensure children with disabilities are reached by immunization programs, and how can these be scaled or improved.

S/N	Subthemes	Authors	Findings
2.1	Enhancing healthcare accessibility and service delivery	Tuckerman et al. (2024) [17]	A focus is placed on adapting information specific to students with disabilities, reassuring parents about safe vaccination spaces and ensuring staff are equipped with basic knowledge to explain the vaccination process.
		Ong et al. (2023) [18]	The parents wished that services were provided closer to their residential area, which suggests that there is a need for temporally or mobile clinics.
		UNICEF and Leonard Cheshire Disability (2020) [25]	Encouragement for incorporating disability-inclusive policies into national immunization programs in order to guarantee that healthcare facilities are accessible and equipped to serve children with different disabilities.
		Fong et al. (2024) [20]	Administering the vaccine in a low-sensory environment, decreasing wait time for vaccination, and ensuring clinic staff have experience in caring for children with special needs.
		Okoro et al. (2015) [22]	Planners and implementers of immunization programs must make greater efforts to understand the sociodemographic factors affecting immunization of children in order to extend coverage to unreached children, reduce dropout rates, and build sustainable programs.
2.2	Implementing tailored interventions for children with disabilities	Tuckerman et al. (2024) [17]	On vaccination day, a safe and structured environment should be created with distraction techniques, individualized spaces, and support staff to assist students.
		Ong et al. (2023) [18]	Distraction and sedation techniques should be included in difficult to vaccinate strategies with the aim of reducing the anxiety among children with disabilities during immunization.
		Bray (2022) [21]	The American Academy of Pediatrics (AAP) recommends vaccinating children with special needs following the same CDC immunization schedule as healthy children unless medically contraindicated. However, health-care providers may consider specific physical and psychosocial challenges when immunizing children with special needs to employ various distraction technics, including but not limited to using handheld devices for entertainment, music therapy, or squeezing soft objects, as they have proven effective in reducing anxiety.
		Okoro et al. (2015) [22]	Parental involvement in the immunization program enhances the immunization program, as it helps to reduce children's anxiety by boosting children's security and contributing toward an informed decision process for the parents.
		UNICEF and Leonard Cheshire Disability (2020) [25]	Collaboration with local disability-focused groups and non-governmental organizations can boost the consideration of a child's unique physical, cognitive, or sensory needs, providing a more inclusive approach to healthcare.
		UNICEF (2024) [26]	Reasonable adjustments appropriate to the age of the child with a disability need to be made to ensure that they are given physical access to services and support for psychosocial disabilities. Also, careful identification of the need for vaccination and fighting stigma that children with disabilities or their parents may face is required.
		UNICEF (2023) [28]	The child with disabilities requires special accommodations to access the health services.
2.3	Addressing societal factors like stigma and education	Tuckerman et al. (2024) [17]	Providing information and consent forms in multiple languages and simplifying communication for parents with culturally and linguistically diverse backgrounds using visuals and tailored formats. Schools are encouraged to better educate parents on the importance of vaccination through resources, information sessions, and school communication channels like newsletters.
		Okoro et al. (2015) [22]	Healthcare workers may identify some signs and symptoms as contradictions for vaccination. Measures to reduce socioeconomic disparities also need to be taken, as they influence vaccination uptake.
		UNICEF (2013) [27]	Including children with disabilities in promotion materials, like posters for immunization programs, can raise awareness and enhance the understanding of the community on the need for vaccination uptake among children with disabilities.
		UNICEF (2023) [28]	Involvement of civil society, community members, children with disabilities, and organizations advocating for people with disabilities is instrumental in ensuring that the policies are inclusive and respond to the stigma.

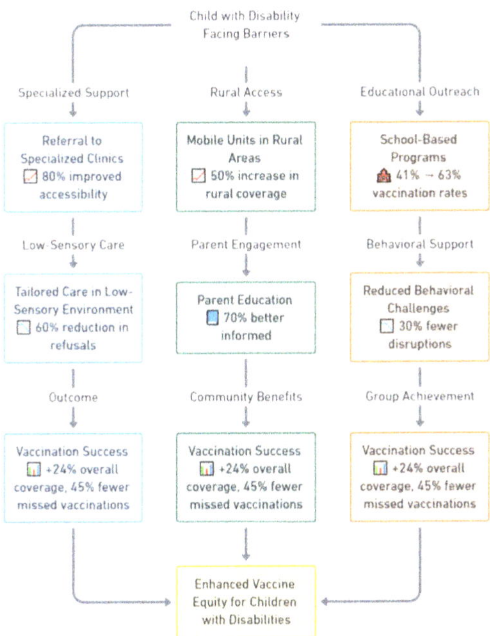

Figure 2. The flowchart illustrates the tailored immunization pathways for children with disabilities, starting with the central challenge, "Child with Disability Facing Barriers". It features three main pathways: Specialized Support, Rural Access, and Educational Outreach. The Specialized Support pathway includes referrals to specialized clinics with 80% improved accessibility, leading to tailored care in low-sensory environments, which reduces vaccination refusals by 60%, and culminates in vaccination success, marked by + 24% overall coverage and 45% fewer missed vaccinations. The Rural Access pathway utilizes mobile units in rural areas, achieving a 50% increase in rural vaccination coverage, followed by parent education initiatives, where 70% of parents report being better informed, resulting in similar vaccination success outcomes. The Educational Outreach pathway employs school-based programs, improving vaccination rates in specialist schools from 41% to 63%, coupled with behavioral support that reduces disruptions by 30%, ultimately leading to vaccination success. The pathways converge on the goal of Enhanced Vaccine Equity for Children with Disabilities. Icons enhance clarity, such as a hospital symbol for specialized clinics, a book for parent education, and a school for school-based programs. Metrics, such as "80% improved accessibility" and "70% better informed", are based on study findings. At the same time, the color coding—blue for specialized support, green for rural access, and orange for educational outreach—helps differentiate pathways visually. The outcome emphasizes significant improvements in coverage and equity for children with disabilities.

A. Enhancing healthcare accessibility and service delivery

The first theme, enhancing healthcare accessibility and service delivery, highlights the importance of creating systems that accommodate the specific needs of children with disabilities. The included studies emphasized the need for better service infrastructure, particularly in underserved and rural areas. Tuckerman (2024) suggests that creating individualized approaches for children, including supporting parents to navigate the vaccination process, can help address gaps in follow-up services [17]. Similarly, Ong et al. (2024) highlight the value of mobile units or temporary vaccination clinics to bring services closer to families, thereby overcoming logistical barriers to accessing immunization [18]. This is complemented by Fong (2024) [20], who recommends administering vaccines in low-sensory environments to minimize anxiety and discomfort. These strategies ensure that children with disabilities are not excluded from immunization programs due to geographical, logistical, or environmental challenges.

B. Implementing tailored interventions for children with disabilities

The second theme, implementing tailored interventions for children with disabilities, focuses on making the vaccination process more manageable for children and parents. Several studies propose using distraction and sedation techniques to reduce anxiety and pain during vaccination. Ong et al. (2024) describe a "Difficult to Vaccinate" clinical pathway, which includes these strategies and ensures that children with disabilities are not excluded due to their unique needs [18]. Bray (2022) also identifies various distraction techniques, such as using handheld devices for entertainment, music therapy, or squeezing soft objects, which have proven effective in reducing anxiety [21]. Moreover, the involvement of parents in the vaccination process can significantly improve outcomes. Parental involvement, as emphasized in both Bray (2022) [21] and Okoro (2015) [22], not only provides emotional security for children but also empowers parents to make informed decisions about vaccination, such as whether to use sedatives or other techniques.

C. Addressing societal factors like stigma and education

Addressing societal factors like stigma and education, the third theme emphasizes tackling misconceptions and promoting understanding about disabilities and vaccines. Okoro (2015) suggests that healthcare workers should be trained to avoid misclassifying disabilities as contraindications to vaccination, which often leads to missed opportunities for immunization [22]. Regular health education campaigns are also recommended to dispel myths and build trust in vaccination programs. Tuckerman (2024) further underscores the need for accessible and understandable information for parents, especially those with low literacy or intellectual disabilities, to ensure they can navigate the vaccination process [17]. Additionally, addressing socioeconomic disparities, as highlighted by Okoro (2015), is crucial in ensuring equitable access to immunization for all children [22]. Policies that promote maternal education and provide financial support can help improve vaccine uptake, particularly in families with lower incomes or those from disadvantaged backgrounds [16].

3.4. Lessons Learned in Ensuring Equitable Access for Children with Disabilities

The included studies highlighted several vital lessons that were grouped into three key themes: creating supportive and inclusive environments, empowering families and children, and tailoring immunization services to individual needs (Table 5).

A. Creating supportive and inclusive environments

The first theme, creating supportive and inclusive environments, emphasizes ensuring vaccination settings are accessible and welcoming for children with disabilities. Tuckerman (2024) highlights that involving school staff in the vaccination process can create a supportive environment, as schools are often seen as "safe spaces" by both parents and children, making them an ideal setting for vaccinations [17]. The physical environment also plays a crucial role, as children with disabilities, particularly those with sensory sensitivities, can experience heightened anxiety during vaccinations. Creating a calm, quiet, and non-threatening space is essential to reduce this anxiety. Bray (2022) underscores the significance of offering comforting techniques, such as allowing a parent to be present or using engaging distractions like toys or music, to alleviate stress and encourage vaccination [21]. Additionally, Ong et al. (2024) stress the importance of flexible and individualized care, where the needs of the child, such as sensory sensitivities or past negative experiences, are considered when designing vaccination procedures [18]. This approach ensures that children are more likely to undergo successful vaccinations without unnecessary distress.

Table 5. Lessons learned in ensuring equitable access for children with disabilities.

S/N	Subthemes	Authors	Findings
3.1	Creating supportive and inclusive environments	Tuckerman et al. (2024) [17]	Children with disabilities are very sensitive to environment, and anything that goes wrong can turn things around easily. The right physical environment with adequate infrastructure and distraction toys for children has a positive impact on the day of vaccination. The necessary efforts must be implemented to ensure that vaccination is successful at the first visit, as repeating the procedure requires extra effort. Some parents request information about alternative information that is outside the knowledge of school staff.
		Ong et al. (2023) [18]	The seduction pathway needs to be implemented in case vaccination with the distraction method is unsuccessful.
		Bray (2022) [21]	Positive techniques exist to assist the pediatric provider. It is essential to consider positioning and restraining the child with special needs during immunization procedures. Rather than lying down, sitting upright during immunizations increases a child's comfort level and sense of control.
		UNICEF and Leonard Cheshire Disability (2020) [25]	Healthcare facilities should be inclusive to take into consideration adolescents and children in the immunization program, and the message delivered for immunization need to be disability friendly to minimize the stigma that children with disabilities frequently confront.
		UNICEF (2023) [28]	The integration of immunization services for children with disabilities among the usual immunization programs that take place at school contributed to the uptake of vaccination among children with disabilities in Indonesia. Further children with disabilities need to be considered in health-sector plans and budgets at the national and sub-national levels.
3.2	Empowering families and children	Tuckerman et al. (2024) [17]	Parents need to be informed about the vaccination date and given the opportunity to attend, fostering a more inclusive and supportive immunization process. Anxiety is common, and some adolescents are scared before being vaccinated.
		Ong et al. (2023) [27]	Having a positive experience among the parents through involvement led to empowerment of these children.
		Okoro et al. (2015) [22]	There is a need to sustain regular health education aimed at emphasizing the benefits of vaccination and dispelling false concerns about the side effects of immunizations.
		Lin et al. (2010) [16]	Health income influenced the uptake level of vaccination, and sensitivity toward the families of children with disabilities is essential for ensuring that they are aware of the benefits of vaccination.
		Bray (2022) [21]	Adequate communication with clear and concise information from healthcare professionals for parents is fundamental in highlighting and convincing the parent to ensure that their child with disabilities adheres to the CDC-recommended immunization schedule.
		UNICEF (2024) [26]	Communicating the rights of children with disabilities to access health services, including immunization, is important to boost the immunization uptake.
3.3	Tailoring immunization services to individual needs	Tuckerman et al. (2024) [17]	The need for more parent information sessions about options and additional support for vaccination outside of the school program was raised by the parents. The immunization program in special schools was perceived as convenient; however, preparing students for vaccination day and catering to individual student needs were important for the vaccination outcome.
		Ong et al. (2023) [18]	Children with needle phobias were prepared through discussion to help them deal with anxiety, and this led to a good outcome. This was complimented by a mock trial with a nitrous mask to sedate the child, and the preparation of the parents through adequate information sharing was taken into consideration a priori. This shows how individual needs were employed.
		Bray (2022) [21]	Healthcare providers, like pediatric providers, need to have knowledge related to the specific needs of children with conditions such as autism to ensure that they are given sufficient information and vaccinated.
		UNICEF and Leonard Cheshire Disability (2020) [25]	Girls with disabilities are less likely to access health services in comparison to boys with disabilities; therefore, additional attention is required to tailor the immunization program to facilitate an increase in uptake in the mentioned group.
		UNICEF (2013) [27]	Immunization services for children with disabilities require special consideration to ensure their inclusiveness.
		UNICEF (2023) [28]	The MoH Regulation No. 25/2014 on Child Health Efforts covers the provision of health services for children with disabilities, whereby they may receive healthcare beyond the healthcare facilities in place, including specialized schools, inclusive education schools, households, and other institutions. In this regulation, the health centers near specialized schools are obliged to provide immunization services at those schools.

B. Empowering families and children

The findings of this review revealed that empowering families and children, focusing on the importance of involving parents in the vaccination process, and providing them with the tools and knowledge to advocate for their children's needs were key to the program's success. Ong et al. (2024) note that parental empowerment is a key strategy, where parents feel more confident and capable when they are provided with clear information and involved in decision-making, especially when it comes to the use of techniques like distraction or sedation [18]. This empowerment helps address vaccine hesitancy, as parents are better informed and more comfortable with the vaccination process. Bray (2022) also highlights the value of communication, noting that honest and transparent conversations between healthcare providers and parents are essential for building trust and reducing anxiety [21]. Parents can feel better equipped to manage their child's healthcare needs in the long term when provided with ongoing support and addressing concerns about future vaccinations. This sense of empowerment can also extend to the children themselves, as preparing them with appropriate information and expectations can help them cope better with the vaccination process [16,18,21].

C. Tailoring immunization services to individual needs

This review also revealed that tailoring immunization services to individual needs emphasizes the necessity of adapting healthcare practices to accommodate the unique challenges faced by children with disabilities and is key to program success. Bray (2022) advocates for a neurodiversity-sensitive approach, where healthcare providers are educated about the specific needs of children with conditions such as autism or ADHD [21]. This ensures that healthcare providers respect individual differences and provide care that is not only effective but also compassionate. Tailoring immunization strategies, such as distraction techniques or providing sensory-friendly environments, can help children with neurodevelopmental disorders feel more comfortable and less anxious. Furthermore, both Tuckerman (2024) and Ong et al. (2024) point out that individualized planning, including offering multiple preparation options for both parents and children, increases the likelihood of successful vaccination [17,18]. These personalized approaches, whether through social stories or flexibility in the vaccination setting, ensure that children with disabilities are not excluded from immunization programs due to their unique needs.

4. Discussion

This review identifies key barriers and strategies for improving immunization coverage among children with disabilities and reducing zero-dose children, particularly in underserved and marginalized communities. The findings highlight the complex, multifaceted nature of the issue and offer valuable insights into how immunization programs can be designed and improved to ensure that children with disabilities are not excluded.

The barriers identified in this review emphasize the critical gaps in healthcare systems, social support, and societal attitudes toward disabilities. These barriers include inadequate healthcare resources, lack of staff training, and inconsistencies in healthcare service delivery, especially in rural areas. Misunderstandings about disabilities and their medical implications can lead to misclassification as vaccine contraindications, further discouraging vaccination efforts [17,22]. Furthermore, inadequate follow-up care and logistical challenges like unclear clinic locations and access issues contribute to missed vaccinations. These barriers underscore the need for comprehensive strategies at multiple health system levels. Strategies to address these barriers focus on enhancing accessibility and service delivery, particularly in underserved regions. Mobile vaccination units and strengthening infrastructure in rural areas are essential for reaching remote communities [18]. Logistical support, including clear signage and support for parents to navigate the vaccination process, is critical for reducing barriers to vaccination [21]. Moreover, creating low-sensory environments for vaccination, which alleviate anxiety for children with disabilities, is another essential strategy for improving immunization outcomes [18].

At the health facility level, offering individualized care through distraction and sedation techniques and the involvement of parents in decision-making can significantly increase vaccination uptake [21].

Designing immunization programs to reduce zero-dose children and ensure equitable access requires addressing the systemic and social factors that prevent children with disabilities from receiving vaccines [6]. The findings suggest that creating supportive and inclusive environments is key to improving immunization rates. Involving school staff in vaccination planning can help provide a safe and trusted space for both children and parents, making vaccination efforts more accessible [17]. Schools can be critical in ensuring a supportive environment, especially when parents perceive them as safe spaces [28,29]. Health systems should adapt to provide calm, non-threatening vaccination spaces, especially for children with sensory sensitivities, and use comforting techniques like toys or music to reduce anxiety [30].

This review revealed empowering families, particularly parents, as another critical strategy. Similarly, earlier work highlighted that providing parents with the knowledge and support to navigate the vaccination process, alongside involving them in decision-making regarding vaccination techniques, can reduce vaccine hesitancy and increase confidence in vaccination programs [31]. Transparent communication addresses concerns and ensures families feel supported throughout the vaccination journey [32]. The need for tailored, individualized care was a recurrent theme in this review. This includes designing personalized vaccination pathways considering each child's medical, psychological, and developmental needs. Previous research by Leask 2006 and Helps 2019 highlighted the need for healthcare providers to receive training on neurodiversity to offer more respectful and accommodating care for children with neurodevelopmental disorders like autism or ADHD [33,34]. Tailoring immunization strategies to address the specific needs of these children is essential for improving vaccination outcomes.

4.1. Intersecting Stigma, Socioeconomic Disparities, and Disability

According to our review, stigma and socioeconomic disparities might intersect with disability to create compounded barriers to immunization. Stigma associated with disability often results in social exclusion, which limits access to healthcare services, including vaccination programs. Families of children with disabilities may face discrimination within their communities, further deterring them from seeking healthcare. This stigma is amplified in lower socioeconomic settings, where families may lack the financial resources to navigate systemic barriers or afford transportation to healthcare facilities. Additionally, limited parental education and cultural misconceptions about both disability and vaccines exacerbate these challenges, leading to reduced awareness of immunization benefits. For example, families living in poverty may prioritize immediate financial needs over healthcare, while stigma can prevent them from accessing community-based interventions. Addressing these intersecting issues requires a multi-faceted approach that includes anti-stigma campaigns, socioeconomic support programs, and culturally tailored community engagement initiatives. Such efforts can promote inclusive environments where families feel supported and empowered to seek immunization for their children, regardless of disability or economic status.

The intersection of disability with other identities, such as gender and ethnicity, compounds barriers to immunization access. Girls with disabilities, for instance, often face heightened discrimination due to societal biases that prioritize male children for healthcare resources in specific cultural contexts. Similarly, ethnic minority groups, such as Indigenous populations in Latin America or tribal communities in South Asia, may experience systemic exclusion from healthcare services. When combined with disability, these factors exacerbate inequities, leading to lower vaccination rates among these subgroups. Language barriers, geographic isolation, and mistrust in healthcare systems further hinder access for ethnically marginalized children with disabilities. For example, Indigenous children with disabilities may lack access to culturally tailored immunization programs, reinforcing health disparities. Addressing these intersecting barriers requires intersectional approaches that account for these populations' unique needs and experiences, such as culturally sensitive outreach campaigns, gender-inclusive policies, and partnerships with community leaders to foster trust and inclusivity.

4.2. *Practical Implementation, Scaling, and Evaluation of Identified Strategies*

4.2.1. Tailored Interventions

To implement tailored interventions, healthcare providers can adopt strategies such as individualized vaccination plans and low-sensory environments in clinics. Training workshops and simulation exercises for healthcare workers can ensure sensitivity to the needs of children with disabilities. These interventions can be scaled through partnerships with organizations specializing in disability care, enabling consistent support across multiple regions.

4.2.2. Mobile Vaccination Units

Mobile units can address geographic barriers by bringing vaccines directly to underserved communities. These units should be equipped with accessibility features, such as ramps and quiet areas, and staffed by personnel trained in disability-inclusive care. Government funding and donor partnerships can help expand such programs nationally, with clear targets for reaching rural and marginalized populations.

4.2.3. Community Engagement

Local leaders, disability advocacy groups, and parent associations can co-design culturally sensitive education campaigns. These initiatives should include testimonials, visual aids, and multilingual materials to combat stigma and misconceptions. Pilot programs can test effectiveness before scaling to larger communities, with adjustments based on feedback from local stakeholders.

4.2.4. School-Based Vaccination Programs

Schools are ideal settings for reaching children with disabilities, particularly in specialized education environments. Policies supporting routine vaccination days, with individualized care plans and consent protocols, can streamline implementation. Scaling such programs requires collaboration between health and education ministries, alongside regular evaluations of student and caregiver satisfaction.

4.2.5. Adapting High-Income Country Strategies for Low- and Middle-Income Countries

High-income countries (HICs) have successfully implemented school-based vaccination programs, digital health records, and targeted outreach campaigns to improve immunization coverage among children with disabilities. For instance, school-based vaccination in specialist education settings in Australia has shown significant success by addressing behavioral challenges and reducing access barriers [28,35]. Similarly, using electronic health records in countries like Denmark and the United States enables efficient tracking of vaccine coverage and identification of under-vaccinated groups [36,37]. However, these approaches require adaptation to fit the unique challenges of LMICs. Resource limitations, infrastructural gaps, and cultural differences necessitate cost-effective modifications, such as using mobile vaccination units to reach underserved areas and employing community health workers for targeted outreach. By adopting lessons from HICs while incorporating the local context, LMICs can develop scalable, sustainable immunization programs that address the needs of children with disabilities effectively.

4.2.6. Monitoring and Evaluation (M&E)

The success of immunization programs in high-income and low- and middle-income countries underscores the importance of robust M&E frameworks. For instance, Australia's school-based vaccination programs incorporate real-time electronic tracking systems that monitor vaccine coverage rates among students with disabilities, providing actionable data for targeted interventions [28,38]. In contrast, Uganda's community health worker (CHW) model includes regular household surveys to assess immunization uptake and identify gaps in rural and underserved areas [39]. Metrics used in these programs include vaccination completion rates, caregiver satisfaction levels, and reductions in missed vaccination appointments. Additionally, participatory approaches, such as involving caregivers and disability advocates in program evaluations, ensure that M&E systems address the specific needs of children with disabilities. Incorporating these practices into future frameworks can enhance accountability and guide continuous improvement, particularly in resource-constrained settings.

4.2.7. Funding and Policy Advocacy

Securing sustainable funding is critical for scaling. Policymakers should allocate specific budget lines for disability-inclusive immunization programs, with international agencies offering technical and financial support. Advocacy campaigns can build momentum for inclusive immunization policies, leveraging the documented benefits of these strategies to demonstrate value.

4.3. Limitations of the Study

A. Addressing data gaps

This review identified several critical data gaps that hinder a comprehensive understanding of immunization barriers for children with disabilities in LMICs. Notably, there is a lack of longitudinal studies that track vaccination coverage and health outcomes over time, making it difficult to assess the long-term effectiveness of interventions. Additionally, certain disability types, such as sensory impairments or rare developmental conditions, are underrepresented in the literature. This underrepresentation limits the generalizability of findings and may result in overlooked barriers or ineffective strategies for these subgroups. Furthermore, geographic disparities in research focus exist, with limited data from rural settings where systemic challenges are often more pronounced. To address these gaps, future research should prioritize inclusive study designs that encompass diverse disability types and settings, incorporate longitudinal methodologies, and focus on equity-driven outcomes to inform targeted and effective immunization policies.

Bridging the identified data gaps requires adopting innovative methodologies and forging strategic partnerships. Participatory action research (PAR) offers a promising approach, actively involving children with disabilities, their caregivers, and community stakeholders in designing and implementing studies [40]. This approach ensures that research questions and interventions are informed by lived experiences, fostering relevance and inclusivity. Additionally, longitudinal cohort studies can provide insights into the long-term effectiveness of strategies, such as tracking vaccination uptake and health outcomes across different disability types and settings. Partnerships with disability advocacy organizations, community health workers, and international agencies like WHO and UNICEF can facilitate resource sharing and capacity building, particularly in low- and middle-income countries. Leveraging technology, such as digital health records and geospatial mapping, can improve data collection, monitor immunization disparities, and identify underserved populations. By adopting these methodologies and partnerships, researchers can generate robust evidence to inform policy and practice, advancing equitable immunization coverage for all children.

B. Methodological limitations and potential biases

The reviewed studies revealed several methodological limitations that may have influenced our findings. A significant issue was the reliance on convenience sampling, which often led to unrepresentative study populations, a lack of standard error measures, and selection bias. For example, families with greater access to healthcare or higher awareness of vaccination programs may have been more likely to participate, potentially overestimating vaccination coverage and underrepresenting those facing severe barriers. Additionally, many studies relied on self-reported data from caregivers, which is prone to recall bias and social desirability bias. Caregivers might overstate vaccine uptake to align with perceived social norms or expectations, especially when vaccination campaigns are highly promoted. Furthermore, variations in data collection methods and outcome definitions across studies make it challenging to compare results or draw generalizable conclusions. Addressing these biases in future research will require rigorous sampling techniques, standardized data collection tools, and the inclusion of diverse perspectives, particularly from underrepresented disability groups (i.e., sampling design).

Since only articles published in English were reviewed, it is possible that useful articles in other languages were excluded. It is important to note that this review did not examine whether vaccines were provided free of charge or if parents had to pay for them at the health facility. Additionally, only electronically available manuscripts were included in this review.

Another notable limitation is that this review utilized a search strategy that included only two electronic databases, PubMed and Google Scholar. While these databases are widely recognized for their extensive coverage of health-related literature, limiting the search to them may have excluded relevant studies indexed in other databases. Additionally, while efforts were made to enhance the robustness of the search by including gray literature from reputable organizations such as UNICEF and the World Health Organization, some pertinent studies may have been overlooked. Future reviews could benefit from a more comprehensive search strategy that includes multiple databases and a wider range of information sources to capture the full spectrum of relevant literature. Finally, a formal assessment of the risk of bias was not conducted due to the limited number of studies retrieved. This limitation suggests that the findings should be interpreted cautiously, as unexamined biases may influence the reported outcomes.

C. Broader methodological discussion

A critique of the methodologies used in the reviewed studies reveals several notable limitations and biases within the field. Many studies relied heavily on cross-sectional designs, which provide only a snapshot of immunization barriers and outcomes. While helpful in identifying immediate issues, these designs fail to capture longitudinal trends, such as vaccine uptake changes over time or interventions' long-term impacts. Additionally, the reliance on convenience sampling was prevalent, often resulting in unrepresentative study populations. For instance, children with severe or less-visible disabilities might have been underrepresented, as caregivers facing significant barriers may not participate in studies.

Another methodological limitation is information bias, which lies in inconsistent data collection tools and metrics. Studies varied widely in how they measured outcomes, such as vaccine coverage rates or caregiver perceptions, complicating comparisons across findings. Some studies used self-reported data from caregivers, which may introduce recall bias, while others lacked standard definitions for key concepts like "accessibility" or "barriers".

Lastly, geographic and cultural contexts were often insufficiently addressed. Many studies conducted in LMICs lacked region-specific adaptations to account for unique barriers such as cultural stigma or infrastructural deficits. Similarly, limited participatory research approaches meant that the perspectives of children with disabilities and their families were not always incorporated into study designs or analyses. Addressing these methodological issues is crucial for developing robust, generalizable evidence for inclusive immunization programs.

D. Inconsistencies in definitions

The variability in the definition of "disability" across the included studies posed challenges for both inclusion and analysis. Some studies defined disability narrowly, focusing on specific conditions such as intellectual disabilities or autism spectrum disorders, while others used broader definitions that included physical, sensory, and developmental disabilities. This inconsistency affected the comparability of findings, as interventions effective for one subgroup may not apply to others. For example, studies targeting children with physical disabilities emphasized environmental accessibility, whereas those involving neurodevelopmental disorders often focused on behavioral support and family engagement. These differing definitions also influenced the inclusion process; studies that lacked a clear or comprehensive definition of disability were excluded to maintain methodological rigor. Addressing this variability required careful thematic analysis to synthesize findings while acknowledging the heterogeneity in the study populations and outcomes.

4.4. Future Research Directions

Despite the insights gained from this review, multiple knowledge gaps hinder the development of inclusive immunization strategies for children with disabilities in LMICs. Addressing these gaps requires a concerted effort to expand the scope and improve the rigor of future research:

A. Longitudinal and Rigorous Study Designs

Long-term impact: Current evidence on the effectiveness of interventions often relies on cross-sectional or short-term studies. Future studies should adopt longitudinal designs (e.g., cohort or panel studies) that track children over time, assessing how immunization uptake and caregiver attitudes evolve as children progress through various stages of the vaccination schedule.

Rigorous sampling: Many studies rely on convenience or opportunistic sampling methods, potentially excluding the most marginalized populations. Probability-based sampling and targeted outreach strategies (e.g., partnering with community health workers) can help capture more diverse participants, including those in remote rural settings.

B. Understudied Disability Types

Visual and hearing impairments: Most existing studies focus on intellectual or physical disabilities, while sensory impairments, such as blindness or deafness, remain underexplored. These populations may face unique barriers to immunization, including communication challenges, inaccessible health education materials, and stigma or misconceptions.

Complex/multiple disabilities: Children with co-occurring conditions (e.g., autism spectrum disorder plus a physical disability) often have complex healthcare needs but are rarely included in research. Future investigations should aim to capture the intersectional experiences of these children, offering a more detailed understanding of how overlapping disabilities multiply barriers to immunization.

C. Participatory and Community-Engaged Methods

Participatory action research (PAR): Engaging caregivers, children (where appropriate), community leaders, and disability advocates in designing and implementing studies can yield richer, more context-specific insights. This approach can also foster community ownership, improving the likelihood that recommended interventions are both practical and culturally acceptable.

Stakeholder involvement: Collaboration with local health authorities, schools, and NGOs specializing in disability services can ensure that interventions are feasible and sustainable within specific cultural and resource contexts.

D. Standardization of Definitions and Outcome Measures

Adoption of the WHO ICF: Building on the work of this review, future studies should use the International Classification of Functioning, ICF, to operationalize disability consistently, thereby improving comparability across different research settings.

Aligned reporting of outcomes: Standardizing immunization coverage metrics (e.g., consistently defining "fully immunized", "zero-dose", and "dropout") facilitates meta-analyses and cross-study comparisons. Clear outcome reporting also supports better monitoring and evaluation of interventions over time.

By prioritizing longitudinal research, inclusive sampling, standardized definitions, and participatory methods, the field can generate a more robust evidence base to inform policy and practice. These steps will not only deepen our understanding of immunization barriers experienced by children with diverse disability types but also drive the development of targeted, equitable, and sustainable solutions in low- and middle-income contexts.

5. Conclusions

In conclusion, the strategies to improve immunization coverage for children with disabilities include healthcare system reforms, tailored interventions, and societal awareness campaigns. Enhancing accessibility to services, adapting vaccination procedures to meet the needs of children with disabilities, and addressing stigma and education gaps were identified as essential strategies to ensure immunization programs can be more inclusive and effective in reaching children with disabilities. Scaling these strategies requires a concerted effort to adapt healthcare systems, train healthcare providers, and engage communities in creating a supportive environment for children with disabilities.

Call to Action for Inclusive Immunization

This study underscores the urgent need for governments, non-governmental organizations (NGOs), and researchers to prioritize inclusive immunization programs for children with disabilities. Governments should enact policies mandating disability-inclusive practices, allocate dedicated funding for tailored interventions, and incorporate accessibility metrics into national health surveys. NGOs can play a key role in implementing community-based programs, conducting caregiver education campaigns, and advocating for systemic change at local and global levels. Researchers must address data gaps by designing longitudinal studies, developing standardized definitions of disability, and ensuring the representation of under-served populations, including those with sensory impairments or living in rural areas.

Collaboration between these stakeholders is critical to scaling successful strategies, such as mobile vaccination units, low-sensory environments, and school-based programs, while promoting an evidence-based culture of continuous improvement. By taking these steps, the global health community can advance equitable vaccine access and strengthen healthcare systems to serve all children, regardless of their abilities.

Author Contributions: Conceptualization, G.M.; methodology, P.G.I. and O.M.; software, D.F.C. and F.D.M.; validation, O.M. and T.D. (Tapiwa Dhliwayo); writing—original draft preparation, G.M., D.F.C. and Z.M.; writing—review and editing, T.D. (Tapiwa Dhliwayo), P.G.I., O.M. and T.D. (Tafadzwa Dzinamarira); supervision, T.D. (Tafadzwa Dzinamarira). All authors have read and agreed to the published version of the manuscript.

Funding: This research received no external funding.

Institutional Review Board Statement: Not applicable.

Informed Consent Statement: Not applicable.

Data Availability Statement: No new data were created or analyzed in this study. Data sharing is not applicable to this article.

Acknowledgments: Authors acknowledge Pierre Gashema and Eric Saramba for their support with database searches.

Conflicts of Interest: The authors declare no conflicts of interest.

References

1. Feikin, D.R.; Karron, R.A.; Saha, S.K.; Sparrow, E.; Srikantiah, P.; Weinberger, D.M.; Zar, H.J. The full value of immunisation against respiratory syncytial virus for infants younger than 1 year: Effects beyond prevention of acute respiratory illness. *Lancet Infect. Dis.* **2024**, *24*, e318–e327. [PubMed]
2. Zhu, J.; Cole, C.B.; Fihman, J.; Adjagba, A.; Dasic, M.; Cernuschi, T. Opportunities to accelerate immunization progress in middle-income countries. *Vaccine* **2024**, *42*, S98–S106.
3. Thaheem, A.K.; Qureshi, A.U.; Sarkar, A.; Liu, G. The Ripple Effect of Vaccines: Health, Economic, and Social Dimensions. *J. Soc. Inform. Glob. Health* **2023**, *2*, 40–48.
4. Rice, I.; Opondo, C.; Nyesigomwe, L.; Ekude, D.; Magezi, J.; Kalanzi, A.; Kerac, M.; Hayes, J.; Robello, M.; Halfman, S. Children with disabilities lack access to nutrition, health and WASH services: A secondary data analysis. *Matern. Child Nutr.* **2024**, *20*, e13642.
5. Mwangi, L.W.; Abuga, J.A.; Cottrell, E.; Kariuki, S.M.; Kinyanjui, S.M.; Newton, C.R. Barriers to access and utilization of healthcare by children with neurological impairments and disability in low-and middle-income countries: A systematic review. *Wellcome Open Res.* **2022**, *6*, 61.
6. O'Neill, J.; Newall, F.; Antolovich, G.; Lima, S.; Danchin, M. Vaccination in people with disability: A review. *Hum. Vaccines Immunother.* **2020**, *16*, 7–15.
7. Thota, A.B.; Mogo, E.I.; Igbelina, C.D.; Sheaf, G.S.; Mustafa, R.; Bakrania, S.; Encalada, A.V.; Wood, G.A. *Inclusion Matters: Inclusive Interventions for Children with Disabilities—An Evidence and Gap Map from Low-and Middle-Income Countries*; UNICEF Office of Research-Innocenti: Florence, Italy, 2022.
8. Emerson, E.; Robertson, J.; Baines, S.; Hatton, C. Vaccine coverage among children with and without intellectual disabilities in the UK: Cross sectional study. *BMC Public Health* **2019**, *19*, 748.
9. Shamseer, L.; Moher, D.; Clarke, M.; Ghersi, D.; Liberati, A.; Petticrew, M.; Shekelle, P.; Stewart, L.A. Preferred reporting items for systematic review and meta-analysis protocols (PRISMA-P) 2015: Elaboration and explanation. *BMJ* **2015**, *349*, g7647.
10. Akers, J.; Aguiar-Ibáñez, R.; Baba-Akbari, A. *Systematic Reviews: CRD's Guidance for Undertaking Reviews in Health Care*; Centre for Reviews and Dissemination, University of York: York, UK, 2009.
11. Robertson-Malt, S. JBI's systematic reviews: Presenting and interpreting findings. *AJN Am. J. Nurs.* **2014**, *114*, 49–54.
12. Kostanjsek, N.F.I. Use of The International Classification of Functioning, Disability and Health (ICF) as a conceptual framework and common language for disability statistics and health information systems. *BMC Public Health* **2011**, *11*, S3.
13. Leonardi, M.; Lee, H.; Kostanjsek, N.; Fornari, A.; Raggi, A.; Martinuzzi, A.; Yáñez, M.; Almborg, A.-H.; Fresk, M.; Besstrashnova, Y. 20 years of ICF—International classification of functioning, disability and health: Uses and applications around the world. *Int. J. Environ. Res. Public Health* **2022**, *19*, 11321. [CrossRef]
14. Team, T.E. *EndNote, EndNote X9*; Clarivate: Philadelphia, PA, USA, 2013.
15. Covidence Systematic Review Software, Veritas Health Innovation, Melbourne, Australia. Available online: www.covidence.org (accessed on 3 January 2025).
16. Lin, J.-D.; Lin, P.-Y.; Lin, L.-P. Universal hepatitis B vaccination coverage in children and adolescents with intellectual disabilities. *Res. Dev. Disabil.* **2010**, *31*, 338–344.
17. Tuckerman, J.; Mohamed, Y.; Justice, F.; Andersson, T.; Wyatt, K.; Broun, K.; Bastable, A.; Overmars, I.; Kaufman, J.; Danchin, M. Stakeholder perspectives of immunisation delivery for adolescents with disability in specialist schools in Victoria, Australia:'we need a vaccination pathway'. *BMC Public Health* **2024**, *24*, 1973.
18. Ong, N.; Brogan, D.; Lucien, A.; Wolman, S.; Campbell, D.; Deng, L.; Koirala, A.; Garg, P.; Sharma, K. The development and evaluation of a vaccination pathway for children with intellectual and developmental disability and needle fear. *Paediatr. Neonatal Pain* **2024**, *6*, 1–9. [PubMed]
19. Rosenberg, R.E.; Law, J.K.; Anderson, C.; Samango-Sprouse, C.; Law, P.A. Survey of vaccine beliefs and practices among families affected by autism spectrum disorders. *Clin. Pediatr.* **2013**, *52*, 871–874.

20. Fong, E.; Adil, D.; Mesterman, R. 28 Vaccination experiences for children with special needs-An examination of the impact of behaviours on vaccine uptake. *Paediatr. Child Health* **2024**, *29*, e12.
21. Bray, A. Vaccination Strategies to Keep Children with Special Needs Healthy. 2022. Available online: https://www.clinicaladvisor.com/features/vaccinating-children-with-special-needs/ (accessed on 1 December 2024).
22. Okoro, J.; Ojinnaka, N.; Ikefuna, A.; Onyenwe, N. Sociodemographic influences on immunization of children with chronic neurological disorders in Enugu, Nigeria. *Trials Vaccinol.* **2015**, *4*, 9–13. [CrossRef]
23. O'Neill, J.; Newall, F.; Antolovich, G.; Lima, S.; Danchin, M. The uptake of adolescent vaccinations through the school immunisation program in specialist schools in Victoria, Australia. *Vaccine* **2019**, *37*, 272–279. [CrossRef]
24. Mactaggart, I.; Kuper, H.; Murthy, G.V.; Sagar, J.; Oye, J.; Polack, S. Assessing health and rehabilitation needs of people with disabilities in Cameroon and India. *Disabil. Rehabil.* **2016**, *38*, 1757–1764. [CrossRef]
25. United Nations Children's Fund and Leonard Cheshire Disability and Inclusive Development Centre. *Disability Prevention Efforts and Disability Rights: Finding Common Ground on Immunization Efforts*; UNICEF: New York, NY, USA, 2020; Available online: https://www.unicef.org/sites/default/files/2022-10/GIP02115_UNICEF_Children-with-Disabilities-Factsheet-final%20-%20accessible.pdf (accessed on 3 January 2025).
26. United Nations Children's Fund. UNICEF Humanitarian Action for Children 2024 Overview. Available online: https://www.unicef.org/media/149906/file/Humanitarian-Action-for-Children-2024-Overview.pdf (accessed on 15 January 2025).
27. United Nations Children's Fund. Children with Disabilities: UNICEF Data 2013. Available online: https://data.unicef.org/wp-content/uploads/2015/12/SOWC_2013_75.pdf (accessed on 15 January 2025).
28. United Nations Children's Fund. The State of World's Children 2023. Available online: https://www.unicef.org/eca/reports/sowc2023-eca (accessed on 15 January 2025).
29. Wang, E.; Clymer, J.; Davis-Hayes, C.; Buttenheim, A. Nonmedical exemptions from school immunization requirements: A systematic review. *Am. J. Public Health* **2014**, *104*, e62–e84.
30. Elias, E.R.; Murphy, N.A.; Liptak, G.S.; Adams, R.C.; Burke, R.; Friedman, S.L.; Houtrow, A.; Kalichman, M.; Kuo, D. Home care of children and youth with complex health care needs and technology dependencies. *Pediatrics* **2012**, *129*, 996–1005.
31. Ashfield, S.; Donelle, L. Parental online information access and childhood vaccination decisions in North America: Scoping review. *J. Med. Internet Res.* **2020**, *22*, e20002.
32. Healy, C.M.; Pickering, L.K. How to communicate with vaccine-hesitant parents. *Pediatrics* **2011**, *127*, S127–S133. [PubMed]
33. Leask, J.; Chapman, S.; Hawe, P.; Burgess, M. What maintains parental support for vaccination when challenged by anti-vaccination messages? A qualitative study. *Vaccine* **2006**, *24*, 7238–7245.
34. Helps, C.; Leask, J.; Barclay, L.; Carter, S. Understanding non-vaccinating parents' views to inform and improve clinical encounters: A qualitative study in an Australian community. *BMJ Open* **2019**, *9*, e026299.
35. Ward, K.; Quinn, H.E.; Bachelor, M.A.; Bryant, V.; Campbell-Lloyd, S.; Newbound, A.; Scully, M.; Webby, R.J.; McIntyre, P.B. Adolescent school-based vaccination in Australia. *Commun. Dis. Intell. Q. Rep.* **2013**, *37*, E156–E167.
36. Krause, T.G.; Jakobsen, S.S.; Haarh, M.; Mølbak, K. The Danish vaccination register. *Euro Surveill. Bull. Eur. Sur Les Mal. Transm. Eur. Commun. Dis. Bull.* **2012**, *17*, 20155.
37. Murthy, N.C.; Rodgers, L.E.; Pabst, L.J.; Fiebelkorn, A.P.; Ng, T. Progress in Childhood Vaccination Data in Immunization Information Systems—United States, 2013–2016. *Morb. Mortal. Wkly. Rep.* **2017**, *66*, 1178–1181.
38. Carter, A.; Klinner, C.; Young, A.; Strnadová, I.; Wong, H.; Vujovich-Dunn, C.; Newman, C.E.; Davies, C.; Skinner, S.R.; Danchin, M. "I Thought It Was Better to Be Safe than Sorry": Factors Influencing Parental Decisions on HPV and Other Adolescent Vaccinations for Students with Intellectual Disability and/or Autism in New South Wales, Australia. *Vaccines* **2024**, *12*, 922. [CrossRef]
39. Bruce, J.; Chantler, T.; Kumakech, E.; Mawanda, A.; Olorunsaiye, C.Z.; Schmucker, L.; Kiapi, L.; Landegger, J.; Webster, J. Evaluation of a data-informed community engagement strategy to increase immunisation coverage in northern Uganda: A cluster-randomised controlled trial with an embedded process evaluation. *Lancet Glob. Health* **2018**, *6*, S15.
40. van der Mark, E.J.; Zuiderent-Jerak, T.; Dedding, C.W.M.; Conradie, I.M.; Broerse, J.E.W. Connecting relational wellbeing and participatory action research: Reflections on 'unlikely' transformations among women caring for disabled children in South Africa. *J. Glob. Ethics* **2023**, *19*, 80–104. [CrossRef]

vaccines

MDPI

Article

Routine Immunization Microplanning Challenges and Opportunities in Low- and Middle-Income Countries: A Mixed-Method Landscape Analysis

Nicole Salisbury [1], Iqbal Hossain [2], Parysa Oskouipour [2], Audry Hong [1], Elan Ebeling [1], Jessica C. Shearer [1] and Emily Grapa [1,*]

1 PATH, Seattle, WA 98121, USA; nsalisbury@path.org (N.S.); eebeling@path.org (E.E.); jess.shearer@gmail.com (J.C.S.)
2 JSI Research and Training Institute, Arlington, VA 22202, USA; iqbal_hossain@jsi.com (I.H.); parysa_oskouipour@jsi.com (P.O.)
* Correspondence: egrapa@path.org

Abstract: Background: Microplanning is widely recognized as a critical tool for improving immunization coverage and equity and is considered a core component of routine immunization. However, there is limited evidence on how microplans are developed and implemented and the effectiveness of microplanning. As such, this study sought to review the existing evidence on implementation and institutionalization of microplanning; identify strategies to improve microplanning; and document evidence on new approaches to microplanning, including digitally enhanced and integrated microplanning. Methods: We employed a three-stage mixed-method approach. First, we conducted a literature review on microplanning for routine immunization. Second, we administered an online survey to gather insights into the factors that constrained and enabled microplanning in low-resource settings. Third, we conducted key informant interviews to better understand the barriers and enablers. Results: We found a paucity of published literature describing the drivers and effectiveness of microplanning and how to sustain it over time. Our review indicates that factors at both the development and implementation stages influence implementation and whether the process is sustained over time. These include the level of community engagement and health care worker ownership, access to data, the complexity of the microplanning tools, and the extent to which supervisors follow up on the plans. Conclusion: Our review indicates that microplanning is successful when health care workers and communities are engaged in the development process. While these findings highlight the benefits of a 'bottom-up' approach to microplanning, this may be more resource-intensive, and there remains a need for more research on the costs and benefits.

Keywords: immunization; vaccine; microplanning; microplan; LMIC

1. Introduction

Microplanning is widely recognized as a critical tool for improving routine immunization coverage and equity. Microplanning is an intervention used to systematically define the activities, resources, timing, and location of immunization services, particularly to reach underserved or under-immunized populations. Initially introduced to immunization programs as a component of polio eradication activities, microplanning was incorporated into global guidance for routine immunization with the introduction of the Reaching Every District (RED) approach in 2002 [1].

The RED approach was developed by WHO, UNICEF, Gavi, and other technical partners with the aim of improving immunization coverage in poorer-performing health districts and facilities [1]. The RED approach outlines operational components that immunization program staff can follow to improve immunization systems. Key among these components is the development and implementation of a comprehensive microplan using local data to map the target population, plan appropriate activities to reach the target population, monitor the data, and work with the community to track children who have missed routine immunization doses.

Microplanning is a core component of routine immunization and has been incorporated into several iterations of global guidelines [2,3]. However, there is limited evidence on whether and how these guidelines are followed in practice, particularly in resource-constrained settings. Most low- and middle-income countries (LMICs) have adopted microplanning through the RED approach, but there is a lack of rigorous studies measuring its effectiveness for increasing routine immunization coverage [4]. Moreover, there is a lack of evidence about whether and how microplanning processes have been institutionalized (or routinized) over time, with microplans being updated at regular intervals and implementation being adjusted as needed. Anecdotal evidence suggests that even where developed, microplans are still suboptimally implemented and institutionalized in routine immunization programs.

MOMENTUM Routine Immunization Transformation and Equity (hereafter referred to as "the project") applies best practices and explores innovations to address entrenched obstacles in immunization and increase equitable immunization coverage. The project is USAID's flagship technical assistance mechanism for immunization in more than 20 countries and seeks to contribute to the global evidence base on interventions to improve routine immunization coverage. The project led this study to the following:

1. Review the existing evidence on the implementation and institutionalization of microplanning for routine immunization;
2. Identify strategies to improve microplanning for routine immunization;
3. Document evidence on new approaches to microplanning which could be applicable for routine immunization contexts, including digitally enhanced microplanning and integrated microplanning.

2. Materials and Methods

2.1. Study Design

The project employed a three-stage mixed-method approach to investigate factors affecting microplanning implementation and institutionalization in LMICs. First, the team conducted a literature review of peer-reviewed and gray literature on microplanning for routine immunization. Second, the team administered an online survey designed to gather insights into the drivers of microplanning from national and subnational immunization program staff and technical partners. Third, the team conducted in-depth key informant interviews with a subset of stakeholders identified in the survey to better understand the enablers and barriers to successful implementation and institutionalization of microplanning. The project employed the Consolidated Framework for Implementation Research (CFIR) throughout the research process to guide the analysis [5].

2.1.1. Literature Review

The team searched three databases (PubMed, CABO Web of Science, and Proquest) for relevant articles using the following search strings: ("vaccine" OR "immunization" OR "immunization program" OR "routine immunization") AND ("microplan" OR "micro plan"). The team reviewed only English language articles and did not restrict articles by date of publication. To augment the search, the team reviewed references of relevant articles to identify additional sources and performed a Google search to identify relevant gray literature.

The literature review was conducted from June to July 2023. Initial searches yielded a total of 117 results. After screening based on exclusion criteria and using a double review on a random selection of abstracts to minimize exclusion bias, the team included 39 articles, reports, or briefs for full-text review (Figure 1). Of these sources, 27 described experiences with microplanning in Africa, 10 in Asia, and 2 in Latin America and the Caribbean. Articles were coded using Excel according to the six domains of the CFIR framework (innovation, outer setting, inner setting, individuals, implementation process, and implementation outcomes) to distill the factors that constrained and enabled microplanning implementation.

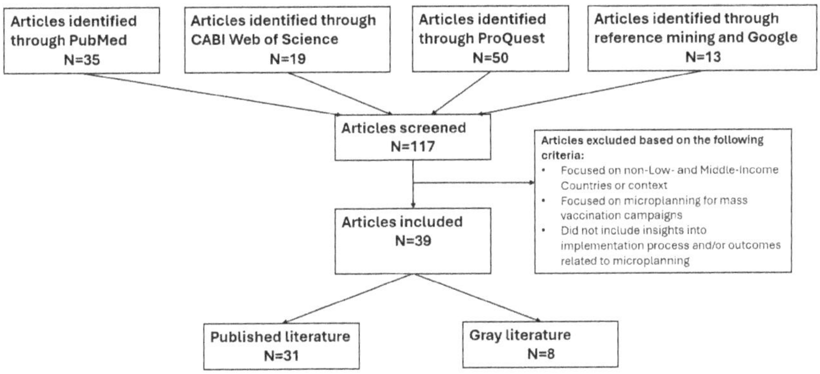

Figure 1. Flow chart diagram of article selection.

2.1.2. Online Survey

To better understand the factors that influence microplanning implementation, the project developed and administered an 11-question online survey targeting stakeholders with experience implementing microplanning in LMICs. The survey tool (Google Forms) included three sections based on the crucial stages of the microplanning process: development, implementation, and institutionalization. The survey was disseminated from June to August 2023 via three online forums (Boost Community Network, Zero-Dose Community of Practice, and TechNet-21 Forum) whose reach includes immunization program managers from LMICs at national and subnational levels. Respondents were given the option to provide their name and contact information if they were open to being interviewed but were not required to do so. Survey results were exported to Excel. Summary statistics were analyzed, and open-ended questions were coded according to the CFIR framework. Survey results were primarily used to (i) identify key respondents for interviews and (ii) inform the development of topic areas for the interview guides used in the third step of the research process.

2.1.3. Key Informant Interviews

As a third step, the team conducted in-depth semi-structured key informant interviews with stakeholders to learn more about their experiences with microplanning implementation and institutionalization. From the countries represented in online survey responses, the project employed a purposive sampling approach to select a subset of countries with varying levels of partner support for routine immunization to reflect different resource contexts within immunization programs. The key informants included technical partners and national or subnational immunization program staff.

Drawing from themes gathered in the online survey responses, the project developed a semi-structured interview guide with the aim of probing further into the factors constraining and enabling implementation and institutionalization of routine immunization microplanning. Interviews were conducted remotely in English or French by project staff and lasted up to one hour. Interviews were recorded with participant consent. Interview transcripts were uploaded to a password-protected folder and coded in Dedoose according to the six CFIR domains.

2.2. Root Cause Analysis

To triangulate and synthesize findings from across the research steps, the project conducted a root cause analysis (RCA) using data collected from the literature review, online survey, and key informant interviews. Due to the paucity of evidence on microplan implementation in the published literature, RCA drew primarily from key informant interview data, triangulated where possible with insights from the literature review and online survey. RCA is an analytic process to identify underlying causes of key process challenges, often by developing a visual diagram that elucidates the causal chain between the challenge and underlying root cause(s) [6]. Project staff who led the data collection and analysis for each research step participated in an iterative RCA process. Coded data on the constraints and enablers of microplanning implementation from all data sources were synthesized and revised iteratively upon review by the technical team. Through the iterative RCA process, the team identified root causes affecting the microplanning process, visualized the relationships between root causes, and organized the root causes based on the following: (1) whether they were related to the development or implementation of microplans and (2) whether they were enablers or barriers of these processes.

2.3. Ethics

IRB exemption was obtained from PATH IRB, as this was determined to be research on non-human subjects. The online survey was voluntary, and participants were informed of the survey's purpose and how the data they provided would be used. Survey respondents provided informed consent and were provided the option to include their contact information if they consented to participate in follow-up interviews. Interview participants provided verbal consent to participate. All study data that contained identifiable information were stored in a password-protected folder only accessible to the study team to ensure the privacy and confidentiality of participants.

3. Results

3.1. Description of Sample

The online survey was completed by 63 individuals from 24 countries (Figure 2). The survey included respondents from all six WHO regions (Africa, Americas, Eastern Mediterranean, Europe, Southeast Asia, Western Pacific), with the majority of responses from the Africa region. The team conducted 14 interviews with individuals from seven countries who are involved in microplanning implementation, including eight technical partners, two national-level routine immunization program staff, and four subnational immunization program staff (Table 1).

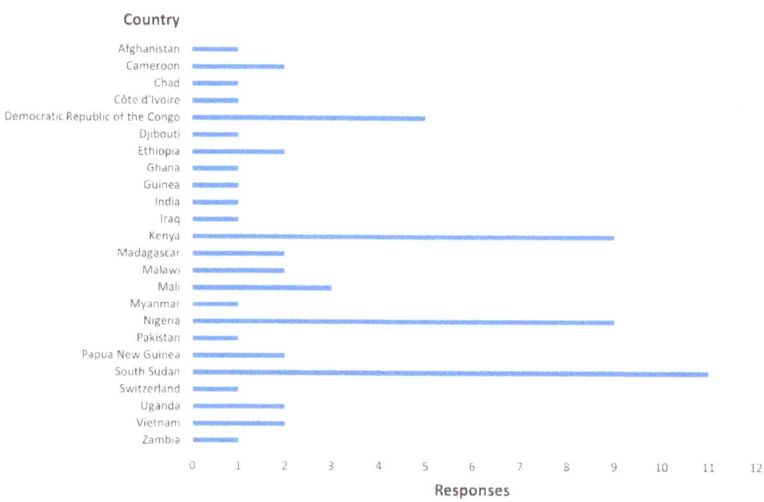

Figure 2. Survey respondents by country.

Table 1. Interviews conducted by country and stakeholder type.

Country	Number of Interviews	Types of Stakeholders Interviewed
DRC	3	Technical partner, National level EPI staff, District health staff
Ethiopia	2	Technical partner
Kenya	2	District health staff
Nigeria	2	Technical partner
Uganda	2	National level EPI staff, District health staff
USA	1	Technical partner
Vietnam	2	Technical partner
Total	14	

3.2. Key Findings

Through the RCA, the project identified two broad categories of factors which constrain and enable the implementation and institutionalization of microplanning processes in routine immunization programs: (1) the process of developing microplans and (2) the implementation of microplans. In addition, digitally enhanced microplanning and integrated approaches to microplanning emerged as two cross-cutting approaches to strengthen both microplanning development and implementation.

3.2.1. Microplan Development

Tools and Templates

RED global guidelines provide tools and guidance to support microplan development at the health facility level. The guidelines begin with a table to analyze data on target populations and immunization coverage in order to categorize and prioritize challenges related to access and utilization. This is used to inform other tools, including an operational map, a session plan, a quarterly work plan, a stock record, a drop-out tracking system, and a monitoring chart. Microplanning tools and templates provide guidance on the information required to develop high-quality microplans. However, according to the literature and key informants, users often find the tools to be complicated. One key informant summarized the following:

> "Tools are not friendly for the lower levels. They need simplification for health care workers (HCWs); making tools friendly for HCWs is important." (Technical partner, Ethiopia)

The literature and key informants indicated that challenges stem from the length and number of tools and templates, the detailed information required to populate them, and the Excel-based format of some templates.

> "Challenges related to microplanning were related to the templates. They are Excel-based, and for those staff who were not used to Excel, it was difficult for them to use. Nothing was automated on the Excel templates, they were just using it as a table. So it was not as useful as it has the power to be." (Technical partner, Ethiopia)

Challenges using microplanning tools can have consequences for the quality of microplans. For instance, a qualitative assessment of the microplanning process in two districts in Uganda found that the complex and bulky nature of the microplanning tool contributed to only 57 percent of health facilities having an updated microplan [7].

To address this challenge, the team found evidence in the literature and in key informant interviews of adaptations made to guidelines, tools, and templates to enhance their user-friendliness and contextual relevance. For example, in Tanzania, microplanning tools were adapted and integrated with other council-level planning tools [8]. In Uganda, one key informant described how microplanning tools and processes have been simplified over time to minimize health worker burden.

Access to High Quality and Timely Data

Microplanning requires accurate, timely data on target populations and catchment areas. However, accessing high-quality denominator data was a commonly cited challenge. According to key informants,

> "During microplanning, the problem is the denominator. Most places use the census for population estimations, but the census is old. And anyway, there is massive population movement. So having the right denominator for planning is one factor that enables or hinders microplanning." (Technical partner, Ethiopia)

As another key informant noted, those developing the microplan may be compelled to use the often outdated and inaccurate census population estimates because they are the official data used by the health system. This may lead to inaccurate estimates of vaccines and other supplies needed, poor quality coverage data, or failing to reach underserved populations [7].

Local enumeration activities can provide up-to-date, high-quality data on target populations, but this process can be time- and resource-intensive. For example, a study in Kaduna State, Nigeria, found that the number of children <1 year of age identified through microplanning household enumeration was 84 percent higher than the estimates based on census data [9]. The authors concluded that periodic household-based microplanning is useful for more accurate denominators but noted that the process required significant manpower and resources from many partners and government agencies.

Digital tools, especially geospatial technologies, are another potential strategy to map target populations for more accurate estimates. However, some key informants cautioned that digital tools may support the microplanning process but should not replace community engagement. Digital tools, without community insights, cannot accurately capture migration patterns, community movement, or perspectives on the timing and location of outreach services (see Section Digitally Enhanced Microplanning).

Health Worker Capacity

Evidence from the literature and key informants pointed to a lack of training, supportive supervision, and mentoring on microplanning as a key challenge to the development and implementation of high-quality microplans. Key informants noted that health care workers (HCWs) often have limited experience in immunization, and training in microplanning is variable or insufficient for HCWs to effectively use the microplanning tools.

> "The majority of staff are new employees and have no immunization background and no experience in microplanning, and [there are] no operational-level trainings for the majority of facilities. We need to build the capacity of our health care workers... Part of the job contract should actually be development and implementation of microplans." (Subnational immunization program staff, Kenya)

Additionally, high staff turnover was commonly mentioned as a challenge that creates microplanning knowledge gaps in facilities. Key informants in Uganda, DRC, and Vietnam provided examples of capacity strengthening activities, such as cascade training, peer exchanges, and mentoring activities implemented by donor-funded projects. However, the sustainability of many of these programs was cited as an ongoing challenge as they remained dependent on partner support and/or donor funding. Engaging HCWs and health facility managers in the process of developing plans and thoughtful capacity strengthening activities was reported to increase motivation to actually implement the activities in the plan (see Section Health Worker Capacity).

Community Engagement

Over time, approaches to microplanning have evolved. In the early days of RED implementation, microplans were often developed through a top-down approach, where ministries of health and technical partners convened workshops for facility and district-level immunization program managers. As the focus of immunization programming has shifted toward reaching missed communities and zero-dose children, a new approach to microplanning, sometimes referred to as "bottom-up microplanning", has emerged. The bottom-up approach starts at the health facility level and emphasizes community engagement in mapping target populations and identifying barriers to immunization. This is consistent with the increased emphasis on community engagement in the microplanning process in the 2017 RED guide from the WHO Regional Office for Africa [3].

The engagement of community members and other non-traditional stakeholders was broadly acknowledged as being critical to the development of high-quality microplans. Key informants reported that the participation of community stakeholders resulted in microplans that were more reflective of local needs and priorities, particularly in the location and timing of immunization sessions. In addition, the participation of local stakeholders encouraged greater local buy-in into microplanning implementation, including local efforts to mobilize resources to support immunization planning. However, engaging communities in the microplanning process requires additional resources, such as reimbursement for transportation costs, which immunization programs may not have.

According to a key informant in Nigeria,

> "Successful microplans need to involve community members and community-based organizations to help with outreach. Have people come to a selected place, whether it's the health facility or the leader's home. However, you need transportation, preparation, and meals–resources in general–to involve the community." (Technical partner, Nigeria)

3.2.2. Microplan Implementation

Health Worker Ownership

Cultivating ownership was found to be an important factor for motivating health workers to develop and implement microplanning. For example, JSI supported microplanning implementation in 25 districts in Uganda from 2014 to 2019 and found that HCWs experienced a higher degree of ownership over the microplans when they were engaged in the process of developing the plans [10]. Conversely, Mafigiri et al. found that HCWs in Uganda who were not involved in the microplan development process did not understand how to implement them, despite recognizing the value of microplanning to improve immunization services [7].

> "Being committed to carry out a plan that people themselves developed wound up being really important. And we also found that it was important to involve the clinic managers in some aspects of the microplanning process because ultimately, they could control where some of the resources went, and played a really important role in implementation." (Global technical partner)

Supportive Supervision, Mentorship, and Accountability

Other factors that key informants indicated enhance health worker ownership, and motivation for implementing microplans were supportive supervision and mentorship, coupled with monitoring and accountability mechanisms from higher levels of the health system. One best practice cited by key informants for monitoring microplanning was creating a WhatsApp group to send reminders to immunization focal persons at the subnational level. The WhatsApp groups provided a venue for higher level authorities to encourage microplan development and use. Conversely, a lack of follow-up from higher levels was mentioned as a constraint, particularly for institutionalizing microplanning.

> "Microplanning has not been advocated very well... it still needs follow up from the high levels to be institutionalized. It is not well aligned with existing mechanisms like district-based plans. There are competing tools that sometimes the higher levels use instead of microplans." (Technical partner, Ethiopia)

Resources to Support Implementation

Survey respondents and key informants both indicated that the implementation of microplans has been constrained by a consistent shortfall in operational funds for immunization programs at the subnational level to support planned activities, such as outreach, to provide services to unreached populations and zero-dose children. This challenge is not specific to microplanning but reflects larger resource constraints for immunization in many countries.

To mitigate this challenge, the 2017 RED guide from the WHO Regional Office for Africa suggests preparing budgets to carefully balance the resources needed with the resources available to implement strategies to reach zero-dose children. Key informants also emphasized the importance of advocacy to generate political will for making operational funds and other resources available for the implementation of the activities outlined in microplans. Key informants suggested addressing the shortfalls of government funding by mobilizing other sources (such as donors, the community, or the private sector) and by prioritizing critical activities to reach zero-dose children. For instance, in Tanzania, bottom-up microplanning was performed in the context of the annual Comprehensive Council Health Plan (CCHIP) process, which was documented as a promising approach for aligning the funds required for outreach and vaccine distribution with the available budget [11].

Several key informants mentioned a lack of funds to even print the final microplan, limiting HCWs' ability to implement the plans:

> "The health facilities were compelled to send their microplans to the district level without any copy left for their own reference. They were not sent back. The facilities that had developed their microplans and that were committed to carrying them out, that knew what they were going to do with them, it left them without those microplans." (Technical partner, Uganda)

3.2.3. Adaptations to Microplanning

This study aimed to learn more about what adaptations to traditional microplanning may be taking place and whether and how those adaptations may be strengthening development, implementation, or institutionalization of microplans. Throughout the course of the study, two cross-cutting adaptations in particular came up during both the literature review and key informant interviews.

Digitally Enhanced Microplanning

Digitally enhanced microplanning includes the utilization of tools such as digital mapping, mobile applications, online training forums, and electronic registries. These tools are used to help map catchment areas, identify target estimates, train health care workers, develop budgets, and monitor vaccine status. Geo-enabled microplanning was the most commonly cited form of digitally enhanced microplanning in the literature review. Geo-enabled microplanning entails using geospatial data to develop digital maps that capture information like the location of settlements, infrastructure, roads, and geographic terrain [12].

Key informants reaffirmed the benefits of digitally enhanced microplanning, citing that such activities result in improved mapping, better estimation of target populations, optimization of staffing assignments, and more efficient resource allocation. However, key informants were also clear in outlining barriers to widespread use of digitally enhanced microplanning, which can include poor technological infrastructure and internet connectivity, limited information technology (IT) capacity of HCWs and other staff, the high costs of making updates to microplans, and continued reliance on technical assistance from partners. In Vietnam, the national immunization information system uses digitized microplanning forms and processes. However, key informants described scenarios at the subnational level wherein health care workers lack the IT skills necessary to make use of these tools. As a result, some HCWs complete paper-based forms for data entry, which must be later manually reconciled with the digitized national immunization system. Despite these occasional incongruencies, the key informants still perceived digitally enhanced microplanning to contribute to more accurate microplans that reduce wastage of vaccines and other materials. Critically, key informants also made note that digital tools should ideally serve as enhancements to the microplanning process and should not replace the role of community engagement in setting priorities and identifying missed communities.

Integrated Microplanning

Integrated microplanning presents an appealing prospect in resource-constrained settings because, theoretically, it has the potential to reduce costs by combining multiple necessary interventions into one microplanning process. The peer-reviewed literature review yielded only two articles that described an integrated approach to microplanning. In Mongolia, microplans were developed for immunization and maternal and child health (MCH) services [13]. While the study did conclude that microplanning was well-suited to other interventions beyond immunization, it did not provide details of any specific barriers or enablers to taking an integrated approach or any measure of the effectiveness of the approach. A study in Uganda reported on efforts to integrate maternal health, nutrition, and child health into a single microplanning tool but cautioned that doing so could make the process more cumbersome and, therefore, increase the workload of HCWs who are already stretched thin [7].

Key informants expressed a growing readiness to adapt integrated approaches to microplanning, particularly in the context of efforts to strengthen primary health care (PHC). PHC is widely considered as a critical pathway to universal health coverage, and immunization is typically identified as a necessary component of robust PHC systems. Given this relationship, there is interest in identifying opportunities for better integration between immunization and other PHC services from program planning to service delivery since it may represent a more holistic use of resources than each health program operating in isolation. This appeared to be the case in Nigeria, where key informants reported increased emphasis on working toward integrated microplanning for PHC. In Uganda, one key informant described how this type of integrated microplanning manifests between immunization and nutrition services, such as Vitamin A supplementation for children aged one year old. In others, the scope is wider, comprising broader MCH services and family planning.

Limited human and financial resources were commonly reported by key informants as barriers to integration, particularly in the implementation phase. A key informant in Uganda reported that identifying zero-dose and missed communities for immunization microplanning provides an entry point to offer additional services (including MCH and nutrition services), but implementation requires additional resources. They noted,

> "...we are grappling with finding additional resources in delivering the integrated packages, because when I deliver an integrated package I'm going to need more health workers, I'll need additional transport. I need additional vaccine carriers. So you need more resources, the resources almost double because of the integrated package." (Technical partner, Uganda)

Another global technical partner noted in their interview that, while many perceived microplanning to be a window of opportunity for more holistic planning for immunization as part of PHC, this approach was not presently being leveraged to the extent it could be. The key informant attributed this in part to siloed funding sources and distinct measurement and reporting requirements by health area.

4. Discussion

The project found very little published and gray literature on microplanning in the context of routine immunization programs. Where microplanning was discussed, it was often as one component of the broader RED approach to improve immunization coverage and equity, without mention of factors that specifically constrained or enabled the microplanning process. Therefore, the team relied primarily on key informant interviews to explore the enablers and barriers to microplan development and implementation. Moreover, the review of the literature confirmed a lack of evidence on whether, how, and why microplanning contributes to immunization outcomes. This is consistent with a recently published evidence review of pro-equity interventions, which found microplanning to be a promising intervention, but noted the lack of rigorous analysis of the effectiveness of microplanning on immunization outcomes [14].

Many implementation constraints identified, such as a lack of HCW ownership, accountability, and operational resources, are not specific to microplanning and instead more broadly reflect barriers to implementation of routine immunization programming [15]. As such, the sub-optimal implementation of microplans should not necessarily be interpreted as shortcomings of microplanning alone but rather as a reflection of broader weaknesses in routine immunization systems.

This review indicates that microplanning is most successful when HCWs are engaged in the development process, thereby increasing their ownership over the process and the likelihood of the plans being implemented. Likewise, community participation was found to contribute to the enhanced recognition of the barriers missed communities face in accessing immunization services, and to better inform the development of remedial strategies. While these findings highlight the benefits of a "bottom-up" approach to microplanning, key informants cautioned that it is resource-intensive, and there remains a need for robust research and documentation on the costs and benefits of this approach.

A concerted and ongoing effort is required for strengthening the capacity of those HCWs responsible for developing, updating, and improving the quality of microplans. The tools and templates for developing a microplan were widely considered to be complicated, and key informants highlighted a need to simplify the microplan templates and guidance. Without proficiency among HCWs and district managers in using the tools and templates, key informants reported that the resulting microplans did not well reflect community needs or the most effective strategies to reach zero-dose children and missed communities. However, it was also emphasized that identifying missed communities and zero-dose children is inherently complex and resource-intensive, so comprehensive tools are necessary to support this process. Therefore, it is important to strike a careful balance between an appropriate level of simplification while also providing ample information and level of detail actually required to identify zero-dose children, understand their barriers to immunization, and reach those communities with high-quality immunization services.

The project found a growing emphasis on digitally enhanced microplanning, especially the use of digital tools and applications to map catchment areas, identify high-risk populations, and estimate populations. Although there is some evidence to support the effectiveness of this approach in arriving at more accurate estimates, they must not be viewed as a replacement for community engagement, as communities may not accept figures if they are not engaged in the process of developing those estimates. Furthermore, digital tools may produce estimates that are inconsistent with officially sanctioned figures that are typically generated using census data and used by different programs across the health system. HCWs must also be sufficiently capacitated to use the digital tools. As such, in order to use digital tools, there is a need for higher level policy decisions. Finally, while digitally enhanced microplanning can address some of the challenges identified through this review, it cannot address all and may in fact exacerbate some without careful evaluation of the costs and benefits.

Due to the widespread uptake of and adherence to the normative framework laid out through the RED guidance starting over 20 years ago, microplanning is broadly acknowledged to be part and parcel of immunization programming for both campaigns and routine immunization. Ministries of Health, and country Expanded Programs on Immunization (EPIs), have reinforced this to varying degrees by requiring that health districts and facilities engage in microplanning. The sub-optimal implementation of those plans is a direct consequence of insufficient resources to both develop microplans, and then to implement the activities therein.

5. Conclusions

In conclusion, the project found that the level of implementation and institutionalization of microplanning for routine immunization was highly variable from setting to setting (between and within countries) and, in many, still highly dependent on partner resources. It is, therefore, important to advocate for increased government recognition of the purpose and value of immunization in improving child health, as well as for adequate resources. Such government endorsement will also contribute to a virtuous cycle, whereby microplans are developed and implemented and the process is institutionalized, as an essential component of achieving equity in immunization.

6. Limitations

This study has several limitations that should be acknowledged. First, although a systematic literature search was conducted, some relevant articles may have been overlooked, particularly those found in gray or unpublished sources or not published in English. Second, the identified literature had limited details about the drivers of microplanning, and microplanning was often discussed as one component of RED/REC guidance and programming, making it difficult to disentangle the drivers of microplanning from those affecting routine immunization more broadly. Third, due to the limited evidence in the literature focused specifically on microplan development and implementation, the project relied heavily on key informant interviews. Due to time and resource constraints, the team interviewed a limited number of key informants, which was insufficient to achieve theoretical saturation. Although the team selected key informants from nine countries who offered valuable insights, these perspectives may not fully capture the range of experiences across countries and do not include the perspectives of community members. Despite these limitations, this review offers practical insights into the factors that facilitate or hinder effective microplanning in varied contexts, which can help to inform stakeholders involved in designing and implementing microplanning.

Author Contributions: Conceptualization, N.S., I.H., P.O. and J.C.S.; Data curation, N.S., P.O. and A.H.; Formal analysis, N.S. and P.O.; Investigation, N.S., I.H., P.O. and A.H.; Methodology, N.S., I.H. and J.C.S.; Project administration, J.C.S. and E.G.; Supervision, J.C.S. and E.G.; Writing—original draft, N.S., I.H., P.O., E.E. and E.G.; Writing—review and editing, N.S., I.H., P.O., E.E., J.C.S. and E.G. All authors have read and agreed to the published version of the manuscript.

Funding: MOMENTUM Routine Immunization Transformation and Equity and this research was funded by the U.S. Agency for International Development (USAID) as part of the MOMENTUM suite of awards and implemented by the JSI Research & Training Institute, Inc. with partners PATH, Accenture Development Partnerships, Results for Development, CORE Group, and The Manoff Group under USAID cooperative agreement #7200AA20CA00017. For more information about MOMENTUM, visit usaidmomentum.org (accessed on 2 December 2024). The contents of this journal article are the sole responsibility of the JSI Research & Training Institute, Inc., and do not necessarily reflect the views of USAID or the United States Government.

Institutional Review Board Statement: IRB exemption was obtained from PATH IRB (Research Record: RES-00597; 22 June 2023), as this was determined to be research on non-human subjects.

Informed Consent Statement: Informed consent was obtained from all subjects involved in this study.

Data Availability Statement: The data presented in this study are available upon request from the corresponding author.

Conflicts of Interest: The authors declare no conflicts of interest.

References

1. Vandelaer, J. The reaching every district (red) approach as a way to improve immunization performance. *Bull. World Health Organ.* **2008**, *86*, 240. [CrossRef] [PubMed]
2. WHO Africa Regional Office. *Implementing the Reaching Every District Approach: A Guide for District Health Management Teams*; WHO AFRO: Brazzaville, Congo, 2008. Available online: https://www.mchip.net/sites/default/files/AFRO-RED_Aug2008.pdf (accessed on 31 October 2024).
3. WHO Africa Regional Office. *Reaching Every District (RED)—A Guide to Increasing Coverage and Equity in All Communities in the African Region*; WHO AFRO: Brazzaville, Congo, 2017; Available online: https://www.afro.who.int/publications/reaching-every-district-red-guide-increasing-coverage-and-equity-all-communities (accessed on 31 October 2024).
4. FHI 360. *Microplanning: Evidence on Pro-Equity Interventions To Improve Immunization Coverage for Zero-Dose Children and Missed Communities*; FHI 360: Durham, UK, 2023; Available online: https://zdlh.gavi.org/sites/default/files/2023-09/9._microplanning_evidence_brief.pdf (accessed on 31 October 2024).
5. Damschroder, L.J.; Reardon, C.M.; Widerquist, M.A.O.; Lowery, J. The Updated Consolidated Framework for Implementation Research Based on User Feedback. *Implement. Sci.* **2022**, *17*, 75. [CrossRef] [PubMed]
6. PATH. *Evaluative Tools for Improving Campaign Effectiveness: Root Cause Analysis Toolkit*; PATH: Seattle, WA, USA, 2019. Available online: https://www.path.org/resources/evaluative-tools-improving-campaign-effectiveness/ (accessed on 31 October 2024).
7. Mafigiri, D.K.; Iradukunda, C.; Atumanya, C.; Odie, M.; Mancuso, A.; Tran, N.; McGrath, J.; Luzze, H. A Qualitative Study of the Development and Utilization of Health Facility-Based Immunization Microplans in Uganda. *Health Res. Policy Syst.* **2021**, *19*, 52. [CrossRef] [PubMed]
8. Maternal and Child Survival Program (MCSP). Increasing Immunization Coverage Through Strengthening Comprehensive Council Health Planning (Cchp) in Kagera, Tanzania; MCSP; 2019. Available online: https://mcsprogram.org/resource/increasing-immunization-coverage-through-strengthening-comprehensive-council-health-planning-cchp-in-kagera-tanzania/ (accessed on 31 October 2024).
9. Umeh, G.C.; Madubu, D.M.; Korir, C.; Loveday, N.; Ishaku, S.; Iyal, H.; Omoleke, S.A.; Nomhwange, T.I.; Aliyu, A.; Musa, A.; et al. Micro-Planning for Immunization in Kaduna State, Nigeria: Lessons Learnt, 2017. *Vaccine* **2018**, *36*, 7361. [CrossRef] [PubMed]
10. JSI. Experience in Building the Capacity of Health Facility Managers in Uganda on Leadership, Management and Accountability: A Missing Link in RI Service Delivery. Available online: https://www.jsi.com/resource/experience-in-building-capacity-of-health-facility-managers-in-uganda-on-leadership-management-and-accountability-a-missing-link-in-routine-immunization-service-delivery/ (accessed on 31 October 2024).
11. Maternal and Child Survival Program (MCSP). Strengthening Comprehensive Council Health Planning to Increase Immunization Coverage: A Pilot Activity in Kagera Region, Tanzania. Available online: https://www.jsi.com/resource/strengthening-comprehensive-council-health-planning-to-increase-immunization-coverage-a-pilot-activity-in-kagera-region-tanzania/ (accessed on 31 October 2024).
12. World Health Organization. Guidance on Operational Microplanning for COVID-19 Vaccination: Revised 2 May 2023; WHO: 2023. Available online: https://iris.who.int/bitstream/handle/10665/367267/WHO-2019-nCoV-vaccination-microplanning-2023.1-eng.pdf?sequence=1 (accessed on 31 October 2024).
13. Enkhtuya, B.; Badamusuren, T.; Dondog, N.; Khandsuren, L.; Elbegtuya, N.; Jargal, G.; Surenchimeg, V.; Grundy, J. Reaching Every District—Development and Testing of a Health Micro-Planning Strategy for Reaching Difficult to Reach Populations in Mongolia. *Rural Remote Health* **2009**, *9*, 1045. [CrossRef] [PubMed]
14. Gavi, The Vaccine Alliance. *Pro-Equity Evidence Map. Reaching the Underserved with Immunization: Map of Pro-Equity Interventions*; Gavi: Geneva, Switzerland, 2023; Available online: https://www.equityevidencemap.org/sites/default/files/document/9._microplanning_evidence_brief.pdf (accessed on 31 October 2024).
15. MOMENTUM Routine Immunization Transformation and Equity. Addressing Insufficient Operational Funding to Reach Zero-Dose Children and Missed Communities. October 2022. Available online: https://usaidmomentum.org/resource/addressing-insufficient-operational-funding-to-reach-zero-dose-children-and-missed-communities/ (accessed on 31 October 2024).

vaccines MDPI

Systematic Review

Integrated Approaches for the Delivery of Maternal and Child Health Services with Childhood Immunization Programs in Low- and Middle-Income Countries: Systematic Review Update 2011–2020

Monica P. Shah [1], Christopher J. Morgan [2,3,4,*], James G. Beeson [4,5,6], Elizabeth Peach [4,7], Jessica Davis [4], Barbara McPake [3] and Aaron S. Wallace [1]

1 Global Immunization Division, Global Health Center, Centers for Disease Control and Prevention, Atlanta, GA 30333, USA; mshah2@cdc.gov (M.P.S.); ccu7@cdc.gov (A.S.W.)
2 Jhpiego, a Johns Hopkins University Affiliate, Baltimore, MD 21231, USA
3 Melbourne School of Population and Global Health, University of Melbourne, Melbourne, VIC 3053, Australia; barbara.mcpake@unimelb.edu.au
4 Burnet Institute, Melbourne, VIC 3004, Australia; james.beeson@burnet.edu.au (J.G.B.); e.peach@unsw.edu.au (E.P.)
5 Department of Infectious Diseases, University of Melbourne, Melbourne, VIC 3053, Australia
6 School of Translational Medicine, Monash University, Melbourne, VIC 3800, Australia
7 Rural Clinical Campuses, University of New South Wales Medicine and Health, Sydney, NSW 2052, Australia
* Correspondence: christopher.morgan@jhpiego.org

Abstract: Background: The integration of maternal and child health services (MCH) with routine immunization is an important global health strategy, particularly in low- and middle-income countries (LMICs). However, evidence is lacking regarding the best practices for service integration and the effect of integration on immunization and linked health service outcomes. **Methods**: We searched publication databases and gray literature for articles published between 2011 and 2020 that include approaches to integrating MCH services with immunizations during the first two years of life in LMICs. Abstracts and full-text articles were screened for eligibility. For the included articles, data extraction and analysis examined the descriptive characteristics of studies, outcomes, and implementation considerations. **Results**: Among the 16,578 articles screened, 44 met the criteria for inclusion, representing 34 studies, of which 29 were from Africa. The commonly linked MCH services were family planning (24%), human immunodeficiency virus (HIV) diagnosis or care (21%), and malaria prevention or control (21%). Multiple integration strategies were typically used; the co-location of linked services (65%), the provision of extra services by immunization staff (41%), and/or the provision of extra information by immunization staff (41%) were the most common. In general, integration improved MCH service outcomes (76%) and was either beneficial (55%) or neutral for immunization (35%), with some examples in family planning, malaria, and HIV where integrated services were not beneficial. Important implementation considerations included the careful matching of target populations in service re-design, ensuring support from policy, logistics, and information systems, the provision of adequate training and support of staff to avoid overload, clear client communication regarding service integration, and the need to address community concerns. **Conclusions**: Integrating MCH services with routine immunization can expand linked services and improve immunization coverage. This study has identified key implementation considerations relevant to both childhood and adult vaccination programs. More research is needed regarding costs and client preferences.

Keywords: integration; vaccination; immunization; service delivery; systematic review; maternal and child health; infant; HIV; malaria; family planning

1. Introduction

The integration of other health and development interventions with immunization services has long been viewed as a cornerstone of global immunization strategies. The latest global framework, known as Immunization Agenda 2030 (IA2030), states the strategic priority of ensuring that all people benefit from recommended immunizations, integrated with essential health services, across the life course [1]. Integrating other health interventions with immunization services can contribute to the goal of universal health coverage, where all people have access to the full range of quality health services they need, when and where they need them [2].

Several rationales exist for integrating other health interventions with immunization services. Providing a package of care in a single visit to eligible individuals and accompanying family members can address individual health needs more comprehensively than vertical or single-disease-focused practices, while also reducing the individual's time and financial costs of seeking care. Childhood immunization services have among the highest and most equitable coverage of any childhood health service [3]. Therefore, immunization visits may provide an important platform for increasing the coverage of other health interventions, particularly in low- and middle-income countries (LMICs) where the coverage of other health interventions may be substantially lower. Integration has the potential to also increase health system efficiency, which can facilitate expanded program reach. Increased efficiency and reach can reduce mortality and morbidity from both vaccine-preventable and non-vaccine-preventable diseases.

However, integrating services is not without concern, as a lack of sufficient investment could lead to overburdened health workers and a decreased quality of service, with potential impacts on service coverage and acceptability [4]. Additional concerns exist regarding the feasibility of service integration due to differing service delivery requirements for considerations such as privacy, delivery time, and the target age range [5,6].

To inform global recommendations, 2 previous systematic reviews, published in 2009 and 2012, comprehensively examined 59 studies integrating maternal and child health (MCH) interventions with immunization services to synthesize the lessons learned and best practices [4,6]. The reported outcomes in the studies reviewed indicated the need for increased coverage for the linked services, although not necessarily to the same levels as seen for immunization services. However, most studies did not report outcomes for immunization services. The reviews noted continuing evidence gaps regarding the cost efficiency of integrating services and the impact of integration on immunization outcomes. Despite these evidence gaps, these reviews provided sufficient evidence to support the development of the 2018 World Health Organization (WHO) technical guidance on the integration of immunization services, entitled "Working Together: an integration resource guide for immunization services throughout the life course" [7]. This WHO guidance, aimed at national immunization programs within Ministries of Health, provides an overview of integration approaches and opportunities, as well as considerations of how to best integrate other health services with immunizations.

Since 2012, when the last systematic review on this topic was published [6], the interest in integrating services has continued to increase, due in large part to a focus on achieving universal healthcare. The 2023 Lusaka Agenda outlines a framework for how global health initiatives (GHIs), which generally focus on supporting a single health program such as immunization, can support a more coordinated approach to strengthening primary healthcare in the integrated delivery of services at a high and equitable level of coverage [8]. Additionally, since 2012, new vaccines have been introduced, and many LMICs have additional doses in the second year of life, providing new opportunities to examine how to integrate health services for these age groups [9]. Meanwhile, efforts to 'catch children up' on earlier missed vaccines—such as the Big Catch-Up during the COVID-19 pandemic—have focused on how to opportunistically integrate immunization into other health services [10]. This new context places a greater emphasis on understanding how best to integrate immunization services, tracking the latest evidence that has emerged across studies.

To inform global, regional, and country-level strategies with the new evidence on the integrated delivery of MCH interventions with immunization services, we undertook an update from the last systematic review on this topic, which reflected studied published up through 2010 [6]. In this review update, we synthesized published and unpublished literature from 2011 to 2020 on integrated approaches for the delivery of MCH services along with childhood immunization programs in LMICs. The objectives of this review were to describe the types of intervention, immunization service delivery platform (fixed, outreach, campaign, mixed), and service change (such as the co-location of services, the provision of extra information or counseling provided, the provision of extra services) used to integrate other services with immunization services provided in the first two years of life. We qualitatively summarized the effect of integration on linked MCH service and immunization outcomes (if measured and reported) and described implementation considerations for integrated service delivery changes.

2. Materials and Methods

The methodology used to conduct this systematic review update draws from the standardized guidelines developed by the Cochrane Collaboration's Effective Practice and Organization of Care group [11]. Detailed information about the methods is described in a protocol registered with the International Prospective Registry of Systematic Reviews [12]; a brief summary is provided here.

2.1. Search Methods

Electronic searches: The following databases were searched on 13 May 2016; 15 May 2020; and 10 March 2023 for articles published between January 2011 and June 2020 (covering the next decade since the previous review [6]) in the English language using a search strategy combining terms for service types (e.g., antenatal, malaria, vitamin A, etc.), similar to a previous review on this topic [6], with additional search terms using integration terminology (full list of terms provided in PROSPERO protocol CRD42016045876 [12]: MEDLINE (via Ovid), EMBASE (via Ovid), CABI Global Health (via EBSCOhost), CINAHL (via EBSCOhost), Cochrane Central Register of Controlled Trials, and the Cochrane Database of Systematic Reviews. **Searching other resources:** Additional publications were identified from the gray literature search of documents from the following agencies: World Health Organization (WHO), UNICEF, BASICS, Family planning—EPI integration working group, Knowledge4Health, POPLINE, John Snow Incorporated, Family Health International, USAID-supported programs, DfID, and the Nigerian Urban Reproductive Health Initiative.

2.2. Criteria for Inclusion and Exclusion

All study designs reporting empirical data were included, while articles from mathematical modeling studies were excluded. Additionally, expert opinions (e.g., perspective articles) and studies that did not focus on the operational impact of integrated service delivery were excluded. Other systematic reviews were excluded, although their reference lists were reviewed to identify any additional eligible studies. We included studies that integrated health services with childhood immunization programs for children aged two years or younger. The review was limited to data from LMICs, as defined by the World Bank for 2016 [13]. Studies were eligible for inclusion if they included one or more linked service and one or more immunization service that had been integrated during pregnancy, postnatally, or in childhood (including the first two years of life) as a function of health service innovation. Studies reporting on missed opportunities for vaccination, where the contact point for integration was health services other than immunization delivery, were not included in this review.

We included studies that involved comparisons with a non-integration population group or pre–post integration comparisons. We excluded studies that had no comparator population group or timeframe. For inclusion in outcome synthesis, studies had to report one or more of the following outcomes for at least one immunization or linked health service: vaccination coverage, vaccination drop-out rates (e.g., first dose of diphtheria-tetanus-pertussis-containing vaccine [DTP1] to DTP3, first dose of pentavalent vaccine [DTP + hepatitis B + Haemophilus influenzae type B; penta1] to penta3), the coverage of a linked MCH service, the number or uptake of services provided (e.g., doses administered, number of tests administered, etc.), the quality of care, the equity of access or coverage, or costs.

2.3. Selection of Studies

Two review authors screened all titles and abstracts for inclusion and assessed full-text articles for eligibility. For studies included at the full-text stage, two review authors extracted data from each article in a pre-tested standardized excel template. Any discrepancies were resolved through discussion or by a third reviewer. Covidence systematic review software (Veritas Health Innovation; Melbourne, Australia) was used to manage the independent assessment of articles across authors at the title/abstract and full-text stages.

During title and abstract screening, multiple publications from the same study were included as individual articles. At the full-text stage, multiple articles from the same study were collated as a single study. Additionally, studies that did not meet inclusion criteria at the full-text stage were listed in a table with their reasons for exclusion. The study selection process was summarized using a Preferred Reporting Items of Systematic reviews and Meta-Analyses (PRISMA) diagram [14].

2.4. Data Extraction

The data extraction template included the following variables: the descriptive characteristics of the study (e.g., geographic location(s), the year of publication, the timing of data collection, etc.); the study design, including comparison groups; the immunization platform selected for integrated service delivery (e.g., either routine or campaign, and further described by fixed, outreach, mobile, or mixed delivery routes); a description of the integration strategy, including the immunization service (e.g., specific vaccines) and additional health service being linked; outcome measures for both the immunization and linked service; and implementation determinants, considering the perspectives of providers of care and recipients of care, health systems, and the social and political context.

The quality of the evidence was assessed using frameworks derived from GRADE assessments [15] for quantitative data and from the Clinical Appraisal Skills Program (CASP) tools [16] for qualitative data. Since meta-analyses were not conducted and the risk of bias was not a consideration affecting inclusion, the results of the risk of bias assessment are not presented here.

2.5. Data Synthesis

Narrative summaries were compiled for key results, following standard practices [17,18], based on the consensus among three authors (C.J.M., M.P.S., A.S.W.). As part of data synthesis, integration strategies were categorized as one or more of the following: a. extra services provided by immunization staff (i.e., testing, treatment, referrals, etc.); b. extra information and/or counseling provided by immunization staff (i.e., one-on-one consultation, providing informational materials, etc.); c. the co-location of services (e.g., same timing or same physical location of immunization delivery and linked health service); d. vaccination provided by non-immunization staff; and e. extra information and/or counseling provided by non-immunization staff (i.e., screening, health education, or immunization promotion, etc.). The results are summarized in a table that is arranged by EPI platform (campaign versus routine), linked health service(s), and study (designated by first author's last name and year of publication).

A single qualitative summary was used to summarize the direction of effect of the integration for the primary outcome(s) for immunization and for the linked MCH service separately. The terms used are defined as follows: "not measured"—there was no outcome measured or no non-integration comparison group available; "negative"—there was lower coverage or service provision in the integration compared to the non-integration group; "mixed negative"—some outcomes were lower in the integration compared to the non-integration group, but others remained static; "static"—no meaningful difference in coverage or service provision between integration and non-integration groups; "mixed positive"—some outcomes were higher in the integration compared to the non-integration group, but others remained static; or "positive"—higher coverage or service provision in the integration compared to the non-integration group. The results are summarized in a table that is arranged by EPI platform (campaign versus routine), linked MCH service(s), integration strategy, and study.

A narrative synthesis was undertaken to synthesize study findings related to the implementation considerations that affected service integration. Implementation considerations affecting service integration were collected into pre-defined categories, including policy and governance topics; the design of integrated service delivery; human resources for health; management, logistics, and costs; operational tools, reporting, and recording; and community and client topics [19].

Data were managed, summarized, and synthesized in Microsoft Excel.

3. Results

3.1. Results of Search

A total of 21,894 records were identified via database searching and, after removing duplicates, 16,578 titles and abstracts were screened (Figure 1). Among these, 471 full-text articles (from 467 studies) were reviewed and 44 articles (from 34 studies) met the eligibility criteria for inclusion; a full list of full-text articles (n = 427) that did not meet eligibility criteria and the reason for exclusion is provided as in the Supplementary Materials as Table S1, List of studies excluded on full-text review and reason for exclusion (n = 427). The most common reasons for full-text exclusion were wrong study design (34%), wrong publication type (27%), or articles not reporting on service delivery integration as the intervention (25%).

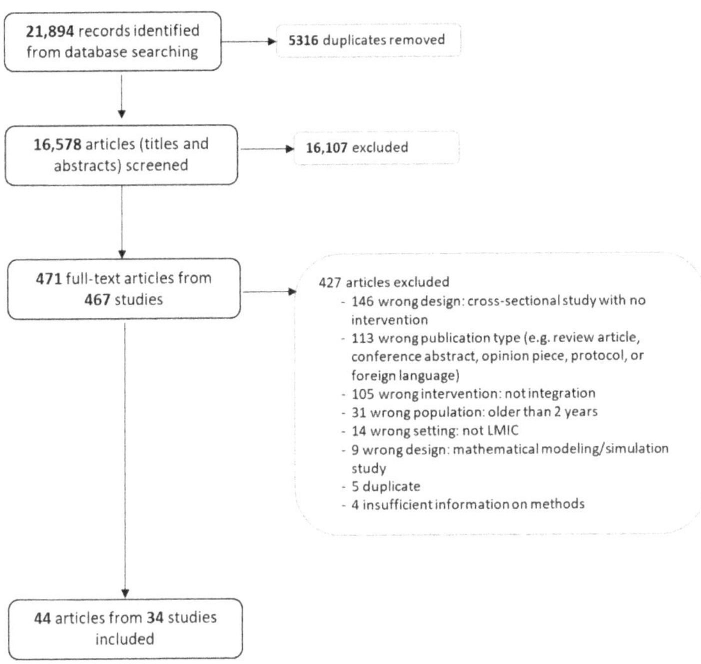

NOTE: PRISMA = Preferred Reporting Items of Systematic reviews and Meta-Analyses

Figure 1. Study flow diagram (PRISMA Diagram), systematic review update 2011–2020.

At the title and abstract screening stage, reviewers A and B had substantial agreement (Cohen's kappa: 0.71), while reviewers A and C had fair agreement (Cohen's kappa: 0.22). At the full-text stage, reviewers A and B and B and C had fair agreement (Cohen's kappa 0.31 and 0.33, respectively), while reviewers A and C had a level of agreement no better than what would be expected by chance (Cohen's kappa: 0).

3.2. Description of Included Studies

Of the 34 studies included on integrated service delivery (Tables 1–4), 29 (85%) were conducted in Africa (Benin, Burkina Faso, Cameroon, Gambia, Ghana, Kenya, Liberia, Malawi, Mali, Madagascar, Nigeria, Rwanda, Sierra Leone, South Africa, South Sudan, Tanzania, and Zambia), 4 (12%) were conducted in Asia (Afghanistan, India, Lao PDR, and Pakistan), and 1 (3%) was conducted in the Americas (Mexico). A majority of included studies reported about the integration of services with routine immunizations (88%) delivered at either health facilities ($n = 20$), outreach sessions ($n = 3$), mobile sites ($n = 2$), or a combination of sites ($n = 5$), while the remaining ($n = 4$, 12%) studies reported about the integration health services within immunization campaigns (Table 1). To summarize further, Tables 1–4 are grouped by immunization delivery platform and/or linked health service; Table 1 describes studies that were integrated into campaigns and includes 4 studies, performed in Lao PDR, Madagascar, Nigeria, and Pakistan. Table 2 describes studies integrating child health screening or family planning advice and services into routine immunizations and includes 10 studies performed in Benin, Burkina Faso, Ghana, India, Liberia, Malawi, Nigeria, Rwanda, South Africa, and Zambia. Table 3 reports studies integrating HIV and malaria services into routine immunizations and includes 7 HIV studies from Cameroon, Kenya, Malawi, Nigeria, Tanzania, and Zambia, and 7 malaria studies from Gambia, Ghana, Mali, Malawi, Rwanda, and Tanzania. Finally, Table 4 describes the integration of primary healthcare (PHC) services; nutrition, water, sanitation, and hygiene (WASH); or a combination of services into routine immunizations and includes 7 studies conducted in Afghanistan, Kenya, Mexico, Nigeria, Sierra Leone, and South Sudan.

Linked health services included child health, hearing, or vision screening (Table 2); family planning (Table 2); HIV prevention, diagnosis, and treatment (Table 3); malaria prevention, control, and treatment (Table 3); packages of MCH and/or other PHC services, including antenatal care (ANC), prenatal care (PNC), and the integrated management of childhood illnesses (IMCI) (Table 4); nutrition; WASH services (Table 4); or a combination of these (e.g., PHC and nutrition; family planning and nutrition; malaria, PHC, nutrition, and WASH; this is shown in Table 4). Of these, the most commonly reported linked health services were family planning (24%; of which, there were $n = 7$ in Africa and $n = 1$ in India), HIV (21%; of which, there was $n = 7$ in Africa [100%]), and malaria (21%; of which, $n = 7$ in Africa [100%]). Only four studies reported the integration of multiple health services with routine immunization service delivery (Table 4), and this was observed in Bawa, 2019 (malaria, PHC, nutrition, and WASH) [20,21]; Edmond, 2020 (PHC and nutrition) [22]; Habib, 2017 (PHC and nutrition) [23]; and Hodges, 2015 (family planning and nutrition) [24].

The risk of bias was assessed as described in the Materials and Methods Section; most studies were rated as having a high risk of bias due to the implementation science framework of many study designs. As a result, the risk of bias assessment result was not considered as a criterion for inclusion in the review.

Table 1. Characteristics of included studies (n = 4) on integration into immunization campaigns by linked health service, systematic review update 2011–2020.

Study [a]	Country (Study Year	Immunization Delivery Platform	Linked Maternal and Child Health Service(s)	Integration Strategy	Description of Integration Strategy	Study Design: Outcome Comparison	Immunization Outcomes Measured (Primary Outcome in Bold)	Linked Health Service Outcomes Measured (Primary Outcome in Bold)
Goodson (2012) and Kulkarni (2010) [25,26]	Madagascar [2007–2008]	Campaign—mixed	Malaria	a. Extra services by immunization staff c. Co-location	Integrated delivery of ITNs, deworming tablets, vit A and measles vaccine to <5-year-olds during a national health campaign.	Post only; two groups [integration = ITNs distributed in campaign package of services; comparison = ITNs were not included]	**Measles vaccination coverage (higher in integration group compared to non-ITN control group, including in poorest households)**	**Proportion of households with at least one ITN (higher in integration compared to non-integration areas)**
Habib (2017) [23]	Pakistan [2013–2014]	Campaign—mixed (fixed and mobile camps)	Nutrition, PHC	b. Extra information and/or counseling by immunization staff c. Co-location	MCH camps alongside polio campaign, offered counseling on hygiene and nutrition, routine immunizations, micronutrient supplements, and general MCH assessments.	Pre/post; three groups: comparison = OPV with routine immunizations; integration 1 = OPV with routine immunizations and other interventions; integration 2 = OPV with routine immunizations, other interventions, and IPV	**-OPV coverage (higher in integration groups versus comparison) -Other routine immunization coverage (higher in integration groups versus comparison)**	**Updates of PHC services noted but were not quantifiable due to lack of comparison data.**
Boselli (2011) [27]	Lao PDR [2007]	Campaign—mixed	Nutrition	a. Extra services by immunization staff	Integrated deworming tablets, vit A and polio vaccine to <5-year-olds. Deworming tablets with tetanus toxoid vaccine to women	Only examined cost effectiveness of integrated vit A and deworming tablet delivery compared to non-integrated delivery	**Not measured**	**Not measured**
Birukila (2017) [28]	Nigeria [2013]	Campaign—mixed (fixed and temporary sites)	PHC	c. Co-location	During polio campaigns, health camps were organized for settlements with high vaccine refusal rates in which other health services were offered with OPV.	Historical comparison 2013 with 2014; integration group = settlements with integrated health camps (polio and other primary healthcare services) in 2013.	**Number of children who received OPV (14,000 in 2013 round with integrated health camps and 7000 in 2014 round without integrated health camps)**	**Not measured**

[a] the last name of the first author and the publication year; studies are ordered by linked maternal and child health service, and then alphabetically by author. Notes: ITN = insecticide-treated bednet; IPV = inactivated polio vaccine; MCH = maternal and child health; OPV = oral polio vaccine; PHC = primary healthcare; vit A = vitamin A supplementation.

Table 2. Characteristics of included studies (n = 10) on integration of child health or family planning into routine immunizations, systematic review update 2011–2020.

Study [a]	Country (Study Year(s))	Immunization Delivery Platform	Linked Maternal and Child Health Service(s)	Integration Strategy	Description of Integration Strategy	Study Design: Outcome Comparison	Immunization Outcomes Measured (Primary Outcome in Bold)	Linked Health Service Outcomes Measured (Primary Outcome in Bold)
Integration into routine immunization—child hearing screening								
Friderichs (2012) [29]	South Africa [2008–2010]	Routine—facility	Child health (hearing screening)	a. Extra services by immunization staff	EPI staff administered a hearing screening test; no non-integration comparison.	Not applicable/no relevant outcomes compared: feasibility study only.	**Not measured**	Proportion of infants that underwent hearing screening. No comparator.
Jac-Okereke (2020) [30]	Nigeria [ND]	Routine—facility	Child health (vision screening)	c. Co-location	Infants attending immunization clinics randomly selected for vision screening.	Not applicable/no relevant outcomes compared: descriptive study only.	**Not measured**	**Not measured**
Integration into routine immunization—family planning (FP) advice and services								
Balasubramaniam (2018) [31]	India [2012]	Routine—outreach	FP	b. Extra information and/or counseling by immunization staff	Providers applied a screening tool to assess for FP; both intervention and control areas updated in post-partum FP.	Mid-point/end-line; two groups [integration group = use of FP screening tool in intervention areas]	**DTP3 coverage (similar increases in intervention and control)**	**Percentage of women receiving FP services (no change in intervention, control decreased). FP methods (increased in intervention, but no change in control)**
Cooper (2015) [32]	Liberia [2012]	Routine—facility	FP	b. Extra information and/or counseling by immunization staff c. Co-location	Pilot of FP counseling by immunization staff at routine immunization visits and same-day referral to a co-located FP service.	Pre/post; two groups [integration group = pilot facilities comparator non-pilot facilities and pre-intervention data]	**-Provision of DTP1 and DTP3 (increase from pre to post and higher in pilot vs non-pilot in one site, but no differences in other sites)** -DTP1—3 drop-out rate (increased from pre to post and higher in pilot facilities compared to non-pilot at both sites).	**-New contraceptive users (increased from pre- to post-intervention in both sites)**

Table 2. *Cont.*

Study [a]	Country (Study Year(s))	Immunization Delivery Platform	Linked Maternal and Child Health Service(s)	Integration Strategy	Description of Integration Strategy	Study Design: Outcome Comparison	Immunization Outcomes Measured (Primary Outcome in Bold)	Linked Health Service Outcomes Measured (Primary Outcome in Bold)
Cooper (2020) [33]	Malawi [2016–2017]	Routine—mixed (facility and outreach)	FP	a. Extra services by immunization staff c. Co-location e. Extra information and/or counseling by non-immunization staff	Same-day family planning services offered by nurses and health surveillance assistants to mothers seeking routine immunization services; screening of vaccination status for infants of family planning clients.	Pre/post; one group	**-Number of DTP1 doses (no change)** **-Number of DTP3 doses (increase from pre to post)**	**Number of women accessing FP services (increase from pre to post)**
Dulli (2016) [34]	Rwanda [2010–2011]	Routine—facility	FP	b. Extra information and/or counseling by immunization staff c. Co-location	Immunization staff provided information on FP and referral for counseling to co-located services. Compared to health facilities not using integrated approach.	Pre/post; two groups [integration group = health facilities implementing integrated family planning and immunization services]	**-Monthly trends in measles vaccinations (similar in integration and non-integration health facilities)** -Monthly trends in DTP1, 2, and 3 collected but not reported	**Proportion of women using a modern contraceptive method (higher in integration health facilities compared to non-integration group)**
Erhardt-Ohren (2020) [35]	Benin [2016–2017]	Routine—facility	FP	b. Extra information and/or counseling by immunization staff	Immunization staff provided information on FP and referral for FP counseling.	Not applicable/no relevant outcomes compared: qualitative process evaluation.	**Not measured**	**Not measured**
Nelson (2019) [36]	Liberia [2016–2017]	Routine—facility	FP	b. Extra information and/or counseling by immunization staff c. Co-location e. Immunization counselling by non-immunization staff	Immunization staff provided information on FP and referral for counseling to co-located services. Compared to matched facilities not using integration.	Pre/post; two groups [integration group = health facilities implementing integrated family planning and immunization services]	**-DTP1–3 drop-out rates (similar in integration and non-integration health facilities)**	**-FP referral (increased over time, higher in integration than non-integration)** **-Contraceptive acceptance (higher in integration than non-integration facilities)**

Table 2. *Cont.*

Study [a]	Country (Study Year(s))	Immunization Delivery Platform	Linked Maternal and Child Health Service(s)	Integration Strategy	Description of Integration Strategy	Study Design: Outcome Comparison	Immunization Outcomes Measured (Primary Outcome in Bold)	Linked Health Service Outcomes Measured (Primary Outcome in Bold)
Vance (2014) [37]	Ghana and Zambia [2009–2010]	Routine—facility	FP	b. Extra information and/or counseling by immunization staff c. Co-location	Immunization staff provided information on FP and referral for services at nine-month visit at intervention health facilities. Outcomes compared to non-intervention (control) facilities.	Pre/post; two groups [integration group = health facilities where vaccinators were trained to provide FP messages and referrals to women presenting for child immunization services]	**Not measured**	**-Non-condom contraceptive use (no changes in intervention compared to control)** **-Women's knowledge of LAM (no differences)** **-Referrals for FP services (non-significant changes across groups)**
Yugbare Belemsaga (2018) [38–40]	Burkina Faso [2013–2015]	Routine—facility	FP	a. Extra services by immunization staff b. Extra information and/or counseling by immunization staff c. Co-location	Provision of maternal-infant post-partum care checks and FP counseling at same time as immunization visits, by co-located staff.	Pre/post; one group	**-Monthly number of doses of DTP administered (no change over time)**	**-Uptake of post-partum care at immunization visits (no pre–post changes overall, some increase during the early post-natal period)**

[a] the last name of the first author and the publication year; studies are ordered by linked maternal and child health service, and then alphabetically by author. Notes: DTP = diphtheria, pertussis, and tetanus vaccine; EPI = expanded program on of immunizations; FP = family planning; LAM = lactational amenorrhea method.

Table 3. Characteristics of included studies (n = 13) on integration of human immunodeficiency virus (HIV)prevention, testing, and treatment or malaria into routine immunizations, systematic review update 2011–2020.

Study [a]	Country (Study Year(s))	Immunization Delivery Platform	Linked Maternal and Child Health Service(s)	Integration Strategy(ies)	Description of Integration Strategy	Study Design: Outcome Comparison	Immunization Outcomes Measured (Primary Outcome in Bold)	Linked Health Service Outcomes Measured (Primary Outcome in Bold)
Integration into routine immunization—HIV services								
Dube 2012 [41]	Malawi [2008–2010]	Routine—facility	HIV	c. Co-location	Testing, counseling, and treatment for EID of HIV offered at 6-week EPI visit.	Not applicable/no relevant outcomes compared: feasibility study to describe completion of EID process during routine EPI visits.	**Not measured**	-Measured, but no non-integration comparator -71.6% of HEIs had early diagnosis, 87.3% of mothers informed of infants' results, ART started in 58% of infants with confirmed infection.
Goodson (2013) and Wallace (2014) [42,43]	Tanzania [2009–2010]	Routine—facility	HIV	a. Extra services by immunization staff b. Extra information and/or counseling by immunization staff c. Co-location	EPI staff identified HEIs offered testing, counseling and care in selected sites. Compared to remaining sites in district (control).	For immunization outcome: pre/post; two groups [integration group] For linked service: not applicable/no relevant outcomes compared—feasibility study only.	**-Monthly vaccine doses [OPV1, OPV3, Penta1, Penta3, Measles] (results differed by urban/rural and by antigen; overall either no change or a decrease in monthly doses)**	**-Measured, but no non-integration comparator** -HIV service uptake increased in all sites
McCollum (2012) [44]	Malawi [2011]	Routine—facility	HIV	b. Extra information and/or counseling by immunization staff c. Co-location	Testing and counseling for EID of HIV offered at EPI clinic. Compared to EID offered at pediatric clinic.	Post only; two groups [integration group = infants attending EPI clinic where EID service was co-located]	**Not measured**	**-Proportion of infants receiving provider initiated HIV testing and counseling for EID (higher in EPI than pediatric clinic)**
Odafe (2020) [45]	Nigeria [2016–2017]	Routine—facility	HIV	c. Co-location	Targeted HIV testing of infants in immunization clinics compared to in TB clinics, inpatient wards, outpatient clinics, and through a family registry system.	Post only; five platforms/groups [integration group = immunization clinics]	**Not measured**	**-Proportion of all tests by platform (testing at immunization clinics low [0.9%] compared to others: pediatric outpatients [49.7%], family registry [38.0%], pediatric inpatient [10.5%], or tuberculosis [0.8%] clinics)**

Table 3. *Cont.*

Study [a]	Country (Study Year(s))	Immunization Delivery Platform	Linked Maternal and Child Health Service(s)	Integration Strategy(ies)	Description of Integration Strategy	Study Design: Outcome Comparison	Immunization Outcomes Measured (Primary Outcome in Bold)	Linked Health Service Outcomes Measured (Primary Outcome in Bold)
Ong'ech (2012) [46]	Kenya [2008–2010]	Routine—facility	HIV	c. Co-location	Services for HEIs (infant feeding support, prophylactic medicines, and HIV diagnosis) offered at MCH clinics with EPI services co-located compared to specialized HIV clinic.	Post only; two groups [integration group = infants seeking care at MCH clinic offering EPI and HEI services]	**-Measles vaccine coverage at 9 months (higher in integrated MCH clinic than specialized HIV clinic)** **-Completion of vaccinations by 12 months (higher in integrated MCH clinic than specialized HIV clinic)**	**-Odds of attending scheduled post-natal visits (higher in integrated MCH clinic than specialized HIV clinic)** **-Proportion of infants attending follow-up (higher in integrated MCH clinic than specialized HIV clinic)**
Tejiokem (2011) [47]	Cameroon [2007–2009]	Routine—facility	HIV	c. Co-location	Testing, counseling, and treatment for EID of HIV offered at 6-, 10-, and 14-week EPI visit and linkage to HAART.	Not applicable/no relevant outcomes compared: feasibility study only.	**Not measured**	-Measured, but no non-integration comparator -Completeness of follow-up of HEIs (83.9% completed)
Wang (2015) [48]	Zambia [2012–2014]	Routine—facility	HIV	a. Extra services by immunization staff b. Extra information and/or counseling by immunization staff c. Co-location	EPI and co-located staff, with commodity support, offered HIV testing and counseling.	Pre/post; three groups [control, simple intervention = re-supply of HIV commodities, integration group = integration of HIV testing with routine immunization]	**-Monthly DTP1 doses (similar change in both intervention arms and matched control sites)** -Qualitative finding: HIV services did not deter families from immunization.	**-Monthly HIV tests administered (higher in integration compared to simple intervention and control)**
Integration into routine immunization—malaria prevention								
Bojang (2011) [49]	Gambia [2006]	Routine—outreach	Malaria	a. Extra services by immunization staff	IPTc during outreach by community-based VHWs) compared to outreach by reproductive and child health trekking teams (EPI staff).	Post only; two groups [integration group = RCH teams (EPI staff) delivery]	**% children ≥ 12 months who were fully vaccinated (lower in RCH teams compared to non-integrated VHW delivery)**	**-Coverage of three courses of IPTc (lower in RCH teams delivery compared to non-integrated VHW)** -Cost of delivery at least first dose of IPTc (more expensive to deliver by RCH teams compared to VHWs)

Table 3. *Cont.*

Study [a]	Country (Study Year(s))	Immunization Delivery Platform	Linked Maternal and Child Health Service(s)	Integration Strategy(ies)	Description of Integration Strategy	Study Design: Outcome Comparison	Immunization Outcomes Measured (Primary Outcome in Bold)	Linked Health Service Outcomes Measured (Primary Outcome in Bold)
Dicko (2011) [50,51]	Mali [2006–2007]	Routine—facility	Malaria	a. Extra services by immunization staff	IPTi services and counseling by staff at EPI clinics in intervention sites. Compared to sites not offering IPTi.	Pre/post; two groups [integration group = randomized areas where IPTi was delivered with routine vaccinations]	**Coverage of fully vaccinated children 9–23 months [BCG, 3 doses of DTP, 3 doses of polio, measles, and yellow fever vaccines] (increase in coverage in intervention compared to control and baseline)**	**-Coverage of IPTi (higher in intervention compared to control)** -Coverage of vitamin A (higher in intervention compared to control) -ITN use (similar in intervention compared to control)
Patouillard (2011) [52]	Ghana [2006]	Routine—outreach	Malaria	a. Extra services by immunization staff b. Extra information and/or counseling by immunization staff	IPTc delivery by VHWs compared to facility-based staff (at outpatient departments or EPI outreach clinics).	Post only; two groups [integration group = facility-based delivery]	**Not measured**	**-Coverage of IPTc (similar in VHW delivery and facility-based delivery)** -Cost of delivering full course of IPTc (more expensive to deliver by EPI nurses compared to VHWs)
Scates 2020 [53]	Ghana, Mali, Tanzania [2015–2016]	Routine—mixed (facility in Ghana, Tanzania, and Mali; community and facility in Zanzibar)	Malaria	a. Extra services by immunization staff	Continuous distribution of insecticide-treated bednets (ITNs) by immunization staff through ANC, EPI, schools, and mass distribution campaign.	Not applicable/no relevant outcomes compared: descriptive study of costs associated with various ITN continuous distribution delivery platforms.	**Not measured**	**Not measured**
Schellenberg (2011) and Willey (2011) [54,55]	Tanzania [2005–2007]	Routine—facility	Malaria	a. Extra services by immunization staff	IPTi services and counseling by staff at EPI clinics in intervention sites. Compared to no IPTi control sites.	Pre/post for infant survival and post only for other outcomes; two groups [integration group = randomized areas where IPTi was delivered with routine vaccinations compared to no IPTi control]	**-DTP3 and measles vaccination coverage (similar in IPTi vs no IPTi groups)**	**-Coverage of three doses of IPTi (higher in intervention compared to control)** -Infant mortality (decrease over time, but no difference between intervention and control groups)

Table 3. *Cont.*

Study [a]	Country (Study Year(s))	Immunization Delivery Platform	Linked Maternal and Child Health Service(s)	Integration Strategy(ies)	Description of Integration Strategy	Study Design: Outcome Comparison	Immunization Outcomes Measured (Primary Outcome in Bold)	Linked Health Service Outcomes Measured (Primary Outcome in Bold)
Theiss-Nyland (2016b) and (2017) [56,57]	Kenya, Malawi, Mali, Rwanda [2014]	Routine—mixed	Malaria	a. Extra services by immunization staff	Continuous distribution of LLINs through ANC and EPI	Not applicable/no relevant outcomes compared: feasibility study of continuous distribution.	**Not measured**	**Not measured**

[a] the last name of the first author and the publication year; studies are ordered by linked maternal and child health service, and then alphabetically by author. Notes: ANC = antenatal care; ART = antiretroviral therapy; BCG = bacille Calmette–Guerin vaccine; DTP = diphtheria, pertussis, and tetanus vaccine; EID = early infant diagnosis; EPI = expanded program of immunizations; HEI = HIV-exposed infant; HIV = human immunodeficiency virus; IPTc/i = intermittent preventive treatment for malaria during infancy/in children; ITN = insecticide-treated bednet; LLIN = long-lasting insecticidal nets; MCH = maternal and child health; OPV = oral polio vaccine;Penta = pentavalent vaccine; VHW = village health worker.

Table 4. Characteristics of included studies ($n = 7$) on the integration of primary healthcare services, nutrition, water, sanitation, and hygiene (WASH), or a combination of services with routine immunizations, systematic review update 2011–2020.

Study [a]	Country (Study Year(s))	Immunization Delivery Platform	Linked Maternal and Child Health Service(s)	Integration Strategy	Description of Integration Strategy	Study Design: Outcome Comparison	Immunization Outcomes Measured (Primary Outcome in Bold)	Linked Health Service Outcomes Measured (Primary Outcome in Bold)
Integration into routine immunization—maternal depression screening								
Bakare (2014) and (2017) [58,59]	Nigeria [2012]	Routine—facility	PHC—maternal depression	c. Co-location	Depression screening service co-located with EPI clinic visits.	Not applicable/no relevant outcomes compared: feasibility study only.	**Not measured**	**Not measured**
Integration into routine immunization—nutrition activities								
Monterrosa (2013) [60]	Mexico [2011]	Routine—mixed	Nutrition	b. Extra information and/or counseling by immunization staff	EPI nurses and radio communications delivered scripted nutrition counseling messages. Behavior change among women with children 6–24 months compared between with and without messages.	Pre/post; two groups [integration group = sites receiving nutrition communications from EPI nurses and via radio]	**Not measured**	**-Frequency of breast feeding (higher in integration group compared to sites not receiving nutrition communications)** -Self-reported feeding (mixed results but some healthier consumption in integration group)

Table 4. *Cont.*

Study [a]	Country (Study Year(s))	Immunization Delivery Platform	Linked Maternal and Child Health Service(s)	Integration Strategy	Description of Integration Strategy	Study Design: Outcome Comparison	Immunization Outcomes Measured (Primary Outcome in Bold)	Linked Health Service Outcomes Measured (Primary Outcome in Bold)
Oladeji (2019) [61]	South Sudan [2017]	Routine—mixed (nutrition treatment centers and community outreach)	Nutrition	c. Co-location e. Extra information and/or counseling by non-immunization staff	Immunization services offered to children visiting nutrition treatment clinics and nutrition community outreach. Nutrition volunteers provide messages on immunization, screen vaccination status and track children. Compared to immunization atPHCs.	Post only; two groups [integration group = immunization delivery at nutrition treatment clinics and community outreach]	-Proportion of children vaccinated in nutrition treatment clinics compared to standard PHC clinics [BCG, OPV 0–3, Penta 1–3, IPV, and measles] (data insufficient for comparison) **-Drop-out Penta1 to Penta3 (lower drop-out in nutrition treatment clinics compared to PHCs)**	**Not measured**
Integration into routine immunization—water, sanitation, and hygiene interventions (WASH)								
Briere (2012) and (Ryman) 2012 [62,63]	Kenya [2009]	Routine—facility	WASH	a. Extra services by immunization staff b. Extra information and/or counseling by immunization staff c. Co-location	During routine immunization visits, health workers offered water treatment, soap and related education to caregivers children aged <1 yr old.	Pre/post; two groups [integration group = district randomly selected to integrate WASH interventions at routine immunization visits]	**-Percent of children 2–20 months who received all vaccine doses [penta, OPV, and measles] (higher in intervention compared to control)** **-Percent of children 2–20 months who received all age-appropriate vaccines (higher in intervention compared to control)**	**-Awareness of water treatment options (increase in both intervention and control from pre to post)** **-Uptake of water treatment (significant pre–post increase in intervention, not control)** **-Percentage of households with soap (pre–post increase in intervention, not control)**
Integration into routine immunization—multiple primary healthcare and disease control interventions								
Bawa (2019) [20,21]	Nigeria [2014–2015]	Routine—mobile	Malaria, PHC, Nutrition, WASH	c. Co-location	Package of MCH services (antenatal care, malaria prevention, iron folate, deworming, child health, WASH, vitamin A, nutrition screening, and routine immunizations) delivered to women and children during mobile outreach visits.	Pre/post; one group	**-Coverage of measles vaccination (increased from pre to post)**	**-Provision of multiple MCH interventions (increase from pre to post)**

Table 4. *Cont.*

Study [a]	Country (Study Year(s))	Immunization Delivery Platform	Linked Maternal and Child Health Service(s)	Integration Strategy	Description of Integration Strategy	Study Design: Outcome Comparison	Immunization Outcomes Measured (Primary Outcome in Bold)	Linked Health Service Outcomes Measured (Primary Outcome in Bold)
Edmond (2020) [22]	Afghanistan [2013]	Routine—mobile	PHC, Nutrition	c. Co-location	Integrated outreach services for ANC, PNC, and immunization by mobile health teams (MHTs).	Post only; two groups [integration group = recent MHT integrated outreach delivery, comparator = areas without recent visits]	**-Measles first dose coverage (higher in areas with recent MHT integrated outreach compared to non-recent)** **-Penta 3 coverage (higher in areas with recent MHT integrated outreach, but not statistically significant)**	**-Coverage of at least one ANC visit (higher in areas with recent MHT integrated outreach)** **-Coverage of at least one PNC visit (no difference)** **-Coverage of facility-based delivery (no difference)** **-Coverage of at least one IMCI visit (higher in areas with recent MHT integrated outreach)**
Hodges (2015) [24]	Sierra Leone [2012–2013]	Routine—facility	Family planning, Nutrition	c. Co-location e. Extra information and/or counseling by non-immunization staff	Extra co-located staff provided vit A and either IYCF counseling or IYCF and FP services, alongside routine and catch-up vaccination, during visits from 6 months of age onwards. Extra staff also gave information on catch-up vaccination.	Post only; three groups [integration group 1 = revised vaccination card with vit A + IYCF + FP counseling, integration group 2 revised vaccination card with vit A, control group = revised vaccination card with vit A]	**-Proportion of fully vaccinated children (similar in all groups)** **-Proportion of infants receiving catch-up vaccination [OPV 2 or 3, penta and/or PCV] (higher in both integration groups compared to control)**	**-Coverage of vit A supplement (higher in both integration groups compared to control)** **-Provision of FP counseling and commodities (higher in both integration groups compared to control)**

[a] the last name of the first author and the publication year; studies are ordered by linked maternal and child health service, and then alphabetically by author. Notes: ANC = antenatal care; BCG = bacille Calmette–Guerin vaccine; EPI = expanded program of immunizations; FP = family planning; IMCI = integrated management of childhood illnesses; IPV = inactivated polio vaccine; IYCF = infant and young child feeding; MCH = maternal and child health;; OPV = oral polio vaccine; PHC = primary healthcare; PCV = pneumococcal conjugate vaccine; Penta = pentavalent; PNC = prenatal care; vit A = vitamin A supplementation; WASH = water, sanitation, and hygiene.

3.3. Integration Strategies

Almost half (44%) of the included studies reported the use of multiple strategies for integrated service delivery (Table 4). The most frequently described strategies were the co-location of services (n = 23 studies, 68%), the provision of extra services by immunization staff (n = 14, 41%), the provision of extra information and/or counseling by immunization staff (n = 14, 41%), and the provision of extra information and/or counseling by non-immunization staff (n = 4, 12%). No studies reported on vaccination services provided by staff whose job description did not usually include vaccination.

In general, there was no clear pattern in the types of strategy used to integrate particular linked MCH services (Tables 1–4). However, it was noted that the provision of 'extra services by immunization staff' was one of the integration strategies described in 88% (7 of 8) of malaria studies [25,26,49–57] and the provision of 'extra information and/or counselling by immunization staff' was one of the strategies described in 78% (7 of 9) of family planning studies [31,32,34–40].

3.4. Effect of Integration on Outcomes for Immunization and Linked Service

Most of the included studies (n = 25, 74%) reported at least one immunization (n = 20) and/or linked health service outcome (n = 21) that could be compared across groups with and without the implementation of integrated service delivery (Table 5). Data on immunization outcomes included vaccination coverage for one or more antigens or the proportion of children who were fully vaccinated (n = 11, 55%), the number of doses for one or more antigen (n = 7, 35%), and drop-out rates (n = 2, 10%). For linked MCH services, the reported outcomes either described the coverage of the service (n = 14, 67%) or the number of participants accessing/using the service (n = 7, 33%). Overall, the effect of integration was beneficial (mixed positive or positive) for most (76%) studies reporting linked MCH service outcomes and nearly half (55%) of studies reporting immunization outcomes.

Table 5. A qualitative summary of the effect of integrated service delivery on immunization and linked service outcomes (n = 25 *) by immunization delivery platform, linked health service, and a combination of integration strategies, systematic review update 2011–2020.

				Qualitative Summary [1] of the Effect of Integrated Service Delivery											
				Immunization Outcome [2,3]						Linked MCH Service Outcome [2,3]					
Study	**Country**	**EPI Platform**	**Linked Health Service(s)**	**NOT MEASURED**	**NEG**	**M-NEG**	**STATIC**	**M-POS**	**POS**	**NOT MEASURED**	**NEG**	**M-NEG**	**STATIC**	**M-POS**	**POS**
Goodson 2012 & Kulkarni 2010 [25,26]	Madagascar	Campaign—mixed	Malaria						A C						A C
Birukila 2017 [23]	Nigeria	Campaign—mixed	PHC						C	C					
Habib 2017 [26]	Pakistan	Campaign—mixed	Nutrition, PHC						B C	B C					
Balasubramaniam 2018 [31]	India	Routine—outreach	FP				B							B	
Cooper 2015 [32]	Liberia	Routine—facility	FP				B C								B C
Dulli 2016 [34]	Rwanda	Routine—facility	FP				B C								B C
Vance 2014 [37]	Ghana, Zambia	Routine—facility	FP	B C									B C		
Cooper 2020 [33]	Malawi	Routine- mixed	FP					A C E							A C E
Nelson 2019 [36]	Liberia	Routine—facility	FP				B C E								B C E
Yugbare Belemsaga 2018 [38]	Burkina Faso	Routine—facility	FP				A B C						A B C		
Odafe 2020 [45]	Nigeria	Routine—facility	HIV	C							C				
Ong'ech 2012 [46]	Kenya	Routine—facility	HIV						C						C
McCollum 2012 [44]	Malawi	Routine—facility	HIV	B C											B C
Goodson 2013 &Wallace 2014 [42,43]	Tanzania	Routine—facility	HIV			A B C				A B C					
Wang 2015 [48]	Zambia	Routine—facility	HIV				A B C								A B C
Bojang 2011 [49]	Gambia	Routine—outreach	Malaria		A						A				
Dicko 2011 [50]	Mali	Routine—facility	Malaria						A						A
Schellenberg 2011 & Willey 2011 [54,55]	Tanzania	Routine—facility	Malaria				A								A

Table 5. *Cont.*

				Qualitative Summary [1] of the Effect of Integrated Service Delivery											
				Immunization Outcome [2,3]						Linked MCH Service Outcome [2,3]					
Study	**Country**	**EPI Platform**	**Linked Health Service(s)**	**NOT MEASURED**	**NEG**	**M-NEG**	**STATIC**	**M-POS**	**POS**	**NOT MEASURED**	**NEG**	**M-NEG**	**STATIC**	**M-POS**	**POS**
Patouillard 2011 [52]	Ghana	Routine—outreach	Malaria	**A B**									**A B**		
Monterrosa 2013 [60]	Mexico	Routine—mixed	Nutrition	**B**											**B**
Oladeji 2019 [61]	South Sudan	Routine—mixed	Nutrition						**C E**	**C E**					
Briere 2012& Ryman 2012 [62,63]	Kenya	Routine—facility	WASH						**A B C**						**A B C**
Bawa 2019 [21]	Nigeria	Routine—mobile	Malaria, PHC, Nutrition, WASH						**C**						**C**
Edmond 2020 [22]	Afghanistan	Routine—mobile	Nutrition, PHC						**C**					**C**	
Hodges 2015 [25]	Sierra Leone	Routine—facility	FP, Nutrition					**C E**							**C E**

Notes: EPI = expanded program of immunizations; HIV = human immunodeficiency virus; FP = family planning; MCH = maternal and child health; PHC = primary healthcare; WASH = water, sanitation, and hygiene. * studies that reported at least one immunization and/or linked health service outcome. [1] primary outcomes that were considered in this qualitative summary are designated in bold in Table 1. [2] a single qualitative summary was used to describe the direction of effect of integration for the primary outcome(s) for immunization and for the linked health service separately. The terms used were defined as follows: "not measured"—no outcome measured or no non-integration comparison group available; "negative"—lower coverage or service provision in the integration compared to the non-integration group; "mixed negative"—some outcomes were lower in the integration compared to the non-integration group but others remained static; "static"—no meaningful difference in coverage or service provision between integration and non-integration groups; "mixed positive"—some outcomes were higher in the integration compared to the non-integration group, but others remained static; or "positive"—higher coverage or services in the integration compared to the non-integration group. [3] integration strategies were categorized in one or more of the following ways: A. extra services provided by immunization staff (i.e., testing, treatment, referrals, etc.); B. extra information and/or counseling provided by immunization staff (i.e., one-on-one consultation, the provision of informational materials, etc.); C. the co-location of services (e.g., same timing or same physical location of immunization delivery and linked health service); D. vaccination provided by non-immunization staff; E. extra information and/or counseling provided by non-immunization staff (i.e., screening, health education, or immunization promotion, etc.).

For most studies that reported both immunization service and linked health service outcomes (n = 16), the relative boost in coverage or uptake obtained for the linked MCH service was generally the same or better than the effect on the immunization outcome. No clear relationship was observed between the integration strategy and the effect when grouped by immunization delivery platform and linked health service (Table 5).

Among studies that integrated service delivery during immunization campaigns (n = 3), groups receiving integrated services had significantly higher vaccination coverage for measles [25,26] and oral polio vaccine (OPV) [23,28], and significantly higher long-lasting insecticide-treated (ITN) bednet coverage [25,26], compared to non-integrated service delivery groups (Table 5).

For studies of the integration of family planning services with routine immunization service delivery (n = 7), the effect on vaccination coverage was static. The exception was the work of Cooper, 2020 [33], which showed a mixed positive effect based on the static coverage of DTP1 but elevated coverage of DTP3. Across the same studies [31–34,36–40], the effect on family planning service outcomes ranged from static to positive (Table 5).

The effect on outcomes was more variable in the seven studies integrating HIV services with routine immunization service delivery [42–46,48]. The three studies reporting immunization outcomes showed mixed negative [42,43], static (48), or positive [46] effects on either vaccination coverage or the number of doses administered. The four studies reporting linked health service outcomes indicated mostly positive effects [44,46,48], but one negative (45) effect, on outcomes related to early infant diagnosis of HIV (Table 5).

Among the six studies integrating malaria interventions with routine immunization service delivery [49–52,54,55], the direction of the effect on outcomes varied. However, within studies, there was some consistency in the outcome effects on both the immunization and linked MCH services. Bojang (2011) [49] reported the negative effects of integration on both fully vaccinated coverage and the coverage of intermittent preventative treatment for malaria in children (IPTc) and Dicko (2011) [50,51] reported positive effects on both fully vaccinated coverage and the coverage of IPT during infancy (IPTi). Schellenberg (2011) and Wiley (2011) [54,55] reported a static effect on DTP3 and measles vaccination coverage, but a positive effect on IPTi. Patouillard (2011) [52] did not measure immunization outcomes and reported a static effect of integration on IPTc (Table 5).

Two studies of the integration of nutrition services with routine immunization service delivery only reported outcomes related to either immunization or linked health services. Monterrosa (2013) [60] reported the positive effect of integration on the frequency of breastfeeding and Oladeji (2019) [61] reported a positive improvement in from Penta 1 to Penta 3 drop-out rates in the integrated group (Table 5).

Two studies focused on the integration of WASH services with immunization services. Briere (2012) and Ryman 2012 [62,63] both reported statistically significant increases in the proportion of fully vaccinated children, and increases in WASH outcomes such as awareness and the uptake of water treatment options in the integrated service delivery group compared to the non-integrated delivery group (Table 5).

For the four studies integrating multiple services with routine immunization service delivery [20–24], the effects of integration on immunization outcomes and linked service outcomes were either mixed positive or positive (Table 5).

3.5. Implementation Considerations

The processes, enablers, and barriers affecting service integration, as described by the included studies, are shown in Table 6.

Table 6. Implementation considerations reported for integrated service delivery of maternal and child health services with immunization programs, systematic review update 2011–2020.

Category	Processes, Enablers, and Barriers Affecting Service Integration	References
Policy and governance topics	Consistency of leadership support	[25,26,28,34,37,48]
	Governments and donors seeking efficiency amidst multiple priorities	[23,33]
	Reducing financial access barriers to the integration of other primary healthcare services with immunization	[23,33,38–40]
Design of integrated service delivery	Optimize co-location of additional staff, especially if extra tasks require more time (e.g., counseling) or skills	[32,33,36,37,61]
	Ensure good matches in terms of of cadence, target groups, and types of services (e.g., preventive rather than curative services may more amenable to integration with immunization)	[38–40,44]
	Ensure additional service requirements do not compromise uptake or quality	[41–43]
	Use integration as an opportunity to provide services to areas/populations that are difficult to reach	[20,21,23,25,26,61]
Human resources for health	Managing workload and time demands for extra tasks	[22,29,36–40,49–53,56,57,60,62,63]
	Additional and skilled staff may be needed (e.g., counseling)	[20–22,28,35–40,44,49,52]
	Motivation and empowerment of healthcare staff to provide expanded care, which healthcare workers generally perceive as better in quality and responsiveness	[32,33,36,48,50,51]
	Training that is (a) harmonized for vaccinators and for providers of linked health service; (b) includes client communications/mobilization; and (c) includes integration processes and tools	[20,21,23,24,27,29,32–34,36–40,45,46,49–51,54–56,61–63]
	Involving community-based health workers to support integrated service delivery	[20,21,24,33,44–46,48,49,52,61–63]
	Ensuring that staff are willing to collaborate in providing additional services	[37–40]
Management, logistics, and costs	Coordinated program planning across program managers and between staff	[32,33,44,48,49]
	Consistency of supplies (particularly for linked service) and coordinated logistics	[20,21,30,32,35,36,46,48–52,56,57,62,63]
	Efficiency may lower costs of integrated service	[27,34,38–40,52,62,63]
	Integrating professional staff may increase costs	[49]
	Ensuring infrastructure is supportive (e.g., privacy)	[29,32,35,36,42,43]
Operational tools, reporting and recording	Consolidation of information systems and reporting, including home-based records	[20,21,31–34,36,56,57]
	Ensuring time for documentation of extra services	[36,56,57]
	Job aids and other tools to support implementation of linked service and referral between programs	[29,31–34,36–40,45,57]
Community and client topics	Promote care seeking, with perceptions of integrated services as more responsive and client-focused	[23,24,27,28,31,36,49–51,57,61–63]
	Ensuring stigma/sensitivity does not hamper uptake	[23,32–36,41–43,46,58,59]
	Ensuring family time and travel costs do not increase	[22,38–43,46,62,63]
	Account for need to involve spouse in care decisions	[32,35,41]
	Ensuring integrated services address common barriers to uptake	[22,27,28,32–36,38–44,46,61–63]
	Ensuring multiple channels of communication on integrated health services	[25,26,33,38–40]

Note: this table outlines the implementation considerations extracted from studies, reporting contributors to the degree to which service integration affected outcomes for the linked service or immunization.

In relation to policy and governance, the key themes that emerged were the consistency of national government support and policies for integration [25,26,28,34,37,48]; the pursuit of efficiency in the delivery of health services by governments and donors, in particular for campaigns [23,33]; and the expansion of policies to minimize the financial burden of integration within primary healthcare services [38–40] (Table 6).

Several studies discussed the re-design of services in a way best suited to promote integration. One frequently mentioned consideration was the need for the co-location in place and time of additional staff, particularly if the linked service was time-consuming or needed specialized skills [32,33,36,37,61]. Additionally, studies also noted that integrated approaches should consider the compatibility of cadence for services, target groups, and types of services [38–40,44]; McCollum (2012) [44] noted that the integration of HIV preventative services with immunization may be more beneficial than treatment due to the better prognoses obtained when initiating care as early as possible. Studies also reported that the process of integration should not compromise the uptake or quality of services [6,41,42]. Integration was also sometimes viewed as an opportunity to provide services, especially with the help of community health workers, to areas or communities that are hard to reach, thus expanding the reach of services [20,21,23,25,26,61] (Table 6).

Most studies mentioned one or more considerations relating to human resources for health that affect the success of integrated service delivery. The training needs highlighted included the benefit of harmonized combined training for vaccinators and linked health services providers [20,21,23,24,27,29,32,34,36–40,46,49–51,54,55], additional training on communications to improve community understanding and the uptake of integrated activities [23,32–34,36,56,61–63], and training focused on integration processes and tools [32–34,36,45]. The management of staff workloads and the time required for additional tasks were also major concerns reported in many studies [22,29,36–40,49–53,56,57,60,62,63]. There was recognition that integration may require additional staff with specific skillsets [20–22,28,35–40,44,49,52]. Other considerations mentioned were the importance of involving community-based health workers in efforts to support integrated service delivery [20,21,24,33,44–46,48,49,52,61–63], improved motivation, the empowerment of healthcare staff to provide expanded care, which healthcare workers generally perceived as better in terms of quality and responsiveness [32,33,36,48,50,51], and ensuring that staff involved in integration were willing to collaborate in order to provide the additional services [37–40] (Table 6). In terms of management, logistics, and costs, the consistent availability of supplies and commodities, particularly for the linked service, and coordinated logistics were mentioned frequently, with some studies noting that stockouts could be a deterrent for clients returning for care or services [20,21,30,32,35,36,46,48–52,56,57,62,63]. Particularly for more sensitive linked services, such as HIV or family planning, studies noted that it was important to ensure that infrastructure for service delivery was supportive and appropriate regarding considerations such as privacy needs [29,32,35,36,42,43]. Additionally, although some studies suggested that improving efficiencies could reduce the costs of integrated service delivery [27,34,38–40,52,62,63], one study noted that integration involving professional staff may, in fact, increase costs [49] (Table 3). Studies noted the need for new systems for reporting and recording integrated service delivery. Other considerations included new tools, such as job aids to support staff in providing integrated care or other operational aspects of integration [20,21,31–34,36,56,57]. There were also reports of the need to account for the additional workload in expanded information and reporting systems [29,31–34,36–40,45,57], including home-based records, and ensure adequate time is taken to record and report additional services [36,56,57] (Table 6).

Many studies reported the importance of addressing community and client considerations during service re-design; specifically, there was a need for some consideration of how integrated services would be perceived and the degree to which they would be seen as more responsive to clients' needs [23,24,27,28,31,36,49–51,57,61–63]. The need for clear communications through multiple channels was reported in some studies [25,26,33,38–40]. In scenarios where linked services were potentially sensitive, such as for HIV diagnosis or care, integration efforts needed to address potential stigma [23,32–36,41–43,46,58,59], and for some, like family planning, they needed consider how to account for clients' preferences in terms of involving a spouse in decision-making [32,35,41]. Clients, like providers, were concerned that integrating services should not unreasonably increase the time or costs of care seeking [22,38–43,46,62,63]. Many studies did consider the degree to which more integrated services could address common constraints on care seeking, and this was reported as an important motivator for pursuing health service integration [22,27,28,32–36,38–44,46,61–63] (Table 6).

4. Discussion

In this systematic review update of the integration of MCH services with childhood immunization services, we synthesized evidence from 34 relevant studies, which were identified between 2011 and 2020, following the publication of the last review on this topic in 2012 [6]. In comparison to previous reviews [4,6], there were fewer articles included reporting on the integration of service delivery within immunization campaigns. With more recent global strategies calling for a shift towards integrated campaigns beyond the co-delivery of multiple vaccine antigens [64], evidence from integrated service delivery in campaigns will be important for informing these approaches. Although a similar range of linked services was observed in this review as in the previous reviews [4,6], the current review included a larger proportion of family planning studies. Additionally, despite recent global initiatives calling for integrated service delivery within primary healthcare structures [1,2,8], most included studies focused on malaria, family planning, and HIV, suggesting that the implementation of integrated service delivery may be driven by specific programs or funded initiatives rather than by a push towards achieving universal health coverage. The considerable heterogeneity of study designs reflects the challenges of conducting real-world implementation research into modifications to service delivery, especially in low-resource settings.

Our review assessed the effect of integrated service delivery on outcomes for immunization and/or linked health services. Among 16 included studies where both outcomes were reported, the effect of integration on the linked health service was generally equal to or showed greater benefit than the effect on immunization; additionally, the effect on immunization was only negative in one study where both outcomes were reported. This result supports previous observations that the coverage of other health services could be expanded through integrated service delivery with immunization programs. This was described, for example, in reviews from 2015 relating to interventions for HIV [65] and family planning [66]. In these, and in our synthesis, the extent of benefit was likely to depend on the strength of the immunization platform prior to integration [6] and on the successful management of implementation considerations. Positive outcomes were not universal: we found two studies in which integrated service delivery had poorer outcomes for the linked service when compared to alternatives for both HIV [45] and malaria [49]; immunization outcomes were not reported in either of these studies. For both studies, there were different processes contributing to the lack of benefit to linked health services from integration. In the HIV study [45], immunization clinics yielded the lowest percentage of eligible children for pediatric HIV testing in comparison with other points of service, possibly due to the lower overlap of the target age range for immunization clinics and pediatric HIV testing (0–14 years). In the malaria study [49], the coverage of IPTc was higher when delivered by village health workers compared to monthly delivery by reproductive and child health trekking teams, which included EPI staff. This may have been due to the convenience of community-based antimalarial delivery, which is available any day of the month rather than on scheduled EPI delivery days. In one study, which integrated family planning with immunization [37] and did not see increased contraceptive uptake, a lack of fidelity in implementation was assessed as the likely cause. Community perceptions appear to play an important role, with caution seen when HIV service referrals are integrated with immunization visits [43], and enthusiasm seen when immunization is linked to malaria control [51].

The previous reviews [4,6] highlighted challenges with integration including, logistical difficulties, concerns with harming existing services, target age group differences, and pre-existing low immunization coverage. Key lessons learned for service delivery integration included the importance of establishing intervention compatibility, considering the current immunization program's strength when choosing to integrate, and ensuring strong planning for integration. In this review, almost all studies noted the critical importance of the details of implementation in determining whether an attempt to integrate services proves beneficial. The considerations summarized in Table 3 provide a framework that can be drawn on by planners wishing to promote greater service integration. Our synthesis suggests that three key areas determine how easy it is to integrate services, and thus contribute to improved service delivery: firstly, whether there is a good alignment of the new linked services' target population and the need for skills and supplies with the capacities of the service platform already in use for immunization; secondly, whether investments are in place to adequately support staff in terms of the guidance, training, time, supplies, and workforce needed to deliver the expanded package of care; and thirdly, whether clients' expectations (for example privacy or timely care) are met and community perceptions are well understood, which can be achieved through formative assessment if necessary. These areas were not demonstrated in all included studies, and relatively fewer studies fully accounted for the client perspective; therefore, this represents our synthesis of the factors that correlated with beneficial outcomes.

In this review, we observed a range of integration processes, such as child health screening; the provision of referrals, counseling, or testing; and the distribution of commodities or medicines. We broadly classified these into types of strategies, such as the provision of extra services or information by immunization or non-immunization staff, and the co-location or timing of service delivery. Most studies reported the use of a combination of these strategies in the integration process, with co-location and the provision of extra services by immunization staff being the most common. The feasibility of the integration strategy depends on the complexity of the linked health service and the EPI platform used for delivery; for instance, easy-to-administer commodities such as ITNs or medicines such as de-worming treatment may be more conducive to extra service provision by immunization staff, either during immunization campaigns or at routine immunization contact points, but more time-intensive and potentially sensitive processes such as counseling for HIV testing and treatment may be better suited to delivery during routine immunization services [5]. Our evidence also suggests that the integration of complex tasks, especially those involving counseling or curative care, may be better handled by the co-location of additional staff at the same time and place as immunization services, rather than via the addition of these tasks to the work of vaccinators.

To enable a focus on integration outcomes, this review was limited to studies reporting on intentional efforts to implement and measure an explicit change to service delivery with the prime purpose of integrating other services with childhood immunization programs. We could not include broader approaches such as the integrated management of childhood illnesses, for which integration is one approach amongst several, as part of primary healthcare-strengthening initiatives; these may also provide valuable examples. Additionally, given this review's focus on integrated service delivery at immunization program contact points, we excluded studies reporting on missed opportunities for vaccination and integrated approaches to community health education, which are other key focus areas for integration with potential benefits to immunization coverage. Additionally, given the wide range of study designs and the heterogeneity of outcomes reported, we were unable to conduct a quantitative synthesis of effect measures.

Our review identified new articles published since the previous review on this topic [6], but several evidence gaps remain. First, there were few studies from LMICs outside of Africa; additional studies from a wider range of LMICs are needed, particularly from

Asian and Pacific nations, given their large populations and/or the knowledge gaps. Second, many studies reporting on integrated campaigns did not include a non-integration comparator, thus limiting our ability to evaluate the effect of integrated service delivery; there is a pressing need to expand the documentation of integrated health campaigns, especially regarding their cost-effectiveness [64,67]. Third, although the cost-saving benefits of integrated services in general are sometimes cited [1], there were few studies reporting on the cost of integrated service delivery compared to the use of non-integrated approaches. Fourth, evidence gaps persist surrounding the role of client preferences for integrated service delivery, including which services to integrate, at what contact points, and how, in the design of integrated approaches. Relatively few of the studies we reviewed included community members' preferences in the design of integrated services. Finally, future implementation research should focus on integrated service delivery in the context of new vaccine introduction, in particular for older age groups beyond the first two years of life. More recently introduced vaccines a in adolescence, such as those against the human papillomavirus (HPV), present a new range of opportunities for integrating other services; these vary considerably by service delivery platform, with different options for integration during school-based vaccination to those available from facility- or community-based services [68].

5. Conclusions

Approaches to integrating MCH services with immunization programs have the potential to expand access to and the utilization of linked services and, in some cases, improve immunization coverage. The strategies and processes for integration varied across studies, and were typically determined by the nature of the linked health service. The details of service design and implementation were found to be critical determinants of the success of integration. Integrated services continue to play an important role in achieving more client-centered services in primary healthcare and progress towards IA2030. Future implementation research should expand the focus of integrated service delivery by taking a life-course approach that examines opportunities for expanded care during immunization services offered at broader age ranges.

Supplementary Materials: The following supporting information can be downloaded at https://www.mdpi.com/article/10.3390/vaccines12121313/s1. Table S1: List of studies excluded on full-text review and reason for exclusion (n = 427).

Author Contributions: Conceptualization, C.J.M. and A.S.W., with input from J.G.B. and B.M.; methodology, C.J.M. and A.S.W., with input from J.G.B. and B.M.; validation, C.J.M., M.P.S. and A.S.W.; formal analysis, M.P.S., C.J.M. and A.S.W.; investigation, C.J.M., E.P., J.D., M.P.S. and A.S.W.; data curation, M.P.S. and C.J.M.; writing—original draft preparation, M.P.S., C.J.M. and A.S.W.; writing—review and editing, all authors (A.S.W., B.M., C.J.M., E.P., J.D., J.G.B. and M.P.S.); visualization, M.P.S. and C.J.M.; supervision, J.G.B. and B.M.; funding acquisition, C.J.M. All authors have read and agreed to the published version of the manuscript.

Funding: Partial support was received by CJM from a National Health and Medical Research Council of Australia Postgraduate Scholarship [1075065]. J.G.B. is supported by a NHMRC Investigator Grant, and Burnet Institute is supported by the NHMRC Independent Research Institutes Infrastructure Support Scheme and Victorian Government Operational Infrastructure Support grant.

Institutional Review Board Statement: Not applicable.

Data Availability Statement: The original contributions presented in this study are included in the article/Supplementary Materials. Further inquiries can be directed to the corresponding author(s).

Acknowledgments: The authors would like to dedicate this article to Vance Dietz and his lifelong work in immunizations, including his support for and expertise on integration. Dietz was the senior author for both of the previous publications on this topic and his contributions to this field will be greatly missed. The authors also gratefully acknowledge early contributions to the design of this review from Beverley Biggs, Patrick Condron, Freya Fowkes, Kathleen Fox, Tracey Goodman,

John Stanback, Margaret Watkins and Emily Wootton. Burnet Institute is located on the traditional lands of the Boon Wurrung people of the Kulin Nations and we pay our respects to their elders past and present.

Conflicts of Interest: The authors declare no conflicts of interest. The findings and conclusions in this report are those of the authors and do not necessarily represent the views of the Centers for Disease Control and Prevention.

References

1. Immunization Agenda Partners. Immunization agenda 2030: A global strategy to leave no one behind. *Vaccine* **2024**, *42* (Suppl. 1), S5–S14. [CrossRef] [PubMed]
2. Universal Health Coverage (UHC): World Health Organization: Geneva. Updated 5 October 2023. Available online: https://www.who.int/news-room/fact sheets/detail/universal-health-coverage-(uhc) (accessed on 16 August 2024).
3. WHO & UNICEF. *Tracking Progress Towards Universal Coverage for Reproductive, Newborn and Child Health: The 2017 Report*; World Health Organization: Geneva, Switzerland, 2017.
4. Wallace, A.; Dietz, V.; Cairns, K.L. Integration of immunization services with other health interventions in the developing world: What works and why? Systematic literature review. *Trop. Med. Int. Health* **2009**, *14*, 11–19. [CrossRef] [PubMed]
5. Wallace, A.; Ryman, T.; Mihigo, R.; Ndoutabe, M.; Tounkara, B.; Grant, G.; Anya, B.; Kiawi, E.C.; Kone, S.; Tesfaye, H.; et al. Strengthening evidence-based planning of integrated health service delivery through local measures of health intervention delivery times. *J. Infect. Dis.* **2012**, *205* (Suppl. 1), S40–S48. [CrossRef] [PubMed]
6. Wallace, A.S.; Ryman, T.K.; Dietz, V. Experiences integrating delivery of maternal and child health services with childhood immunization programs: Systematic review update. *J. Infect. Dis.* **2012**, *205* (Suppl. 1), S6–S19. [CrossRef] [PubMed]
7. *Working Together: An Integration Resource Guide for Immunization Services Throughout the Life Course*; Contract No.: Licence: CC BY-NCSA 3.0 IGO; World Health Organization: Geneva, Switzerland, 2018.
8. The Lusaka Agenda: Conclusions of the Future of Global Health Initiatives Process. In Proceedings of the Future Global Health Initiatives, Addis Ababa, Ethiopia, 14 June 2024.
9. Wallace, A.S.; Ryman, T.K.; Privor-Dumm, L.; Morgan, C.; Fields, R.; Garcia, C.; Sodha, S.V.; Lindstrand, A.; Nic Lochlainn, L.M. Leaving no one behind: Defining and implementing an integrated life course approach to vaccination across the next decade as part of the immunization Agenda 2030. *Vaccine* **2024**, *42* (Suppl. 1), S54–S63. [CrossRef]
10. *The Big Catch-Up: An Essential Immunization Recovery Plan for 2023 and Beyond*; WHO: New York, NY, USA, 2023.
11. Cochrane Effective Practice and Organisation of Care (EPOC). Available online: https://epoc.cochrane.org/ (accessed on 9 September 2024).
12. Morgan, C.J.; Davis, J.; Watkins, M.; Wallace, A.; Fox, F.; Goodman, T.; Stanback, J.; Fowkes, F.; Condron, P.; Biggs, B.; et al. Integration of Immunisation Services and Other Health Services in Low- and Middle-Income Countries: Protocol for an Updated Systematic Review: CRD420160458762016. Available online: https://www.crd.york.ac.uk/prospero/display_record.php?ID=CRD42016045876 (accessed on 15 November 2024).
13. The World by Income and Region, 2016: The World Bank Group. Available online: https://datatopics.worldbank.org/world-development-indicators/the-world-by-income-and-region.html (accessed on 9 September 2024).
14. Page, M.J.; McKenzie, J.E.; Bossuyt, P.M.; Boutron, I.; Hoffmann, T.C.; Mulrow, C.D.; Shamseer, L.; Tetzlaff, J.M.; Akl, E.A.; Brennan, S.E.; et al. The PRISMA 2020 statement: An updated guideline for reporting systematic reviews. *BMJ* **2021**, *372*, n71. [CrossRef]
15. Balshem, H.; Helfand, M.; Schünemann, H.J.; Oxman, A.D.; Kunz, R.; Brozek, J.; Vist, G.E.; Falck-Ytter, Y.; Meerpohl, J.; Norris, S.; et al. GRADE guidelines: 3. Rating the quality of evidence. *J. Clin. Epidemiol.* **2011**, *64*, 401–406. [CrossRef]
16. *Critical Appraisal Skills Programme (CASP) Qualitative Checklist*; Critical Appraisal Skills Programme: Oxford, UK, 2014.
17. Mays, N.; Pope, C.; Popay, J. Systematically reviewing qualitative and quantitative evidence to inform management and policy-making in the health field. *J. Health Serv. Res. Policy* **2005**, *10* (Suppl. 1), 6–20. [CrossRef]
18. Snilstveit, B.; Oliver, S.; Vojtkova, M. Narrative approaches to systematic review and synthesis of evidence for international development policy and practice. *J. Dev. Effect.* **2012**, *4*, 409–429. [CrossRef]
19. *SURE Guides for Preparing and Using Evidence-Based Policy Briefs*; SURE Collaboration; Norwegian Knowledge Center for the Health Services: Oslo, Norway, 2011.
20. Bawa, S.; McNab, C.; Nkwogu, L.; Braka, F.; Obinya, E.; Galway, M.; Mirelman, A.J.; Hammanyero, K.I.; Safiyanu, G.; Chukwuji, M.; et al. Using the polio programme to deliver primary health care in Nigeria: Implementation research. *Bull. World Health Organ.* **2019**, *97*, 24–32. [CrossRef]
21. Bawa, S.; Shuaib, F.; Saidu, M.; Ningi, A.; Abdullahi, S.; Abba, B.; Idowu, A.; Alkasim, J.; Hammanyero, K.; Warigon, C.; et al. Conduct of vaccination in hard-to-reach areas to address potential polio reservoir areas, 2014-2015. *BMC Public Health* **2018**, *18* (Suppl. 4), 1312. [CrossRef] [PubMed]
22. Edmond, K.; Yousufi, K.; Naziri, M.; Higgins-Steele, A.; Qadir, A.Q.; Sadat, S.M.; Bellows, A.L.; Smith, E. Mobile outreach health services for mothers and children in conflict-affected and remote areas: A population-based study from Afghanistan. *Arch. Dis. Child.* **2020**, *105*, 18–25. [CrossRef] [PubMed]

23. Habib, M.A.; Soofi, S.; Cousens, S.; Anwar, S.; Haque, N.U.; Ahmed, I.; Ali, N.; Tahir, R.; Bhutta, Z.A. Community engagement and integrated health and polio immunisation campaigns in conflict-affected areas of Pakistan: A cluster randomised controlled trial. *Lancet Glob. Health* **2017**, *5*, e593–e603. [CrossRef]
24. Hodges, M.H.; Sesay, F.F.; Kamara, H.I.; Nyorkor, E.D.; Bah, M.; Koroma, A.S.; Kandeh, J.N.; Ouédraogo, R.; Wolfe, A.C.; Katcher, H.I.; et al. Integrating Vitamin A Supplementation at 6 months into the Expanded Program of Immunization in Sierra Leone. *Matern. Child Health J.* **2015**, *19*, 1985–1992. [CrossRef]
25. Goodson, J.L.; Kulkarni, M.A.; Eng, J.L.V.; Wannemuehler, K.A.; Cotte, A.H.; Desrochers, R.E.; Randriamanalina, B.; Luman, E.T. Improved equity in measles vaccination from integrating insecticide-treated bednets in a vaccination campaign, Madagascar. *Trop. Med. Int. Health* **2012**, *17*, 430–437. [CrossRef] [PubMed]
26. Kulkarni, M.A.; Eng, J.V.; Desrochers, R.E.; Cotte, A.H.; Goodson, J.L.; Johnston, A.; Wolkon, A.; Erskine, M.; Berti, P.; Rakotoarisoa, A.; et al. Contribution of integrated campaign distribution of long-lasting insecticidal nets to coverage of target groups and total populations in malaria-endemic areas in Madagascar. *Am. J. Trop. Med. Hyg.* **2010**, *82*, 420–425. [CrossRef]
27. Boselli, G.; Yajima, A.; Aratchige, P.E.; Feldon, K.E.; Xeuatvongsa, A.; Phounphenghak, K.; Sihakhang, K.; Chitsavang, C.; Phengkeo, S.; Gabrielli, A.F.; et al. Integration of deworming into an existing immunisation and vitamin A supplementation campaign is a highly effective approach to maximise health benefits with minimal cost in Lao PDR. *Int. Health* **2011**, *3*, 240–245. [CrossRef]
28. Birukila, G.; Babale, S.M.; Epstein, H.; Gugong, V.; Anger, R.; Corkum, M.; Nebanat, A.J.; Musoke, F.; Alabi, O. Reducing resistance to polio immunisation with free health camps and Bluetooth messaging: An update from Kaduna, Northern, Nigeria. *Glob. Public Health* **2017**, *12*, 19–30. [CrossRef]
29. Friderichs, N.; Swanepoel, D.; Hall, J.W., 3rd. Efficacy of a community-based infant hearing screening program utilizing existing clinic personnel in Western Cape, South Africa. *Int. J. Pediatr. Otorhinolaryngol.* **2012**, *76*, 552–559. [CrossRef]
30. Jac-Okereke, C.A.; Ezegwui, I.R.; Okoye, O. Vision Screening in Infants Attending Immunization Clinics in a Developing Country. *J. Prim. Care Community Health* **2020**, *11*, 2150132720907430. [CrossRef]
31. Balasubramaniam, S.; Kumar, S.; Sethi, R.; Charurat, E.; Lalchandani, K.; Schuster, A.; Sood, B. Quasi-experimental Study of Systematic Screening for Family Planning Services among Postpartum Women Attending Village Health and Nutrition Days in Jharkhand, India. *Int. J. Integr. Care* **2018**, *18*, 7. [CrossRef] [PubMed]
32. Cooper, C.M.; Fields, R.; Mazzeo, C.I.; Taylor, N.; Pfitzer, A.; Momolu, M.; Jabbeh-Howe, C. Successful proof of concept of family planning and immunization integration in Liberia. *Glob. Health Sci. Pract.* **2015**, *3*, 71–84. [CrossRef] [PubMed]
33. Cooper, C.M.; Wille, J.; Shire, S.; Makoko, S.; Tsega, A.; Schuster, A.; Hausi, H.; Gibson, H.; Tappis, H. Integrated Family Planning and Immunization Service Delivery at Health Facility and Community Sites in Dowa and Ntchisi Districts of Malawi: A Mixed Methods Process Evaluation. *Int. J. Environ. Res. Public Health* **2020**, *17*, 4530. [CrossRef]
34. Dulli, L.S.; Eichleay, M.; Rademacher, K.; Sortijas, S.; Nsengiyumva, T. Meeting Postpartum Women's Family Planning Needs Through Integrated Family Planning and Immunization Services: Results of a Cluster-Randomized Controlled Trial in Rwanda. *Glob. Health Sci. Pract.* **2016**, *4*, 73–86. [CrossRef]
35. Erhardt-Ohren, B.; Schroffel, H.; Rochat, R. Integrated Family Planning and Routine Child Immunization Services in Benin: A Process Evaluation. *Matern. Child Health J.* **2020**, *24*, 701–708. [CrossRef] [PubMed]
36. Nelson, A.R.; Cooper, C.M.; Kamara, S.; Taylor, N.D.; Zikeh, T.; Kanneh-Kesselly, C.; Fields, R.; Hossain, I.; Oseni, L.; Getahun, B.S.; et al. Operationalizing Integrated Immunization and Family Planning Services in Rural Liberia: Lessons Learned from Evaluating Service Quality and Utilization. *Glob. Health Sci Pract.* **2019**, *7*, 418–434. [CrossRef]
37. Vance, G.; Janowitz, B.; Chen, M.; Boyer, B.; Kasonde, P.; Asare, G.; Kafulubiti, B.; Stanback, J. Integrating family planning messages into immunization services: A cluster-randomized trial in Ghana and Zambia. *Health Policy Plan.* **2014**, *29*, 359–366. [CrossRef]
38. Belemsaga, D.Y.; Goujon, A.; Bado, A.; Kouanda, S.; Duysburgh, E.; Temmerman, M.; Degomme, O. Integration of postpartum care into child health and immunization services in Burkina Faso: Findings from a cross-sectional study. *Reprod. Health* **2018**, *15*, 171. [CrossRef]
39. Yugbaré Belemsaga, D.; Goujon, A.; Degomme, O.; Nassa, T.; Duysburgh, E.; Kouanda, S.; Temmerman, M. Assessing changes in costs of maternal postpartum services between 2013 and 2014 in Burkina Faso. *Int. J. Equity Health* **2019**, *18*, 154. [CrossRef]
40. Yugbaré Belemsaga, D.; Goujon, A.; Tougri, H.; Coulibaly, A.; Degomme, O.; Duysburgh, E.; Temmerman, M.; Kouanda, S. Integration of maternal postpartum services in maternal and child health services in Kaya health district (Burkina Faso): An intervention time trend analysis. *BMC Health Serv. Res.* **2018**, *18*, 298. [CrossRef]
41. Dube, Q.; Dow, A.; Chirambo, C.; Lebov, J.; Tenthani, L.; Moore, M.; Heyderman, R.; Van Rie, A. Implementing early infant diagnosis of HIV infection at the primary care level: Experiences and challenges in Malawi. *Bull. World Health Organ.* **2012**, *90*, 699–704. [CrossRef] [PubMed]
42. Goodson, J.L.; Finkbeiner, T.; Davis, N.L.; Lyimo, D.; Rwebembera, A.; Swartzendruber, A.L.; Wallace, A.S.; Kimambo, S.; Kimario, C.J.; Wiktor, S.Z.; et al. Evaluation of using routine infant immunization visits to identify and follow-up HIV-exposed infants and their mothers in Tanzania. *J. Acquir. Immune Defic. Syndr.* **2013**, *63*, e9–e15. [CrossRef] [PubMed]
43. Wallace, A.; Kimambo, S.; Dafrossa, L.; Rusibamayila, N.; Rwebembera, A.; Songoro, J.; Arthur, G.; Luman, E.; Finkbeiner, T.; Goodson, J.L. Qualitative assessment of the integration of HIV services with infant routine immunization visits in Tanzania. *J. Acquir. Immune Defic. Syndr.* **2014**, *66*, e8–e14. [CrossRef]

44. McCollum, E.D.; Johnson, D.C.; Chasela, C.S.; Siwande, L.D.R.; Kazembe, P.N.M.; Olson, D.; Hoffman, I.P.; van der Horst, C.; Hosseinipour, M.C. Superior uptake and outcomes of early infant diagnosis of HIV services at an immunization clinic versus an "under-five" general pediatric clinic in Malawi. *J. Acquir. Immune Defic. Syndr.* **2012**, *60*, e107–e110. [CrossRef]
45. Odafe, S.; Onotu, D.; Fagbamigbe, J.O.; Ene, U.; Rivadeneira, E.; Carpenter, D.; Omoigberale, A.I.; Adamu, Y.; Lawal, I.; James, E.; et al. Increasing pediatric HIV testing positivity rates through focused testing in high-yield points of service in health facilities-Nigeria, 2016–2017. *PLoS ONE* **2020**, *15*, e0234717. [CrossRef]
46. Ong'ech, J.O.; Hoffman, H.J.; Kose, J.; Audo, M.; Matu, L.; Savosnick, P.; Guay, L. Provision of services and care for HIV-exposed infants: A comparison of maternal and child health clinic and HIV comprehensive care clinic models. *J. Acquir. Immune Defic. Syndr.* **2012**, *61*, 83–89. [CrossRef] [PubMed]
47. Tejiokem, M.C.; Faye, A.; Penda, I.C.; Guemkam, G.; Ndongo, F.A.; Chewa, G.; Rekacewicz, C.; Rousset, D.; Kfutwah, A.; Boisier, P.; et al. Feasibility of early infant diagnosis of HIV in resource-limited settings: The ANRS 12140-PEDIACAM study in Cameroon. *PLoS ONE* **2011**, *6*, e21840. [CrossRef]
48. Wang, P.C.; Mwango, A.; Moberley, S.; Brockman, B.J.; Connor, A.L.; Kalesha-Masumbu, P.; Mutembo, S.; Bweupe, M.; Chanda-Kapata, P.; Biemba, G.; et al. A Cluster Randomised Trial on the Impact of Integrating Early Infant HIV Diagnosis with the Expanded Programme on Immunization on Immunization and HIV Testing Rates in Rural Health Facilities in Southern Zambia. *PLoS ONE* **2015**, *10*, e0141455. [CrossRef]
49. Bojang, K.A.; Akor, F.; Conteh, L.; Webb, E.; Bittaye, O.; Conway, D.J.; Jasseh, M.; Wiseman, V.; Milligan, P.J.; Greenwood, B. Two strategies for the delivery of IPTc in an area of seasonal malaria transmission in the Gambia: A randomised controlled trial. *PLoS Med.* **2011**, *8*, e1000409. [CrossRef]
50. Dicko, A.; Konare, M.; Traore, D.; Testa, J.; Salamon, R.; Doumbo, O.; Rogier, C. The implementation of malaria intermittent preventive trialtreatment with sulphadoxine-pyrimethamine in infants reduced all-cause mortality in the district of Kolokani, Mali: Results from a cluster randomized control. *Malar. J.* **2012**, *11*, 73. [CrossRef]
51. Dicko, A.; Toure, S.O.; Traore, M.; Sagara, I.; Toure, O.B.; Sissoko, M.S.; Diallo, A.T.; Rogier, C.; Salomon, R.; de Sousa, A.; et al. Increase in EPI vaccines coverage after implementation of intermittent preventive treatment of malaria in infant with Sulfadoxine-pyrimethamine in the district of Kolokani, Mali: Results from a cluster randomized control trial. *BMC Public Health* **2011**, *11*, 573. [CrossRef] [PubMed]
52. Patouillard, E.; Conteh, L.; Webster, J.; Kweku, M.; Chandramohan, D.; Greenwood, B. Coverage, adherence and costs of intermittent preventive treatment of malaria in children employing different delivery strategies in Jasikan, Ghana. *PLoS ONE* **2011**, *6*, e24871. [CrossRef] [PubMed]
53. Scates, S.S.; Finn, T.P.; Wisniewski, J.; Dadi, D.; Mandike, R.; Khamis, M.; Greer, G.; Serbantez, N.; Segbaya, S.; Owusu, P.; et al. Costs of insecticide-treated bed net distribution systems in sub-Saharan Africa. *Malar. J.* **2020**, *19*, 105. [CrossRef]
54. Schellenberg, J.R.; Maokola, W.; Shirima, K.; Manzi, F.; Mrisho, M.; Mushi, A.; Alonso, P.; Mshinda, H.; Tanner, M.; Schellenberg, D.M. Cluster-randomized study of intermittent preventive treatment for malaria in infants (IPTi) in southern Tanzania: Evaluation of impact on survival. *Malar. J.* **2011**, *10*, 387. [CrossRef]
55. Willey, B.A.; Armstrong Schellenberg, J.R.; Maokola, W.; Shirima, K.; Chemba, M.; Mshinda, H.; Alonso, P.; Tanner, M.; Schellenberg, D. Evaluating the effectiveness of IPTi on malaria using routine health information from sentinel health centres in southern Tanzania. *Malar. J.* **2011**, *10*, 41. [CrossRef]
56. Theiss-Nyland, K.; Ejersa, W.; Karema, C.; Koné, D.; Koenker, H.; Cyaka, Y.; Lynch, M.; Webster, J.; Lines, J. Operational challenges to continuous LLIN distribution: A qualitative rapid assessment in four countries. *Malar. J.* **2016**, *15*, 131. [CrossRef]
57. Theiss-Nyland, K.; Koné, D.; Karema, C.; Ejersa, W.; Webster, J.; Lines, J. The relative roles of ANC and EPI in the continuous distribution of LLINs: A qualitative study in four countries. *Health Policy Plan.* **2017**, *32*, 467–475. [CrossRef] [PubMed]
58. Bakare, M.O.; Bello-Mojeed, M.A.; Munir, K.M.; Duduyemi, O.O.; Orovwigho, A.O.; Odetunde, O.I.; Taiwo, O.G.; Olofinlade, J.A.; Omotoso, O.N.; Famurewa, O.H.; et al. Improving access to interventions among mothers screened positive for post-partum depression (PPD) at National Programme on Immunization (NPI) clinics in south-western and south-eastern Nigeria—A service development report. *Matters* **2017**, *2017*. [CrossRef]
59. Bakare, M.O.; Okoye, J.O.; Obindo, J.T. Introducing depression and developmental screenings into the national programme on immunization (NPI) in southeast Nigeria: An experimental cross-sectional assessment. *Gen. Hosp. Psychiatry* **2014**, *36*, 105–112. [CrossRef]
60. Monterrosa, E.C.; Frongillo, E.A.; de Cossío, T.G.; Bonvecchio, A.; Villanueva, M.A.; Thrasher, J.F.; Rivera, J.A. Scripted messages delivered by nurses and radio changed beliefs, attitudes, intentions, and behaviors regarding infant and young child feeding in Mexico. *J. Nutr.* **2013**, *143*, 915–922. [CrossRef]
61. Oladeji, O.; Campbell, P.; Jaiswal, C.; Chamla, D.; Oladeji, B.; Ajumara, C.O.; Minguiel, L.M.; Senesie, J. Integrating immunisation services into nutrition sites to improve immunisation status of internally displaced persons' children living in Bentiu protection of civilian site, South Sudan. *Pan Afr. Med. J.* **2019**, *32*, 28. [CrossRef] [PubMed]
62. Briere, E.C.; Ryman, T.K.; Cartwright, E.; Russo, E.T.; Wannemuehler, K.A.; Nygren, B.L.; Kola, S.; Sadumah, I.; Ochieng, C.; Watkins, M.L.; et al. Impact of integration of hygiene kit distribution with routine immunizations on infant vaccine coverage and water treatment and handwashing practices of Kenyan mothers. *J. Infect. Dis.* **2012**, *205* (Suppl. 1), S56–S64. [CrossRef] [PubMed]

63. Ryman, T.K.; Briere, E.C.; Cartwright, E.; Schlanger, K.; Wannemuehler, K.A.; Russo, E.T.; Kola, S.; Sadumah, I.; Nygren, B.L.; Ochieng, C.; et al. Integration of routine vaccination and hygiene interventions: A comparison of 2 strategies in Kenya. *J. Infect. Dis.* **2012**, *205* (Suppl. 1), S65–S76. [CrossRef] [PubMed]
64. *Collaborative Action Strategy (CAS) for Health Campaign Effectiveness, 2024–2028;* Health Campaign Effectiveness Coalition: Decatur, GA, USA, 2023.
65. Chamla, D.; Luo, C.; Adjorlolo-Johnson, G.; Vandelaer, J.; Young, M.; Costales, M.O.; McClure, C. Integration of HIV infant testing into immunization programmes: A systematic review. *Paediatr. Int. Child Health* **2015**, *35*, 298–304. [CrossRef] [PubMed]
66. Cleland, J.; Shah, I.H.; Daniele, M. Interventions to Improve Postpartum Family Planning in Low- and Middle-Income Countries: Program Implications and Research Priorities. *Stud. Fam. Plan.* **2015**, *46*, 423–441. [CrossRef]
67. Ahmed, S.T.; Haider, S.S.; Hanif, S.; Anwar, H.B.; Mehjabeen, S.; Closser, S.; Bazant, E.; Sarker, M. A scoping review on integrated health campaigns for immunization in low- and middle-income countries. *Health Policy Plan.* **2023**, *38*, 1198–1224. [CrossRef]
68. Morgan, C.; Giattas, M.R.; Holroyd, T.; Pfitzer, A.; Engel, D.; Sidibe, A.; Holloway, M.; Bloem, P.; Fields, R.; Shimp, L.; et al. Integration of other services with human papillomavirus vaccination; lessons from earlier in the life course highlight the need for new policy and implementation evidence. *Vaccine* **2022**, *40* (Suppl. 1), A94–A99. [CrossRef]

vaccines

MDPI

Opinion

Epidemiology of Pertussis After the COVID-19 Pandemic: Analysis of the Factors Involved in the Resurgence of the Disease in High-, Middle-, and Low-Income Countries

Lucia F. Bricks [1,*], Juan C. Vargas-Zambrano [2] and Denis Macina [2]

[1] Sanofi Vaccines Medical, Av Nações Unidas, São Paulo 14401, Brazil
[2] Sanofi Vaccines Medical, 14 Espace Henri Vallee, 69007 Lyon, France; juan.vargas@sanofi.com (J.C.V.-Z.); denis.macina@sanofi.com (D.M.)
* Correspondence: lucia.bricks@sanofi.com

Abstract: Pertussis is a highly contagious bacterial disease of the respiratory tract that can be prevented by vaccination. Before the COVID-19 pandemic, the vaccine coverage rate for the third dose of a DPT-containing vaccine was 86%, with large disparities among countries. Since 2022, many high-income countries have reported a resurgence of pertussis, especially in the European region, but the disease has also caused outbreaks in middle- and low-income countries, despite their less extensive disease surveillance capacities. This paper aims to review the incidence rates (IRs) of pertussis in high-, middle-, and low-income countries following the COVID-19 pandemic and to discuss the most relevant factors associated with the resurgence of the disease. The epidemiology of pertussis is highly variable and is influenced not only by the type of vaccine used but also by the specific characteristics of the disease, vaccine coverage rates, vaccination schedules, and the quality of surveillance. Since the cessation of COVID-19 measures, there have been significant pertussis outbreaks that could have been partially mitigated with higher coverage rates and more comprehensive pertussis vaccination throughout life.

Keywords: pertussis; vaccines; epidemiology; diagnosis; surveillance

1. Introduction

Pertussis, commonly known as whooping cough, is a highly contagious respiratory disease caused by *Bordetella pertussis*, a Gram-negative bacillus that exclusively infects humans. The bacterium has a limited survival time outside its host, contributing to its human-specific transmission. Pertussis occurs globally in both endemic and epidemic forms, affecting individuals of all ages. However, its incidence is highest among unvaccinated or incompletely vaccinated infants and young children, who are particularly vulnerable to severe disease and complications. Infants under six months old, particularly those who are premature or have low birth weight, face the greatest risk, with an elevated likelihood of complications, hospitalization, and even death [1–4].

Transmission occurs through respiratory secretions and the disease is known for its high infectivity, with a basic reproduction number (R_0) ranging from 12 to 17, comparable to that of measles. This high infectivity, combined with a low infectious dose, makes pertussis highly transmissible, particularly in crowded environments such as schools and universities [1–3].

The peak period of transmissibility occurs within the first three weeks after the onset of coughing, during which the risk of transmission is highest. Although breakthrough infection in previously vaccinated individuals generally proceeds to milder symptoms, complications can still arise in up to 25% of cases [1–3]. Importantly, recent studies suggest that asymptomatic carriers may also contribute to the spread of the disease, further complicating diagnosis and control efforts [5,6].

Despite the availability of vaccines, pertussis is not considered eradicable due to its high transmissibility and the waning of immunity that follows both natural infection and vaccination. Vaccines provide incomplete and non-sterilizing immunity, making booster doses necessary throughout life to maintain protection [1,2,7]. The primary aim of vaccination is to reduce the disease burden in young infants, with the World Health Organization (WHO) recommending three primary doses in infancy followed by periodic boosters. Since 2015, maternal vaccination during pregnancy has been advised to protect newborns under three months of age [2].

Globally, vaccine coverage rates (VCRs) have improved over the past two decades, reaching 86% for the third dose of diphtheria-, tetanus-, and pertussis-containing vaccines (DPT) in 2018. However, the COVID-19 pandemic disrupted immunization programs, causing a decline to 83% by 2021. In 2023, the VCR for the third dose of DTP was 84%, but 14.5 million infants did not receive an initial dose of a DTP vaccine and an additional 6.5 million are partially vaccinated. Of these 21 million, just under 60% of these children live in 10 countries: Afghanistan, Angola, the Democratic Republic of the Congo, Ethiopia, India, Indonesia, Nigeria, Pakistan, Sudan, and Yemen [3]. In several of these countries, VCRs remain below 90% [8] and in some, booster doses after the first year of life are not routinely administered [9]. Interestingly, despite lower VCRs in many low- and middle-income countries, most recent pertussis outbreaks have been reported in developed nations [8,10].

This paper aims to review the incidence of pertussis following the COVID-19 pandemic and explore key factors contributing to its resurgence, based on the WHO and Ministry of Health websites of countries that reported pertussis outbreaks and the most recent literature available in PUBMED.

2. Results

2.1. Global Epidemiology of Pertussis Pre- and Post-COVID-19 Pandemic

Between 2019 and 2022, during the COVID-19 pandemic, there was a marked reduction in the incidence rate (IR) of pertussis. This decrease has been attributed to widespread public health measures, such as the use of masks, social isolation, enhanced hygiene practices, and disruptions in healthcare access and disease reporting [3]. According to the WHO, the global pertussis IR fell four-fold from 16.1 per million in 2016 (pre-pandemic) to 4.6 per million in 2021. However, starting in 2023, the global IR began to rise again, reaching 10.2 per million. Notably, this resurgence was not uniform across all regions. In Europe, the IR increased 30-fold between 2021 and 2023, although significant variation was observed across regions (Table 1) and countries (Table 2) [10].

Table 1. Pertussis incidence rates by WHO region, 2014 to 2024 [10].

WHO Region	2023	2022	2021	2020	2019	2018	2017	2016	2015	2014
African	8.4	7.3	6.2	4.9	8.6	16.4	10.5	3.1	11.6	**17.6**
Eastern Mediterranean	5.5	2.3	**8.8**	1	3.2	5.4	3.3	3.3	2.6	3.9
European	**104.4**	6.8	3.4	23.7	74.7	66.1	68.1	81.1	67.1	72.2
American	6	3.2	6.6	20.1	11.5	23.5	29.4	28.6	32.9	**48.4**
South-east Asia	5.8	4.7	0.4	6.3	6	8.7	17.1	21.3	17.7	**28.5**
Western Pacific	26.4	21.7	5.8	6.1	**33.2**	27.9	14.6	16.2	18.5	10.3

Note: Incidence rates refer to the IR per 1,000,000 in total population. In bold the highest pertussis IR from 2014 to 2024.

Table 2. Pertussis incidence rates in selected HIC in the last 10 years, 2014–2023.

	Pertussis Incidence Rates Post-COVID-19 Pandemic						Pertussis Incidence Rates Pre-COVID-19 Pandemic			
Country	**2023**	**2022**	**2021**	**2020**	**2019**	**2018**	**2017**	**2016**	**2015**	**2014**
Australia	92.3	18.3	21.2	134.3	471.7	499.8	489.8	823.6	939.9	501.9
Austria	305.6	18.1	14.4	73.4	251.4	**248.5**	160.4	145.3	67	43.3
Belgium	89.3	6.9	1.4	10.7	95.6	118.5	134.9	185.7	106.7	133.9
Canada	36.5	5.4	0.8	25	67.3	45	108.6	107.2	97.6	42.9
Croatia	1233.6	0.5	1.8	2.5	14	**31.8**	19.6	19.1	13.6	-
Czechia	45.7	8.8	4.8	66	137	71.3	63.3	59.5	55.6	239.7
Denmark	1018.6	8.8	13.7	490.8	635.8	177.4	187.5	**364.9**	169.3	151.5
Netherlands	156.3	7.2	4.2	53.5	346.6	270.4	260.2	205.9	383.8	526.1
Spain	53.4	4.5	1.2	5.1	64.8	77.8	98.9	104.7	-	-
UK	13.7	1.2	0.8	18.2	68.7	51.3	76.8	107.5	79.6	62.4

Note: Incidence rates refer to the IR per 1,000,000 in total population. All countries adopted acellular pertussis vaccines before 2014. In bold, the highest pertussis IR reported before COVID-19 pandemic and in red, the highest IR reported in the last 10 years.

2.2. Pertussis Incidence Rates in High-Income Countries

High-income countries (HICs) consistently report higher incidence rates than middle-income countries (MICs) and low-income countries (LICs) [10].

Table 2 shows the incidence rates of pertussis in HICs that experienced an increase in cases during the post-pandemic period. All of these countries use acellular pertussis (aP) vaccines, albeit with different vaccination schedules, and report high vaccine coverage rates (VCRs) [8–10]. The pertussis IRs in Austria, Croatia, and Denmark were the highest in the last 10 years. In Belgium and Croatia, the pertussis VCRs were not impacted by the COVID-19 pandemic, and in Austria, since 2018, before the COVID-19 pandemic, the VCRs varied between 84–86% [8].

According to the European Centre for Disease Prevention and Control (ECDC), pertussis cases surged dramatically in Europe, with over 32,000 cases and 19 deaths reported between January and April 2024. However, the rise in cases was uneven across the continent, initially affecting Austria, Denmark, and Norway in the second half of 2023 [11]. Variations in incidence across age groups were influenced by factors such as vaccination schedules (2 + 1 versus 3 + 1 in the primary series), the timing and frequency of booster doses, availability of laboratory diagnostics, and the surveillance strategies in place [7,11–19].

In Europe, the USA, and Australia, the majority of cases were recorded among adolescents, adults, and elderly populations [7,11–22]. In Canada [23,24], Spain [15], and Czechia [17], outbreaks primarily affected children over five years of age and adolescents, particularly in areas where VCRs were below 90%.

Additionally, in some communities, particularly those with vaccine hesitancy, outbreaks occurred despite high national VCRs. For instance, in Israel, where national VCR exceeds 90%, an outbreak occurred in a religious community that refuses vaccination, primarily affecting infants under one year of age [25].

Partial data from 2024 indicate that pertussis continues to spread in developed countries. Notable outbreaks were recorded in the UK (10,493 cases) [14], Czechia (7898) [17], the USA (22,273) [20], France (>34,000 cases) [17,18], and Australia (30,544 cases) [21].

Despite most cases occurring among older individuals, the highest mortality rates were seen in young infants. In Europe, 19 deaths were recorded between January and March 2024, with 58% in infants and 42% in people aged $\geq$ 60 years [11]. The case-fatality rate was very low (0.056%). In HICs, where the VCR for the third dose of DTP-containing vaccines is high, there is an increasing emphasis on vaccinating pregnant women with Tdap to protect infants under three months of age [11–14].

2.3. Pertussis Incidence Rates in Middle- and Low-Income Countries

In many MICs and LICs, a resurgence of pertussis was also noted after the COVID-19 pandemic. Most LICs use whole-cell pertussis (wP) vaccines with few or no booster doses, and there are limited data available on pertussis incidence in these regions. Some MICs, while still primarily using wP vaccines, have introduced aP vaccines in their schedules. Table 3 presents data on MICs and LICs that reported higher pertussis IRs during the post-pandemic period. Afghanistan, Bolivia, China, Ecuador, Indonesia, Malaysia, Papua New Guinea, the Russian Federation, and Serbia reported their highest pertussis IRs since 2014 [9,10].

Table 3. Pertussis incidence rates in MICs and LICs, pre- and post-COVID-19 pandemic, in selected countries, 2014 to 2023 [10].

	Pertussis Incidence Rates Post-COVID-19 Pandemic				Pertussis Incidence Rates Pre-COVID-19 Pandemic					
Country	2023	2022	2021	2020	2019	2018	2017	2016	2015	2014
Afghanistan (wP)	36.9	8.2	2.7	-	-	**13.3**	0	0	12.8	0
Argentina (wP)	13.3	4.3	3.8	3.6	21.7	20.2	19.5	38.4	22.4	13
Bolivia (wP)	67.5	18.5	0	1	2.5	1.8	0.6	2.4	1	**6.9**
Chile (wP/aP) [1]	21.6	0	1.5	3.2	18.5	36.1	45.7	41.2	40.7	63
China (aP) [2]	28.9	26.9	6.7	3.1	21.2	**15.5**	7.4	4	4.8	2.5
Costa Rica (aP)	4.3	1	0.4	2	10.2	7.3	**11.8**	4.7	4.2	6.5
Ecuador (wP)	10.3	3.2	0	0.5	3.3	1.8	**3.6**	1	0.4	0.6
India (wP)	3.4	3.1	0.4	9	8.5	9.6	17.5	27.7	19	35.6
Indonesia (wP)	**7.7**	1.5	-	0.1	0.1	0.1	3.9	3.1	-	**8**
Malaysia (aP)	34.2	2.9	0.3	4	27.4	27.1	10.9	9.4	**30.1**	16.3
Mexico (aP)	1.4	0.5	0.2	2	6.9	6.3	6.7	8.4	**9.1**	8
Papua New Guinea (wP)	177.1	0.8	1	5.2	**48.1**	0	0	0	0	0
Peru (wP)	3.9	0.1	1.1	1.4	12.8	15.1	**19.5**	4.6	39	7.8
Russian Fed. (wP/aP) [3]	**362.9**	21.9	7.6	41.5	**96.3**	71.2	37	56.5	44.4	32.5
Serbia (wP)	**209.8**	0.7	0.7	9	-	50	40.3	20.8	12.4	**38.9**
South Africa (aP)	4.2	**12.6**	9.1	1.7	9.3	**16.3**	1.8	0.7	1.8	4.1
Ukraine (wP)	18.7	0.8	2.1	23.3	51.5	49	54.6	**68.7**	53	-

Notes: Incidence rates refers to incidence 1 per 1,000,000 in total population. In bold, the year with the highest IR reported before the COVID-19-pandemic. In red, the highest IR reported in the last 10 years; [1] Chile introduced aP in routine schedule in 2018; [2] China introduced aP co-purified vaccines in routine schedule in 2015; [3] Russian Federation introduced aP in routine schedule 2022.

The situation of LICs and MICs is diverse and detailed data are not available for most countries; however, some pertussis outbreaks were reported in several of these countries, independently of the type of pertussis vaccine used in routine [9,10].

Among these countries using aP vaccines, South Africa was one of the first countries to report a resurgence of pertussis after the COVID-19 pandemic. A total of 818 pertussis cases were reported between June 2022 and January 2023, mostly in Cape Town [26], but the highest IRs were observed in Russia and Serbia [10,27,28]. Serbia reported more than 1400 pertussis cases, the highest number the last two decades [28]. China, where aP co-purified vaccines have been used since 2015, recorded a dramatic increase in pertussis cases over the past two years [29,30]. In April 2024, China recorded 91,272 cases of whooping cough and seven deaths [30].

Pertussis outbreaks were also registered in countries using wP vaccines. Despite the limited information about pertussis in the poorest countries, it is evident that even in some of these countries, pertussis is resurging. Two examples are Afghanistan and Papua New Guinea. In Afghanistan, in 2023, 1531 pertussis cases were registered, more than 10 times greater in comparison with 2021 (108 cases) [10]. Other countries reported regional pertussis outbreaks. Bolivia recorded 693 pertussis cases in 2023, mostly in Santa

Cruz Province [31,32]. In Argentina, 605 cases were reported in 2023, most of which were concentrated in the province of Salta [33]. In Peru, despite the low IR, the number of pertussis deaths in 2023 was 144 with 6 deaths, a case-fatality rate (4.2%) higher than that observed in HICs [34]. In Brazil, despite the high number of children that did not receive any pertussis-containing vaccine in recent years, until 2023, the pertussis IR was only 1 per 1,000,000 in the population. However, since January 2024, pertussis outbreaks have been registered in many cities, with a total of 2954 confirmed pertussis cases and 12 deaths as of November 2024 [35].

3. Discussion

The high incidence rates of pertussis recorded in Europe (Table 1) might surprise those unfamiliar with the diagnostic criteria and vaccination strategies used across different regions. Many European countries use acellular pertussis vaccines, maintain high VCRs, and recommend booster doses for various groups, including schoolchildren, adolescents, adults, pregnant women, and healthcare professionals [8,9]. In contrast, lower IRs are observed in countries that primarily use whole-cell pertussis vaccines and often report lower VCRs and fewer boosters [8,9]. Several factors contribute to the resurgence of pertussis; notably, the specific characteristics of the disease, the type of vaccine used, VCRs, vaccination schedules, and the quality of epidemiological surveillance.

3.1. Specificities of the Disease

Pertussis is a highly transmissible disease that persists in both endemic and epidemic forms, with outbreaks occurring every 3–5 years, regardless of vaccination type or VCR [1–3]. The introduction of wP vaccines in the 1940s significantly reduced the peaks and frequency of epidemics, but these outbreaks never fully disappeared [1,2]. Similarly, countries that adopted aP vaccines following decreased acceptance of wP vaccination in the late 1970s saw continued outbreaks [7]. Pertussis is not eradicable because neither natural infection nor vaccination provides lifelong protection. Immunity wanes over time, and unless regular boosters perpetuate protection, the growing pool of susceptible individuals increases the likelihood of outbreaks [1–3,7,10,20,23].

3.2. Vaccine Coverage Rates and Vaccination Schedules

Globally, the highest IRs of pertussis are observed in unvaccinated or incompletely vaccinated infants. However, the age distribution of pertussis cases varies depending on VCRs and vaccination schedules. In HICs with high VCRs, most cases occur among adolescents and adults, including the elderly, but serious cases and deaths occurs more frequently in infants too young to receive the first doses of pertussis-containing vaccines [11,13–24]. In countries or areas with lower VCRs, children under five years of age are predominantly affected [1,2,8,9,36–39].

While HICs have maintained high VCRs for over two decades, they still experience periodic pertussis outbreaks [1,2,7]. Variable pertussis incidence rates were observed in MICs that adopted aP vaccines in their routine schedules, and this can be associated with VCRs. In Mexico, which reported a 72% VCR for the third dose of a DPT vaccine after the COVID-19 pandemic, there was a smaller increase in pertussis cases compared to Chile, which maintained VCRs above 90% even during the pandemic [10]. In China, where no booster vaccination is available beyond toddler age, most pertussis cases were observed in school-aged children [29,30]. Similarly, Russia, despite VCRs above 90% for the primary series, does not recommend booster doses for preschool children and has seen a surge in cases among school-aged children [27].

In MICs and LICs that primarily use wP vaccines, lower VCRs and low pertussis IRs might suggest that these vaccines offer better protection, but this is not the case. Underreporting is a big challenge in these countries where pertussis is still primarily viewed as a childhood disease and diagnostic capabilities are limited [10,36–39]. For example, countries like Angola, Bangladesh, Haiti, and Venezuela, which report low VCRs for diphtheria–tetanus–pertussis (DTP) vaccines (Table S1 in Supplementary Material), rarely report pertussis, despite experiencing other vaccine-preventable disease outbreaks, such as diphtheria or polio [8,10]. India and Indonesia have reported increases in pertussis IRs, but these figures are much lower than expected, given the number of unvaccinated children in these countries [10]. Argentina and Bolivia reported regional outbreaks despite the low VCRs in the entire country, showing that other factors, such as awareness and surveillance, are relevant factors related to epidemiologic information. In Brazil, in 2014 there was a pertussis outbreak with 8338 cases (IR = 41.7); from 2015 to 2019, the IRs varied from 6.9 to 14.5, despite the substantial reduction in VCR observed since 2015 (Table S1 Supplementary Material). From 2020 to 2023, the pertussis IRs ranged from 0.7 (2021) to 1.2 in 2022, but in 2024 the number of confirmed pertussis cases increased by almost 30 times (2954) as compared to 2023 (124), with large variation among the states. Parana State reported the highest number of cases (1108) and deaths (4 from 12), followed by São Paulo State (766). In these states, about 70% of cases were confirmed by laboratorial tests (culture and/or PCR) and more than 20% by clinical–epidemiological linkage. In the north and north-east region, low numbers of pertussis cases were reported (73), the majority were registered in children and those less than one year, and only 50% of pertussis cases have been confirmed by laboratory tests [35].

These examples demonstrate that pertussis resurgence is not solely dependent on the type of vaccine used (wP or aP). The WHO has emphasized that both vaccines are effective in preventing pertussis in the first year of life, but neither provides lifelong protection. Booster doses are essential to maintaining immunity and vaccination coverage should exceed 90% to reduce transmission risks [2].

3.3. *Characteristics of Epidemiological Surveillance*

There is considerable heterogeneity in the pattern of pertussis resurgence, not only related to heterogeneity in immunization and VCR practices, but also to the characteristics of epidemiological surveillance. Pertussis transmission is highest in the first two weeks after cough onset, a period when it is easily confused with other viral or bacterial respiratory diseases. This complicates both diagnosis and the timely application of preventive measures, such as chemoprophylaxis, when there is no or limited access to laboratory resources [1–3].

The WHO and CDC recommend that pertussis diagnosis should be confirmed through laboratory testing, including culture, polymerase chain reaction (PCR), and serology [40,41]. However, many MICs and LICs lack the resources necessary to implement these tests, contributing to the significant underreporting of the disease.

PCR has greatly improved the diagnosis of pertussis, especially in HICs and some MICs, where its introduction has led to more accurate epidemiological data [36–39,42–44]. Countries like Costa Rica, Argentina, and Brazil saw sharp increases in reported pertussis cases following the introduction of PCR-based diagnostic methods [37–39,42,43]. A similar situation was observed in other countries, like Russia and China. In Russia, in 2013 the PCR was used in 33 (38.8%) regions, increasing to 64 regions (75.3%) in 2017 [44]. In China, the introduction of nationwide guidance on PCR use for pertussis diagnosis in December 2023 may also be contributing to the observed increase in the identification of pertussis cases [29,30].

The improvement of the surveillance of community-acquired pneumonias (CAPs) was responsible for the better detection of pertussis in Egypt and South Africa. In Egypt, a study carried out between August 2014 and September 2017, with 400 children hospitalized for CAP, showed that *B. pertussis* was detected in 7.7% of infants under 4 months of age [45]. In South Africa, an increase in pertussis was also noted after the improvement of hospital surveillance of pneumonia and most cases occurred in children too young to receive the vaccine [46].

Since 1990s, serologic tests have been used in many HICs, especially to confirm pertussis diagnosis in adolescents and adults, even before the introduction of aP vaccines [47–50].

Berber et al. (2021) showed through a seroepidemiological study performed in European countries that pertussis was very common in adults (40–50 years) [51]. In MICs and LICs, serological tests are rarely used to confirm pertussis, but there is evidence that pertussis is common in adolescents and adults [52–59].

New diagnostic tests (multiplex PCR) capable of identifying multiple bacteria and viruses have been introduced in some countries, facilitating the rapid diagnosis of the causative agents of CAP. Through these tests, it is possible to verify that co-infections are common, particularly in children. In young infants, co-infection with RSV is the most common [60–67], and there is evidence that co-infection between *B. pertussis* and RSV may even worsen the clinical picture. Many pertussis cases may be ignored if physicians only search for RSV [60]. Other virus and bacteria can also cause co-infections in children and adults. In adults, co-infections with *B. pertussis* and influenza and other viruses also have been reported, but the detection of co-infections will depend on the seasonality, occurrence of outbreaks of pertussis, and capacity to detect viral and bacterial agents. Multiplex PCR tests are little used due to their high cost, but it is expected that in the future they may be more accessible for the early diagnosis of outbreaks and epidemics.

3.4. Characteristics of the Type of Vaccine Used in Primary Series

The analysis of these data clearly shows that pertussis resurgence was not related only to the type of vaccine used (wP or aP).

The latest WHO position paper on pertussis states that both wP and aP vaccines are effective in preventing the disease in the first year of life and that the vaccination of pregnant women should also be prioritized to protect infants too young to receive the first dose of the vaccine [2]. However, the assertion that "wP vaccines have greater efficacy and duration of protection compared to aP vaccines" should be revised.

The efficacy data for wP vaccines analyzed in the WHO position paper refer to vaccines that are no longer available and have been replaced in the last decades by wP vaccines never tested in efficacy trials. Additionally, even the old wP vaccines had variable efficacy, ranging from 36% to 96%, while the efficacy of aP vaccines has been consistently higher than 80% [2].

Several studies have been published in recent years showing that there are clear differences in the immune response to wP and aP vaccines. Although wP vaccines induce an immune response that appears closer in nature to that induced by natural infection and may have a greater impact on reducing respiratory tract colonization, according to data in non-human primate infection models, it is still unclear what the real role of this in the epidemiology of the disease. In an excellent review on the subject, Domenech de-Celles et al. (2024) [68] addressed the challenges related to the understanding of the immune response and the models used to assess the impact of different types of vaccines on the epidemiology and emergence of outbreaks. Many biases have been found in the studies that support the claims of greater protection and longer duration of protection offered by wP vaccines, such as different designs, use of different vaccines, lack of unvaccinated controls in efficacy studies, and heterogeneity of the populations and laboratory tests used to evaluate immune responses, among others. Immunity to pertussis is still little known and even natural infection does not protect for life. For these reasons, booster doses are necessary regardless of the vaccine used (wP or aP). More than preventing infection, it is crucial to reduce morbidity and mortality from pertussis. Acellular pertussis vaccines have proven their efficacy and effectiveness and can maintain protection until preschool age [1,2,7,69,70].

Although the wP vaccines currently in use can reduce the burden of the disease, there are few studies on their immunogenicity and effectiveness. The limited evidence on the immunogenicity of wP vaccines suggests that the duration of immunity is short, probably less than five years [71]. In one of the rare studies on the effectiveness of wP vaccines, conducted in Africa, the effectiveness was much lower than that offered by aP vaccines [72].

The concept that wP vaccines can induce long-duration protection also needs to be revised. The acellular pertussis vaccines for use in adolescents and adults were developed to protect these age groups that became more vulnerable to pertussis when HICs achieved high VCRs. These age groups obviously did not receive aP in their infancy. Serologic studies performed in HICs clearly showed that pertussis reinfections occur in adolescents and adults (47–51). In the last decade, several seroepidemiological surveys have also been carried out in MICs, such as Mexico, Russia, China, Iran, Cambodia, and Indonesia, which have revealed that asymptomatic pertussis infections occur 3 to 5 years after the last dose of wP vaccines, showing that the duration of protection offered by these vaccines also decreases over time [52–58]. Among these studies, the most interesting was carried out in Poland, because it was conducted in a population where half of the children had been vaccinated with a wP vaccine and the other half with an aP vaccine in the basic series. The reduction in anti-pertussis antibody titers occurred similarly in both groups, at five years after the preschool booster dose, indicating that the duration of protection provided by both vaccines was quite similar [73].

Data from Latin American countries demonstrated that adolescents and adults can be sources of pertussis infection to young infants [33,39,59]. Despite the limited access to serologic tests in this region, in Brazil, the largest use of PCR in some states showed that, in 2024, 38% of confirmed pertussis cases occurred in adolescents and 29% in adults. All 12 confirmed pertussis deaths registered in 2024 occurred in infants less than six months of age; from these, 75% were in infants of one or two months of age [35]. Besides the necessity to improve the VCR for children, health authorities have also emphasized the necessity to improve the Tdap VCR for pregnant women and health care professionals who have contact with infants.

4. Conclusions

The epidemiology of pertussis is extremely variable and is not related solely to the type of vaccine used (wP or aP). Incidence rates are influenced by multiple factors inherent to the bacteria (high transmissibility and silent circulation), vaccination schedules (number of doses and boosters), vaccination coverage, and access to laboratory resources to diagnose and implement control measures to prevent the rapid spread of the disease.

Periodic epidemics occur at intervals of 2 to 5 years, whenever there is an accumulation of susceptible individuals. The last pertussis epidemics occurred more than five years ago. During and immediately after the COVID-19 pandemic, a reduction in vaccination coverage was observed and millions of children did not receive the primary series and booster doses. In 2022, incidence rates increased in several countries. Apparently, countries that use aP vaccines have higher incidence rates of the disease, but it is not possible to compare the epidemiological data of countries with differing surveillance capacities and different criteria for the clinical and laboratory diagnosis of pertussis.

HICs offer better access to health services and laboratory resources that facilitate diagnosis in different age groups. In these countries, most pertussis cases are recorded in adolescents and adults and deaths are rare, occurring mainly in very young infants whose mothers did not receive Tdap during pregnancy. In MICs/LICs, although pertussis incidence rates are generally lower, only more severe cases are diagnosed and the number of deaths is much higher than that recorded in HICs.

Infant protection is a priority to reduce the risk of hospitalizations and deaths. It is essential to achieve a VCR > 90% in the first year of life and to vaccinate pregnant women with Tdap in each pregnancy. All children should be vaccinated without delay and booster doses are necessary, regardless of the vaccine used (wP or aP).

Children who were not vaccinated during the COVID-19 epidemic should receive booster doses to prevent outbreaks in daycare centers/schools.

Up-to-date and accurate epidemiological information is essential for taking immediate action. Therefore, it is essential to improve epidemiological surveillance by making highly sensitive tests available for diagnosing the disease, as well as educating doctors and laypeople about the risk of pertussis epidemics after the COVID-19 pandemic. Unfortunately, in the poorest regions, there is a lack of reliable data on the epidemiology of the disease and there is a delay in the investigation and dissemination of information. It is precisely in these regions that pertussis causes the most deaths.

Supplementary Materials: The following supporting information can be downloaded at: https://www.mdpi.com/article/10.3390/vaccines12121346/s1, Table S1: Vaccine coverage rates (%) for the third dose of pertussis vaccines in selected MICs/LICs, 2014–2023 [8].

Author Contributions: All authors made substantial contributions to the development of the work and the analysis and interpretation of the data. L.F.B. prepared the first draft. D.M. and J.C.V.-Z. reviewed it critically and contributed with the selection of papers and discussion. All authors approved the final version to be published and are fully accountable for all aspects of the work. All authors have read and agreed to the published version of the manuscript.

Funding: This research received no external funding.

Data Availability Statement: All data were based in the references mentioned in the paper.

Conflicts of Interest: L.F.B., J.C.V.-Z. and D.M. are employees of Sanofi and may hold shares and/stock options in the company.

References

1. Edwards, K.M.; Decker, M.D. Pertussis vaccines. In *Vaccines*, 7th ed.; Plotkin, S.A., Orenstein, W.A., Offit, P.A., Eds.; Elsevier: Philadelphia, PA, USA, 2018; pp. 711–761.
2. Anonymous. Pertussis vaccines: WHO position paper—September 2015. *Wkly. Epidemiol. Rec.* **2015**, *90*, 433–458.
3. Available online: http://www.who.int/immunization/diseases/pertussis/en/ (accessed on 14 August 2024).
4. Chiappini, E.; Petrolini, C.; Sandini, E.; Licari, A.; Pugni, L.; Mosca, F.A.; Marseglia, G.L. Update on vaccination of preterm infants: A systematic review about safety and efficacy/effectiveness. Proposal for a position statement by Italian Society of Pediatric Allergology and Immunology jointly with the Italian Society of Neonatology. *Expert Rev. Vaccines* **2019**, *18*, 523–545. [CrossRef] [PubMed]
5. Craig, R.; Kunkel, E.; Crowcroft, N.S.; Fitzpatrick, M.C.; de Melker, H.; Althouse, B.M.; Merkel, T.; Scarpino, S.V.; Koelle, K.; Friedman, L.; et al. Asymptomatic Infection and Transmission of Pertussis in Households: A Systematic Review. *Clin. Infect. Dis.* **2020**, *70*, 152–161. [CrossRef]
6. Gill, C.J.; Gunning, C.E.; MacLeod, W.; Mwananyanda, L.; Thea, D.; Pieciak, R.; Kwenda, G.; Mupila, Z.; Rohani, P. Asymptomatic *Bordetella pertussis* infections in young African infants and their mothers identified within a longitudinal cohort. *eLife* **2021**, *10*, e65663. [CrossRef] [PubMed] [PubMed Central]
7. Folkhasolmybdighaten. Pertussis Surveillance in Sweden (folkhalsomyndigheten.se). Available online: https://www.folkhalsomyndigheten.se/contentassets/975cc036216b48a39b7bf34319d4ecee/pertussis-surveillance-sweden-23rd-annual-report.pdf (accessed on 22 August 2024).
8. Immunization Coverage Estimates (who.int). Available online: https://www.who.int/data/gho/data/themes/topics/immunization-coverage (accessed on 14 October 2024).
9. Vaccination Schedule for Pertussis (who.int). Available online: https://immunizationdata.who.int/global/wiise-detail-page/vaccination-schedule-for-pertussis?TARGETPOP_GENERAL=GENERAL (accessed on 14 October 2024).
10. Pertussis Reported Cases and Incidence (who.int). Available online: https://immunizationdata.who.int/global/wiise-detail-page/pertussis-reported-cases-and-incidence?GROUP=WHO_REGIONS&YEAR= (accessed on 12 August 2024).
11. Available online: https://www.ecdc.europa.eu/sites/default/files/documents/Increase%20in%20pertussis%20cases%20in%20the%20EU-EEA%20-%20May%202024%20FINAL.pdf (accessed on 8 May 2024).
12. Khalil, A.; Samara, A.; Campbell, H.; Ladhani, S.N.; Amirthalingam, G. Recent increase in infant pertussis cases in Europe and the critical importance of antenatal immunizations: We must do better. . .now. *Int. J. Infect. Dis.* **2024**, *146*, 107148. [CrossRef] [PubMed]
13. Nordholm, A.C.; Emborg, H.D.; Nørgaard, S.K.; Nygaard, U.; Ronayne, A.; Nielsen, L.B.; Søborg, B.; Andersen, P.H.; Dalby, T. Pertussis Epidemic in Denmark, August 2023 to February 2024. *Eurosurveillance* **2024**, *29*, 2400160. [CrossRef]
14. Confirmed Cases of Pertussis in England by Month—GOV.UK. Available online: www.gov.uk (accessed on 21 August 2024).
15. Instituto de Salud Carlos III. Brote de Tos Ferina en España 2023/2024. Tosferina—CNE—ISCIII Portal Web (Data as of 11 July 2024). Available online: https://cne.isciii.es/en/tosferina (accessed on 14 August 2024).
16. Current figures on whooping cough in the Netherlands | RIVM. Available online: https://www.rivm.nl/en/whooping-cough/current-figures-on-whooping-cough-in-netherlands (accessed on 26 March 2023).
17. Pertussis outbreak in Czech Republic—The Lancet Infectious Diseases. Available online: https://www.thelancet.com/journals/laninf/article/PIIS1473-3099(24)00291-3/fulltext (accessed on 7 May 2024).

18. Coqueluche en France. Coqueluche en France. Point au 18 Septembre 2024. (santepubliquefrance.fr). Available online: https://www.santepubliquefrance.fr/maladies-et-traumatismes/maladies-a-prevention-vaccinale/coqueluche/documents/bulletin-national/coqueluche-en-france.-point-au-18-septembre-2024 (accessed on 27 September 2024).
19. Centre National de Référence de la Coqueluche et Autres Bordetelloses. Institut Pasteur. Available online: http://www.pasteur.fr/fr/sante-publique/CNR/les-cnr/coqueluche-et-autres-bordetelloses (accessed on 30 September 2024).
20. Weekly Cases* of Notifiable Diseases, United States, U.S. Territories, and Non-U.S. Residents Week Ending November 2, 2024 (Week 44). Available online: https://wonder.cdc.gov/nndss/static/2024/44/2024-44-table990.html (accessed on 21 November 2024).
21. Australian National Notificable Dashboard Surveillance System Dashboard·NINDSS Portal (health.gov.au). Available online: https://nindss.health.gov.au/pbi-dashboard/ (accessed on 25 September 2024).
22. Jayasundara, D.; Randall, D.; Sheridan, S.; Sheppeard, V.; Liu, B.; Richmond, P.C.; Blyth, C.C.; Wood, J.G.; Moore, H.C.; McIntyre, P.B.; et al. Estimating the excess burden of pertussis disease in Australia within the first year of life, that might have been prevented through timely vaccination. *Int. J. Epidemiol.* **2023**, *52*, 250–259. [CrossRef]
23. Pertussis Outbreak Now Zone-Wide in South Zone | Alberta Health Services. 27 April 2023. Available online: https://www.albertahealthservices.ca/news/Page17295.aspx (accessed on 12 November 2024).
24. Whooping Cough Cases in Alberta on Track for One of the Worst Years in a Decade. *CBC News*. 12 August 2024. Available online: https://www.cbc.ca/news/canada/calgary/whooping-cough-pertussis-alberta-1.7065298 (accessed on 13 November 2024).
25. Stein-Zamir, C.; Shoob, H.; Abramson, N.; Brown, E.H.; Zimmermann, Y. Pertussis outbreak mainly in unvaccinated young children in ultra-orthodox Jewish groups, Jerusalem, Israel 2023. *Epidemiol. Infect.* **2023**, *151*, e166. [CrossRef] [PubMed]
26. Available online: https://www.nicd.ac.za/wp-content/uploads/2023/01/NICD-Communique-JAN-2023.pdf (accessed on 15 September 2024).
27. Basov, A.A.; Vysochanskaya, S.O.; Tsvirkun, O.V.; Belova, T.R.; Aduguzelov, S.E.; Zhernov, Y.V.; Yatskovsky, K.A. Criteria for assessing the epidemiologic situation for pertussis in Russian Federation. *Epidemiol. Vaccine Prev.* **2024**, *23*, 4–13. [CrossRef]
28. Ristić, M.; Medić, S.; Vuković, V.; Rajčević, S.; Koprivica, M.; Banjac, J.; Ljubičić, S.; Petrović, V. Pertussis Epidemiology in the Autonomous Province of Vojvodina, Serbia, 1948–2023. *Vaccines* **2024**, *12*, 525. [CrossRef]
29. Mengyang, G.; Yahong, H.; Qinghong, M.; Wei, S.; Kaihu, Y. Resurgence and Atypical Patterns of Pertussis in China. *J. Infect.* **2024**, *88*, 106140. [CrossRef] [PubMed]
30. Murphy, F. Whooping cough: Doctors urge Chinese authorities to review vaccine strategy as cases surge. *BMJ* **2024**, *385*, q12744. [CrossRef] [PubMed]
31. Available online: https://www.minsalud.gob.bo/es/7154-gobierno-llama-a-autoridades-de-santa-cruz-a-que-vuelquen-sus-esfuerzos-en-atender-y-controlar-brote-de-tos-ferina (accessed on 23 January 2023).
32. Alerta Sobre Surto de Coqueluche na Bolívia 21/08/2023. Disponível em: ALERTA-05-COQUELUCHE-final.pdf (apecih.org.br). Available online: https://www.apecih.org.br/down/ALERTA-05-COQUELUCHE-final.pdf (accessed on 25 April 2024).
33. Salta. Boletin_202023.pdf (salta.gov.ar). Available online: http://saladesituacion.salta.gov.ar/web/inicio/boletines/documentos/boletin_202023.pdf (accessed on 19 March 2024).
34. Peru Centro Nacional de Epidemiologia, Prevención y Control de Enfermedades—MINSA. tosf.pdf (dge.gob.pe). Available online: https://www.dge.gob.pe/portal/docs/vigilancia/sala/2024/SE04/tosf.pdf (accessed on 25 July 2024).
35. Brasil. Ministério da Saúde. Epidemiologia da Coqueluche, 2014–2024. Access at TabNet Win32 3.3: COQUELUCHE—Casos confirmados Notificados no Sistema de Informação de Agravos de Notificação—Brasil. Available online: http://tabnet.datasus.gov.br/cgi/tabcgi.exe?sinannet/cnv/coquebr.def (accessed on 11 November 2024).
36. Jog, P.; Memon, I.A.; Thisyakorn, U.; Hozbor, D.; Heininger, U.; von König, C.H.W.; Tan, T. Pertussis in Asia: Recent country-specific data and recommendation. *Vaccine* **2022**, *40*, 1170–1179. [CrossRef] [PubMed]
37. Gentile, A.; Bricks, L.; Ávila-Agüero, M.L.; Kfouri, R.A.; Torres, J.P.; Ulloa-Gutierrez, R.; Glover, R.E.; Sarti, E. Pertussis in Latin America and the Hispanic Caribbean: A systematic review. *Expert Rev. Vaccines* **2019**, *18*, 829–845. [CrossRef] [PubMed]
38. Gentile, Á.; Torres-Torreti, J.P.; López-López, P.; Ulloa-Gutierrez, R. Epidemiologic changes, and novelties on vaccination against *Bordetella pertussis* in Latin America. *Rev. Chil. Infectol.* **2021**, *38*, 232–242. [CrossRef]
39. Avila-Agüero, M.L.; Camacho-Badilla, K.; Ulloa-Gutierrez, R.; Espinal-Tejada, C.; Morice-Trejos, A.; Cherry, J.D. Epidemiology of pertussis in Costa Rica and the impact of vaccination: A 58-year experience (1961–2018). *Vaccine* **2022**, *40*, 223–228. [CrossRef] [PubMed]
40. World Health Organization. *Laboratory Manual for the Diagnosis of Whooping Cough Caused by Bordetella Pertussis/Bordetella Parapertussis*; WHO: Geneva, Switzerland, 2014. Available online: http://apps.who.int/iris/bitstream/10665/127891/1/WHO_IVB_14.03_eng.pdf (accessed on 16 July 2024).
41. CDC. Laboratory Testing for Pertussis | Pertussis (Whooping Cough) | CDC. Available online: https://www.cdc.gov/pertussis/php/laboratories/index.html (accessed on 13 August 2024).
42. Pinell-McNamara, V.A.; Acosta, A.M.; Pedreira, M.C.; Carvalho, A.F.; Pawloski, L.; Tondella, M.L.; Briere, E. Expanding Pertussis Epidemiology in 6 Latin America Countries through the Latin American Pertussis Project. *Emerg. Infect. Dis.* **2017**, *23*, S94–S100. [CrossRef]

43. Fernandes, E.G.; Sartori, A.M.C.; de Soárez, P.C.; Carvalhanas, T.R.M.P.; Rodrigues, M.; Novaes, H.M.D. Challenges of interpreting epidemiologic surveillance pertussis data with changing diagnostic and immunization practices: The case of the state of Sao Paulo, Brazil. *BMC Infect. Dis.* **2018**, *18*, 126. [CrossRef] [PubMed] [PubMed Central]
44. Pimenova, A.S.; Borisova, A.B.; Gauda, N.T.; Borisova, O.U.; Afanasieve, S.S.; Petrova, M.S.; Mironov, A.Y.; Aleshkin, V.A. PCR-based diagnosis of whooping cough in the Russian Federation. *Klin. Lab. Diagn.* **2021**, *66*, 52–58, English. [CrossRef] [PubMed]
45. El Basha, N.R.; Shaaban, H.H.; El Atroush, H.A.; Sherif, M.M.; El Kholy, A.A. The use of multiplex PCR for the detection of atypical pathogens in Egyptian children with CAP: A high rate of *Bordetella pertussis* in early infancy. *J. Egypt. Public Health Assoc.* **2019**, *94*, 5. [CrossRef]
46. Izu, A.; Nunes, M.C.; Solomon, F.; Baillie, V.; Serafin, N.; Verwey, C.; Moore, D.P.; Laubscher, M.; Ncube, M.; Olwagen, C.; et al. All-cause and pathogen-specific lower respiratory tract infection hospital admissions in children younger than 5 years during the COVID-19 pandemic (2020–22) compared with the pre-pandemic period (2015-19) in South Africa: An observational study. *Lancet Infect. Dis.* **2023**, *23*, 1031–1041. [CrossRef] [PubMed] [PubMed Central]
47. Vincent, M.; Rodeghiero, C.; Eylenbosch, R.; Mans, Y.; Swalus-Steenhouwer, J.; Piérard, D.; Huygen, K.; Vanhoof, R. Pertussis serodiagnosis in Belgium from 1990 to 2009. *Clin. Vaccine Immunol.* **2011**, *18*, 588–594. [CrossRef] [PubMed] [PubMed Central]
48. Dalby, T.; Andersen, P.H.; Hoffmann, S. Epidemiology of pertussis in Denmark, 1995 to 2013. *Eurosurveillance* **2016**, *21*, 30334. [CrossRef] [PubMed] [PubMed Central]
49. Rendi-Wagner, P.; Paulke-Korinek, M.; Stanek, G.; Khanakah, G.; Kollaritsch, H. Impact of a pertussis booster vaccination program in adolescents and adults on the epidemiology of pertussis in Austria. *Pediatr. Infect. Dis. J.* **2007**, *26*, 806–810. [CrossRef] [PubMed]
50. Bhagat, D.; Saboui, M.; Huang, G.; Domingo, F.R.; Squires, S.G.; Salvadori, M.I.; Li, Y.A. Pertussis epidemiology in Canada, 2005–2019. *Can. Commun. Dis. Rep.* **2023**, *49*, 21–28. [CrossRef] [PubMed] [PubMed Central]
51. Berbers, G.; van Gageldonk, P.; Kassteele, J.V.; Wiedermann, U.; Desombere, I.; Dalby, T.; Toubiana, J.; Tsiodras, S.; Ferencz, I.P.; Mullan, K.; et al. Circulation of pertussis and poor protection against diphtheria among middle-aged adults in 18 European countries. *Nat. Commun.* **2021**, *12*, 2871. [CrossRef] [PubMed] [PubMed Central]
52. Kurova, N.; Timofeeva, E.V.; Guiso, N.; Macina, D. A cross-sectional study of *Bordetella pertussis* seroprevalence and estimated duration of vaccine protection against pertussis in St. Petersburg, Russia. *Vaccine* **2018**, *36*, 7936–7942. [CrossRef] [PubMed]
53. Noel, G.; Borand, L.; Leng, C.; Keang, C.; Botr, C.; Dim, B.; Kerleguer, A.; Peng, Y.S.; Sreng, N.; Ork, V.; et al. Circulation of *Bordetella pertussis* in vaccinated Cambodian children: A transversal serological study. *Int. J. Infect. Dis.* **2021**, *106*, 134–139. [CrossRef] [PubMed]
54. Echaniz-Aviles, G.; García-Cisneros, S.; Sánchez-Alemán, M.A.; Olamendi-Portugal, M.; Romero-Martinez, M.; Deantonio, R.; Cervantes-Apolinar, M.Y.; Ortega-Barria, E.; Cortes-Alcala, R.; Alpuche-Aranda, C.M. Estimating *Bordetella pertussis* seroprevalence in adolescents and young adults in Mexico using the 2012 National Health and Nutrition Survey (ENSANUT). *Vaccine* **2021**, *39*, 5839–5844. [CrossRef] [PubMed]
55. Noel, G.; Badmasti, F.; Nikbin, V.S.; Zahraei, S.M.; Madec, Y.; Tavel, D.; Aït-Ahmed, M.; Guiso, N.; Shahcheraghi, F.; Taieb, F. Transversal sero-epidemiological study of *Bordetella pertussis* in Tehran, Iran. *PLoS ONE* **2020**, *15*, e0238398. [CrossRef] [PubMed] [PubMed Central]
56. Yao, N.; Zeng, Q.; Wang, Q. Seroepidemiology of diphtheria and pertussis in Chongqing, China: Serology-based evidence of *Bordetella pertussis* infection. *Public Health* **2018**, *156*, 60–66. [CrossRef] [PubMed]
57. Zhu, Y.; Zhang, W.; Hu, J.; Luo, S.; Zhou, Y.; Tang, X.; Yan, R.; Deng, X.; He, H. Seroprevalence of IgG antibodies against pertussis toxin in the Chinese population: A systematic review and meta-analysis. *Hum. Vaccines Immunother.* **2024**, *20*, 2341454. [CrossRef] [PubMed] [PubMed Central]
58. Hartanti, M.D.; Panjaitan, N.S.D.; Sunarno, S.; Ningrum, N.; Hasugian, A.R.; Dewi, R.M.; Handayani, S.; Maha, M.S.; Fairuza, F.; Sari, M.; et al. Seroprevalence of *Bordetella pertussis* infection in children 1-14 years old: Indonesia basic health research (Riskesdas) 2013 and 2018 data. *PLoS ONE* **2024**, *19*, e0311362. [CrossRef] [PubMed] [PubMed Central]
59. Nunes, A.; Abreu, A.; Furtado, B.; Soares da Silva, A.; Coelho, E.B.; de Barros, E.N. Epidemiology of pertussis among adolescents, adults, and older adults in selected countries of Latin American: A systematic review. *Hum. Vaccines Immunother.* **2021**, *17*, 1733–1746. [CrossRef] [PubMed] [PubMed Central]
60. Mihara, Y.; Yoshino, S.; Nakatani, K.; Nishimura, T.; Kan, H.; Yamamura, Y.; Tanaka, E.; Ishii, S.; Shimonodan, H.; Okada, K.; et al. *Bordetella pertussis* is a common pathogen in infants hospitalized for acute lower respiratory tract infection during the winter season. *J. Infect. Chemother.* **2021**, *27*, 497–502. [CrossRef] [PubMed]
61. Lamrani Hanchi, A.; Guennouni, M.; Rachidi, M.; Benhoumich, T.; Bennani, H.; Bourrous, M.; Maoulainine, F.M.R.; Younous, S.; Bouskraoui, M.; Soraa, N. Epidemiology of Respiratory Pathogens in Children with Severe Acute Respiratory Infection, and Impact of the Multiplex PCR Film Array Respiratory Panel: A 2-Year Study. *Int. J. Microbiol.* **2021**, *2021*, 2276261. [CrossRef] [PubMed] [PubMed Central]
62. Tao, Y.; Tang, M.; Luo, L.; Xiang, L.; Xia, Y.; Li, B.; Cao, Q.; Mo, X. Identification of etiologic agents and clinical characteristics for patients suspected of having pertussis in a large Children's Hospital in China. *Ann. Transl. Med.* **2019**, *7*, 443. [CrossRef] [PubMed] [PubMed Central]

63. Efendiyeva, E.; Kara, T.T.; Erat, T.; Yahşi, A.; Karbuz, A.; Kocabaş, B.A.; Özdemir, H.; Karahan, Z.C.; İnce, E.; Çiftçi, E. The incidence and clinical effects of Bordetella pertussis in children hospitalized with acute bronchiolitis. *Turk. J. Pediatr.* **2020**, *62*, 726–733. [CrossRef] [PubMed]
64. Ferrari, A.; Schiavetti, I.; Ogliastro, M.; Minet, C.; Sibilio, R.; Giberti, I.; Costa, E.; Massaro, E.; Lai, P.L.; Mosca, S.; et al. Co-detection of respiratory pathogens among ILI patients: Characterization of samples collected during the 2018/19 and 2019/20 pre-pandemic seasons. *BMC Infect. Dis.* **2024**, *24*, 881. [CrossRef] [PubMed] [PubMed Central]
65. Yang, S.; Li, H.; Tang, Y.; Yu, F.; Ma, C.; Zhang, H.; Pang, L.; Zhao, H.; Wang, L. Multiplex Tests for Respiratory Tract Infections: The Direct Utility of the FilmArray Respiratory Panel in Emergency Department. *Can. Respir. J.* **2020**, *2020*, 6014563. [CrossRef] [PubMed] [PubMed Central]
66. He, F.; Xia, X.; Nie, D.; Yang, H.; Jiang, Y.; Huo, X.; Guo, F.; Fang, B.; Hu, B.; Jiang, H.; et al. Respiratory bacterial pathogen spectrum among COVID-19 infected and non-COVID-19 virus infected pneumonia patients. *Diagn. Microbiol. Infect. Dis.* **2020**, *98*, 115199. [CrossRef] [PubMed] [PubMed Central]
67. Krumbein, H.; Kümmel, L.S.; Fragkou, P.C.; Thölken, C.; Hünerbein, B.L.; Reiter, R.; Papathanasiou, K.A.; Renz, H.; Skevaki, C. Respiratory viral co-infections in patients with COVID-19 and associated outcomes: A systematic review and meta-analysis. *Rev. Med. Virol.* **2023**, *33*, e2365. [CrossRef] [PubMed] [PubMed Central]
68. Domenech de Cellès, M.; Rohani, P. Pertussis vaccines, epidemiology, and evolution. *Nat. Rev. Microbiol.* **2024**, *22*, 722–735. [CrossRef]
69. Sánchez-González, G.; Luna-Casas, G.; Mascareñas, C.; Macina, D.; Vargas-Zambrano, J.C. Pertussis in Mexico from 2000 to 2019: A real-world study of incidence, vaccination coverage, and vaccine effectiveness. *Vaccine* **2023**, *41*, 6105–6111, Erratum in *Vaccine* **2024**, 42, 126085. [CrossRef] [PubMed]
70. Calvo, A.E.; Urrutia, A.G.; Vargas-Zambrano, J.C.; Castillo, H.C. Pertussis vaccine effectiveness following country-wide implementation of a hexavalent acellular pertussis immunization schedule in infants and children in Panama. *Hum. Vaccines Immunother.* **2024**, *20*, 2389577. [CrossRef]
71. Bagattini, A.M.; Quarti, M.M.; Martinez-Silveira, M.S.; Policena, G.; Coelho, L.E.; Luz, P.M.; Russell, L.B.; Toscano, C.M. Systematic review of immunogenicity and duration of immunity of currently licensed pertussis wP vaccines in children. *Gates Open Res.* **2022**, *6*, 101. [CrossRef]
72. Kalthan, E.; Lakei-Abdon, C.; Wol-Wol, P.; Pamatika, C.M.; Belizaire, M.R. Case study of a 2022 pertussis epidemic in the Baoro sub-prefecture (Central African Republic). *Infect Dis. Now.* **2023**, *53*, 104778. [CrossRef] [PubMed]
73. Paradowska-Stankiewicz, I.; Rumik, A.; Bogusz, J.; Zbrzeźniak, J.; Rastawicki, W.; Śmietańska, K.; Vargas-Zambrano, J.C.; Macina, D. Duration of protection against Bordetella pertussis infection elicited by whole-cell and acellular vaccine priming in Polish children and adolescents. *Vaccine* **2021**, *39*, 6067–6073. [CrossRef] [PubMed]

vaccines

MDPI

Review

Seasonal Influenza Vaccination Programs in the Americas: A Platform for Sustainable Life-Course Immunization and Its Role for Pandemic Preparedness and Response

Francisco Nogareda [1,*,†], Margherita Ghiselli [1,*,†], Martha Velandia-González [1], Bremen de Mucio [2], Jorge Jara [1], Paula Couto [3], Angel Rodriguez [3], Marc Rondy [3], Andrea Vicari [3], Murat Hakan Ozturk [4], Shoshanna Goldin [5], Alba Vilajeliu [6], Eva Leidman [7], Jaymin Patel [8], Julie Carlton [8], Ashley L. Fowlkes [9], Eduardo Azziz-Baumgartner [9], Daniel Salas Peraza [1] and Alba Maria Ropero [10]

1 Special Program Comprehensive Immunization, Pan American Health Organization (PAHO)/World Health Organization (WHO), Washington, DC 20037, USA; velandiam@paho.org (M.V.-G.); jarajor@paho.org (J.J.); salasdan@paho.org (D.S.P.)
2 Women and Reproductive Health, Latin American Center for Perinatology, Pan American Health Organization (PAHO)/World Health Organization (WHO), Washington, DC 20037, USA; demuciob@paho.org
3 Health Emergencies Department, Pan American Health Organization (PAHO)/World Health Organization (WHO), Washington, DC 20037, USA; coutopau@paho.org (P.C.); rodrigueza@paho.org (A.R.); rondymar@paho.org (M.R.); vicarian@paho.org (A.V.)
4 Revolving Fund for Access to Vaccines, Pan American Health Organization (PAHO)/World Health Organization (WHO), Washington, DC 20037, USA; ozturkmur@paho.org
5 World Health Emergencies Program, World Health Organization (WHO), 1211 Geneva, Switzerland; goldins@who.int
6 Immunization, Vaccines and Biologicals, World Health Organization (WHO), 1211 Geneva, Switzerland; avilajeliu@who.int
7 Coronavirus and Other Respiratory Viruses Division, National Center for Immunization and Respiratory Diseases, US Centers for Disease Control and Prevention, Atlanta, GA 30333, USA; wzu0@cdc.gov
8 Global Immunization Division, Global Health Center, US Centers for Disease Control and Prevention, Atlanta, GA 30333, USA; isr0@cdc.gov (J.P.); wvd9@cdc.gov (J.C.)
9 Influenza Division, National Center for Immunization and Respiratory Diseases, US Centers for Disease Control and Prevention, Atlanta, GA 30333, USA; ahl4@cdc.gov (A.L.F.); eha9@cdc.gov (E.A.-B.)
10 Country Office for the Dominican Republic, Pan American Health Organization (PAHO)/World Health Organization (WHO), Ensanche La Fé, Santo Domingo 10514, Dominican Republic; roperoal@paho.org
* Correspondence: nogaredfra@paho.org (F.N.); ghisellmar@paho.org (M.G.)
† These authors contributed equally to this work.

Abstract: Background: Vaccination is one of the most effective measures to prevent influenza illness and its complications. Since the 1980s, countries and territories in the Americas have progressively implemented influenza vaccination operations in high-risk priority groups—such as older adults, pregnant persons, persons with comorbidities and health workers. **Methods:** In this review, we present the history and progress of the seasonal influenza program in the Americas, how the program contributed to the efficient and timely roll-out of the COVID-19 vaccines during the pandemic, and how the program can be used to promote immunization operations across the life span for existing and future vaccines. **Results:** The influenza A(H1N1)pdm09 pandemic in 2009 and the COVID-19 pandemic in 2020–2023 underscored the importance of having a robust seasonal influenza vaccination program for pandemic preparedness and response. Overall, countries with existing seasonal influenza vaccination programs were better prepared and rolled out the delivery of COVID-19 vaccines more quickly and effectively compared to other countries where the influenza vaccination platform was weak or non-existent. **Conclusions:** Traditionally, national immunization programs of developing countries have been predominately focused on newborns, children younger than five years and school-aged children while often limiting their investment in effective adult vaccination programs; these programs are typically isolated to high-income countries. Countries in Latin America have been the exception, with strong influenza vaccination programs for adults regardless of national income level. The presence of functional and effective adult influenza vaccination programs can also facilitate the acceptance and uptake of other adult vaccines targeting priority groups at higher risk for severe illness or complications.

Keywords: influenza; COVID-19; respiratory syncytial virus; vaccines; immunization; outbreaks; maternal vaccination; vaccination week in the Americas; pandemic preparedness and response; life-course immunization

1. Introduction

Seasonal influenza epidemics pose a substantial burden of disease, affecting individuals of all ages and causing substantial morbidity and mortality. The World Health Organization (WHO) estimates that each year influenza causes 1 billion infections, including 3–5 million severe illnesses and 290,000–650,000 influenza-related deaths globally [1]. In the Americas, data reported from member states to SARI*net* plus—a Pan American Health Organization (PAHO) integrated respiratory illness surveillance network created in 2014 to monitor influenza and other respiratory viruses in the Americas—indicate that influenza contributes significantly to the respiratory disease burden in the Region [2]. It is estimated that between 716,000 and 829,000 influenza-associated respiratory hospitalizations and 41,007 to 71,710 influenza-associated deaths occur every year in the Region [3,4]. Preliminary findings from a 2022–2023 analysis covering 70% of the population, estimate approximately 55 million annual cases of mild influenza in the Americas. In 2020, SARI*net* plus was expanded to integrate COVID-19 surveillance into existing sentinel-based severe acute respiratory infection (SARI)/influenza-like illness (ILI) surveillance systems [5,6].

Vaccination is one of the most effective measures to prevent influenza illness and its complications. Safe and effective influenza vaccines are available and are routinely used globally [7]. Historically, the Americas has been one of the regions with the highest seasonal influenza vaccination coverage in the world [8], yet some countries struggled to sustain routine immunization services during the COVID-19 pandemic [9]. The first seasonal influenza vaccine was developed in the 1930s and introduced in the United States in 1945. Since 1980, countries and territories in the Americas have been progressively implementing and expanding influenza vaccination activities in priority groups—such as older adults, pregnant persons, children 6–23 months of age, persons with comorbidities and health workers—and integrating this vaccine into their national immunization programs [8,10,11]. The influenza A(H1N1)pdm09 pandemic in 2009 and the COVID-19 pandemic in 2020–2023 underscored the importance of having a robust influenza vaccination program for pandemic preparedness and response [12,13]. Countries with existing seasonal influenza vaccination programs targeting adult populations were better prepared and rolled out the COVID-19 vaccines more quickly in comparison to other countries where the influenza vaccination program was weak or non-existent [14–16]. Also, high-performing influenza vaccination programs have been shown to facilitate the acceptance and uptake of other vaccines among high-risk priority groups, such as pregnant persons, health workers and older adults [14,17,18].

In this review, we describe the progress of the seasonal influenza vaccination in the Americas and the lessons learned about building robust, sustainable life-course approach immunization programs and assess their role in facilitating the rollout of novel or existing vaccines during public health emergencies. Its purpose is to describe the key lessons learned about sustainable vaccine introduction, as well as examine how the program contributed to a timely roll-out of COVID-19 vaccines during the recent pandemic. We discuss how these experiences can serve as a blueprint for the introduction of new vaccines—for example, against the respiratory syncytial virus (RSV) or during preparedness and response operations to new epidemics and pandemics—for similar adult priority groups. We intend this review to be useful in delineating the next steps for advancing influenza vaccination programs in the Americas and in supporting other WHO regions in improving their own programs to reduce the burden of influenza morbidity and mortality globally through a life-course immunization approach.

2. Influenza Vaccination Program in the Americas

2.1. Influenza Vaccine Introduction

Seasonal influenza vaccination in the Americas was first introduced in the United States in 1945 [19] and in Canada and Chile in 1980 with a focus on older adults. Since then, countries in the Americas have been progressively introducing the vaccine to risk groups and expanding the vaccination activities to other priority groups. While in 2002 only seven countries in the Americas were vaccinating priority groups, in 2023, 41 (93%) out of the 44 countries and territories that report their data through the PAHO/WHO and the United Nations Children's Fund (UNICEF) electronic Joint Reporting Form (eJRF) were using the vaccine in at least one priority group. Only Guyana, Haiti and Saint Vincent and the Grenadines do not have a seasonal influenza vaccination program targeting any priority group. Older adults and health workers were targeted for vaccination in 40 (98%) countries and territories, persons with chronic diseases in 36 (88%), pregnant persons in 35 (85%), and children older than 6 months in 30 (73%) countries [8,10,11] (Table 1 and Figure 1).

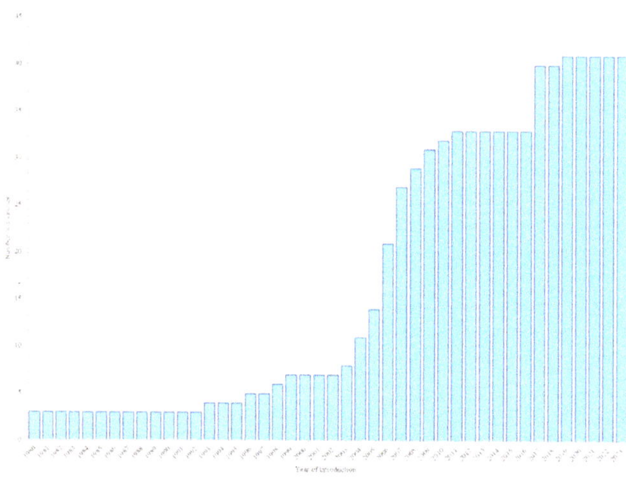

Figure 1. Cumulative number of countries with seasonal influenza vaccination by year, Region of the Americas, 1980–2023. Source: eJRF.

Table 1. Seasonal influenza vaccination in the Americas, year of introduction, vaccine formulation and priority groups by country, 2023 (n = 44).

Country/Territory †	Seasonal Influenza Vaccination * (n = 44)	Year of Introduction	Vaccine Formulation &	Priority Groups ±				
				HCW °	Older Adults	Pregnant Persons	Persons with Chronic Diseases	Children
North America								
Canada	•	1980	NH	•	•	•	•	•
Mexico	•	2004	NH	•	•	•	•	•
United States of America	•	1980	NH	•	•	•	•	•
Caribbean								
Anguilla	•	2017	NH	•	•			
Antigua and Barbuda	•	2007	NH	•	•	•	•	•
Aruba	•	2017	NH	•	•	•	•	•
Bahamas	•	2005	NH	•	•	•	•	•
Barbados	•	2006	NH	•				
Belize	•	2008	NH	•	•	•		•
Bermuda	•	2017	NH	•	•	•	•	•
British Virgin Islands	•	2017	NH	•	•	•	•	
Cayman Islands	•	2017	NH	•	•	•	•	•
Cuba	•	1998	SH	•	•	•	•	•
Curaçao	•	2006	NH		•			
Dominica	•	2011	NH	•	•	•	•	•
Dominican Republic	•	2006	NH	•	•	•	•	•
Grenada	•	2006	NH	•	•	•	•	•
Guyana								

Table 1. *Cont.*

Country/Territory †	Seasonal Influenza Vaccination * (n = 44)	Year of Introduction	Vaccine Formulation &	Priority Groups ±				
				HCW °	Older Adults	Pregnant Persons	Persons with Chronic Diseases	Children
Haiti								
Jamaica	•	2006	NH	•	•	•	•	•
Montserrat	•	2017	NH	•	•			
Saint Kitts and Nevis	•	2019	NH	•	•	•	•	
Saint Lucia	•	2006	NH	•	•	•	•	
Saint Vincent and the Grenadines								
Sint Maarten	•	2009	NH	•	•	•	•	
Suriname	•	2009	NH	•	•		•	
Trinidad and Tobago	•	2007	NH	•	•	•	•	•
Turks and Caicos Islands	•	2017	NH	•	•	•	•	•
Central America								
Costa Rica	•	2004	SH	•	•	•	•	•
El Salvador	•	2004	SH	•	•	•	•	•
Guatemala	•	2007	NH	•	•	•	•	•
Honduras	•	2003	SH	•	•	•	•	•
Nicaragua	•	2007	SH	•	•	•	•	
Panama	•	2005	SH	•	•	•	•	•
Andean								
Bolivia	•	2010	SH	•	•	•	•	•
Colombia	•	2007	SH	•	•	•	•	•
Ecuador	•	2006	NH	•	•	•	•	•
Peru	•	2008	SH	•	•	•	•	•

Table 1. *Cont.*

Country/Territory †	Seasonal Influenza Vaccination * (n = 44)	Year of Introduction	Vaccine Formulation &	Priority Groups ±				
				HCW °	Older Adults	Pregnant Persons	Persons with Chronic Diseases	Children
Venezuela	•	2007	NH	•	•		•	
Southern Cone								
Argentina	•	1993	SH	•	•	•	•	•
Brazil	•	1999	SH	•	•	•	•	•
Chile	•	1980	SH	•	•	•	•	•
Paraguay	•	2005	SH	•	•	•	•	•
Uruguay	•	1996	SH	•	•	•	•	•
Number of countries—n (%)	41 (93%)	41 (93%)	41 (93%)	40 (98%)	40 (98%)	35 (85%)	36 (88%)	30 (73%)

Each grey cell represents the exclusion of the population group from the list of priority persons in each country to whom influenza vaccination should be offered. † Countries and territories reporting to PAHO/WHO. Additional seven countries/territories in the Americas Region do not report to PAHO/WHO: Bonaire, French Guiana, Guadeloupe, Martinique, Puerto Rico, Saba, and St. Eustatius. * In at least one priority group, either private or public sector. & Vaccine formulation NH: Northern Hemisphere; SH: Southern Hemisphere. ± Target groups and eligible age groups for vaccination (e.g., older adults, people with comorbidities and children) vary across countries. Percentage calculated based on 41 countries with influenza vaccination. ° HCW = health workers.

2.2. Influenza Vaccine Formulations

Seasonal influenza vaccine composition is updated every year for both hemispheres to optimize the effectiveness of the vaccine with the circulating strains. In 2023, 27 (66%) countries/territories with a seasonal influenza vaccination program used the Northern Hemisphere vaccine formulation, while 14 (34%) used the Southern Hemisphere vaccine formulation (Table 1) [8]. To date, no country/territory in Latin America and the Caribbean has reported the public-sector use of live attenuated influenza vaccines (LAIV) to PAHO/WHO. These countries use only inactivated influenza vaccines. However, LAIV has been used in Canada for individuals aged 2–59 years [20] and in the United States for healthy non-pregnant people aged 2–49 years [21]. Since 2024, most of the countries in the Region are using trivalent vaccines (composed of two influenza A strains and one influenza B) following the recommendations of the WHO influenza vaccine composition advisory committee [22].

2.3. Procurement Through the PAHO Revolving Fund for Vaccines in the Americas

While Argentina, Brazil, Canada, Curaçao, Chile, Mexico, Sint Marteen, USA, and Venezuela produce or purchase influenza vaccines directly from manufacturers, 32 of the 41 (78%) countries/territories with seasonal influenza vaccination programs access influenza vaccines through the PAHO Revolving Fund for Access to Vaccines (RFV) [23]. This technical cooperation mechanism provides timely access to quality-assured vaccines and immunization supplies at affordable prices for countries and territories in Latin America and the Caribbean. By consolidating requirements from National Immunization Programs and orchestrating pooled procurement, the RFV leverages economies of scale to improve member states' purchasing power and supports all procurement and logistics processes. The RFV has been instrumental in enabling rapid and equitable access to new vaccines and in supporting regional goals for disease elimination. Annually, more than 30 million doses of seasonal influenza vaccines are procured through the RFV mechanism. The RFV facilitated the distribution of vaccines for routine immunization programs and emergencies, including COVID-19 vaccines during the pandemic in collaboration with the COVAX facility.

2.4. Quality of Influenza Vaccination Monitoring Data

Despite significant improvements in influenza vaccination program efforts in recent years, the completeness and timeliness of influenza vaccination data remain suboptimal in many countries across the Region [8,11]. First, countries often rely on outdated census data, health workforce statistics, or rough estimations to determine the size of different target groups, such as pregnant persons or people with chronic conditions. Also, countries in Latin America and the Caribbean inconsistently report the number of vaccinated persons per season to PAHO—leaving gaps in the regional estimates of disease burden and vaccination coverage rates. Moreover, merging data from different sources—such as national vaccination registries, healthcare provider registers and surveys—can be challenging due to variations in data formats, definitions and collection methods within the same country. Finally, the demand for vaccination fluctuates each year, complicating efforts to monitor instances of stockout. On the other hand, regional-level information systems are designed to support interoperability between various systems. For example, great strides have been made in facilitating the joint analysis of seasonal influenza surveillance information systems and vaccination registration platforms to calculate regional vaccine effectiveness estimates.

2.5. Seasonal Influenza Vaccination Coverage by Priority Group

It is estimated that every year, more than 100 million doses of influenza vaccine are administered in the Americas using different strategies (e.g., primary care and health-based immunization, door-to-door outreach activities, vaccination campaigns). Target groups and eligible age groups considered for vaccination (e.g., older adults, people with comorbidities and children) vary across countries, which makes comparisons difficult. For instance, some countries target older adults aged 60 years and older, while others focus on persons aged 65 years or older. Countries and territories systematically report data on influenza vaccination programs and vaccination coverage on an annual basis to PAHO, WHO and the United Nations Children's Fund (UNICEF) via the eJRF [8]. These data are then published annually in publicly accessible "Immunization in the Americas" brochures [11]. While the reported PAHO influenza vaccine coverage rate is the highest by any WHO Region, the Americas still fall short of global goals. According to the 2023 eJRF report, only Colombia, Cuba, Dominican Republic and Mexico achieved the 75% target coverage rate set by WHO for older adults. Regional median vaccination coverage achieved in 2023 among high-risk priority groups in the Region are presented in Table 2 [21].

Table 2. Regional median influenza vaccination coverage reported by priority groups in the Americas, 2023.

Priority Groups *	Countries/Territories Targeting The Priority Groups	Countries/Territories Reporting to PAHO eJRF °	Median Vaccination Coverage	Interquartile Range (IQR)
Health workers	40	18	61%	34–99%
Older adults	40	17	56%	15–74%
Pregnant persons	35	19	60%	40–81%
Persons with chronic diseases	36	11	85%	43–100%
Children aged ≥6–12 months †	30	19	47%	26–70%
Children aged 12–23 months †	30	15	72%	41–91%

Source: PAHO/UNICEF eJRF 2023. † Vaccinated with two doses or a single dose if previously vaccinated with two doses. * Different target populations and age groups are considered by the countries. ° eJRF = WHO/UNICEF electronic Joint Reporting Form.

2.6. Vaccination Week in the Americas

Vaccination Week in the Americas (VWA) is a yearly regional initiative that promotes the benefits of vaccination to all persons in the Region. In its 22-year history, more than 40 countries and territories reached 1.15 billion people during the VWA, according to country-level tallies compiled by PAHO. The initiative aims to close the most urgent immunity gaps and contribute to disease elimination efforts in the Americas, all while offering versatile plans for operational execution, communication, and political advocacy that can be adapted to each country's priorities.

To date, more than 502 million doses of influenza vaccine have been delivered through this initiative across the Americas, with 47 million doses in 2023 alone [24]. Many countries in the Southern Hemisphere use the VWA platform to kick off their seasonal influenza vaccination activities. Also, between 2021 and 2023, approximately 150 million COVID-19 vaccine doses were administered across the Region under the umbrella of the VWA.

2.7. Vaccine Effectiveness and Impact Evaluation of Influenza Vaccination

Established in 2013, the Network for the Evaluation of the Effectiveness of the Vaccine in Latin America and the Caribbean-influenza (REVELAC-I) uses the test-negative design approach to estimate the vaccine effectiveness of influenza vaccines [25]. It leverages sentinel surveillance systems for severe acute respiratory infections (SARIs) at the country level to produce semiannual regional and national estimates of influenza vaccine effectiveness. It also evaluates the impact of the vaccination expressed as the number of influenza illnesses averted through vaccination. Such estimates can be used as inputs for economic analyses to evaluate the value of currently licensed and future vaccines to prevent viral respiratory illnesses. This well-established and flexible platform was expanded to estimate the effectiveness of other respiratory viruses' vaccines, including those to prevent COVID-19. For the 2024 season, five countries (Argentina, Brazil, Chile, Paraguay, Uruguay) are collecting and analyzing SARI sentinel surveillance and immunization data to generate influenza and COVID-19 vaccines effectiveness against hospitalization. Estimates are stratified by vaccine type, age group and by circulating subtype of influenza virus and variant of SARS-CoV-2 [26]. Interim 2024 vaccine effectiveness estimates against influenza-associated hospitalization are 34.5% (95% confidence interval (CI): 26.4, 41.7) for any type of influenza, 37.2% (95% CI: 22.0, 49.5) for influenza A(H1N1)pdm09 and 36.5% (95% CI: 25.6, 45.7) for influenza A(H3N2) [27]. Mid-season and end-of-season influenza vaccine effectiveness estimates are reported twice a year to the Global Influenza Vaccine Effectiveness (GIVE) working group and presented at the meeting on the Composition of Influenza Virus Vaccines contributing to the recommendation for the viral composition of the next season's influenza vaccine. Since January 2024, the network has been expanded further to generate effectiveness estimates on preventing severe disease in infants for the maternal RSV vaccine and for the infant receipt of RSV monoclonal antibodies (i.e., laboratory-made proteins that are administered to newborns to protect them against severe RSV disease).

2.8. Partnerships

PAHO maintains strong partnerships with the Ministries and Departments of Health of all 51 countries and territories of the Americas. In the context of influenza vaccination, PAHO is working closely with most member states to maintain the high performance of their existing program or prepare for the introduction of the seasonal influenza vaccine in the national immunization schedule. This close collaboration is essential for the ongoing collection and collation of complete, timely and reliable surveillance data on SARI and ILI events, which in turn allows the Region to assess viral circulation in both hemispheres and take appropriate action to prevent epidemics. Also, PAHO is in a technical and financial partnership with the U.S. Centers for Disease Control and Prevention (CDC), which has been a supporter of the SARInet and REVELAC-I networks since their inception.

3. Leveraging Seasonal Influenza Vaccination Programs for Pandemic Vaccination in the Americas

3.1. Seasonal Influenza Vaccination for Pandemic Preparedness and Response

The existence of seasonal influenza vaccination programs contributed to the response to both the 2009 influenza A(H1N1)pdm09 pandemic and the COVID-19 pandemic. An analysis of the 2009 pandemic revealed that countries with a pre-existing seasonal influenza vaccination program were able to more quickly roll-out the pandemic influenza A(H1N1)pdm09 vaccine [12]. Similarly, 12 months after the introduction of COVID-19 vaccines, countries with an influenza vaccination program had reached an average vaccination coverage of 47% of the total population with the primary series compared to 22% in countries without influenza programs [14]. During and after the COVID-19 pandemic, several assessments suggested that, among the potential predictors of COVID-19 vaccine introduction and roll-out success (i.e., national maturity levels for childhood, adolescent, and adult vaccinations; experience conducting emergency vaccination; tendency to be early adopters of new vaccines; degree of trust in the vaccine product; availability of human resources; income status) [14,15], only the presence of seasonal influenza vaccination programs were associated with a swift introduction capacity for COVID-19 vaccines and higher coverage levels [13]. These results are compatible with findings from COVID-19 vaccine post-introduction evaluations (c-PIE) conducted in 20 countries globally between 2021 and 2022 and supported by the findings of key-informant interviews with the WHO regional and country-level immunization officers [14,16]. The following factors were identified as essential for the successful introduction of the COVID-19 vaccines, according to the WHO technical guidelines for the National Deployment and Vaccination Plan (NDVP) [28].

3.2. Regulatory Pathways for Authorization, Vaccine Introduction and Roll-Out

Countries with seasonal influenza vaccination programs had more straightforward regulatory approvals or emergency authorization mechanisms for the pandemic COVID-19 vaccines and established procedures for importation and use in the target population. Data collected through standardized COVID-19 post-introduction evaluation conducted at national and subnational levels in LMIC indicated that 29% of countries with influenza vaccination programs encountered barriers to regulatory approval of COVID-19 vaccines compared to 40% of countries without an influenza vaccination program [14]. On the other hand, countries without influenza vaccination programs were often slower in their operations for vaccine introduction, distribution, and administration.

3.3. Vaccination in Priority Groups

Existing seasonal influenza vaccination strategies targeting priority groups in the adult population (i.e., older adults, health workers, pregnant persons, and adults with chronic conditions) played a crucial role in guiding effective operations and achieving high vaccination coverage of COVID-19 vaccines within these populations. For example, the COVID-19 vaccination coverage of at least one dose among health workers was 83% in countries with an influenza vaccination program compared to 69% in countries without health worker vaccination programs. Also, adults with comorbidities had higher COVID-19 vaccine uptake in countries with health worker vaccination programs than in countries without health worker vaccination programs [14]. In addition, influenza vaccination programs for older adults provided sources of data (e.g., nominal electronic immunization registries, collaboration with nursing homes and medical specialists) to identify and locate this population at the time of COVID-19 vaccination. Furthermore, the expertise of advisory committees on how to determine national priority groups for influenza vaccination was leveraged to determine the priority risk groups for COVID-19 vaccination.

3.4. National Technical Advisory Groups

The role of National Immunization Technical Advisory Groups (NITAG) as key experts responsible for providing independent, transparent, evidence-informed and timely recommendations on vaccines and immunizations to health authorities, was pivotal in guiding outbreak responses and aiding in COVID-19 pandemic recovery efforts. Most NITAGs in the Region served as the main advisory body guiding the immunization program on the introduction and use of COVID-19 vaccines. This responsibility included the definition of groups at higher risk for severe illness (or complications) who should be prioritized for vaccination [29]. Operational recommendations for reaching these groups also benefitted from the existing national guidance for influenza vaccination [14,16].

3.5. Experience in Vaccination Campaigns

Health staff already familiar with mass vaccination campaigns for both young children and older adults accelerated the deployment of COVID-19 vaccines. Their experience administering vaccines to multiple age groups facilitated the rapid scale-up of COVID-19 vaccination campaigns on a massive scale and under considerable political and societal pressure. Countries with a seasonal influenza vaccination program reported fewer problems with cold chain capacity (7%) compared to countries with no vaccination program (25%) [14]. Also, experience with influenza vaccination campaigns allowed COVID-19 vaccination events to be tailored to the needs of priority groups (e.g., convenient timing and location of the vaccination sites; transportation; accommodations while waiting). Public awareness and education campaigns on influenza vaccination—targeting both the general population and high-risk priority groups—served as a model for COVID-19 vaccination campaigns, helping to increase acceptance, uptake and coverage [14,16].

3.6. Vaccination Information Systems

The vaccination monitoring and recording systems developed for influenza—especially for the pediatric population—were adapted to track the distribution and administration of COVID-19 vaccines. In fact, some countries without pre-existing systems took advantage of the COVID-19 vaccine introduction to develop and implement nominal electronic immunization registries, use SMS reminders, conduct real-time data collection and reporting, and generate digital vaccination certificates; many of which are now being expanded to include other vaccines in their national immunization program (e.g., influenza, RSV). The introduction of influenza vaccines against influenza pandemic A(H1N1)pdm09 in 2009 and against COVID-19 highlighted the importance of monitoring and reporting adverse events following immunization, especially for new vaccines. PAHO has revised and updated the regional manual for the surveillance of Events Supposedly Attributable to Vaccination or Immunization (ESAVI) and established a regional strategy for conducting permanent and functioning ESAVI surveillance for all vaccines [30].

4. Influenza Vaccination as Part of the Life-Course Approach

The life-course approach to health provides a framework to understand the health and well-being of individuals and populations as the sum of capacities that are built, sustained, and recovered across both life stages and generations. Today, the life-course approach to immunization states that people should receive all recommended doses of vaccines throughout their lives to obtain the maximum benefits of protection against vaccine-preventable diseases at different ages, across generations, and in their communities [31,32]. Integrating vaccination programs for respiratory viruses into routine health services, such as adult scheduled immunization visits or antenatal care visits, can contribute to the lasting sustainability of vaccination programs at large. Below, we report examples of PAHO strategies and operations that contributed to strengthening national political and programmatic frameworks around life-course immunization using the influenza vaccination platform as a starting point.

4.1. Policy Recommendations from the WHO and PAHO Technical Advisory Groups

Since 2004, PAHO's Technical Advisory Group (TAG) and WHO's Strategic Advisory Group of Experts (SAGE) on immunization have built upon each other's recommendations. In the context of COVID-19, the latest recommendations promote prioritization of high-risk groups (i.e., older adults, pregnant persons, persons with comorbidities, immunocompromised persons, health workers) for vaccination against respiratory infections [33–36]. Since 2021, both groups have recommended that the influenza vaccination platform be used to promote the rapid deployment and uptake of COVID-19 vaccinations, thus reducing the rates of severe disease, hospitalization, and death among priority populations. Additionally, coadministration of both influenza and COVID-19 vaccines during the same vaccination encounter, as recommended by WHO SAGE in October 2021 [37], could facilitate the implementation of integrated vaccine programmes, improve vaccination uptake, and decrease the overall burden on health services [38].

In November 2023, the TAG issued a statement where it strongly supported the SAGE recommendation that countries should integrate COVID-19 vaccination operations into their national immunization programs to maintain focus on achieving high vaccination coverage against the SARS-CoV-2 virus among priority groups and promote vaccination among all age groups [39]. During this same meeting, the TAG considered whether to recommend RSV vaccination among pregnant persons at 32–36 weeks of gestation to prevent disease in infants while minimizing the risk of preterm birth. The TAG did not issue comments on the coadministration of this vaccine with other antigens during pregnancy, but the US Centers for Disease Control and Prevention (CDC) states that the "RSVpreF vaccine can be administered to pregnant persons with other recommended vaccines, such as tetanus, diphtheria, and pertussis (Tdap), influenza, and COVID-19 vaccines" [40].

4.2. Addition of RSV to the SARInet Network

SARI*net* plus has long integrated RSV into national sentinel surveillance strategies, proving essential for providing comprehensive monitoring of virologic and epidemiological data to increase situational awareness and guide preventive measures [2,5]. The network improves coordination among national respiratory surveillance systems in both outpatient and hospital settings and incorporates RSV diagnostic testing at National Influenza Centers

(NICs) and National Reference Laboratories (NRLs) contributing to the WHO Global Influenza Surveillance and Response System (GISRS).

SARI*net* plus supports public health decisions aimed at reducing RSV-related morbidity and mortality by analyzing trends, seasonal variations, and regional differences overall and in relation to the disease severity (i.e., RSV-related hospitalizations), focusing on high-risk groups like infants and older adults. Analyses dating back to 2010 have revealed significant regional variations in RSV seasonality, underscoring the need for tailored interventions [41]. Regional and climatic factors are known to influence RSV activity, typically starting in the south and moving northward with differing onset and peak times [42,43]. Understanding these patterns is crucial for optimizing interventions and mitigating the substantial burden of RSV across all age groups.

4.3. Latin American Center for Perinatology, Women and Reproductive Health (CLAP/WR) Network

Since 1983, CLAP/WR has promoted a standardized clinical record for maternal and perinatal care, known as the Perinatal Clinical Record, which includes information about vaccines administered during pregnancy [44]. This record is supported by the Perinatal Information System (SIP), available free of charge to all countries in the Americas. Nineteen health facilities in nine countries that are members of the "CLAP Network for Maternal Health Surveillance" regularly contribute their data to the Perinatal Clinical Record. The network maintains high-quality data on coverage with vaccines recommended for routine use during pregnancy, including COVID-19 vaccines. This platform has enabled the network to follow trends in vaccination coverage among pregnant persons, identify factors associated with the vaccine uptake and to monitor ESAVIs associated with various COVID-19 vaccination platforms used in these countries. More recently, the network has begun monitoring ESAVIs associated with RSV vaccination of pregnant persons in Argentina and Uruguay.

4.4. Behavioral and Social Drivers Studies

Behavioral and Social Drivers (BeSD) of vaccination are defined as beliefs and experiences specific to vaccination that are potentially modifiable to increase vaccine uptake [45]. The WHO developed the BeSD tool to help countries understand the reasons for low vaccine uptake, track trends over time, and reduce coverage inequities by gathering and using data to systematically design, implement, and evaluate tailored interventions [46]. In 2021 and 2022, PAHO used this methodology in countries of the Caribbean and Latin Americas to assess attitudes towards COVID-19 vaccines among health workers. By the end of 2024, PAHO will have implemented the Spanish version of the tool to collect perceptions around vaccination against influenza, COVID-19 and RSV among pregnant persons aged 18 years or older in Argentina. BeSD results can be used to inform the design and implementation of interventions that increase acceptance and confidence in vaccines in the persons at the highest risk of infection and severe disease.

Also, in 2024, PAHO published a performance monitoring tool to support countries in conducting a self-assessment of their national immunization program [47]. Results from these exercises will provide additional information about member states' efforts and challenges in providing vaccination services to high-risk priority groups.

5. Discussion

The strong seasonal influenza vaccination program in the Americas, built over decades, prevents hundreds of thousands of illnesses, hospitalizations and influenza-associated deaths every year [48]. Following the 2009 A(H1N1) influenza and 2020–2023 COVID-19 pandemics, countries of the Americas have continued their efforts to sustain seasonal influenza vaccine uptake among priority groups at higher risk for severe illness (or complications), especially in the adult population and among pregnant persons. Countries have also continued strengthening their influenza surveillance systems, immunization platforms, and information systems—efforts which indirectly bolster preparedness for future pandemics [6,9,49]. Furthermore, influenza vaccination efforts have greatly contributed to the successful expansion of life-course immunization beyond childhood vaccines. It has facilitated the introduction of COVID-19 vaccines in the Americas and progressively reduced mortality due to vaccine-preventable diseases. Below, we outline six key recommendations that could support other WHO Regions in strengthening their seasonal influenza vaccination strategies.

1. Promote high-level advocacy and collaboration between Ministries of Health, PAHO Immunization Program and Revolving Fund for Access to Vaccines, and their partners to promote and consistently finance seasonal influenza vaccination for the general population and among high-risk priority groups.
2. Strengthen technical cooperation between these stakeholders to develop updated guidance and tools and to strengthen national capacities for timely vaccination in priority groups. These materials supported member states in their decision-making to strengthen national policies and programs for influenza vaccination and improved the reach and quality of their seasonal programs [50].
3. Expand the seasonal influenza vaccination program to persons aged 6 months or older, with a focus on young children, older adults, pregnant persons, people with comorbidities and health workers. Such an approach of vaccinating multiple age groups concomitantly allowed countries to implement and promote the concept of immunization across the life course well before it was included as a strategic priority of the Immunization Agenda 2030. As more vaccines come through the pipeline to address more diseases and conditions, these lessons learned about how to facilitate vaccine acceptance and delivery across the life course will become more and more critical.
4. Document lessons learned from the introduction and roll-out of the COVID-19 vaccines during the pandemic. Employing existing structures of the seasonal influenza vaccination programs—such as regulatory pathways, vaccination strategies, campaign planning and implementation, cold chain capacities, information systems, public awareness and trained health workers—was essential for a rapid introduction and roll-out of COVID-19 vaccines. Having a strong seasonal influenza vaccination program contributes to better preparedness and would support emergency response operations during the next pandemic.
5. Improve the completeness, timeliness and accuracy of the data flow after vaccines are in use in populations—from needs assessments to data collection, analysis, interpretation and interoperability. This step can strengthen the completeness, timeliness and reliability of the information on influenza vaccination programs and therefore promote the use of evidence to inform policy decisions.
6. Intensify maternal vaccination operations, which can benefit from the existing capacities of the influenza vaccination program to reach this population. For pregnant persons specifically, the option of receiving these additional vaccines in conjunction with the annual dose against influenza or RSV can facilitate acceptance and uptake. The integration of vaccination operations with other essential care and antenatal services is likely to further boost coverage rates.

As part of its ongoing efforts to support immunization operations and reduce the burden of vaccine-preventable diseases, the Americas will continue to improve national immunization programs against respiratory pathogens and contribute to the lasting sustainability of vaccination programs at large.

6. Conclusions

Influenza vaccination protects people at risk from developing severe disease. It reduces the burden of disease, including hospitalization and deaths. It also protects health workers by reducing transmission and helps maintain the health system during influenza epidemics and pandemics. Seasonal influenza vaccination provides a sustainable platform for life course immunization against influenza and other vaccine-preventable diseases and contributes to a foundation for pandemic preparedness and response.

Author Contributions: F.N. and M.G. drafted the manuscript. M.V.-G., B.d.M., J.J., P.C., A.R., M.R., A.V. (Andrea Vicari), M.H.O., S.G., A.V. (Alba Vilajeliu), E.L., J.P., J.C., A.L.F., E.A.-B., D.S.P. and A.M.R. provided detailed comments and suggestions. All authors have read and agreed to the published version of the manuscript.

Funding: This publication was supported by the Grant or Cooperative Agreement Number NU66GH002171, funded by the Centers for Disease Control and Prevention. Its contents are solely the responsibility of the authors and do not necessarily represent the official views of the Centers for Disease Control and Prevention or the Department of Health and Human Services.

Acknowledgments: We express our sincere gratitude for the tireless effort and dedication of the immunization staff. Their commitment to public health remained strong even in the most challenging moments of the pandemic. Their collaboration and commitment have been fundamental to confront this global crisis. The solidarity and cooperation they demonstrated reflect the strength of our Region and are inspiring examples of Pan-Americanism.

Conflicts of Interest: The authors declare no conflicts of interest.

References

1. World Health Organization. Global Influenza Programme. Available online: https://www.who.int/teams/global-influenza-programme/surveillance-and-monitoring/burden-of-disease (accessed on 2 December 2024).
2. Pan American Health Organization. Data | SARINET. Available online: https://sarinet.org/data/ (accessed on 2 December 2024).
3. Palekar, R.S.; Rolfes, M.A.; Arriola, C.S.; Acosta, B.O.; Guidos, P.A.; Vargas, X.B.; Bancej, C.; Ramirez, J.B.; Baumeister, E.; Bruno, A.; et al. Burden of Influenza-Associated Respiratory Hospitalizations in the Americas, 2010–2015. *PLoS ONE* **2019**, *14*, e0221479. [CrossRef] [PubMed]
4. Iuliano, A.D.; Roguski, K.M.; Chang, H.H.; Muscatello, D.J.; Palekar, R.; Tempia, S.; Cohen, C.; Gran, J.M.; Schanzer, D.; Cowling, B.J.; et al. Estimates of Global Seasonal Influenza-Associated Respiratory Mortality: A Modelling Study. *Lancet* **2018**, *391*, 1285–1300. [CrossRef] [PubMed]
5. Pan American Health Organization. *Influenza and Other Respiratory Viruses: Surveillance in the Americas 2021*, 4th ed.; Pan American Health Organization (PAHO): Bloomfield, NJ, USA, 2022; ISBN 978-92-75-12499-4.
6. Vicari, A.S.; Olson, D.; Vilajeliu, A.; Andrus, J.K.; Ropero, A.M.; Morens, D.M.; Santos, I.J.; Azziz-Baumgartner, E.; Berman, S. Seasonal Influenza Prevention and Control Progress in Latin America and the Caribbean in the Context of the Global Influenza Strategy and the COVID-19 Pandemic. *Am. J. Trop. Med. Hyg.* **2021**, *105*, 93–101. [CrossRef] [PubMed]
7. World Health Organization. Vaccines Against Influenza: WHO Position Paper—May 2022. Available online: https://www.who.int/publications/i/item/who-wer9719 (accessed on 3 December 2024).
8. World Health Organization. WHO/UNICEF Joint Reporting Process. Available online: https://www.who.int/teams/immunization-vaccines-and-biologicals/immunization-analysis-and-insights/global-monitoring/who-unicef-joint-reporting-process (accessed on 3 December 2024).
9. Nogareda, F.; Gharpure, R.; Contreras, M.; Velandia, M.; Lucia Pacis, C.; Elena Chevez, A.; Azziz-Baumgartner, E.; Salas, D. Seasonal Influenza Vaccination in the Americas: Progress and Challenges during the COVID-19 Pandemic. *Vaccine* **2023**, *41*, 4554–4560. [CrossRef] [PubMed]
10. World Health Organization. WHO Immunization Data Portal. Available online: https://immunizationdata.who.int/global/wiise-detail-page (accessed on 3 December 2024).
11. Pan American Health Organization. Immunization Brochure—PAHO/WHO | Pan American Health Organization. Available online: https://www.paho.org/en/tag/immunization-brochure (accessed on 3 December 2024).
12. Porter, R.M.; Goldin, S.; Lafond, K.E.; Hedman, L.; Ungkuldee, M.; Kurzum, J.; Azziz-Baumgartner, E.; Nannei, C.; Bresee, J.S.; Moen, A. Does Having a Seasonal Influenza Program Facilitate Pandemic Preparedness? An Analysis of Vaccine Deployment during the 2009 Pandemic. *Vaccine* **2020**, *38*, 1152–1159. [CrossRef] [PubMed]
13. Volkmann, A.-M.; Goldin, S.; McMurren, B.; Gapare, C.; Anne Pratt, B.; Frost, L.; Desai, S. Leveraging Seasonal Influenza Health Worker Vaccination Programmes for COVID-19 Vaccine Introduction: A Global Qualitative Analysis. *Vaccine* **2024**, *42*, 125534. [CrossRef] [PubMed]
14. McCarron, M. Lessons Learned from Leveraging Seasonal Influenza Vaccination Infrastructure in COVID-19 Vaccination. In Proceedings of the Global Exchange Forum on Integrated Immunization Programs and Enhanced Pandemic Preparedness, London, UK, 18–19 October 2023.
15. Chelsey, G. The Impact of an Established Influenza Vaccination Program for Health Workers on COVID-19 Vaccine Rollout and Uptake in Low-, Lower Middle-, and Upper Middle-Income Countries. In Proceedings of the Options XII Conference, Brisbane, Australia, 29 September–2 October 2024.

16. Centers for Disease Control and Prevention (CDC), The Task Force for Global Health Country COVID-19 Vaccine Introduction Evaluations (cPIE): Cross-Country Review of Findings. Available online: https://www.technet-21.org/en/resources/report/country-covid-19-vaccine-introduction-evaluations-cpie-cross-country-review-of-findings (accessed on 3 December 2024).
17. Galanis, P.; Vraka, I.; Siskou, O.; Konstantakopoulou, O.; Katsiroumpa, A.; Kaitelidou, D. Uptake of COVID-19 Vaccines among Pregnant Women: A Systematic Review and Meta-Analysis. *Vaccines* **2022**, *10*, 766. [CrossRef] [PubMed]
18. McCarron, M.; Yau, T.S.; Griffin, C.; Marcenac, P.; Ebama, M.S.; Lafond, K.E.; Igboh, L.S.; Duca, L.M.; Bino, S.; Bettaieb, J.; et al. Do Pregnant Persons Want Influenza Vaccines? Knowledge, Attitudes, Perceptions, and Practices Toward Influenza Vaccines in 8 Low- and Middle-Income Countries. *J. Infect. Dis.* **2024**, jiae340. [CrossRef] [PubMed]
19. Burney, L.E. Influenza Immunization: Statement. *Public Health Rep. Wash. DC 1896* **1960**, *75*, 944. [CrossRef]
20. NACI Recommendations on the Use of Live, Attenuated Influenza Vaccine (FluMist®): Supplemental Statement on Seasonal Influenza Vaccine for 2011–2012. *Can. Commun. Dis. Rep.* **2011**, *37*, 1–77. [CrossRef]
21. Centers for Disease Control and Prevention (CDC). Live Attenuated Influenza Vaccine [LAIV] (The Nasal Spray Flu Vaccine). Available online: https://www.cdc.gov/flu/vaccine-types/nasalspray.html (accessed on 3 December 2024).
22. Recommendations for Influenza Vaccine Composition. Available online: https://www.who.int/teams/global-influenza-programme/vaccines/who-recommendations (accessed on 3 December 2024).
23. Pan American Health Organization. PAHO Revolving Fund—PAHO/WHO | Pan American Health Organization. Available online: https://www.paho.org/en/revolving-fund (accessed on 3 December 2024).
24. Vaccination Week in the Americas 2023: Final Report—PAHO/WHO | Pan American Health Organization. Available online: https://www.paho.org/en/documents/vaccination-week-americas-2023-final-report (accessed on 3 December 2024).
25. Pan American Health Organization. Network for the Evaluation of Vaccine Effectiveness in Latin America and the Caribbean—Influenza, (REVELAC-i)—PAHO/WHO | Pan American Health Organization. Available online: https://www.paho.org/en/network-evaluation-vaccine-effectiveness-latin-america-and-caribbean-influenza-revelac-i (accessed on 3 December 2024).
26. Nogareda, F.; Regan, A.K.; Couto, P.; Fowlkes, A.L.; Gharpure, R.; Loayza, S.; Leite, J.A.; Rodríguez, A.; Vicari, A.; Azziz-Baumgartner, E.; et al. Effectiveness of COVID-19 Vaccines against Hospitalisation in Latin America during Three Pandemic Waves, 2021–2022: A Test-Negative Case-Control Design. *Lancet Reg. Health Am.* **2023**, *27*, 100626. [CrossRef] [PubMed]
27. Zeno, E.E.; Nogareda, F.; Regan, A.; Couto, P.; Rondy, M.; Jara, J.; Voto, C.; Rojas Mena, M.P.; Katz, N.; Del Valle Juarez, M.; et al. Interim Effectiveness Estimates of 2024 Southern Hemisphere Influenza Vaccines in Preventing Influenza-Associated Hospitalization—REVELAC-i Network, Five South American Countries, March–July 2024. *MMWR Morb. Mortal. Wkly. Rep.* **2024**, *73*, 861–868. [CrossRef]
28. World Health Organization. Guidance on Developing a National Deployment and Vaccination Plan for COVID-19 Vaccines. Available online: https://www.who.int/publications/i/item/WHO-2019-nCoV-Vaccine-deployment-2021.1-eng (accessed on 3 December 2024).
29. Henaff, L.; Zavadska, D.; Melgar, M.; Fihman, J.; Steffen, C.; Hombach, J. The Role of NITAGs in Government Decisions on Vaccine Use: Insights from the Fifth Global NITAG Network Meeting. *Lancet Infect. Dis.* **2024**, *24*, e214–e215. [CrossRef]
30. Vacunación Segura En Las Américas. Experiencia Sobre La Vigilancia de Los Eventos Supuestamente Atribuibles a La Vacunación o Inmunización y La Interoperabilidad de Los Datos. Available online: https://iris.paho.org/handle/10665.2/57547 (accessed on 3 December 2024).
31. World Health Organization. Our Work: Life Course. Available online: https://www.who.int/our-work/life-course (accessed on 3 December 2024).
32. Pan American Health Organization. *Building Better Immunity: A Life Course Approach to Healthy Longevity*; PAHO: Durham, NC, USA, 2023; ISBN 978-92-75-12744-5.
33. Pan American Health Organization. 16 TAG Final Report, 2004—PAHO/WHO | Pan American Health Organization. Available online: https://www.paho.org/en/documents/16-tag-final-report-2004 (accessed on 3 December 2024).
34. Vaccines against Influenza WHO Position Paper—November 2012. *Relev. Epidemiol. Hebd.* **2012**, *87*, 461–476.
35. Pan American Health Organization. The Immunization Program in the Context of the COVID-19 Pandemic—PAHO/WHO | Pan American Health Organization. Available online: https://www.paho.org/en/publications/immunization-program-context-covid-19-pandemic (accessed on 3 December 2024).
36. World Health Organization. WHO SAGE Seasonal Influenza Vaccination Recommendations During the COVID-19 Pandemic. Available online: https://www.who.int/publications/m/item/who-sage-seasonal-influenza-vaccination-recommendations-during-the-covid-19-pandemic (accessed on 3 December 2024).
37. World Health Organization. Coadministration of Seasonal Inactivated Influenza and COVID-19 Vaccines. Available online: https://www.who.int/publications/i/item/WHO-2019-nCoV-vaccines-SAGE_recommendation-coadministration-influenza-vaccines (accessed on 3 December 2024).
38. World Health Organization. Considerations for Integrating COVID-19 Vaccination into Immunization. Available online: https://www.who.int/publications/i/item/9789240064454 (accessed on 3 December 2024).
39. Vaccine-Preventable Diseases TAG—PAHO/WHO | Pan American Health Organization. Available online: https://www.paho.org/en/technical-advisory-group-vaccine-preventable-diseases (accessed on 3 December 2024).
40. Fleming-Dutra, K.E.; Jones, J.M.; Roper, L.E.; Prill, M.M.; Ortega-Sanchez, I.R.; Moulia, D.L.; Wallace, M.; Godfrey, M.; Broder, K.R.; Tepper, N.K.; et al. Use of the Pfizer Respiratory Syncytial Virus Vaccine During Pregnancy for the Prevention of Respiratory

Syncytial Virus–Associated Lower Respiratory Tract Disease in Infants: Recommendations of the Advisory Committee on Immunization Practices—United States, 2023. *MMWR Morb. Mortal. Wkly. Rep.* **2023**, *72*, 1115–1122. [CrossRef]
41. Pan American Health Organization. Influenza Situation Report. Available online: https://app.powerbi.com/view?r=eyJrIjoiNDg2ZmU1NWYtZmJkMi00MjlmLThkNTYtOTc4MjNmMjc4YzBjIiwidCI6ImU2MTBlNzljLTJlYzAtNGUwZi04YTE0LTFlNGIxMDE1MTlmNyIsImMiOjR9 (accessed on 3 December 2024).
42. Bloom-Feshbach, K.; Alonso, W.J.; Charu, V.; Tamerius, J.; Simonsen, L.; Miller, M.A.; Viboud, C. Latitudinal Variations in Seasonal Activity of Influenza and Respiratory Syncytial Virus (RSV): A Global Comparative Review. *PLoS ONE* **2013**, *8*, e54445. [CrossRef]
43. Li, Y.; Reeves, R.M.; Wang, X.; Bassat, Q.; Brooks, W.A.; Cohen, C.; Moore, D.P.; Nunes, M.; Rath, B.; Campbell, H.; et al. Global Patterns in Monthly Activity of Influenza Virus, Respiratory Syncytial Virus, Parainfluenza Virus, and Metapneumovirus: A Systematic Analysis. *Lancet Glob. Health* **2019**, *7*, e1031–e1045. [CrossRef]
44. Pan American Health Organization. Latin American Center for Perinatology, Women and Reproductive Health (CLP/WR)—PAHO/WHO | Pan American Health Organization. Available online: https://www.paho.org/en/clap (accessed on 3 December 2024).
45. World Health Organization. Acceptance and Demand. Available online: https://www.who.int/teams/immunization-vaccines-and-biologicals/essential-programme-on-immunization/demand (accessed on 3 December 2024).
46. World Health Organization. *Behavioural and Social Drivers of Vaccination: Tools and Practical Guidance for Achieving High Uptake*, 1st ed.; World Health Organization: Geneva, Switzerland, 2022; ISBN 978-92-4-004968-0.
47. Pan American Health Organization. Performance Monitoring Tool for the National Expanded Program on Immunization—PAHO/WHO | Pan American Health Organization. Available online: https://www.paho.org/en/topics/immunization/performance-monitoring-tool-national-expanded-program-immunization (accessed on 3 December 2024).
48. Pan American Health Organization. Myths and Truths About Seasonal Influenza and the Flu Vaccine—PAHO/WHO | Pan American Health Organization. Available online: https://www.paho.org/en/news/14-5-2019-myths-and-truths-about-seasonal-influenza-and-flu-vaccine (accessed on 3 December 2024).
49. Ropero-Álvarez, A.M.; El Omeiri, N.; Kurtis, H.J.; Danovaro-Holliday, M.C.; Ruiz-Matus, C. Influenza Vaccination in the Americas: Progress and Challenges after the 2009 A(H1N1) Influenza Pandemic. *Hum. Vaccines Immunother.* **2016**, *12*, 2206–2214. [CrossRef] [PubMed]
50. World Health Organization. Influenza Vaccination Toolkit. Available online: https://www.who.int/teams/global-influenza-programme/vaccines/influenza-vaccination-toolbox (accessed on 3 December 2024).

vaccines

MDPI

Review

Scoping Review of Current Costing Literature on Interventions to Reach Zero-Dose Children in Low- and Middle-Income Countries

Ann Levin [1], Teemar Fisseha [2], Heidi W. Reynolds [3], Gustavo Corrêa [3], Tewodaj Mengistu [3] and Nancy Vollmer [2,*]

1 Levin & Morgan, LLC, Bethesda, MD 20817, USA; ann@levinmorgan.com
2 JSI Research & Training Institute, Inc., Arlington, VA 22202, USA; teemar_fisseha@jsi.com
3 Gavi, The Vaccine Alliance, 1211 Geneva, Switzerland; hreynolds@gavi.org (H.W.R.); gcorrea@gavi.org (G.C.); tmengistu@gavi.org (T.M.)
* Correspondence: nancy_vollmer@jsi.com

Abstract: Introduction: A limited number of studies focus on estimating the costs of interventions to increase childhood immunization coverage in low- and middle-income countries (LMICs). Existing reviews often compare estimated costs but lack information on the methods used. The objective of this review is to summarize the methods used in costing studies that assessed interventions to reach zero-dose (ZD) children. **Methods:** We conducted a review of existing studies that estimate the costs of increasing childhood vaccination and reducing prevalence of ZD children in LMICs. We conducted searches of PubMed using terms including "immunization", "cost", "coverage increase", "zero-dose", and "LMIC", and further extended our search to bibliographies and gray literature from organizations working to reach ZD children. We only included articles that estimated the cost of interventions to increase childhood vaccination and/or reach ZD children and not articles about introducing new vaccines or other age groups. We categorized each article according to their costing methods, cost components, types of costs calculated, and presence of uncertainty analysis. **Results:** Eleven articles met our inclusion criteria. Interventions costs varied from USD 0.08 per additional dose for SMS reminders in Kenya to USD 67 per dose for cash transfers in Nicaragua. Most of the studies were from South Asia: India (4), Pakistan (2), and Bangladesh (1). The rest were from Africa (3) and Latin America (1). Most articles did not include a description of their costing methods. Only three described their methods in detail. **Conclusions:** Few studies have estimated the costs of increasing childhood vaccination coverage and reducing the number of ZD children in LMICs. The wide variation in intervention costs underscores the need for standardized costing methodologies to enhance comparability across studies. Only three studies detailed their costing methods, making comparisons challenging. Establishing research principles for costing ZD interventions could strengthen future evidence for policymaking.

Keywords: immunization; cost; coverage increase; zero-dose; vaccination; LMICs

1. Introduction

The Gavi-funded Zero-Dose Learning Hub (ZDLH) is a global project led by JSI working to generate evidence and learning on interventions to identify and reach children that are either under-immunized or zero-dose (ZD) in low- and middle-income countries (LMICs). There are currently four Gavi-funded country learning hubs (Bangladesh, Uganda, Nigeria, and Mali) where the effectiveness of interventions to reach ZD children are being assessed and, in some cases, the costs are recorded and analyzed as well.

Zero-dose children are operationally defined by Gavi, the World Health Organization (WHO IA2030), and the ZDLH, as children who have not received the first dose of the diphtheria–tetanus–pertussis (DTP1)-containing vaccine by the end of their first year of life. While the concept of ZD interventions generally focuses on interventions that increase DTP1 coverage, the broader intent is to identify and reach children that have been missed during routine immunization (RI). Thus, there are various definitions of ZD interventions in the literature, ranging from interventions that increase childhood vaccination coverage to more specific ones such as reaching children that are under-vaccinated and have not received all of their required vaccines in the first year according to WHO recommendations. Interventions that are designed to increase immunization of ZD and under-immunized children often require additional resources and tailoring to the local context and can include a wide range of strategies, including periodic intensification of routine immunization, improvements in micro-planning, demand-side interventions, and systems improvement.

Despite over two decades of progress increasing access to childhood immunization, the number of ZD children in Gavi-supported countries has increased in recent years. ZD children and the communities where they live have been systematically missed by vaccination and other primary healthcare services and tend to suffer multiple forms of socioeconomic deprivation. Gavi is focused on achieving immunization equity and reaching ZD children through its current 5.0 strategy. The emphasis on equity and reaching ZD children requires differentiated, targeted subnational strategies that are tailored to the context. As a result, there is growing interest in understanding how to reliably measure the incremental cost of reaching ZD and under-immunized children as well as the cost-effectiveness of different ZD interventions.

Understanding of the costs of tailored delivery strategies is important, as costs may vary widely across the types of interventions needed to address the immunization barriers in different ZD contexts across countries and populations. Many immunization costing studies have been conducted over the past four decades. These studies have various objectives: (1) informing decision-making regarding new vaccine introduction [1]; (2) evaluating the efficiency and/or effectiveness of immunization programs at different levels [2]; (3) conducting planning and advocacy for resource mobilization [3]; (4) evaluating the cost-effectiveness of different strategies such as routine vs. supplementary immunization activities (SIAs) or for elimination of diseases [4]; and (5) estimating the cost of increasing vaccination coverage [5,6]. Estimating the costs of increasing coverage and reaching ZD children is particularly important because of the challenges associated with reaching marginalized populations and other hard-to-reach groups. Information about the costs of different types of ZD interventions is needed for planning purposes, to advocate for funding with policymakers and program managers, and to evaluate the cost-effectiveness of different interventions. Information on cost-effectiveness can be used in decision-making to improve resource use, i.e., allocative efficiency. It is also important to conduct these studies to ascertain whether it is more costly to reach ZD children and in which contexts.

Costing studies tend to differ in their methods, which makes it difficult to develop a general estimate of the additional costs of reaching ZD and reduces the comparability across studies. Some of the differences are related to whether ingredients or top–down costing is used, the type of sampling employed, the comprehensiveness of cost categories, and types of costs analyzed (e.g., financial and economic, recurrent and capital, startup and implementation). Cost estimates will be more rigorous if a more disaggregated methodology, such as ingredients costing, is used and both startup and implementation costs are included, as this approach increases the likelihood of capturing all resources employed. Analyzing economic costs as well as financial costs is also useful, since it includes opportunity costs (e.g., in-kind and donated items) as well as accounting costs (monetary costs incurred).

This scoping review provides a synthesis of articles that estimated the costs of interventions to reach ZD children using primary data as opposed to modeled estimates. This review differs from earlier reviews since it focuses on methods used in costing of ZD interventions as well as their findings.

2. Methods

Our search strategy aimed to identify peer-reviewed articles and gray literature published after 2005 that reviewed or estimated the costs of interventions targeting ZD or hard-to-reach children, with a focus on increasing overall vaccination coverage in LMICs. We broadened our search to include articles on the costs of increasing childhood immunization coverage rather than focusing specifically on DTP1, as the latter definition was rarely used in studies. In addition, we searched for studies that focused on increasing childhood immunization coverage rather than reducing ZD, since the ZD terminology is relatively new and few studies focus on it. Limiting the review to studies published post-2005 allowed us to build upon earlier systematic reviews without duplicating prior findings. The methods are compliant with PRISMA guidelines for a scoping review.

Our methodology comprised three main approaches:

1. We searched PubMed using the following search terms: immunization, cost, coverage increase, zero-dose, vaccination, LMICs.
2. We reviewed the bibliographies of systematic review articles to identify studies published after 2005 that focused on LMICs and included cost analyses of increasing childhood vaccination.
3. We searched gray literature from organizations that are implementing projects intended to reach ZD children in LMICs, such as Thinkwell, JSI, and International Vaccine Access Center (IVAC), and conducted additional searches on Google.

The inclusion criteria were studies that had the following characteristics: (1) focused on interventions that increased childhood vaccination, (2) estimated the costs of the interventions, (3) were from LMICs, and (4) were conducted after 2005.

We selected search terms pertaining to immunization, cost, and increasing coverage. We also included vaccination, LMIC, and zero-dose in our search terms. Our search included papers on increasing child vaccination as well as reducing ZD children, since the focus on ZD is relatively recent.

For each selected paper that estimated the cost of interventions to increase coverage, we reviewed and documented information on the study context; the methods used, including incremental and/or retrospective methods; financial and economic cost; cost components; and output/outcome variables. The study findings on cost per dose or per child were also documented.

Key Concepts and Terms Used in this Paper

Cost per additional dose for intervention: Additional intervention cost of providing another dose (calculated by dividing the extra cost by additional vaccine doses administered).

Cost per intervention: Total cost of implementing an intervention (calculated by adding the value of the cost categories together).

Cost per percentage change in immunization coverage: Cost divided by additional percent change in immunization coverage.

Cost per person reached: Intervention cost divided by number of persons reached.

Incremental cost-effectiveness ratio (ICER): Measure that summarizes the cost-effectiveness of an intervention (ratio of costs of intervention divided by effectiveness measure—such as deaths or disability-adjusted life years (DALYs) averted).

Zero-dose child: Child that has not received the first dose of the DTP-containing vaccine.

3. Results

3.1. Reviews

We found three systematic reviews that focused on estimating the costs of increasing childhood immunization coverage after 2005. Two of the papers reviewed articles in high-income countries as well as LMICs. Munk's review [5] focused on studies in LMICs. Table 1 summarizes the findings of the three systematic reviews.

Table 1. Description of systematic reviews on estimation of costs of increasing immunization doses delivered in LMICs.

Authors	Year	Title	Findings
Munk, et al. [5]; BMC Health Services Research https://doi.org/10.1186/s12913-019-4468-4	2019	Systematic review of the costs and effectiveness of interventions to increase childhood vaccination coverage in LMICs	14 articles on the costs of increasing coverage with considerable heterogeneity in costing methods. Incremental cost-effectiveness ratios (ICERs) ranged from USD 0.66 to USD 162 per child reached with a dose; vaccines included DTP3 and measles.
Ozawa, et al. [7] Vaccine https://doi.org/10.1016/j.vaccine.2018.05.030	2018	Systematic review of the incremental costs of interventions that increase immunization coverage	42 articles met criteria, 17 of which were in LMICss; intervention cost per dose per percent change in coverage ranged from USD 0.01 to USD 38.16 [mean USD 3.13, SD USD 7.02] for various interventions to increase immunization coverage.
Yemeke, et al. [8] Vaccine https://doi.org/10.1016/j.vaccine.2021.05.075	2021	Promoting, seeking, and reaching vaccination services: A systematic review	57 studies describing information, education and communication (IEC) costs, social mobilization costs, and costs of interventions to increase vaccination demand, 30 of which were in LMICs: mean costs per dose in low-income countries were USD 0.41 (SD USD 0.83) and in middle-income countries they were USD 18.87 (USD 50.65); vaccines included Hepatitis B, meningitis, HPV, measles, and oral cholera.

Munk et al. [5] found 14 articles that included data on the costs of increasing childhood vaccination coverage in LMICs. They found that interventions aimed at improving delivery mechanisms were associated with the largest coverage increases. The intervention cost per person in 2017 ranged from USD 1.38–USD 162.25, with a median value of USD 23.64. The authors found that many of the included studies did not describe the costing methods used in their analyses. Seven of the fourteen articles in Munk's systematic review also met our criteria of the current synthesis, i.e., estimated costs of increasing coverage of childhood vaccination after 2005. Articles were excluded if they focused on vaccines targeting populations over two years of age, did not provide the cost per dose or cost per person, or did not estimate costs (the study authors contacted some of the individual authors to obtain cost data).

Yemeke et al. [8] found 30 articles that reported on the estimated cost of increasing immunization coverage in LMICs. The mean cost per dose of interventions was USD 0.41 in low-income countries and USD 18.86 in middle-income countries. Only five articles from the Yemeke systematic review met our study criteria, i.e., focused on the costs of interventions to increase immunization uptake rather than costs of introducing vaccines or costs of vaccines that targeted older age groups (e.g., oral cholera vaccine and HPV), or did not report on the costs.

Ozawa et al. [7] found 42 articles, of which 17 focused on increasing immunization coverage in LMICs. The study estimated that the intervention cost per 1% increase in coverage (the authors estimated the increase in immunization coverage that occurred after the intervention was introduced and then calculated the cost of increasing coverage by 1%) was USD 0.06 in low-income countries and that the cost increases with baseline immunization coverage level, reflecting the higher cost of reaching under-vaccinated children. This study differs from the other two reviews, since the authors estimated the intervention cost per dose per percent coverage change compared to baseline coverage. It should be noted, however, that the estimates in this cost function combine intervention costs per dose from diverse interventions and these may not be comparable. Six of the articles included in Ozawa [7] meet our study criteria for the current synthesis.

3.2. Search on PubMed

Most of the articles for this study had already been identified in the three previous systematic reviews or did not meet our study inclusion criteria. We found one additional article that was not identified in the three reviews—a study by Chatterjee et al. [6] that focused on estimating the costs of increasing coverage through the Intensified Mission Indradhanush (IMI) Program in India.

3.3. Gray Literature

We identified three articles that examined economic issues related to ZD children [9–11]. Two of the papers focused on the economic benefits of immunization for ZD children and the third paper focused on the insufficiency of funding to reach ZD children. These papers did not focus on the costs of vaccination interventions and therefore, all three were excluded from the review. Figure 1 presents a PRISMA flow diagram of our search strategy.

3.4. Articles on Increasing Coverage of Childhood Vaccination in LMICs

Eleven (note that one additional study [12] utilized Chatterjee's estimates to estimate cost per ZD child reached through the IMI program in India) peer-reviewed articles met our criteria for inclusion: studies that estimated the cost of interventions to increase childhood vaccination coverage from an LMIC. We categorized each article that met the criteria according to the following: descriptions of their costing methods, tables or figures showing the costs by component, the type of costs calculated, and whether uncertainty analysis was conducted. Table 2 provides detailed information about the reviewed studies, including the study methods.

The interventions in the included studies differ in their approaches to increasing childhood vaccination. Three of the studies focus on the education of mothers/caregivers on the benefits of immunization [13–15]; three studies focus on reminding caregivers to take their children for vaccination [16–18]; three papers examine interventions that identify vaccination defaulters and conduct follow-up vaccination [6,19,20]; one article focuses on immunization camps in rural areas [21]; and one article focuses on cash transfers that require children to attend preventative health visits [22].

The costs of the interventions range from USD 0.08 per additional dose for a cellular phone contact to encourage return visits in Kenya [18] to USD 84 for an intervention of immunization camp and incentive intervention in rural villages in India [21]. The median intervention cost per additional dose is USD 3.72 (see Table 2).

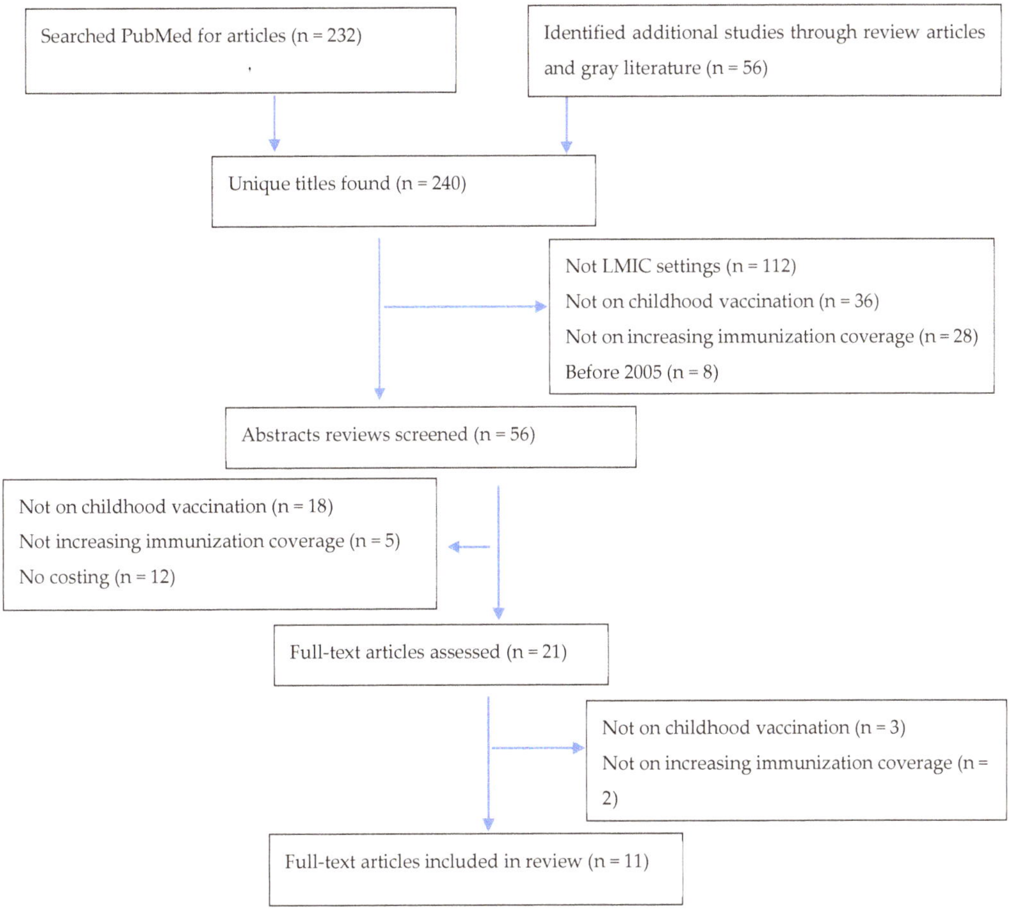

Figure 1. PRISMA flow diagram.

Table 2. List of articles that estimate costs of increasing childhood vaccination coverage in LMICs after 2005.

Author and Journal	Country	Article Name	Description	Outcome of Interest	Intervention Cost (Cost per Dose/Child) (2017 USD)	Intervention Cost per ZD Child Reached	Costing Methods
Andersson [14] *BMC Int Health and Human Rights*	Pakistan	Evidence-based discussion increases childhood vaccination uptake: a randomized cluster-controlled trial of knowledge translation in Pakistan	Costing of structured group discussion education intervention on vaccination benefits with adults in rural communities with low vaccination uptake	DTP3 and measles vaccination status	Estimated government intervention cost was USD 90,000 total (USD 12.63 per dose)	NA	Cost components not described. Notes that the cost of provincial and national coordinators working on the project were excluded.

Table 2. *Cont.*

Author and Journal	Country	Article Name	Description	Outcome of Interest	Intervention Cost (Cost per Dose/Child) (2017 USD)	Intervention Cost per ZD Child Reached	Costing Methods
Banerjee [21] *BMJ*	India	Improving immunization coverage in rural India: clustered randomized controlled evaluation of immunization campaigns with and without incentives	Costing of an immunization camp and incentives intervention in rural villages	Proportion of children aged 1–3 that were partially or fully immunized	USD 41,109 vs. USD 27,420 (USD 84 per child vs. USD 42 per child in 2017 USD)	NA	Methods described and cost components Includes worker salaries, travel, village worker honorarium, training, refrigerators, monitoring, and incentives.
Bangure *BMC Public Health* [16]	Zimbabwe	Effectiveness of short message services reminders on a childhood immunization program in Kadoma, Zimbabwe—a randomized controlled trial	Effectiveness of a short message services (SMS) reminder on a childhood immunization program in Kadoma, Zimbabwe	Pentavalent Immunization coverage at 6, 10, and 14 weeks	NA (USD 0.0.25)	NA	Costs include messages to study participants (USD 57.46) and capturing of data cost (USD 0.33 per message for human resources).
Barham [22] SSRN Electron J.	Mexico and Nicaragua	Beyond 80%: Are there new ways of increasing vaccination coverage?	Cash transfers conditional on children attending preventative health visits and mothers attending health education talks	DTP3 coverage	Mexico: USD 2.3 billion total (USD 44 per child 2017 USD) Nicaragua: USD 5,000,000 (USD 67 per child 2017 USD)	NA	Costs include program and transfer costs.
Chatterjee et al. [6] *Health Policy and Planning*	India	The incremental cost of improving immunization coverage in India through the Intensified Mission Indradhanush Program	Identified missed children and vaccinated them in temporary outreach sites for one week over a consecutive 4-month period	Full immunization coverage	No cost for program as a whole (USD 3.20 per dose) in Uttar Pradesh and highest in Maharashtra (USD 11.35 per dose)	USD 82.88 *	Costs estimated economic and financial incremental costs; Data collected at district and sub-district levels.
Haji [17] *BMC Public Health*	Kenya	Reducing routine vaccination dropout rates: evaluating two interventions in three Kenyan districts	Costing of text message reminder intervention in three districts	Pentavalent3 vaccination	USD 136 (USD 0.33 per child)	NA	Costs include 1488 messages sent to the participants in the SMS, and premium cost of scheduling messages from web for six months (USD 66.70).

Table 2. *Cont.*

Author and Journal	Country	Article Name	Description	Outcome of Interest	Intervention Cost (Cost per Dose/Child) (2017 USD)	Intervention Cost per ZD Child Reached	Costing Methods
Hayford [19] *Vaccine*	Bangladesh	Cost and sustainability of a successful package of interventions to improve vaccination coverage for children in urban slums of Bangladesh	Extended hours at satellite clinics; training; clinic screening tool; volunteer community group	DTP3, full immunization coverage	NA (USD 2.84 per dose; USD 22.15 per fully immunized child	NA	Used document review and stakeholder interviews to collect data. Estimated both financial and opportunity costs of the intervention, including un-compensated time, training and supervision costs.
Mokaya [18] *Pan African Medical Journal*	Kenya	Use of cellular phone contacts to increase return rates for immunization services in Kenya	Costing of a cellphone contact intervention to track defaulters	Pentavalent2, Pentavalent3 status	Aver. cost tracking w/phone (USD 0.07 per child)	NA	Used the monthly post-bills to confirm the cost of the calls and multiplied by the frequency.
Owais [13] *BMC Public Health*	Pakistan	Does improving maternal knowledge of vaccines impact childhood immunization rates?	Three targeted pictorial messages regarding vaccines	DTP3 completion	NA (USD 1.15 per child)	NA	Cost of laminated colored pictorial cards used by CHWs as well as pamphlets; Estimate that cost of national scale-up will be USD 200,000–USD 100,000 for cards and pamphlets and USD 100,000 for training sessions.
Powell-Jackson [15] *PLoS Med*	India	Effect and cost-effectiveness of educating mothers childhood DPT vaccination on immunization uptake, knowledge and perceptions in Uttar Pradesh: A randomized controlled trial	Intervention on educating mothers about childhood DTP vaccination	Proportion of children that received DTP3 vaccination	USD 11,137 (USD 24 per child)	NA	Costs collected through accounting systems and categorized as startup/ implementation; estimated cost of scale-up assuming no change to average cost but double the children reached.

Table 2. *Cont.*

Author and Journal	Country	Article Name	Description	Outcome of Interest	Intervention Cost (Cost per Dose/Child) (2017 USD)	Intervention Cost per ZD Child Reached	Costing Methods
Rainey [20]	India	Providing monovalent oral polio vaccine type 1 to newborns	Identifying and vaccinating newborns with OPV within 72 h of birth	OPV1 vaccination	NA (USD 3.72 per dose)	NA	Cost of motorbikes, per diem, travel allowance, incentives, and delivery kits for traditional birth attendants. Does not include table listing cost components/drivers.

* Estimated in [12]. Figure 2 illustrates the median intervention cost per dose per person for each type of intervention. For the three types of interventions—reminders to caregivers, identification and vaccination of defaulters and maternal education on the benefits of vacation—the median cost was under USD 15 per person per dose. In contrast, immunization camps and cash transfers interventions showed higher median costs, ranging from USD 40–55 per person, making them at least 400% more expensive than the other interventions. It is important to note that these latter interventions provide additional preventative health services beyond immunization, which makes direct comparisons with the first three types of interventions challenging.

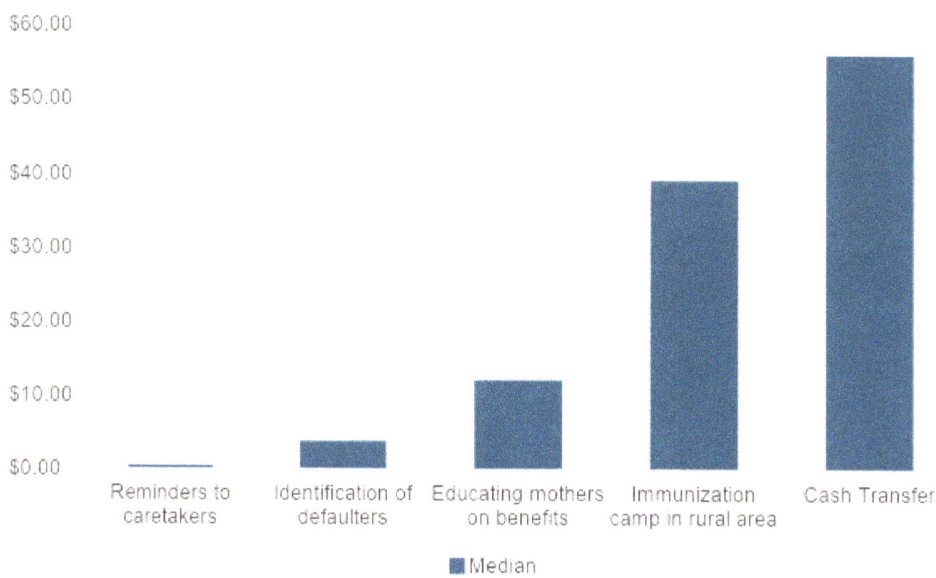

Figure 2. Median intervention cost per dose/person for increasing immunization coverage (2017 USD).

3.5. Description of Costing Methods

Only three of the papers provided detailed descriptions of their costing methods [6,19,21]. Other papers mentioned that they calculated costs but did not go into detail about the cost components and methods of analysis.

Table 3 shows the methods used in these papers. All three papers described their methods and included tables and figures with cost components and percentages of total costs. Two of the three conducted uncertainty analyses to account for uncertainty in the cost values with the use of sensitivity analyses or confidence intervals.

Table 3. Costing methods used in three studies with detailed description.

	Describes Costing Methods	Displays Cost Components with Percentiles	Calculates Economic Costs	Defines Other Types of Costs Used (Recurrent, Fixed)	Uses Uncertainty Analysis
Banerjee [21]	In-study appendix	Yes	No	Fixed, average, and marginal costs	Sensitivity analysis
Chatterjee [6]	Yes	Yes	Yes	Incremental costs	Calculation of confidence intervals
Hayford [19]	Combination of activity-based costing and 'ingredients' approach	Yes	Yes	Recurrent costs	Not available

4. Discussion

This review highlights the scarcity of studies that estimate the costs of interventions aimed at increasing childhood vaccination or reaching ZD in LMICs, as most studies evaluating vaccination interventions in these contexts do not provide detailed cost estimates. The eleven studies included in this review assessed different types of interventions and estimated the cost of increasing childhood vaccination but did not specifically address the cost of reaching ZD children. Median costs varied widely across interventions, from USD 0.30 per person for SMS reminders to caregivers to USD 56 per person for cash transfer programs.

Three studies examined interventions that cost less than USD 15 per person, suggesting that some strategies may be affordable for governments. However, it should be noted that costs and affordability are context-specific and sometimes depend on the baseline coverage levels. For example, the cost of a universal cash transfer program aimed at increasing coverage (in an area that is already close to 100%) cannot be compared to the cost of targeted demand incentive approaches in communities with existing low baseline levels. In addition, the costs may differ substantially depending on the costing methods used.

Geographically, seven of the included studies were from South Asia (India, Pakistan and Bangladesh); three were from African countries; and the remaining study was from Latin America.

Only three papers provided detailed descriptions of their cost estimation methods, including the types of costs estimated (e.g., recurrent and capital costs, or financial and economic costs). Two of the three papers included some analysis of uncertainty in their cost estimates.

Relatively few studies on the cost of reaching ZD children or increasing childhood immunization coverage in LMICs are available. Most studies have focused more on reaching higher DTP3 coverage rather than the reduction in the percentage of ZD children. The paucity of studies may partially stem from the complexity of costing programmatic interventions that target ZD children, as calculating the cost of increasing coverage is often challenging. Defining pre-intervention costs and allocating costs within multi-intervention projects is difficult, especially when some activities may pre-date the project itself. Relatively few of the studies that do exist describe the cost estimation methods used, which complicates efforts to assess the adequacy of their analyses and comparability to other studies.

Limitations

Comparing studies that estimate the cost of increasing vaccination coverage is difficult due to differences in measured outcomes (e.g., cost per child/person exposed vs. cost per dose vs. cost per intervention). Additionally, variations in intervention design make direct comparisons difficult, as each program may use distinct approaches and target populations. Local and regional differences in costs for different categories (e.g., labor and commodities) can also affect the ability to make comparisons among studies.

5. Conclusions

In conclusion, the current literature on the costs of reaching ZD children in LMICs is insufficient to develop a solid evidence base for decision-making. Our review shows that per-dose costs vary widely by intervention type, with cash transfer programs being among the most expensive. However, most studies that have estimated the costs of increasing coverage have not adequately described their methods. Only three studies described the methods that they used to estimate costs. Thus, it is difficult to compare the costs among studies. More information on the intervention costs is needed to provide important insight for understanding the resources incurred for the purposes of improving implementation, planning, and as a component for cost-effectiveness studies.

Ideally, cost studies should be incentivized by global funding agencies whenever an immunization equity approach is implemented. Future studies should prioritize clear and standardized descriptions of costing methods for ZD interventions through referring to guidance documents on immunization costing [2,23,24]. It is also important to prioritize the generation of costing evidence from subnational areas to generate reliable costing data for different zero-dose contexts. Additionally, the national and subnational settings should be described in all costing studies to improve comparability across studies and contexts. Where possible, costing analyses should estimate the additional costs associated with identifying, planning and reaching ZD and under-vaccinated children through tailored delivery strategies. Establishing principles for cost estimation and standardized cost components would strengthen the comparability of ZD intervention studies, allowing for findings to be synthesized across populations and countries. Costing studies aligned with these principles would offer a more comparable evidence base to inform resource allocation and policy decisions aimed at achieving universal immunization coverage in LMICs.

Author Contributions: Conceptualization, A.L., N.V., T.F., H.W.R. and G.C.; methodology, A.L., T.F. and N.V.; writing—original draft preparation, A.L.; writing—review and editing, N.V., T.F., H.W.R., G.C. and T.M. All authors have read and agreed to the published version of the manuscript.

Funding: This research was funded by the Gavi Alliance grant number MEL 11578 6 22. The APC was funded by the Gavi Alliance.

Institutional Review Board Statement: Not applicable.

Informed Consent Statement: Not applicable.

Data Availability Statement: Not applicable.

Conflicts of Interest: Author Ann Levin was employed by the company Levin & Morgan, LLC. Author Teemar Fisseha and Nancy Vollmer were employed by the company JSI Research & Training Institute, Inc. Author Heidi Reynolds, Gustavo Corrêa and Tewodaj Mengistu were employed by the company Gavi, The Vaccine Alliance. The authors declare that the research was conducted in the absence of any commercial or financial relationships that could be construed as a potential conflict of interest.

Acronyms

DALY	Disability-adjusted life years.
DTP	Diphtheria–tetanus–pertussis-containing vaccine.
ICERs	Incremental cost-effectiveness ratios.
IEC	Information, education, and communication.
IVAC	International Vaccine Access Center.
IMI	Intensified Mission Indradhanush.
LMICs	Low- and middle-income countries.
RI	Routine immunization.
WHO	World Health Organization.
ZD	Zero dose.
ZDLH	Zero-Dose Learning Hub.

References

1. Levin, A.; Yeung, K.H.T.; Hutubessy, R. Systematic review of cost projections of new vaccine introduction. *Vaccine* **2024**, *42*, 1042–1050. [CrossRef]
2. Brenzel, L.; Young, D.; Walker, D.G. Costs and financing of routine immunization: Approach and selected findings of a multi-country study (EPIC). *Vaccine* **2015**, *33* (Suppl. 1), A13–A20. [CrossRef] [PubMed]
3. Kamara, L.; Milstein, J.; Patyna, M.; Lydon, P.; Levin, A.; Brenzel, L. Strategies for financial sustainability of immunization programs. A review of the strategies from 50 national immunization program financial sustainability plans. *Vaccine* **2008**, *26*, 6717–6726. [CrossRef] [PubMed]
4. Levin, A.; Burgess, C.; Shendale, S.; Morgan, W.; Hutubessy, R.; Measles-Rubella Eradication Modelling Group; Jit, M. Cost-effectiveness of Measles and Rubella Elimination in Low- and Middle-income Countries. *BMJ Glob. Health* **2023**, *8*, e011425. [CrossRef] [PubMed]
5. Munk, C.; Munk, C.; Portnoy, A.; Portnoy, A.; Suharlim, C.; Suharlim, C.; Clarke-Deelder, E.; Clarke-Deelder, E.; Brenzel, L.; Brenzel, L.; et al. Systematic review of the costs and effectiveness of interventions to increase infant vaccination coverage in low- and middle-income countries. *BMC Health Serv. Res.* **2019**, *19*, 741. [CrossRef] [PubMed]
6. Chatterjee, S.; Das, P.; Pinheiro, A.; Haldar, P.; Ray, A.; Brenzel, L.; Resch, S. The incremental cost of improving immunization coverage in India through the Intensified Mission Indradhanush programme. *Health Policy Plan.* **2021**, *36*, 1316–1324. [CrossRef]
7. Ozawa, S.; Yemeke, T.T.; Thompson, K.M. Systematic review of the incremental costs of interventions that increase immunization coverage. *Vaccine* **2018**, *36*, 3641–3649. [CrossRef]
8. Yemeke, T.T.; Mitgang, E.; Wedlock, P.T.; Higgins, C.; Chen, H.H.; Pallas, S.W.; Abimbola, T.; Wallace, A.; Bartsch, S.M.; Lee, B.Y.; et al. Promoting, seeking, and reaching vaccination services: A systematic review of costs to immunization programs, beneficiaries, and caregivers. *Vaccine* **2021**, *39*, 4437–4449. [CrossRef] [PubMed]
9. International Vaccine Access Center. The Economics and Value of Immunizing Zero-Dose Children: An Advocacy Brief. Baltimore, MD. 2023. Available online: https://publichealth.jhu.edu/ivac/resources/zero-dose-knowledge-summaries-and-advocacy-briefs#economics (accessed on 23 April 2024).
10. Willens, V.; Applegate, J.; Chou, V.B. Summary of Key Evidence related to Economic Benefits of Immunization for Zero-Dose Children. International Vaccine Access Center (IVAC). 2023. Available online: https://publichealth.jhu.edu/sites/default/files/2024-02/61-zd-and-economic-benefitsknowledge-summaryax.pdf (accessed on 9 October 2024).
11. MOMENTUM Routine Immunization Transformation and Equity. Addressing Insufficient Operational Funding to Reach Zero-Dose Children and Missed Communities. What Works Series: Rapid Evidence and Insights to Overcome Entrenched Obstacles to Immunization Coverage & Equity. 2022. Available online: https://usaidmomentum.org/resource/addressing-insufficient-operational-funding-to-reach-zero-dose-children-and-missed-communities/ (accessed on 23 April 2024).
12. Clarke-Deelder, E.; Suharlim, C.; Chatterjee, S.; Portnoy, A.; Brenzel, L.; Ray, A.; Cohen, J.L.; Menzies, N.A.; Resch, S.C. Health impact and cost-effectiveness of expanding routine immunization coverage in India through Intensified Mission Indradhanush. *Health Policy Plan* **2024**, *39*, 583–592. [CrossRef] [PubMed]
13. Owais, A.; Hanif, B.; Siddiqui, A.R.; Agha, A.; Zaidi, A.K. Does improving maternal knowledge of vaccines impact infant immunization rates? A community-based randomized-controlled trial in Karachi, Pakistan. *BMC Public Health* **2011**, *11*, 239. [CrossRef]
14. Andersson, N.; Cockcroft, A.; Ansari, N.M.; Omer, K.; Baloch, M.; Foster, A.H.; Shea, B.; Wells, G.A.; Soberanis, J.L. Evidence-based discussion increases childhood vaccination uptake: A randomised cluster-controlled trial of knowledge translation in Pakistan. *BMC Int. Health Hum. Rights* **2009**, *9* (Suppl. 1), S8. [CrossRef] [PubMed]
15. Powell-Jackson, T.; Fabbri, C.; Dutt, V.; Tougher, S.; Singh, K. Effect and cost-effectiveness of educating mothers about childhood DPT vaccination on immunisation uptake, knowledge and perceptions in Uttar Pradesh, India: A randomised controlled trial. *PLoS Med.* **2018**, *15*, e1002519. [CrossRef] [PubMed]

16. Bangure, D.; Chirundu, D.; Gombe, N.; Marufu, T.; Mandozana, G.; Tshimanga, M.; Takundwa, L. Effectiveness of short message services reminder on childhood immunization programme in Kadoma, Zimbabwe—A randomized controlled trial. *BMC Public Health* **2015**, *15*, 137. [CrossRef]
17. Haji, A.; Lowther, S.; Ngan'ga, Z.; Gura, Z.; Tabu, C.; Sandhu, H.; Arvelo, W. Reducing routine vaccination dropout rates: Evaluating two interventions in three Kenyan districts. *BMC Public Health* **2016**, *16*, 152. [CrossRef] [PubMed]
18. Mokaya, E.; Mugoya, I.; Raburu, J.; Shimp, L. Use of cellular phone contacts to increase return rates for immunization services in Kenya. *Pan Afr. Med. J.* **2017**, *28*, 24. [CrossRef] [PubMed]
19. Hayford, K.; Uddin, M.J.; Koehlmoos, T.P.; Bishai, D.M. Cost and sustainability of a successful package of interventions to improve vaccination coverage for children in urban slums of Bangladesh. *Vaccine* **2014**, *32*, 2294–2299. [CrossRef] [PubMed]
20. Rainey, J.J.; Bhatnagar, P.; Estivariz, C.F.; Durrani, S.; Galway, M.; Sandhu, H.; Bahl, S.; Jafari, H.; Wenger, J. Providing monovalent oral polio vaccine type 1 to newborns: Findings from a pilot birth-dose project in Moradabad district, India. *Bull. World Health Organ.* **2009**, *87*, 955–959. [CrossRef]
21. Banerjee, A.V.; Duflo, E.; Glennerster, R.; Kothari, D. Improving immunisation coverage in rural India: Clustered randomised controlled evaluation of immunisation campaigns with and without incentives. *BMJ* **2010**, *340*, c2220. [CrossRef] [PubMed]
22. Barham, T.; Brenzel, L.; Maluccio, J. Beyond 80%: Are there new ways of increasing vaccination coverage? In *Evaluation of CCT Programs in Mexico and Nicaragua*; HNP Paper; World Bank: Washington, DC, USA, 2007.
23. Levin, A.; Boonstopped, L.; Brenzel, L.; Griffiths, U.; Hutubessy, R.; Jit, M.; Mogasale, V.; Pallas, S.; Resch, S.; Suharlim, C.; et al. WHO-led consensus statement on vaccine delivery costing: Process, methods, and findings. *BMC Med.* **2022**, *20*, 88. [CrossRef] [PubMed]
24. Resch, S.; Menzies, N.; Portnoy, A.; Clarke-Deelder, E.; O'Keefe, L.; Suharlim, C.; Brenzel, L. *How to Cost Immunization Programs: A Practical Guide on Primary Data Collection and Analysis*; Immunizationeconomics.org./Harvard T.H. Chan School of Public Health: Cambridge, MA, USA, 2020.

vaccines

MDPI

Review

Dengue Vaccine Development and Deployment into Routine Immunization

Annelies Wilder-Smith *, Thomas Cherian and Joachim Hombach

World Health Organization, CH-1211 Geneva, Switzerland; cherriant@mmglobalhealth.org (T.C.); hombachj@who.int (J.H.)
* Correspondence: wildersmitha@who.int

Abstract: Dengue has emerged as a significant global health threat. Despite decades of research, only two dengue vaccines—CYD-TDV (Dengvaxia) and TAK-003 (Qdenga)—have been licensed to date, with limited implementation. This paper explores and outlines strategies for integrating dengue vaccines into routine immunization programs, particularly in high-burden regions. TAK-003, a tetravalent live-attenuated vaccine, has demonstrated 61% efficacy against virologically confirmed dengue and 84% efficacy against hospitalizations in endemic settings. However, concerns remain about vaccine-enhanced disease, particularly among seronegative individuals exposed to DENV3 and DENV4. WHO recommends targeted introduction in high-transmission settings without pre-vaccination screening, while ongoing post-introduction studies will further clarify long-term safety and efficacy. Effective vaccine rollout requires a multi-pronged approach, including school-based immunization, integration with adolescent health services, and strong community engagement. Decision-making for vaccine introduction should be guided by National Immunization Technical Advisory Groups (NITAGs), local epidemiological data, and cost-effectiveness assessments. While future vaccines, including mRNA and virus-like particle candidates, are under development, optimizing the use of currently available vaccines is crucial to reducing dengue's public health impact. Given the continued rise in cases, immediate action—combining vaccination with vector control—is essential to prevent further morbidity and mortality.

Keywords: dengue; Qdenga; CYD-TDV; TAK-003; Wolbachia; antibody-dependent enhancement; mRNA vaccines; school-based programs

1. Introduction

Dengue has emerged as one of the leading global health threats, with a significant rise in incidence and geographic spread. Despite decades of research, as of early 2025, only two dengue vaccines have been licensed, neither of which has been widely implemented. This paper examines the key challenges in dengue vaccine development and deployment, including scientific, regulatory, logistical, and policy barriers. It also explores strategies to integrate dengue vaccines into the Essential Programme on Immunization (EPI), ensuring broader access and long-term disease control.

Dengue is caused by any of the four dengue virus (DENV) serotypes, belonging to the family of Flaviviridae, and is primarily transmitted by *Aedes aegypti* and *Aedes albopictus* mosquitoes, which are endemic to most tropical and subtropical regions [1]. The co-circulation of different DENV serotypes varies by region, with some areas experiencing simultaneous outbreaks of multiple serotypes [2,3]. However, one serotype usually dominates at any given time.

https://doi.org/10.3390/vaccines13050483

The clinical spectrum of dengue ranges from asymptomatic, mild, or subclinical illness to more severe and potentially life-threatening forms of the disease. In hyperendemic areas, symptomatic dengue is primarily a disease of younger children. In moderately endemic countries, it affects the full range of children and younger adults. Additionally, in regions with low-to-moderate endemicity, clinical disease is typically also seen among older persons, as reported in ref. [4], with the frequency and types of complications observed reflecting underlying co-morbidities in this group [5]. Diabetes, hypertension, cardiovascular conditions, and sickle cell disease increase the risk of severe dengue. Pregnant women with dengue also face higher risks of adverse outcomes [6].

With proper clinical management, case fatality rates can be reduced to well below 0.1%. However, the absence of reliable prognostic markers for severe dengue progression often leads to the need for hospitalization and close monitoring of many patients [7]. During outbreaks, this places immense pressure on already fragile healthcare systems, resulting in increased case fatality rates.

2. Why Is There a Need for a Dengue Vaccine?

Dengue has experienced an increase in the incidence of cases and number of outbreaks, as well as geographic expansion, and is poised to increase further [8,9]. Approximately 4 billion people are living in regions where *Aedes* mosquitoes are endemic resulting in an estimated 400 million dengue infections annually [10]. The main drivers for the proliferation of *Aedes* mosquitoes and increasing dengue incidence are population growth, rural-to-urban migration, high population densities, unplanned urbanization with substandard water and waste management, global warming, and disorganized and inadequately funded mosquito control programs [8]. Outbreaks are increasing in frequency and magnitude. Regions such as Asia and the Americas are most affected, though recent outbreaks in Africa suggest a larger burden in that continent than previously estimated [11]. Dengue incidence is poised to increase further, both in frequency as well as geographic range. Dengue is also increasingly reported in countries not classically endemic for dengue [12–17].

Dengue control has traditionally focused on mosquito control, but scaling up these efforts remains both complex and costly [18]. The continued rise in dengue cases suggests that existing strategies have largely fallen short, and while innovative approaches like *Wolbachia* show promise [19], they require time for full implementation and will not be enough to achieve complete dengue control on their own [20]. To effectively reduce the disease burden, dengue vaccines should be integrated into routine immunization through the Essential Programme on Immunization (EPI) alongside vector control measures.

3. What Is the Current Status of Dengue Vaccine Development?

Dengue vaccine development has been ongoing for over 50 years, but numerous challenges have made bringing a vaccine to market difficult. One major obstacle has been the lack of an appropriate animal model, along with a limited understanding of the immune correlates needed for both protection and disease enhancement. Controlled human infection models (CHIMs) have been developed; however, they may not provide sufficient answers given that the infecting virus has to be attenuated and, therefore, does not totally mimic real infection. Furthermore, according to the antibody-dependent enhancement hypothesis (ADE), a safety signal would only be seen after an extended period [21]. However, the most significant challenge lies in the complex immunological interactions between the four antigenically distinct dengue serotypes [22,23]. These interactions often lead to imbalanced vaccine performance, which could, in some cases, increase the risk of ADE.

Over the years, various vaccine platforms have been explored, including live-attenuated chimeric recombinant viruses, live-attenuated viruses, inactivated viruses, recombinant proteins, and mRNA-based vaccines. Despite this broad range of approaches, only live-attenuated vaccines have completed Phase 3 trials. Ideally, a tetravalent live-attenuated vaccine would generate strong, independent immune responses to all four serotypes. However, achieving this balance has proven to be a significant challenge.

There are currently two licensed dengue vaccines: CYD-TDV (Dengvaxia, Sanofi) and TAK-003 (Qdenga, Takeda). Both are tetravalent live-attenuated vaccines but differ in the extent of chimerization and the genome backbone. Another tetravalent live-attenuated dengue vaccine (TV003/005) developed at the Laboratory of Infectious Diseases, at the National Institutes of Allergy and Infectious Diseases (NIAID) in the United States, has completed Phase 3 trials in Brazil, but the final data have yet to be released. All three live-attenuated vaccines use chimerization, and these vaccines differ by the extent of chimerization and the backbone used, as well as in efficacy by serotype and safety.

CYD-TDV, a tetravalent live attenuated with a yellow fever 17D backbone, developed by Sanofi Pasteur, known under the trade name of Dengvaxia®, was the first dengue vaccine to be licensed. Phase 3 trials revealed a vaccine efficacy that varied by age, serostatus, and serotype [24]. Although this vaccine has a clear overall population-level benefit, in baseline seronegative persons, this vaccine increases the risk of severe dengue over time when exposed [25,26]. For Dengvaxia®, the World Health Organization (WHO) therefore recommends a pre-vaccination screening strategy, whereby only dengue-seropositive persons are vaccinated [27]. Because of the cost and programmatic hurdles for pre-screening before vaccination, the use of Dengvaxia® in national immunization programs has been very limited. For commercial reasons, the company has therefore decided not to further manufacture this vaccine, and it will be discontinued.

The advantages of TAK-003 and TV003/005 over CYD-TDV are the inclusion of non-structural proteins of the dengue backbone and reduced numbers of doses needed.

TAK-003 was developed by Takeda and is known under the trade name of Qdenga® [28,29]. TAK-003 consists of an attenuated DENV-2 (DEN2-PDK-53) backbone, whereby three chimeric viruses containing the prM and envelope proteins of DENV-1, -3, and -4 are inserted into the DEN2-PDK-53 backbone. The advantage of TAK-003 to CYD-TDV, therefore, is the presence of more non-structural proteins due to the DENV2 backbone. TAK-003 induces high levels of DENV2-neutralizing antibodies against DENV2, but lower levels of DENV1-, DENV3-, and DENV4-neutralizing antibodies [30]. Various studies and Phase 1–3 trials have been published on TAK-003 (Qdenga) [28,31–47]. Of note, no important safety risks were identified, and TAK-003 was well tolerated irrespective of age, gender, or baseline dengue serostatus in recipients aged 4–60 years [48].

In the pivotal trials conducted in dengue endemic countries, the vaccine efficacy (VE) of TAK-003 over 5 years against virologically confirmed dengue (VCD) was 61% (95% CI 56.0, 65.8), and against dengue-related hospitalizations the vaccine efficacy was 84% (77.8–88.6) [28,37]. TAK-003 demonstrated efficacy against all four serotypes among baseline seropositive subjects and against DENV1 and DENV2 in baseline seronegative subjects. There was no efficacy in baseline seronegative subjects against DENV3 and 4.

Modeling indicates that the population-level benefit of this vaccine will be substantial, with the public health impact highest in settings with high seroprevalence (e.g., high proportion of seropositive persons indicating high burden of disease) and in settings where serotype 2 is circulating [49].

The large pivotal Phase 3 trial involving about 20,000 children was not sufficiently powered to definitively rule out a risk of vaccine-enhanced disease in seronegative persons exposed to DENV3 and DENV4 as the number of cases due to DENV3 and DENV4 was relatively small during the trial period. There were higher rates of symptomatic as well as hospitalized DENV3 cases amongst seronegative vaccinated persons than among seronegative unvaccinated persons, but this excess was small and not statistically significant. WHO acknowledges that vaccine-enhanced disease in a subpopulation of seronegative persons exposed to DENV3 and possibly DENV4 is biologically plausible and cannot be excluded from the results of the Phase 3 trial.

Modeling suggests that at a population level, after 10 years of vaccination, seronegative persons will have a net benefit, even in relation to DENV3 and DENV4 [29]. However, statistical uncertainty remains. What is clear is that TAK-003 will have the greatest public health impact and be the most cost-effective in settings with high dengue transmission intensity.

The available trial data indicate that the benefits of this vaccine significantly outweigh the risks. Like many other vaccines, this vaccine is only partially protective. Breakthrough infections can occur in vaccinated persons, in both seropositive and seronegative persons at the time of vaccination, and such breakthrough infections can be associated with mild to severe disease. On an individual basis, breakthrough disease cannot be distinguished from potential cases of enhanced disease. The risk of enhanced disease can only be determined in population-based studies with a long observation time. These data may not become available for at least five years, pending post-introduction studies.

4. How to Use TAK-003 (Qdenga) in Endemic Populations?

The WHO recommends that countries consider introducing the TAK-003 dengue vaccine into routine immunization programs in areas where dengue poses a significant public health burden due to high transmission intensity. Since dengue transmission varies geographically, some countries may opt for a targeted rollout in specific subnational regions with higher transmission rates rather than a nationwide approach.

Seroprevalence is the proportion of seropositive persons in a population and a measure of the force of infection. The higher the force of infection, the higher the seroprevalence at a younger age [50]. Higher seroprevalence at younger ages indicates greater dengue transmission intensity.

To determine whether a region qualifies as a high-transmission setting, countries should assess data on age-specific seroprevalence and/or age-specific dengue hospital admissions. While there is no exact seroprevalence threshold that indicates when vaccination should be introduced, the benefits of the vaccine increase with higher seroprevalence, particularly in individuals who have already been exposed to dengue. As a general guideline, a seroprevalence of more than 60% by the age of 9 years indicates high transmission, while a mean age of peak dengue-related hospitalizations well below 16 years could also serve as an indicator. A map on national and subnational levels of seroprevalence rates was published to guide countries in their decision to introduce TAK-003: https://arbomap.org/ (accessed on 10 February 2025).

In settings with high dengue transmission, pre-vaccination screening to limit vaccination to seropositive individuals is not recommended, as it would significantly reduce the public health impact and increase programmatic costs. Instead, vaccine introduction should be supported by a well-designed communication strategy and strong community engagement to ensure public trust and awareness.

In areas with low-to-moderate dengue transmission, the WHO does not recommend the programmatic use of TAK-003 until more data are available on its efficacy and risk profile in seronegative individuals, particularly for DENV3 and DENV4 [29,51].

5. What About the Reported Cases of Anaphylaxis Post-Vaccination?

Whilst during the clinical Phase 3 trials involving more than 20,000 participants in two continents no cases of anaphylaxis were observed, during vaccine roll-out, cases of anaphylaxis and hypersensitivity reactions were reported. In the initial roll out in Brazil, of 380,358 doses of Qdenga administered, 626 AEFI were reported [52]. Of these, 85 were cases of immediate hypersensitivity, with 24 (63.1 cases per million) being anaphylaxis, including three cases of anaphylactic shock. For 42% of these cases, hypersensitivity reactions began within 15 min after vaccination. In view of these hypersensitivity reactions, the Ministry of Health of Brazil published recommendations for intensifying actions for safe vaccination, including healthcare professional training and post-vaccination observation [52].

The WHO's Global Advisory Committee for Vaccine Safety (GACVS) published in November 2024 that in the vaccine roll-out in Brazil and beyond with more than 2 million doses, between 1 March 2023 and 12 September 2024, 501 hypersensitivity reactions (147.1 per million doses) were reported after vaccination with Qdenga® [53]. Of these, 447 occurred after the first dose (183.1 per million doses), and 24 occurred after the second dose (31.0 per million doses). Of all the reactions, 124 were classified as anaphylaxis (36.4 per million doses), with 117 after the first dose (44.5 per million doses) and 7 after the second dose (9.0 per million doses). In Brazil, immunization outreach activities are being replaced by in-facility vaccination [53]. GACVS states that for children with mild-to-moderate reactions, a supervised second dose can be given [53]. A second dose is contraindicated for those with confirmed anaphylaxis. A research project is under way to investigate risk factors, including possible allergic components of the vaccine and the mechanisms of the reactions [53].

No deaths related to anaphylaxis have been reported to date.

6. What Are the Programmatic Considerations for Including TAK-003 (Qdenga) in Routine Immunization?

To effectively roll out TAK-003, identifying high transmission areas is essential. Conducting seroprevalence studies can guide targeted vaccination strategies, ensuring those at highest risk are prioritized while reducing the risk of adverse events in dengue-naïve individuals. Documenting peak incidence of hospitalization is a further aid.

Education and awareness campaigns are vital to improve vaccine acceptance and build public trust. Transparent communication about the benefits and potential risks—especially the possibility of increased disease severity in certain epidemiological contexts—is critical for informed decision-making.

The vaccine is recommended for school-aged children and adolescents (ages 6–16, per WHO guidance). This requires strong platforms for school- and adolescent-based immunization. Co-administering TAK-003 with other routine vaccines, such as HPV and tetanus-diphtheria, can increase coverage and lower operational costs. Vaccination can be organized by school grade, class, or age to ensure broad access and integration into existing school health services. Schools with dedicated health personnel can more easily incorporate vaccination into routine programming. Facilities must also be equipped to manage anaphylaxis, with extended post-vaccination observation periods to ensure rapid response. For school-based programs, portable emergency kits should be at hand, as well as an effective referral system to higher level care, should it be needed.

To achieve high uptake, it is essential to foster public confidence, supportive social norms, and deliver high-quality services. Introduction strategies should be tailored to local contexts, accounting for epidemiological trends, demographic factors, and available resources. This includes prioritizing areas with high transmission, assessing age-specific seroprevalence, and focusing on regions with high dengue-related hospitalization rates.

Community engagement, risk communication, and context-specific messaging should precede rollout. Studies on behavioral and social drivers of vaccine uptake can help design more effective interventions. Efforts should also reinforce vector control and environmental management to support broader dengue prevention.

For out-of-school children and adolescents—such as those who are homeschooled, older than school age, or in areas without school-based programs—non-school-based strategies are essential. These include outreach campaigns, community clinics, and integration with other adolescent health services like counseling and screenings. Utilizing accessible locations and community networks helps overcome logistical barriers and expand coverage.

Outreach and national vaccination campaigns are particularly important in underserved areas. Mobile health teams can deliver vaccines directly to communities. Strategies like holding two national immunization days three months apart, followed by annual boosters, can quickly increase uptake.

Vaccination through clinics and healthcare facilities provides a safe, monitored environment. Hosting dedicated vaccination days, paired with incentives like shorter wait times and educational sessions, can boost participation. Schools can also host on-site vaccination events, making the process more accessible and less intimidating.

To maximize coverage—especially in rural and underserved areas—a mix of school-based, clinic-based, and outreach approaches is often necessary.

Effective implementation depends on coordinated involvement from all stakeholders. **In brief, government officials** need data-driven evidence to justify national adoption. **Health and education authorities** must align vaccine rollout with broader public health goals. **Schools,** supported by trained staff and adequate resources, play a key role in implementation. **Health workers,** as frontline communicators, must be equipped to address community concerns. **Community organizations,** including professional, religious, and cultural groups, can help tailor messaging to diverse audiences. **Politicians and the media** shape public perception and must be informed advocates for the vaccine.

Tailored engagement with each stakeholder group is critical for successful vaccine uptake and long-term public health impact.

7. What Are the Key Steps in Deciding Whether a Dengue Vaccine Should Be Introduced into a Routine Immunization Program?

A structured and transparent process is essential for making decisions about introducing a dengue vaccine. Governments should be guided by recommendations from the National Immunization Technical Advisory Group (NITAG), input from relevant stakeholders, and an assessment of public health needs and feasibility.

NITAG—or an equivalent advisory body—should conduct an independent, evidence-based review of the vaccine's suitability. This ensures credibility, minimizes external influence, and supports funding decisions. The process, led by the National Immunization Program (NIP), should align with national decision-making frameworks and include the evaluation of the local dengue burden and transmission intensity.

Following established steps (such as those outlined in Box 1) enables a well-coordinated, evidence-informed vaccine introduction that strengthens immunization programs and improves health outcomes.

Box 1. Key Steps in the Decision-Making Process.

- **Engage Key Stakeholders**
  - Involve representatives from **public health, government agencies, and advocacy groups**.
  - High-level advocates, such as government officials or influential figures, can help **drive discussions and secure support**.
- **Consult NITAG**
  - Seek **expert review** of the dengue vaccine's evidence and recommendations.
  - Engage **regional dengue specialists** if additional expertise is needed.
- **Establish a Technical Working Group (TWG)**
  - Form a **multi-sectoral team** of experts in immunization, infectious diseases, and public health to **provide technical guidance and coordination**.
- **Prioritize High-Transmission Regions**
  - Identify **areas with the highest dengue burden** for targeted rollout.
  - Develop a **phased introduction plan** based on subnational needs to **optimize resource allocation**.
- **Integrate into National Strategies**
  - Upon approval, incorporate the vaccine into the **National Immunization Strategy** and **Primary Health Care Strategy**.
  - Define **funding, implementation, and monitoring** frameworks.
- **Develop Vaccination Plans**
  - Create **locally tailored plans** prioritizing **school-age children and adolescents**.
  - Design **micro plans** within existing immunization structures.
- **Leverage Existing Vaccination Platforms**
  - Utilize **school-based and adolescent vaccination programs**.
  - Consider **co-administering with other vaccines** (e.g., **HPV**, **tetanus**) and integrating with **other health initiatives** (e.g., **WASH programs**) to enhance coverage.
- **Establish Governance Structures**
  - Set up **national, subnational, and district-level committees** to oversee vaccine **procurement, distribution, safety, and surveillance**.
- **Set Subnational Targets**
  - Define clear **coverage goals**, aiming for **at least 90% vaccination** in target populations.
  - Integrate with **school-based health programs** and include **catch-up vaccinations** for broader age groups.

8. What Is the Modeled Impact of TAK-003 (QDenga) in Endemic Settings?

A mathematical model developed at Imperial College (London) predicted that TAK-003 would provide high protection against virologically confirmed dengue (VCD) and dengue hospitalizations caused by DENV2 and moderate protection against VCD and hospitalization caused by DENV1 for both seropositive and seronegative children. Simulating 80% routine vaccination coverage at age 6–12 years, the model predicts positive impacts of routine vaccination with TAK-003 at the population level, with clearly larger impacts in higher transmission settings [29]. Overall, the impact is modest with an average proportion of all cases averted not exceeding 15% and 20%, respectively, for VCD and hospitalization [29,49]. Assuming moderate protection against infection gives a higher population impact than assuming no protection, especially in lower transmission settings. Furthermore, a positive average individual-level benefit of vaccination in all strata of the population can be expected, including for baseline seronegative individuals and in cases of primary breakthrough infections. However, the analysis suggests that the 95% range of possible outcomes includes a small probability of negative outcomes associated with DENV3 and DENV4 primary breakthrough infections. Pre-vaccination serological screening could largely, although not completely, remove any potential risk to seronegative individuals;

however, such screening is estimated to halve the population-level impact of vaccination, impose substantially increased programmatic costs, and hamper vaccine uptake. Clearly, with the roll-out of vaccines, empiric data need to be obtained to assess the risk of severe dengue in seronegative persons exposed to DENV3 and 4.

9. What About the Use of Qdenga in Travelers?

Travelers are at risk of dengue and contribute to the global spread of DENV [14,15,54–57]. However, the WHO recommendations focus on how best to use Qdenga in endemic populations rather than travelers [58]. No benefit–risk assessments have been conducted for the use of dengue vaccines in travelers. Nevertheless, the WHO acknowledges its benefit in seropositive travelers visiting highly dengue endemic areas, whilst the benefit in seronegative travelers is lower [50]. Most travelers are seronegative, hence the overall effectiveness of Qdenga in travelers is clearly lower compared to endemic populations with high seropositivity rates. Travelers must be informed that Qdenga has no efficacy against serotypes 3 and 4 if they are seronegative, and a safety signal in such persons has not been proven or disproven. First experiences in the use of Qdenga in travelers have been published [59].

10. Which Other Dengue Vaccines Are in the Pipeline?

The Laboratory of Infectious Diseases at the National Institutes of Health (NIAID), United States, has developed five single-dose live-attenuated tetravalent DENV vaccines, of which TV003 and TV005 are the most promising candidates based on the most optimal immunogenicity and safety profile. A relatively balanced immune response to all four serotypes has been documented [60]. Both TV003 and TV005 have undergone extensive Phase 1 and 2 testing, including human challenge studies [61], and the Instituto Butantan is completing a Phase 3 trial using TV003 in Brazil. TV003 and TV005 share the same four monovalent components; the differences are in the dosing for serotype 2. TV005 has a 10-fold higher dose at 10^4 PFU to potentially overcome the over-attenuated serotype 2 component [61,62]. NIH has licensed out the vaccines to different manufacturers.

Several developers have secured licensure for this vaccine, with Merck having the largest global share. Instituto Butantan owns the licensure for distribution in Brazil. Butantan led the Phase 3 efficacy trial in Brazil in 16 sites, involving 16,235 volunteers aged 2 to 59 years using a single dose schedule. The two-year results have to date only been published in a press release. Over the initial two years, the vaccine was 79.6% effective in preventing dengue (serotypes 1 and 2) [63]. Efficacy in seropositive vs. seronegative persons was 89.2% and 73.5%, respectively. No confidence intervals were provided. The efficacy could only be assessed for serotypes 1 and 2, as serotypes 3 and 4 were not circulating during those initial two years. Efficacy against DENV-1 was higher with 89.5% versus 69.6% for DENV-2. By mid 2025, the results of the 5-year trial observation time are expected to become publicly available. Submission of the regulatory dossier to the European Medicine Agency has already taken place.

Recent advancements in dengue vaccine development have explored several additional innovative platforms beyond traditional live-attenuated vaccines. These include mRNA vaccines, which may offer a scalable and flexible approach to targeting multiple dengue virus serotypes [64]. Virus-like particle (VLP) vaccines mimic the structure of viruses without containing viral genetic material, eliciting strong immune responses while being non-infectious. A study published in 2024 describes the development of a tetravalent dengue VLP vaccine that induced robust immune responses against all four serotypes in animal models, maintaining efficacy for over a year [65]. Subunit vaccines use specific protein fragments of the dengue virus to stimulate immunity. A bioinformatics-driven approach has been proposed to design multi-epitope subunit vaccines targeting conserved regions of dengue virus proteins, aiming to induce comprehensive immune responses [66].

These innovative platforms aim to overcome the imbalanced performance of live-attenuated vaccines by eliciting balanced immunity against all four dengue virus serotypes. However, none of these platforms have moved beyond animal or Phase 1 studies. Ongoing research and clinical trials are crucial to evaluate the safety, efficacy, and scalability of these novel vaccine candidates. Given the enormous costs and complexities of running large Phase 3 trials, there is an urgent need to identify correlates of protection and, perhaps even more importantly in the context of antibody dependent enhance, correlates of enhanced disease [67].

As yet, no single vaccine can fully prevent and eliminate dengue infections. Hence, dengue vaccines will need to be used in conjunction with vector control [9].

Although Zika virus infections are currently rare, the risk of re-emergence with its catastrophic consequences of congenital Zika disease would justify developing a combination vaccine protecting both against dengue and Zika; however, several challenges persist which make such a vaccine less likely, as recently reviewed [68].

11. Conclusions

There is no perfect dengue vaccine, just as there is no vaccine with 100% efficacy for any other disease. The focus should be on optimizing the use of currently licensed dengue vaccines to maximize public health benefits while minimizing risks. Waiting for a perfect dengue vaccine will only result in more dengue morbidity and preventable deaths. Instead, we must act now, using available vaccines—despite their limitations—alongside effective vector control measures to reduce the burden of dengue and save lives. A well-planned vaccine roll-out combined with transparent communication, epidemiological monitoring, surveillance (serotype and genomic surveillance), and post-introduction studies to determine its safety in seronegative persons is needed.

Funding: This research received no external funding.

Conflicts of Interest: The authors declare no conflicts of interest.

References

1. Wilder-Smith, A.; Ooi, E.E.; Horstick, O.; Wills, B. Dengue. *Lancet* **2019**, *393*, 350–363. [CrossRef] [PubMed]
2. Messina, J.P.; Brady, O.J.; Golding, N.; Kraemer, M.U.G.; Wint, G.R.W.; Ray, S.E.; Pigott, D.M.; Shearer, F.M.; Johnson, K.; Earl, L.; et al. The current and future global distribution and population at risk of dengue. *Nat. Microbiol.* **2019**, *4*, 1508–1515. [CrossRef]
3. Messina, J.P.; Brady, O.J.; Pigott, D.M.; Brownstein, J.S.; Hoen, A.G.; Hay, S.I. A global compendium of human dengue virus occurrence. *Sci. Data* **2014**, *1*, 140004. [CrossRef] [PubMed]
4. Rowe, E.K.; Leo, Y.S.; Wong, J.G.; Thein, T.L.; Gan, V.C.; Lee, L.K.; Lye, D.C. Challenges in dengue fever in the elderly: Atypical presentation and risk of severe dengue and hospital-acquired infection [corrected]. *PLoS Negl. Trop. Dis.* **2014**, *8*, e2777. [CrossRef]
5. Woon, Y.L.; Hor, C.P.; Hussin, N.; Zakaria, A.; Goh, P.P.; Cheah, W.K. A Two-Year Review on Epidemiology and Clinical Characteristics of Dengue Deaths in Malaysia, 2013–2014. *PLoS Negl. Trop. Dis.* **2016**, *10*, e0004575. [CrossRef] [PubMed]
6. Vouga, M.; Chiu, Y.C.; Pomar, L.; de Meyer, S.V.; Masmejan, S.; Genton, B.; Musso, D.; Baud, D.; Stojanov, M. Dengue, Zika and chikungunya during pregnancy: Pre- and post-travel advice and clinical management. *J. Travel Med.* **2019**, *26*, taz077. [CrossRef]
7. Lee, Y.H.; Leong, W.Y.; Wilder-Smith, A. Markers of dengue severity: A systematic review of cytokines and chemokines. *J. Gen. Virol.* **2016**, *97*, 3103–3119. [CrossRef] [PubMed]
8. Wilder-Smith, A.; Gubler, D.J. Geographic expansion of dengue: The impact of international travel. *Med. Clin. N. Am.* **2008**, *92*, 1377–1390. [CrossRef]
9. Wilder-Smith, A.; Lindsay, S.W.; Scott, T.W.; Ooi, E.E.; Gubler, D.J.; Das, P. The Lancet Commission on dengue and other Aedes-transmitted viral diseases. *Lancet* **2020**, *395*, 1890–1891. [CrossRef]
10. Bhatt, S.; Gething, P.W.; Brady, O.J.; Messina, J.P.; Farlow, A.W.; Moyes, C.L.; Drake, J.M.; Brownstein, J.S.; Hoen, A.G.; Sankoh, O.; et al. The global distribution and burden of dengue. *Nature* **2013**, *496*, 504–507. [CrossRef]

11. Yang, X.; Quam, M.B.M.; Zhang, T.; Sang, S. Global burden for dengue and the evolving pattern in the past 30 years. *J. Travel Med.* **2021**, *28*, taab146. [CrossRef] [PubMed]
12. Amatya, B.; Schwartz, E.; Biber, A.; Erster, O.; Lustig, Y.; Pradhan, R.; Khadka, B.; Pandey, P. Dengue serotype characterization during the 2022 dengue epidemic in Kathmandu, Nepal. *J. Travel Med.* **2023**, *30*, taad034. [CrossRef] [PubMed]
13. Bijukchhe, S.M.; Hill, M.; Adhikari, B.; Shrestha, A.; Shrestha, S. Nepal's worst dengue outbreak is a wake-up call for action. *J. Travel Med.* **2023**, *30*, taad112. [CrossRef] [PubMed]
14. Diaz-Menendez, M.; Angelo, K.M.; de Miguel Buckley, R.; Bottieau, E.; Huits, R.; Grobusch, M.P.; Gobbi, F.G.; Asgeirsson, H.; Duvignaud, A.; Norman, F.F.; et al. Dengue outbreak amongst travellers returning from Cuba—GeoSentinel surveillance network, January–September 2022. *J. Travel Med.* **2023**, *30*, taac139. [CrossRef] [PubMed]
15. Duvignaud, A.; Stoney, R.J.; Angelo, K.M.; Chen, L.H.; Cattaneo, P.; Motta, L.; Gobbi, F.G.; Bottieau, E.; Bourque, D.L.; Popescu, C.P.; et al. Epidemiology of travel-associated dengue from 2007 to 2022: A GeoSentinel analysis. *J. Travel Med.* **2024**, *31*, taae089. [CrossRef]
16. Lee, S.Y.; Shih, H.I.; Lo, W.C.; Lu, T.H.; Chien, Y.W. Discrepancies in dengue burden estimates: A comparative analysis of reported cases and global burden of disease study, 2010–2019. *J. Travel Med.* **2024**, *31*, taae069. [CrossRef]
17. Salvo, P.F.; Baldin, G.; Raffaelli, F.; Ciccullo, A.; Borghetti, A.; Tamburrini, E.; Ricci, R.; Di Donato, M.; Di Giambenedetto, S.; Torti, C. Autochthonous dengue outbreak in Rome, Italy, in 2023. *J. Travel Med.* **2024**, *31*, taae111. [CrossRef]
18. Achee, N.L.; Gould, F.; Perkins, T.A.; Reiner, R.C., Jr.; Morrison, A.C.; Ritchie, S.A.; Gubler, D.J.; Teyssou, R.; Scott, T.W. A critical assessment of vector control for dengue prevention. *PLoS Negl. Trop. Dis.* **2015**, *9*, e0003655. [CrossRef]
19. Lim, J.T.; Mailepessov, D.; Chong, C.S.; Dickens, B.; Lai, Y.L.; Ng, Y.; Deng, L.; Lee, C.; Tan, L.Y.; Chain, G.; et al. Assessing Wolbachia-mediated sterility for dengue control: Emulation of a cluster-randomized target trial in Singapore. *J. Travel Med.* **2024**, *31*, taae103. [CrossRef]
20. O'Reilly, K.M.; Hendrickx, E.; Kharisma, D.D.; Wilastonegoro, N.N.; Carrington, L.B.; Elyazar, I.R.F.; Kucharski, A.J.; Lowe, R.; Flasche, S.; Pigott, D.M.; et al. Estimating the burden of dengue and the impact of release of wMel Wolbachia-infected mosquitoes in Indonesia: A modelling study. *BMC Med.* **2019**, *17*, 172. [CrossRef]
21. Katzelnick, L.C.; Gresh, L.; Halloran, M.E.; Mercado, J.C.; Kuan, G.; Gordon, A.; Balmaseda, A.; Harris, E. Antibody-dependent enhancement of severe dengue disease in humans. *Science* **2017**, *358*, 929–932. [CrossRef]
22. Izmirly, A.M.; Alturki, S.O.; Alturki, S.O.; Connors, J.; Haddad, E.K. Challenges in Dengue Vaccines Development: Pre-existing Infections and Cross-Reactivity. *Front. Immunol.* **2020**, *11*, 1055. [CrossRef] [PubMed]
23. Waggoner, J.J.; Katzelnick, L.C.; Burger-Calderon, R.; Gallini, J.; Moore, R.H.; Kuan, G.; Balmaseda, A.; Pinsky, B.A.; Harris, E. Antibody-Dependent Enhancement of Severe Disease Is Mediated by Serum Viral Load in Pediatric Dengue Virus Infections. *J. Infect. Dis.* **2020**, *221*, 1846–1854. [CrossRef] [PubMed]
24. Hadinegoro, S.R.; Arredondo-Garcia, J.L.; Capeding, M.R.; Deseda, C.; Chotpitayasunondh, T.; Dietze, R.; Ismail, H.I.; Reynales, H.; Limkittikul, K.; Rivera-Medina, D.M.; et al. Efficacy and Long-Term Safety of a Dengue Vaccine in Regions of Endemic Disease. *N. Engl. J. Med.* **2015**, *373*, 1195–1206. [CrossRef] [PubMed]
25. Wilder-Smith, A.; Flasche, S.; Smith, P.G. Vaccine-attributable severe dengue in the Philippines. *Lancet* **2019**, *394*, 2151–2152. [CrossRef]
26. Flasche, S.; Wilder-Smith, A.; Hombach, J.; Smith, P.G. Estimating the proportion of vaccine-induced hospitalized dengue cases among Dengvaxia vaccinees in the Philippines. *Wellcome Open Res.* **2019**, *4*, 165. [CrossRef] [PubMed]
27. Wilder-Smith, A.; Hombach, J.; Ferguson, N.; Selgelid, M.; O'Brien, K.; Vannice, K.; Barrett, A.; Ferdinand, E.; Flasche, S.; Guzman, M.; et al. Deliberations of the Strategic Advisory Group of Experts on Immunization on the use of CYD-TDV dengue vaccine. *Lancet Infect. Dis.* **2019**, *19*, e31–e38. [CrossRef]
28. Rivera, L.; Biswal, S.; Saez-Llorens, X.; Reynales, H.; Lopez-Medina, E.; Borja-Tabora, C.; Bravo, L.; Sirivichayakul, C.; Kosalaraksa, P.; Martinez Vargas, L.; et al. Three-year Efficacy and Safety of Takeda's Dengue Vaccine Candidate (TAK-003). *Clin. Infect. Dis.* **2022**, *75*, 107–117. [CrossRef]
29. SAGE Background Paper on the Use of TAK-003 Dengue Vaccine 2023. Available online: https://terrance.who.int/mediacentre/data/sage/SAGE_eYB_Sept2023.pdf (accessed on 15 January 2025).
30. White, L.J.; Young, E.F.; Stoops, M.J.; Henein, S.R.; Adams, E.C.; Baric, R.S.; de Silva, A.M. Defining levels of dengue virus serotype-specific neutralizing antibodies induced by a live attenuated tetravalent dengue vaccine (TAK-003). *PLoS Negl. Trop. Dis.* **2021**, *15*, e0009258. [CrossRef]
31. Bengolea, A.; Scigliano, C.; Ramos-Rojas, J.T.; Rada, G.; Catalano, H.N.; Izcovich, A. Effectiveness and safety of the tetravalent TAK-003 dengue vaccine: A systematic review. *Medicina (Buenos Aires)* **2024**, *84*, 689–707.
32. de Silva, A.; White, L. Immunogenicity of a Live Dengue Vaccine (TAK-003). *J. Infect. Dis.* **2022**, *227*, 163–164. [CrossRef] [PubMed]

33. El Hindi, T.; Alera, M.T.; Bravo, L.; Moreira, E.D., Jr.; Dietze, R.; Oliveira, A.L.; Watanaveeradej, V.; Zhao, Y.; Sonderegger, I.; Tricou, V.; et al. Estimated Efficacy of TAK-003 Against Asymptomatic Dengue Infection in Children/Adolescents Participating in the DEN-301 Trial in Asia Pacific and Latin America. *J. Infect. Dis.* **2025**, jiaf145. [CrossRef] [PubMed]
34. Fernando, L.; Kastner, R.; Wickramasinghe, P.; Fernando, A.D.; Gunasekera, D.; Nguyen, V.H.; Liu, M.; LeFevre, I.; Wallace, D.; Folschweiller, N.; et al. Role of the dengue vaccine TAK-003 in an outbreak response: Modeling the Sri Lanka experience. *PLoS Negl. Trop. Dis.* **2024**, *18*, e0012376. [CrossRef]
35. Flacco, M.E.; Bianconi, A.; Cioni, G.; Fiore, M.; Calo, G.L.; Imperiali, G.; Orazi, V.; Tiseo, M.; Troia, A.; Rosso, A.; et al. Immunogenicity, Safety and Efficacy of the Dengue Vaccine TAK-003: A Meta-Analysis. *Vaccines* **2024**, *12*, 770. [CrossRef]
36. LeFevre, I.; Bravo, L.; Folschweiller, N.; Medina, E.L.; Moreira, E.D., Jr.; Nordio, F.; Sharma, M.; Tharenos, L.M.; Tricou, V.; Watanaveeradej, V.; et al. Bridging the immunogenicity of a tetravalent dengue vaccine (TAK-003) from children and adolescents to adults. *NPJ Vaccines* **2023**, *8*, 75. [CrossRef]
37. Lopez-Medina, E.; Biswal, S.; Saez-Llorens, X.; Borja-Tabora, C.; Bravo, L.; Sirivichayakul, C.; Vargas, L.M.; Alera, M.T.; Velasquez, H.; Reynales, H.; et al. Efficacy of a Dengue Vaccine Candidate (TAK-003) in Healthy Children and Adolescents 2 Years after Vaccination. *J. Infect. Dis.* **2022**, *225*, 1521–1532. [CrossRef] [PubMed]
38. Patel, S.S.; Winkle, P.; Faccin, A.; Nordio, F.; LeFevre, I.; Tsoukas, C.G. An open-label, Phase 3 trial of TAK-003, a live attenuated dengue tetravalent vaccine, in healthy US adults: Immunogenicity and safety when administered during the second half of a 24-month shelf-life. *Hum. Vaccin. Immunother.* **2023**, *19*, 2254964. [CrossRef] [PubMed]
39. Petri, E.; Biswal, S.; Lloyd, E.; Tricou, V.; Folschweiller, N. Early onset of protection of the TAK-003 dengue vaccine: Data from the DEN-301 clinical trial. *Vaccine* **2024**, *42*, 126309. [CrossRef]
40. Rauscher, M.; Youard, Z.; Faccin, A.; Patel, S.S.; Pang, H.; Zent, O. Pregnancy outcomes following unintentional exposure to TAK-003, a live-attenuated tetravalent dengue vaccine. *Expert Rev. Vaccines* **2025**, *24*, 221–229. [CrossRef]
41. Saez-Llorens, X.; Biswal, S.; Borja-Tabora, C.; Fernando, L.; Liu, M.; Wallace, D.; Folschweiller, N.; Reynales, H.; LeFevre, I.; Group, T.S. Effect of the Tetravalent Dengue Vaccine TAK-003 on Sequential Episodes of Symptomatic Dengue. *Am. J. Trop. Med. Hyg.* **2023**, *108*, 722–726. [CrossRef]
42. Sirivichayakul, C.; Biswal, S.; Saez-Llorens, X.; Lopez-Medina, E.; Borja-Tabora, C.; Bravo, L.; Kosalaraksa, P.; Alera, M.T.; Reynales, H.; Rivera, L.; et al. Efficacy and Safety of a Tetravalent Dengue Vaccine (TAK-003) in Children With Prior Japanese Encephalitis or Yellow Fever Vaccination. *J. Infect. Dis.* **2024**, *230*, e1214–e1225. [CrossRef] [PubMed]
43. Tricou, V.; Essink, B.; Ervin, J.E.; Turner, M.; Escudero, I.; Rauscher, M.; Brose, M.; Lefevre, I.; Borkowski, A.; Wallace, D. Immunogenicity and safety of concomitant and sequential administration of yellow fever YF-17D vaccine and tetravalent dengue vaccine candidate TAK-003: A phase 3 randomized, controlled study. *PLoS Negl. Trop. Dis.* **2023**, *17*, e0011124. [CrossRef] [PubMed]
44. Tricou, V.; Eyre, S.; Ramjee, M.; Collini, P.; Mojares, Z.; Loeliger, E.; Mandaric, S.; Rauscher, M.; Brose, M.; Lefevre, I.; et al. A randomized phase 3 trial of the immunogenicity and safety of coadministration of a live-attenuated tetravalent dengue vaccine (TAK-003) and an inactivated hepatitis a (HAV) virus vaccine in a dengue non-endemic country. *Vaccine* **2023**, *41*, 1398–1407. [CrossRef]
45. Tricou, V.; Winkle, P.J.; Tharenos, L.M.; Rauscher, M.; Escudero, I.; Hoffman, E.; LeFevre, I.; Borkowski, A.; Wallace, D. Consistency of immunogenicity in three consecutive lots of a tetravalent dengue vaccine candidate (TAK-003): A randomized placebo-controlled trial in US adults. *Vaccine* **2023**, *41*, 6999–7006. [CrossRef] [PubMed]
46. Tricou, V.; Yu, D.; Reynales, H.; Biswal, S.; Saez-Llorens, X.; Sirivichayakul, C.; Lopez, P.; Borja-Tabora, C.; Bravo, L.; Kosalaraksa, P.; et al. Long-term efficacy and safety of a tetravalent dengue vaccine (TAK-003): 4.5-year results from a phase 3, randomised, double-blind, placebo-controlled trial. *Lancet Glob. Health* **2024**, *12*, e257–e270. [CrossRef] [PubMed]
47. Wilder-Smith, A. TAK-003 dengue vaccine as a new tool to mitigate dengue in countries with a high disease burden. *Lancet Glob. Health* **2024**, *12*, e179–e180. [CrossRef]
48. Patel, S.S.; Rauscher, M.; Kudela, M.; Pang, H. Clinical Safety Experience of TAK-003 for Dengue Fever: A New Tetravalent Live Attenuated Vaccine Candidate. *Clin. Infect. Dis.* **2023**, *76*, e1350–e1359. [CrossRef]
49. Daniels, B.C.; Ferguson, N.; Dorigatti, I. Efficacy, public health impact and optimal use of the Takeda dengue vaccine. *MedRxiv* **2025**. [CrossRef]
50. WHO. WHO position paper on dengue vaccines-May 2024. *Wkly. Epidemiol. Rec.* **2024**, *18*, 203–224.
51. WHO. WHO Position Paper on TAK-003 Dengue Vaccine 2024. Available online: https://www.who.int/publications/i/item/who-wer-9918-203-224 (accessed on 15 January 2025).
52. Percio, J.; Kobayashi, C.D.; Silva, R.M.A.; Marinho, A.; Capovilla, L.; Andrade, P.H.S.; da Nobrega, M.E.B.; Cabral, C.M.; de Moraes, M.B.; Werneck, G.L.; et al. Safety signal detected: Anaphylaxis after attenuated dengue vaccine (TAK-003)—Brazil, 1 March 2023–11 March 2024. *Vaccine* **2024**, *42*, 126407. [CrossRef]
53. Update on Safety of the Dengue Vaccine Qdenga®. Available online: https://www.who.int/groups/global-advisory-committee-on-vaccine-safety/topics/dengue-vaccines (accessed on 15 January 2025).

54. Manciulli, T.; Zammarchi, L.; Lagi, F.; Fiorelli, C.; Mencarini, J.; Fognani, M.; Rossolini, G.M.; Pollini, S.; Bartoloni, A.; Spinicci, M. Emergence of dengue fever: Sentinel travellers uncover outbreak in Sharm El-Sheikh, Egypt, May 2024. *J. Travel Med.* **2024**, *31*, taae080. [CrossRef] [PubMed]
55. McGuinness, S.L.; Leder, K. Dengue severity in travellers: Challenges and insights. *J. Travel Med.* **2023**, *30*, taad146. [CrossRef] [PubMed]
56. Sohail, A.; Anders, K.L.; McGuinness, S.L.; Leder, K. The epidemiology of imported and locally acquired dengue in Australia, 2012–2022. *J. Travel Med.* **2024**, *31*, taae014. [CrossRef] [PubMed]
57. Kitro, A.; Imad, H.A.; Pisutsan, P.; Matsee, W.; Sirikul, W.; Sapbamrer, R.; Rapheal, E.; Fernandez, S.; Cotrone, T.S.; Farmer, A.R.; et al. Seroprevalence of dengue, Japanese encephalitis and Zika among long-term expatriates in Thailand. *J. Travel Med.* **2024**, *31*, taae022. [CrossRef]
58. Freedman, D.O. A new dengue vaccine (TAK-003) now WHO recommended in endemic areas; what about travellers? *J. Travel Med.* **2023**, *30*, taad132. [CrossRef]
59. Kopke, C.; Rothe, C.; Zeder, A.; Boecken, G.; Feldt, T.; Janke, C.; Jordan, S.; Kohler, C.; Lobermann, M.; Muller, A.; et al. First clinical experiences with the tetravalent live vaccine against dengue (Qdenga (R)) in travellers: A multicentric TravelMedVac study in Germany. *J. Travel Med.* **2025**, *32*, taaf004. [CrossRef]
60. Nivarthi, U.K.; Swanstrom, J.; Delacruz, M.J.; Patel, B.; Durbin, A.P.; Whitehead, S.S.; Kirkpatrick, B.D.; Pierce, K.K.; Diehl, S.A.; Katzelnick, L.; et al. A tetravalent live attenuated dengue virus vaccine stimulates balanced immunity to multiple serotypes in humans. *Nat. Commun.* **2021**, *12*, 1102. [CrossRef]
61. Wilder-Smith, A. The Dengue-in-Dhaka Initiative: Results from a phase 2 trial evaluating the TV005 tetravalent dengue vaccine in Bangladesh. *Lancet Infect. Dis.* **2024**, *24*, 112–113. [CrossRef]
62. Wilder-Smith, A.B.; Freedman, D.O.; Wilder-Smith, A. Edging towards a third dengue vaccine. *Lancet Infect. Dis.* **2024**, *24*, 1182–1184. [CrossRef]
63. TetraVax-DV (V180) Dengue Vaccine. Available online: https://www.precisionvaccinations.com/vaccines/tetravax-dv-v180-dengue-vaccine (accessed on 15 January 2025).
64. Liu, X.; Salmon, D. Opportunities and challenges of mRNA technologies in the development of dengue vaccines. *arXiv* **2024**. [CrossRef] [PubMed]
65. Thoresen, D.; Matsuda, K.; Urakami, A.; Ngwe Tun, M.M.; Nomura, T.; Moi, M.L.; Watanabe, Y.; Ishikawa, M.; Hau, T.T.T.; Yamamoto, H.; et al. A tetravalent dengue virus-like particle vaccine induces high levels of neutralizing antibodies and reduces dengue replication in non-human primates. *J. Virol.* **2024**, *98*, e0023924. [CrossRef] [PubMed]
66. Saha, O.; Razzak, A.; Sarker, N.; Rahman, N.; bin Zahid, A.; Sultana, A.; Shishir, T.A.; Bahadur, N.M.; Rahaman, M.; Hossen, F.; et al. In silico design and evaluation of multi-epitope dengue virus vaccines: A promising approach to combat global dengue burden. *Discov. Appl. Sci.* **2024**, *6*, 210. [CrossRef]
67. Katzelnick, L.C.; Harris, E. Immune correlates of protection for dengue: State of the art and research agenda. *Vaccine* **2017**, *35*, 4659–4669. [CrossRef] [PubMed]
68. Ostrowsky, J.T.; Katzelnick, L.C.; Bourne, N.; Barrett, A.D.T.; Thomas, S.J.; Diamond, M.S.; Beasley, D.W.C.; Harris, E.; Wilder-Smith, A.; Leighton, T.; et al. Zika virus vaccines and monoclonal antibodies: A priority agenda for research and development. *Lancet Infect. Dis.* **2025**. [CrossRef]

vaccines

MDPI

Systematic Review

Evaluating the Immunogenicity, Efficacy, and Effectiveness of Recombinant Zoster Vaccine for Global Public Health Policy

Lucy R. Williams [1], Joachim Hombach [2] and Melanie Marti [2,*]

[1] MRC Centre for Global Infectious Disease Analysis, School of Public Health, Imperial College London, London W12 0BZ, UK
[2] Immunisation, Vaccines and Biologicals Department, World Health Organisation, Avenue Appia 20, 1211 Geneva, Switzerland
* Correspondence: martim@who.int

Abstract: Background: Herpes zoster (HZ) is a painful neurocutaneous disease caused by the varicella-zoster virus. The recombinant zoster vaccine (RZV) is becoming increasingly incorporated into national vaccination schedules. We aimed to evaluate RZV from a global public health policy perspective. **Methods**: We performed a rapid review of studies evaluating the immunogenicity, efficacy, and effectiveness of RZV for protection against HZ and associated complications. We searched PubMed for English-language studies published between 7 August 2012 and 30 September 2023. Included studies reported vaccine efficacy or effectiveness against HZ and HZ-associated complications. Immunogenicity studies were included if they contributed to the understanding of RZV protection over time and/or co-administration with other vaccines. HZ outcomes were stratified by socio-demographic and clinical variables. **Results**: From 405 identified publications, 33 were eligible for the study. Most studies were conducted in the US (N = 12), across North America (N = 10), and Europe (N = 5), or across multiple locations across North America, Latin America, and Asia–Australia (N = 6). Vaccine efficacy against HZ in immunocompetent populations ranged between 90% and 97%, while effectiveness ranged between 71% and 86%. Protection stayed above 70% for at least 10 years, with no significant differences by age or ethnicity. **Conclusions**: RZV is effective in reducing the risk of HZ and its associated complications. Protection is long-lasting and the vaccine is suitable for older and immunocompromised populations. However, the decision to incorporate the vaccine into national policies depends on additional factors (e.g., cost-effectiveness), which may be difficult to characterize without an understanding of the global disease burden.

Keywords: vaccine; immunization; herpes zoster; varicella zoster virus; health policy

1. Introduction

Herpes zoster (HZ), or shingles, is a painful neurocutaneous disease caused by reactivation of the varicella-zoster virus (VZV) in the dorsal root ganglia [1,2]. It is characterized by a blister-like rash on one side of the body, which is commonly accompanied by radicular pain lasting 2–4 weeks. The pain associated with HZ can be debilitating and lead to depression, social withdrawal, and reduced quality of life, and places a large burden on patients, carers, healthcare systems, and employers [3,4].

A large proportion of the burden of HZ on healthcare systems is from HZ-associated complications, of which post-herpetic neuralgia (PHN) is the most common. PHN is a chronic neuropathic pain that persists after resolution of the acute phase of vesicular rash, which occurs in approximately one in five HZ patients [5]. If VZV reactivates in certain cranial nerves, it can also cause herpes zoster ophthalmicus (HZO) and this may lead to conjunctivitis, keratitis, iritis, uveitis, and vision loss [6]. Other complications include disseminated HZ (rash in ≥3 dermatomes), and neurological, visceral, or vascular diseases, including stroke and myocardial infarction (MI) [7].

Between 20% and 30% of the population are expected to develop HZ in their lifetime [8,9]. An estimated 14.9 million cases of HZ occurred globally in 2020 in individuals aged over 50 years, and this is predicted to increase to up to 19.1 million cases by 2030 [10]. The risk and severity of HZ increases with age, particularly after the age of 50 years, due to age-related decline in immunity [11]. Patients with immunosuppression and other severe comorbidities are also at higher risk of developing HZ than immunocompetent individuals of any age, and they are more likely to suffer from severe disease or HZ-associated complications [12,13]. Data availability on the incidence of HZ and its associated complications varies widely, with most studies conducted in North America and Europe. In a systematic literature review of HZ incidence worldwide in the population over 50 years, van Oorschot et al. found that the incidence of HZ ranged between 5.2 and 10.9 per 1000 person-years across North America, Europe, and the Asia-Pacific region [14], but, consistent with other studies, they found little to no data for the regions of Eastern Europe, the Middle East, South America, or Africa [15–17].

There are over a dozen candidate vaccines in clinical development for the prevention of HZ, and, to date, two vaccines have been licenced: Zoster Vaccine Live (ZVL, Zostavax®, Merck Sharp & Dohme B.V, Haarlem, The Netherlands) and the Recombinant Zoster Vaccine (RZV, Shingrix®, GlaxoSmithKline, Brentford, UK). ZVL demonstrated moderate vaccine efficacy of 51.3% during follow-up lasting a median time of 3.1 years [18,19]. Vaccine effectiveness in real-world settings, particularly over extended follow-up, was low, with one study reporting an effectiveness of 31.8% after 8 years post-vaccination [20]. Additionally, as it contains a weakened form of the VZV, it is contraindicated in immunocompromised individuals [20]. RZV is a recombinant (non-live) vaccine which contains the adjuvant $AS01_B$ and recombinant VZV glycoprotein E (gE). It was licenced under a two-dose regimen by the U. S. Food and Drug Administration (FDA) in 2017 and the European Medicines Agency (EMA) in 2018 for adults 50 years or older and immunocompromised adults over the age of 18 years. ZVL has now been discontinued by the manufacturer, so many countries have already begun, or are currently in the process of transitioning to the use of RZV for their HZ vaccination programmes [3].

This rapid review aims to provide an up-to-date assessment of the evidence on the immunogenicity, efficacy, and effectiveness of RZV and how this differs across key clinical and socio-demographic characteristics. It may help to inform policymakers who are tasked with issuing guidance on RZV use on the benefits and potential risks in different population groups.

2. Materials and Methods

2.1. Search Strategy, Inclusion and Exclusion Criteria

We conducted our literature search in PubMed to identify randomized controlled trials (RCTs) and non-randomized studies evaluating the immunogenicity, efficacy, and effectiveness of RZV from 7 August 2012 to 30 September 2023. This date range was chosen because the first phase 2 trial results were published in August 2012 [21]. One reviewer (LRW) performed the study selection and data extraction. Included studies reported on protection against HZ, PHN, and other HZ-associated complications. Immunogenicity studies were included if they contributed to the understanding of continued vaccine protection over time and/or the breadth of immune response when RZV was co-administered with other vaccines. We allowed for any population characteristics and did not impose an age limit. We compare two doses of RZV to no RZV administration, and we only included publications written in English. Inclusion and exclusion criteria are provided in Table 1 and search terms are provided in Table 2. A systematic review of safety outcomes was beyond the scope of this report; however, we summarized the findings (reactogenicity, adverse events, and serious adverse events) of other reviews on the topic.

Table 1. Inclusion and exclusion criteria for rapid review.

	Inclusion	Exclusion
Population	General population	
Intervention	Two doses of recombinant adjuvanted zoster vaccine	
Comparison	No RZV	
Outcomes	Herpes zoster, postherpetic neuralgia, herpes zoster ophthalmicus, other HZ-associated complications. Humoral and cellular immune response for follow-up ≥ 5 years and/or co-administration with another vaccine	
Study design	RCT or non-randomised	Case reports, case series, reviews, systematic reviews, commentaries, editorials, in vitro only studies, animal studies
Time frame	7 August 2012 to 30 September 2023	
Languages	English	Other languages

The publication date of the RZV phase 2 trial results was 7 August 2012 [21]. RZV = Recombinant zoster vaccine; RCT = randomized controlled trial.

Table 2. PubMed search terms.

Row	Term	Purpose
1	"Herpes Zoster" [Mesh] OR zoster[tiab] OR shingle*[tiab]	Mesh and title/abstract terms for herpes zoster
2	Shingrix[tiab] OR RZV OR HZ/su[tiab] OR "recombinant vaccine"[tiab:~3] OR "subunit vaccine"[tiab:~3] OR "glycoprotein E vaccine"[tiab:~3] OR "gE vaccine"[tiab:~3] OR "inactivated vaccine"[tiab:~3] OR "adjuvant* vaccine"[tiab:~3]	Title/abstract terms for Shingrix
3	("7 August 2012"[Date—Publication]: "30 September 2023"[Date—Publication]	Limit publications to those published when the vaccine was in late-stage development or implementation, up to the date of the literature search
4	(#1 AND #2 AND #3) NOT (case reports[Publication Type] NOT systematic review[Publication Type]	Exclude reviews and case reports

2.2. Data Extraction

Data extracted included the study methodology (design, sample size, location, duration, population characteristics) and study outcomes. Outcomes of interest were the incidence rate, relative risk (RR), and vaccine efficacy/effectiveness against HZ, PHN, hospitalization, and other HZ-associated complications (e.g., HZO, stroke, myocardial infarction). We stratified HZ outcomes by age, geographic ancestry/ethnicity (Asian, Black, Hispanic, White), sex, receipt of previous ZVL, immune status, co-administration with another vaccine, and time since vaccination. Immunogenicity outcomes included humoral and cellular immune responses.

Vaccine efficacy and effectiveness are presented as reported. If only RR was reported, if it had been calculated as the incidence rate ratio or hazard ratio, we calculated efficacy/effectiveness as 1-RR. Odds ratios were not converted to efficacy/effectiveness [22]. Where there were no cases in the vaccinated group, efficacy/effectiveness is given as 100% with no confidence intervals.

2.3. Bias Assessment

One reviewer (MM) independently assessed the quality, level of evidence, and risk of bias of all included studies (Supplementary Methods). The Cochrane Risk of Bias tool (RoB2) was used for RCTs and the Risk of Bias in Non-randomized Studies of Interventions (ROBINS-I) was used for observational studies. All studies, regardless of their methodological quality, underwent data extraction and estimates are presented.

3. Results

3.1. Summary of RZV Study Characteristics

A total of 405 publications were identified from the database search. After titles and abstracts were assessed for eligibility, 88 publications were appraised for eligibility based on the pre-specified inclusion and exclusion criteria. We identified 33 eligible publications from 23 studies evaluating the efficacy [23–35] (Table 3), effectiveness [36–44] (Table 4), and immunogenicity [30,31,45–55] (Table 5) of RZV (Figure 1). Most studies were conducted exclusively in the US (N = 12), across multiple countries in North America and Europe (N = 5), or across multiple locations across North America, Latin America, and Asia–Australia (N = 6). Six studies were randomized controlled trials, eight were open-label randomized trials, eight were cohort studies, and one was case–control. The overall quality of the included RCTs was high and most had a low risk of bias (Supplementary Table S1). While well executed, most of the observational studies had a moderate risk of bias (Supplementary Table S2).

Table 3. Characteristics of studies reporting vaccine efficacy of recombinant zoster vaccine against herpes zoster and its complications.

Author(s), Year	Study Acronym or NCT Number [1]	N Enrolled	Study Design	# Centres /Location	Study Start—Study End Year	Follow-Up	Population	Risk of Bias
Lal et al., 2015 [23] Cunningham et al., 2016 [24] Kovac et al., 2018 [25] Willer et al., 2019 [26] Curran et al., 2021 [27] Dagnew et al., 2021 [28] Kim et al., 2021 [29] Boutry et al., 2022 [30] Strezova et al., 2022 [31] Oostvogels et al., 2019 [32]	ZOE-50	15,411	Phase 3 RCT	248/Europe, North America, Latin America, and Asia	Enrollment: 2010–2011	Mean 3.5 years	Immuno competent adults, 50+ years old	Low

Table 3. *Cont.*

Author(s), Year	Study Acronym or NCT Number [1]	N Enrolled	Study Design	# Centres /Location	Study Start—Study End Year	Follow-Up	Population	Risk of Bias
Cunningham et al., 2016 [24] Kovac et al., 2018 [25] Willer et al., 2019 [26] Curran et al., 2021 [27] Dagnew et al., 2021 [28] Kim et al., 2021 [29] Boutry et al., 2022 [30] Strezova et al., 2022 [31] Oostvogels et al., 2019 [32]	ZOE-70	13,900	Phase 3 RCT	248/Europe, North America, Latin America, and Asia	Enrollment: 2010–2011; Last study visit: 2015	Mean 3.7 years	Immuno competent adults, 70+ years old	Low
Bastidas et al., 2019 [33] Stadtmauer et al., 2021 [34]	ZOE-HSCT	1868	Phase 3 RCT	167/Multi	2010–2017	Median 1.8 years	HSCT recipients, 18+ years old	Low
Dagnew et al., 2019 [35]	Zoster-039	606	Phase 3 RCT	77/Europe, North America, Latin America, and Asia	Enrollment: March 2013–September 2015	Median 11.1 months	Hematological malignancy patients	Some concerns
Boutry et al., 2022 [30] Strezova et al., 2022 [31]	ZOE-LTFU [2]	7413	Phase 3B open-label single arm	248/Europe, North America, Latin America, and Asia	2016-Present	Up to 6 years [3]	Immuno competent adults, 50+ years old	Low
Curran et al., 2021 [27]	ZOE-Frailty [2]	26,976	Phase 3 RCT	248/Europe, North America, Latin America, and Asia	Enrollment: 2010–2011	Mean 4 years	Frail immuno competent adults, 50+ years old	Low

NCT = National clinical trial, ZOE = Zoster efficacy study, LTFU = long-term follow-up. [1] NCT Number is the ClinicalTrials.gov Identifier: KA-03909·NLM Customer Support Center (nih.gov (accessed on 19 February 2025)). [2] ZOE-LTFU (NCT02723773) is a follow-up study and ZOE-Frailty (NCT03563183) is a subgroup analysis of the ZOE-50 (NCT01165177) and ZOE-70 (NCT01165229) studies. [3] Beginning of follow-up was 4 years post-vaccination.

Table 4. Characteristics of studies reporting vaccine effectiveness of Recombinant Zoster Vaccine against herpes zoster and its complications.

Author(s), Year	N Enrolled	Study Design	Location	Study Start—Study End Year	Follow-Up	Population	Risk of Bias
Sun et al., 2021 (A) [36]	78,358	Retrospective cohort	Hawaii	2018–2019	Mean 0.7 years	Immunocompetent adults, 50+ years old	Moderate
Kochhar et al., 2021 [37]	112,220	Retrospective cohort	US	2017–2020	Minimum 9 months	Inflammatory bowel disease patients, 50+ years old	Serious
Izurieta et al., 2021 [38]	15,589,546	Prospective cohort	US	2017–2019	Median 3.1 years	General population, 65+ years old	Moderate
Sun et al., 2021 (B) [39]	4,769,819	Retrospective cohort	US	2018–2019	Median 7 months	Immunocompetent adults, 50+ years old	Moderate
Lu et al., 2021 [40]	4,842,579	Retrospective cohort	US	2018–2019	Median 730 days	Immunocompetent adults, 50+ years old	Moderate
Bruxvoort et al., 2022 [41]	41,251	Retrospective cohort	US	2019–2020	Minimum 1 year	Immunocompetent adults, 50+ years old	Low
Khan et al., 2022 [42]	33,300	Retrospective cohort	US	2018–2020	Mean 1.13 years	Inflammatory bowel disease patients, 50+ years old	Low
Parameswaran et al., 2023, A [44]	2,165,505	Retrospective case–control	US	2010–2020	30 days following HZ infection	General population, 18+ years old	Moderate
Parameswaran et al., 2023, B [43]	2,165,584	Retrospective cohort	US	2015–2020	30 days following HZ infection	General population, 18+ years old	Moderate

Table 5. Characteristics of studies reporting on the immune response to the recombinant zoster vaccine.

Author(s), Year	Study Acronym or NCT Number	N Enrolled	Study Design	# Centres/ Location	Study Start—Study End Year	Follow-Up	Population	Co-Administered Vaccine
				Co-administration				
Schwarz, 2017 [45]	NCT01954251	829	Phase 3 Randomized open label trial	20/Canada, Germany, US	2013–2015	14–16 months	Immuno competent, 50+ years	Quadrivalent seasonal inactivated influenza vaccine (IIV4)
Maréchal, 2018 [46]	NCT02045836	865	Phase 3 Randomized open label trial	9/US, Canada, Estonia	2014–2016	12 months	Immuno competent, 50+ years	23-valent pneumococcal polysaccharide vaccine (PPSV23)
Strezova, 2019 [47]	NCT02052596	904	Phase 3 Randomized open label trial	13/US	2014–2016	12 months	Immuno competent, 50+ years	Diphtheria-tetanus-acellular pertussis vaccine (Tdap)
Min, 2022 [48]	NCT03439657	912	Phase 3B Randomized open label trial	13/Canada, Estonia, Germany, US	2018–2020	12 months	Immuno competent, 50+ years	13-valent pneumococcal conjugate vaccine (PCV13)
Naficy, 2023 [49]	NCT05047770	454	Phase 3 Randomized open label trial	47/US	2021–2022	34 weeks	Immuno competent, 50+ years	Coronavirus Disease 2019 mRNA-1273
Galgani, 2023 [50]	NCT03894969	541	Phase 2a Randomized open label trial	14/Estonia, Finland, France, Italy, Spain	2019–2021	Up to 6 months	Healthy adults 50–80 years with history of smoking	Non-typable Hemophilus influenzae–Moraxella catarrhalis (NTHi-Mcat)
				Long-term (≥5 years) follow-up				
Chlibek, 2016 [51] Schwarz, 2018 [52] Hastie, 2021 [53]	NCT02735915	70	Phase 3B open-label single arm follow-up study	7/Czech Republic, Germany, Sweden	2016–2018 [2]	108 to 120 months after first vaccine dose	Immuno competent adults, 60+ years old	NA
Boutry, 2022 [30] Strezova, 2022 [31]	ZOE-LTFU [1]	7413	Phase 3B open-label single arm	248/Europe, North America, Latin America, and Asia	2016-Present	Up to 10 years after first vaccine dose	Immuno competent adults, 50+ years old	NA
Johnson, 2022 [54] Weinberg, 2023 [55]	NCT02114333	159	Phase 1 RCT	1/US	2014–2020	60 months	Immunocompetent adults, 50–85 years	NA

NCT = national clinical trial, ZOE = zoster efficacy study, LTFU = long-term follow-up. [1] ZOE-LTFU is follow-up study of ZOE-50 and ZOE-70 studies. [2] Original study conducted 2016–2018. This study started after 9 years of follow-up.

3.2. *Immunocompetent Populations*

Vaccine efficacy against HZ was evaluated in two pivotal phase III efficacy trials in immunocompetent populations over 50 years (ZOE-50 [23]) and 70 years (ZOE-70 [24]) (Figure 2). ZOE-50 demonstrated high efficacy against HZ (97.2%, 95% CI 93.7–99.0) after a mean follow-up of 3.5 years, while ZOE-70 demonstrated that protection is maintained in older populations (efficacy against HZ 89.8%, 95% CI 84.2–93.7, mean follow-up 3.7 years). Effectiveness in the real world is typically lower than efficacy in controlled clinical trials, and although this holds for RZV, the protection against HZ has been shown to be substantial. In immunocompetent populations, effectiveness against HZ has ranged between 70.5% (95% CI 69.0–72.0) [38] and 85.5% (95% CI 83.5–87.3) [39] in cohort studies conducted in the US.

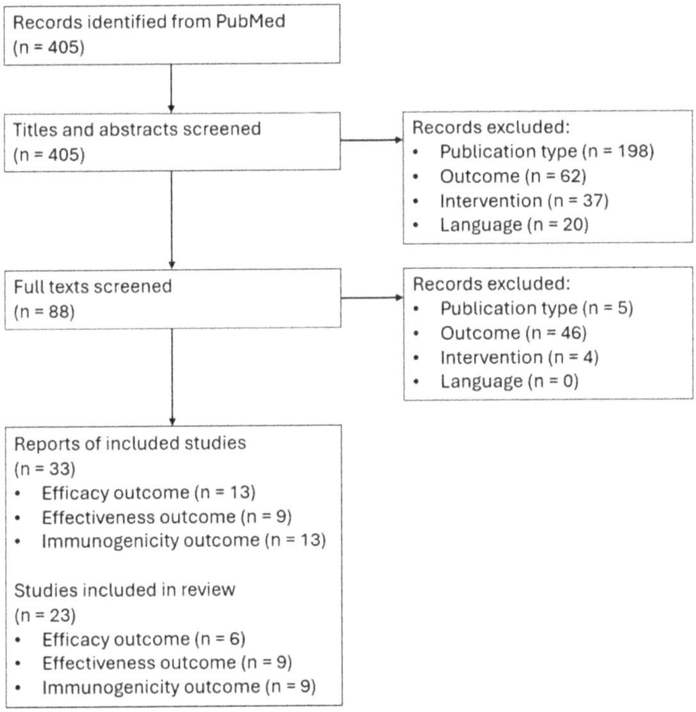

Figure 1. Study flow diagram.

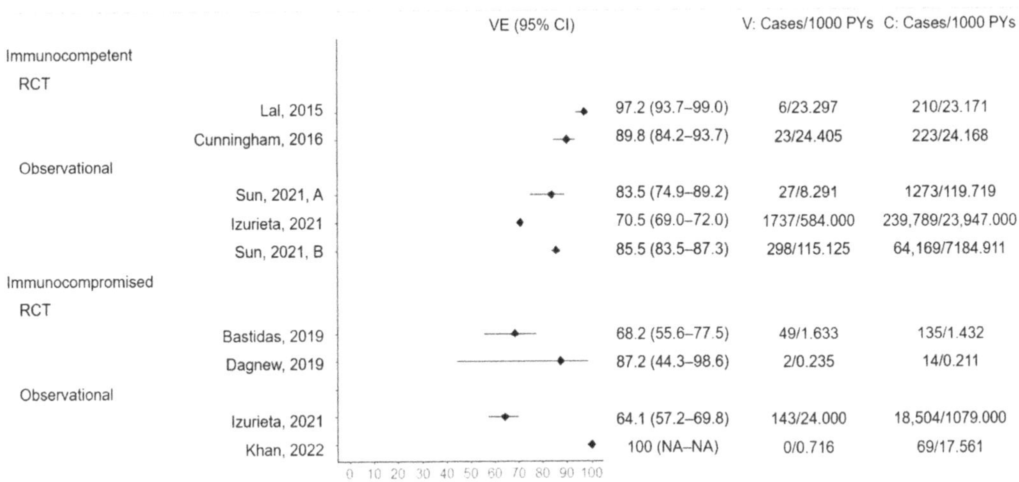

Figure 2. Vaccine efficacy and effectiveness against herpes zoster in immunocompetent and immunocompromised populations. Studies: Lal et al., 2015 (ZOE-50) [23], Cunningham et al., 2016 (ZOE-70 only) [24], Sun et al., 2021 (A) [36], Izurieta et al., 2021 (general immunocompromised status) [38], Sun et al., 2021 (B) [39], Bastidas et al., 2019 (hematopoietic stem cell recipients) [33], Dagnew et al., 2019 (Haematological malignancy patients) [35], Khan et al., 2022 (inflammatory bowel disease patients, 50–60 years age group, vaccine effectiveness calculated from hazard ratio) [42]. V = vaccine arm; C = control arm/unvaccinated; PYs = person-years.

3.3. Immunocompromised Populations

Individuals with an immunosuppressive disease or on immunosuppressive therapy were excluded from the ZOE-50 and ZOE-70 efficacy trials. However, included participants with pre-existing potential immune-mediated diseases (majority psoriasis, rheumatoid arthritis, and spondyloarthropathy) were evaluated in a post hoc analysis [28]. In this population, vaccine efficacy against HZ was 90.5% (95% CI 73.5 to 97.5). Efficacy against HZ in truly immunocompromised populations was evaluated in two RCTs: ZOE-HSCT [33] and ZOE-039 [35]. The ZOE-HSCT study of hematopoietic stem cell transplant recipients found efficacy against HZ to be lower than in the comparative immunocompetent ZOE-50 and ZOE-70 populations. However, the protection was still moderate, with an estimated efficacy of 68.2% (95% CI 55.6–77.5) (Figure 2). In a post hoc analysis stratified by disease, the sample size was moderate for patients with multiple myeloma (n = 472) and non-Hodgkin B-cell lymphoma (n = 237), for which efficacy was estimated at 72.35% (95% CI 54.76–83.71) and 60.46% (95% CI 31.02–78.16), respectively [34]. For all other diseases (non-Hodgkin T-cell lymphoma, Hodgkin lymphoma, acute myeloid leukemia, and solid malignancies and autoimmune diseases), efficacy estimates ranged from 42.5% to 100% with wide confidence intervals (Figure 3). Zoster-039 found greater protection in a population of immunocompromised patients with hematological malignancies but, due to a small number of cases in both trial arms, with low precision (vaccine efficacy = 87.2%, 95% CI 44.3–98.6).

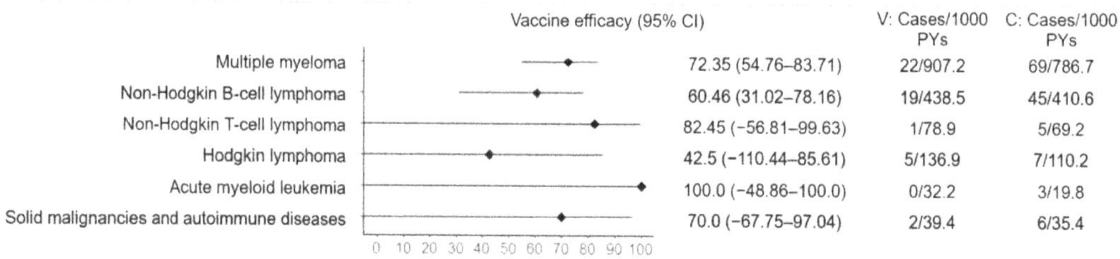

Figure 3. Vaccine efficacy against herpes zoster by disease in an immunocompromised trial population, reported by Stadtmauer et al. [34]. V = vaccine arm; C = control arm/unvaccinated; PYs = person-years.

Vaccine effectiveness in immunosuppressed populations has been assessed in two studies of inflammatory bowel disease (IBD) patients [37,42], and one prospective cohort study of Medicare C beneficiaries [38]. In the Medicare C beneficiaries cohort, vaccine effectiveness was statistically significantly lower in the immunocompromised population (64.1%, 95% CI, 57.2–69.8), compared to the immunocompetent population (70.5%, 95% CI 69.0–72.0). Both studies of IBD patients found a reduction in the risk of HZ. Khan et al. [42] used their 50–60-year age group as a proxy for a population unlikely to have had prior HZ vaccine exposure. In this group, incidence in the vaccinated reduced from 3.93 to 0.00 per 1000 person-years, while in the >60-year age group (proxy for possibility of prior HZ vaccine exposure), incidence reduced from 4.57 to 1.80 per 1000 person-years. This corresponds to 100% (95% CI not calculable) and 61% (95% CI 20–81) effectiveness against HZ in the younger and older age groups, respectively. Among a similar population of IBD patients, Kochhar et al. showed a reduction in the odds of HZ by 64% (95% CI 44–77) [37]. While multiple studies have shown that protection against HZ is lower in immunocompromised populations than immunocompetent ones, protection is still substantial.

3.4. Protection Against HZ Complications and Hospitalization

Pooled analysis of the ZOE-50 and ZOE-70 studies gave a larger sample size in which to investigate protection against PHN and other complications. In the >50-year-old vaccination cohort, PHN occurred at a rate of 0.1 cases per 1000 person-years in the vaccine arm and 0.9 cases per 1000 person-years in the placebo arm, which translated to an efficacy of 91.2% (95% CI 75.9 to 97.7) [24] (Figure 4). Only one non-PHN complication, ophthalmic disease, was recorded in the vaccine arm compared to sixteen in the placebo arm, in over 50,000 person-years of follow-up in each arm [25]. This gave an efficacy of 93.7% (95% CI 59.5 to 99.9) against non-PHN complications. Hospitalizations were also rare, with no cases observed in the RZV arm over 24,440 person-years and 5 in 24,631 years follow-up in the placebo arm. This gave a high estimated vaccine efficacy against hospitalization with wide confidence intervals (100%, 95% CI -9.9–100.0), which is consistent with ZOE-HSCT, in which the hazard ratio of hospitalization was 0.15 (95% CI, 0.03–0.68) [33]. Protection against PHN and HZO have also been shown to be high in real-world settings, with estimates ranging between 66.8% [38] and 93.3% [36] for HZO and one study reporting vaccine effectiveness of 76.0% for PHN. Again, these estimates are similar to the two-dose vaccine effectiveness against HZ (70.1%, 95% CI 68.6–71.5), suggesting negligible additional protection against complications after development of HZ.

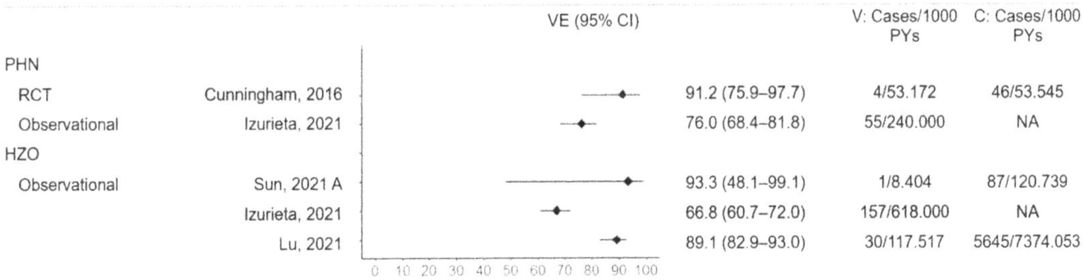

Figure 4. Vaccine efficacy and effectiveness of RZV against post-herpetic neuralgia (PHN) and herpes zoster ophthalmicus (HZO). Studies: Cunningham, 2016 [24], Izurieta, 2021 [38], Sun, 2021 (A) [36], Lu, 2021 [40]. VE = vaccine efficacy/effectiveness; V = vaccine arm; C = control arm/unvaccinated; PYs = person-years.

The risk of myocardial complications is also lower in HZ patients who have previously been vaccinated with RZV. In one retrospective case–control study, the elevated risk of stroke in HZ patients compared to non-HZ patients (OR 1.93, 95% CI 1.57–2.40) was reduced by 43% in those who had previously been vaccinated with RZV (OR vaccinated HZ patient vs. unvaccinated HZ patient 0.57, 95% CI 0.46–0.72) [44]. Increased risk of myocardial infarction in HZ patients was also reduced by 28% in those vaccinated with RZV-vaccinated HZ (OR 0.82 95% CI, 0.74–0.92) [43].

3.5. Differences in Protection Against HZ Across Populations

3.5.1. Age

In pooled ZOE-50/70 analysis, there was a slight decrease in efficacy with age, but it was statistically insignificant and estimates kept above 90% in all age groups (vaccine efficacy 50–59 years = 96.6% (95% CI 93.7–99.0), vaccine efficacy ≥80 years = 91.4 (95% CI 80.2–97.0) [24] (Figure 5). In observational studies, there has been mixed evidence for a slight reduction in people over 80 years. A retrospective cohort study conducted in the US by Sun et al. [39] found effectiveness in the ≥80-year-old population to be slightly lower (vaccine effectiveness = 80.3%, 95% CI 75.1–84.3) than in the population aged 50 to 79 years (vaccine effectiveness = 85.5%, 95% CI 83.5–87.3). Despite this, other observational studies have found no statistically significant difference across age groups [36,38].

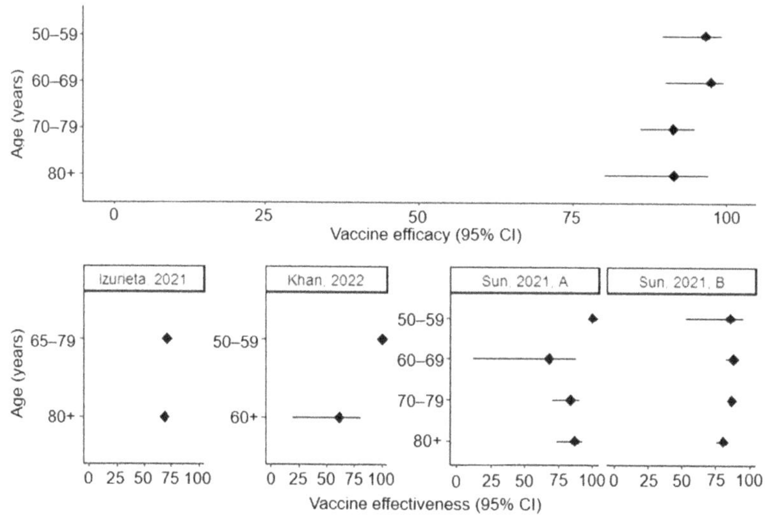

Figure 5. Vaccine efficacy and effectiveness against herpes zoster by age. Vaccine efficacy estimates taken from ZOE-50 study [23] for age groups 50–59 years and 60–69 years, and ZOE-50/70 for age groups 70–79 years and 80+ years [24]. Khan, 2022 vaccine effectiveness calculated from hazard ratio [42]. Other studies: Sun, 2021 (A) [36], Izurieta, 2021 [38], Sun, 2021 (B) [39].

3.5.2. Ethnicity

Post hoc analyses of ZOE-50/70 participants stratifying by geographic region and ethnicity found no statistically significant differences across either metric, although the sample size and therefore precision of estimates was low for some subgroups (Figure 6) [26,29]. Similarly, subgroup analyses of observational studies identified no statistically significant differences by ethnicity, but in some subgroups, there were no cases in the vaccinated cohort so confidence intervals could not be determined [36,39].

3.5.3. Sex

Post hoc analyses of data from the ZOE-50/70 trials demonstrated no impact of sex on efficacy of RZV [26,29]. Efficacy against HZ was >90% in both female and male participants in the ZOE-50/70 populations. In the pooled ZOE-50/70 analysis, efficacy against PHN was 91.5% (95% CI: 65.7–99.1) and 83.3% (95%CI 24.8–98.2) in female and male participants, respectively [26]. Sun et al. [39] reported similar estimates of vaccine effectiveness by sex (adjuvanted vaccine effectiveness in females = 84.7% (95% CI 82.2–87.0) and males = 86.8 (95% CI 83.3–89.6)).

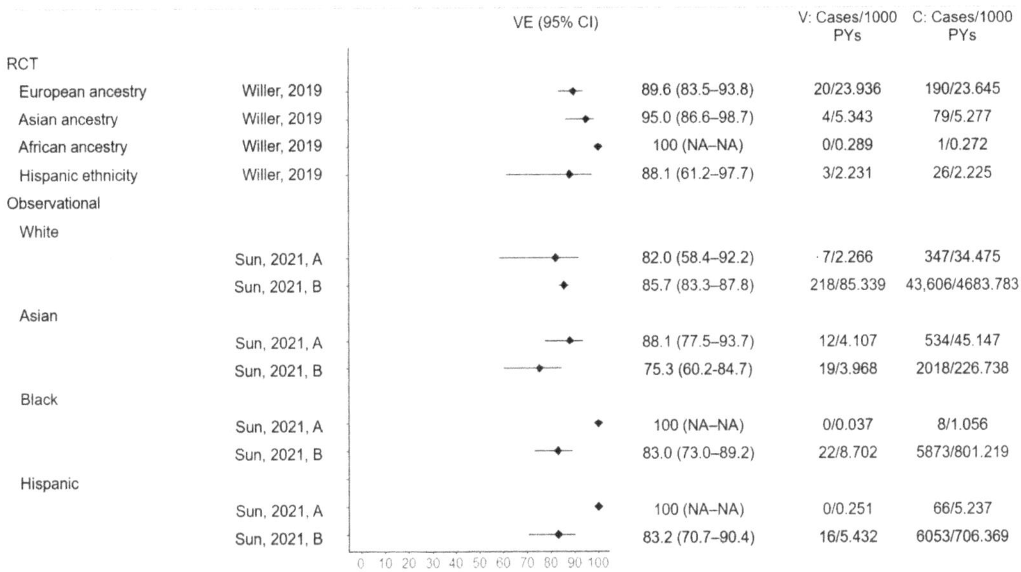

Figure 6. Vaccine efficacy and effectiveness of RZV against herpes zoster by geographic ancestry/ethnicity. RCT results reported in Willer et al. [26], observational results from Sun, 2021 (A) [36], and Sun, 2021 (B) [39]. Confidence intervals were not reported for subgroups with no cases in vaccinated cohort. VE = vaccine efficacy/effectiveness; V = vaccine arm; C = control arm/unvaccinated; PYs = person-years.

3.6. Duration of Protection

In the pooled ZOE-50/70 studies, vaccine efficacy stayed above 89% across the four-year follow-up period [31]. The ZOE-LTFU study is a long-term follow-up study of a subset of the ZOE-50/70 populations that compares the incidence of HZ in the ZOE-50/70 vaccine arm to historical controls from the placebo arm. In the most recent ZOE-LTFU interim analysis, eligible participants had been followed up for a mean of 5.6 years to 9.6 years post-vaccination [31]. The vaccine efficacy against HZ over this time period was 81.6% (95% CI 75.2–86.6). Annual estimates over time showed a gradual decline, from 88.5% (95% CI 74.9–95.6) at Y6 to 84.2% (95% CI 67.9–93.1) at Y8 and 73.2% (95% CI 46.9–87.6) at Y10 (Figure 7). Humoral immune responses were over 5-fold greater than pre-vaccination levels through 10 years post-vaccination. They were relatively constant up to Y8 but decreased slightly into Y9. Cell-mediated immune responses remained stable and over 6-fold above the pre-vaccination level through Y10. This is consistent with other long-term immunogenicity studies which have found humoral and cell-mediated immune responses to stay above pre-vaccination levels for up to 10 years after vaccination [53,55]. No vaccine effectiveness studies that evaluated the change in effectiveness over time were identified, but the study with the longest follow-up (median 3.1 years) found a vaccine effectiveness of 70.1% (95% CI 68.6–71.5) [38].

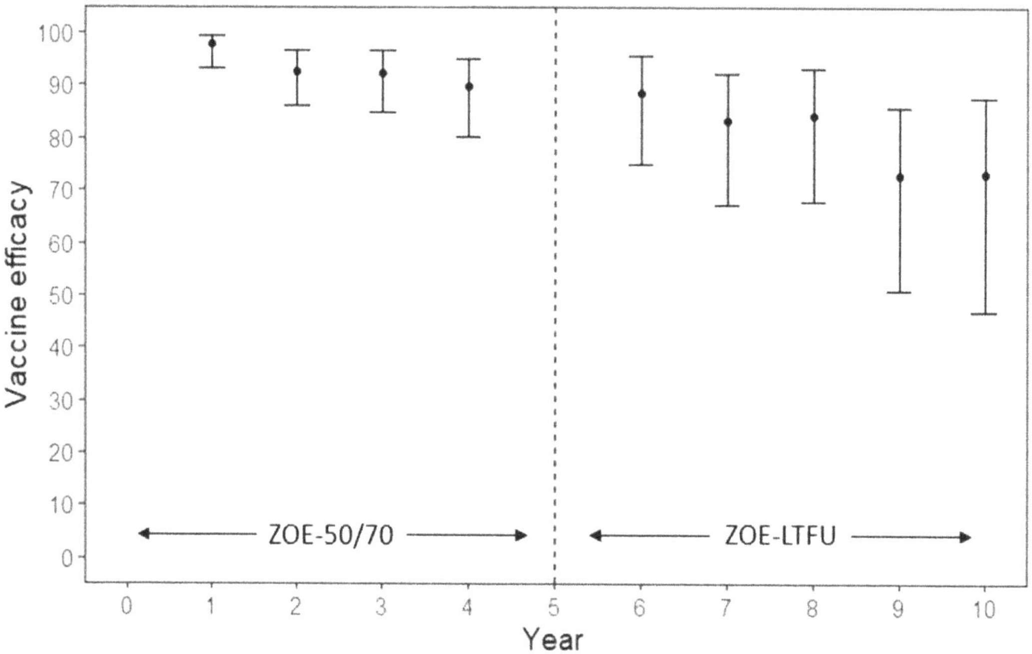

Figure 7. Vaccine efficacy (VE) against herpes zoster in the ZOE-50/70 and ZOE-LTFU studies over time since 1 month post-second dose reported in Strezova et al. [31]. No vaccine efficacy estimate given for year 5 due to switch between studies. In ZOE-50/70, VE was estimated using placebo control as comparator. In ZOE-LTFU, VE was estimated using historic controls from ZOE-50/70 placebo arm.

3.7. Prior Vaccination for HZ

To date, no studies have evaluated efficacy against HZ in participants who have previously experienced HZ or who have been vaccinated with ZVL. Izurieta et al. compared the effectiveness against HZ in Medicare beneficiaries who had and had not received ZVL vaccination within the 5 years leading to study initiation [38]. Beneficiaries unvaccinated with RZV who had previously received ZVL had a lower incidence of HZ than those who had not previously received ZVL (prior ZVL = 8.52 cases per 1000 person-years, no prior ZVL = 10.60 cases per 1000 person-years) (Figure 8). RZV provided a protective effect against HZ regardless of prior ZVL status but had greater impact on those not previously vaccinated with ZVL (effectiveness of RZV in participants with prior ZVL = 63.0%, 95% CI 58.3–67.2), effectiveness of RZV in participants without prior ZVL = 71.1%, 95% CI 69.5–72.6). Sun et al. evaluated RZV effectiveness in study participants with and without vaccination with ZVL in the year before study initiation [36]. The sample size for the population vaccinated with RZV who had received ZVL was small and only one case occurred within this group. This led to wide confidence intervals for the effectiveness estimate, making conclusions from this study on the relative protection of RZV with and without prior ZVL difficult to draw.

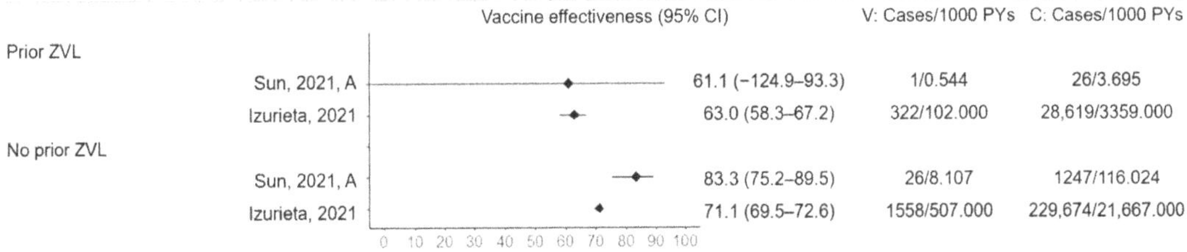

Figure 8. Vaccine effectiveness against herpes zoster in populations who had and had not previously been vaccinated with Zoster Vaccine Live (ZVL, Zostavax). Studies: Sun, 2021 (A) [36], Izurieta, 2021 [38]. V = vaccine arm; C = control arm/unvaccinated; PYs = person-years.

3.8. Co-Administration

RZV is safe and effective when co-administered at different anatomic sites with other adult vaccines. In a cohort study in Southern California [41], RZV was administered to 28,353 and 12,898 individuals with and without co-administration, and the risk of HZ was not significantly different between the groups (HR HZ co-administration vs. no co-administration = 0.75 (95% CI, 0.53–1.08)). The majority of concomitant vaccine recipients only received one other vaccine with RZV (86.6%), with the most common being influenza vaccines (65.9%), pneumococcal vaccines (20.2%), and Td/Tdap (tetanus, diphtheria/tetanus, diphtheria, and pertussis) vaccines (12.3%). This is the only study to date that has evaluated vaccine effectiveness of RZV with concomitant vaccination.

However, the immunogenicity of the RZV and the following vaccines are unaffected by co-administration: 13-valent pneumococcal conjugate vaccine (PCV13) [48], 23-valent pneumococcal polysaccharide vaccine (PPSV23) [46], quadrivalent seasonal inactivated influenza vaccine (IIV4) [45], COVID-19 mRNA-1273 [49], and reduced-antigen-content diphtheria-tetanus-acellular pertussis vaccine (Tdap) (excluding one of the 5 Tdap antigens which did not meet the humoral response non-inferiority criterion) [47] (Table 5). Sequential administration of different vaccines containing the same AS01-adjuvant system was hypothesized to have the potential to cause immune interference [50], but, in a phase 2 study reporting on the immunogenicity of a candidate AS01-adjuvanted vaccine containing four surface proteins from non-typable Hemophilus influenzae and Moraxella catarrhalis (NTHi-Mcat), no evidence was found [50].

4. Discussion

This review found that RZV is both efficacious and effective for the prevention of HZ and its complications. Efficacy in immunocompetent populations was 97% in those over 50 years and 90% in those over 70 years. While protection is lower in immunocompromised populations, it is still substantial, with efficacy estimates ranging between 68% and 87%. There is no clear evidence of a reduction in protection with age or for differences across geographies, sexes, or ethnicities, but more data on subgroups would be valuable to yield more precise estimates. The vaccine provides protection when ZVL had previously been administered and vaccine efficacy remains over 70% through at least 10 years of follow-up.

Our findings are consistent with other reviews of RZV [56–62]. Xia et al. performed a systematic review and meta-analysis to directly compare both the RZV and ZVL vaccines [56]. They found RZV to be highly efficacious in a population over 60 years, and superior to ZVL across age and genders (relative vaccine efficacy: 84%, 95% CI: 53–95, and relative vaccine effectiveness: 49%, 95% CI: 21–67). Mbinta et al. found a conservative real-world effectiveness of ZVL against HZ of 46%, 95% CI: 42–49) and a higher post hoc estimate for RZV effectiveness of 79·2% (95% CI: 57·6–89·7) [58]. However, at the time of writing, few studies had evaluated the effectiveness of RZV for protection against HZ and its complications. In a more recent systematic review and meta-analysis, Zeevaert et al. illustrated high efficacy and effectiveness of RZV for HZ in immunocompetent and immunocompromised populations (VE immunocompetent 94%, 95% CI: 79–98, VE immunocompromised 70%, 95% CI: 53–81) [61]. Yet, they note that even with high levels of protection, the number needed to vaccinate in immunocompetent populations is high for HZ, and higher still for PHN. This is an important consideration in areas where the incidence of HZ is low or unknown, such as Eastern Europe, the Middle East, South America, and Africa [14]. In these areas, more targeted vaccination campaigns for immunocompromised and older populations at greater risk may be favourable, also from a perspective of cost-effectiveness.

Our review adds to these studies by providing the most up to date and comprehensive evaluation of the efficacy, effectiveness, and immunogenicity of RZV. No reviews have included an analysis of vaccine efficacy or immunogenicity for longer than 7 years post-vaccination [61], and we provide in-depth looks at key considerations for policymakers, such as the differences in protection across age groups, ethnicities, and immunocompromising conditions.

As the incidence and risk of complications for HZ increases with age, long-term protection is an important feature of a vaccine. Vaccine efficacy and humoral and cell-mediated immune responses gradually declined over time, but the evidence presented in this review supports protection for at least 10 years after vaccination. Furthermore, the decline in immune responses is slow and modelling of immunogenicity data suggests that both cellular and humoral immune responses may persist as long as 20 years after initial vaccination [53]. To add, a recently published abstract (See Abstracts at CIDSCON 2024. Journal of Clinical Infectious Diseases Society. 2(3):163–292, Jul-Sep 2024. ABSTRACT 100: Sammya Bhowmick et al. 2024. Adjuvanted Recombinant Zoster Vaccine—The First Vaccine to Provide Durable Protection against HZ in All Age Ranges $\geq$50 Years: Final Efficacy and Safety Analysis after 11 Years of Follow-up) suggests annual vaccine efficacy against HZ at Y11 being 82.0% (95% CI 63.0–92.2) in participants $\geq$50 years and 72.0% (95% CI 33.4–89.8) in those $\geq$70 years. While this suggests a booster dose may not be necessary for many individuals, a single booster dose does elicit strong humoral and cell-mediated immune responses [53]. This may be beneficial for subpopulations that experience a higher rate of immune waning. In the ZOE-50/70 trials, there was a faster decay of gE-specific cell-mediated immunity with older age in the first four years after vaccination [24], and in a study comparing the longevity of immune responses in RZV and ZVL recipients over 5 years post-vaccination, older age had a negative effect on the persistence of anti-gE antibody levels and avidity after 2 years post-vaccination [55]. RZV-induced protection against HZ is long lasting but continued research into the duration of protection and differences across populations will be useful for informing vaccination policies.

We did not identify any publications reporting on the efficacy or effectiveness of RZV in people who had previously experienced an HZ episode. However, the immunogenicity of RZV in patients $\geq$50 years after prior HZ disease was studied in an observational study in Canada and Russia [63]. Over 90% of participants reached the primary outcome of a four-fold increase in anti-gE antibodies one month after the second vaccination. Considering this immunogenicity evidence and the additional protection provided by RZV for patients who had previously received ZVL, vaccination regardless of prior infection status is likely to be beneficial.

Strengths of this review include the broad scope, including both RCTs and observational studies without limitation on the populations included. We went into depth on stratification by immune status, age, ethnicity, sex, and prior receipt of ZVL and considered additional outcomes such as hospitalization, PHN, HZO, and myocardial complications.

These are important features for policymakers to consider when making vaccine recommendations. Limitations of our review include the small sample size for some stratifications of protection against HZ. For example, there were no vaccinated cases in people of Black or Hispanic ethnicity in observational studies evaluating vaccine effectiveness and few vaccinated cases in people of non-European ancestry in clinical trials evaluating vaccine efficacy. This makes differences in protection across ethnicities difficult to assess, and therefore an area in which further research would be valuable. Furthermore, estimates for immunocompromised populations are for a small subset of conditions, and we did not stratify by other specific comorbidities, such as HIV or rheumatoid arthritis. Finally, as we performed a rapid review, it does not comply fully with the PRISMA guidelines.

A systematic review of the reactogenicity and safety of RZV was beyond the scope of this review, but other reviews have found RZV to be safe in both RCTs and observational studies [56,57,60,61]. In the ZOE-50 and ZOE-70 trials, local reactions such as pain, redness, and swelling were more common in RZV recipients (74–82%) than placebo recipients (10–12%), but most were short-lived and lasted for a median of 2 days [61]. In RCTs of immunocompromised populations, the frequency of local reactions was similar to immunocompetent populations. Systemic reactions such as headache and myalgia were also more frequent in the vaccine than the placebo arm in trials of both immunocompetent and immunocompromised populations (RR 2.28, 95% CI: 1.45–3.65) [60]. Across trials of immunocompetent and immunocompromised populations, no differences in severe adverse events have been observed between RZV and placebo [33,35,64–66]. One cohort study on community-dwelling Medicare beneficiaries found an increased risk of Guillain–Barré syndrome in the RZV group compared to ZVL (RR 2.34, 95% CI 1.00–5.41) [67]. However, early monitoring and post-licensure safety surveillance have not confirmed this, nor identified any other SAE signals [61]. Overall, although RZV is a reactogenic vaccine, it is safe, the duration of symptoms is typically short, and it does not translate to reduced uptake of the second dose [61].

Another consideration for policymakers will be the cost effectiveness of the vaccine. The current list price in the US for RZV is $215.51 per dose [68], making it one of the most expensive vaccines available. Despite this, multiple cost-effectiveness modelling studies have shown that its long-term benefits in reducing the incidence and severity of HZ and its complications result in substantial cost savings, directly from reductions in healthcare costs and indirectly from a reduction in productivity losses. A systematic review of cost-effectiveness modelling studies found that 15 of 18 studies showed RZV to be cost effective compared to no vaccination or vaccination with ZVL, and cost-effective when revaccinating cohorts previously vaccinated with ZVL. However, all studies were conducted in North America, Europe, or Asia. Where the vaccine is considered by policymakers, context-specific economic evaluations are critical in order to take informed decisions. The cost-effectiveness will depend on the local epidemiology, healthcare systems, and potential support from non-governmental organizations in reducing the cost of vaccination for lower-income countries. In areas of Africa and South America, where there is a known high burden of disease of other life-threatening vaccine-preventable diseases such as dengue, malaria, and tuberculosis, RZV vaccination is currently unlikely to be a priority for policymakers, particularly given the high cost. RZV has the potential for great public health benefits, but without wider access to affordable vaccines it also has the potential for driving inequality both nationally and internationally.

With this being said, life-course vaccination is recognized as a global health priority, with the Immunization Agenda 2030 (IA2030) calling for the strengthening of immunization policies and service delivery throughout the life-course and for new collaborations and private-sector partnerships to mobilize financing for vaccination of older age groups.

HZ vaccination should be considered in the context of an over-all life-course approach of immunization. Ultimately, in developing policy, the results of this review should be considered jointly with local burden of disease data, given that age of disease onset may vary based on temperate or tropical climate, on current VZV policy, and vaccination uptake.

In conclusion, our comprehensive review underscores the significant protection provided by RZV against HZ and its associated complications. It highlights the good safety profile as well as the considerable efficacy and effectiveness of the vaccine, including in individuals with underlying conditions and comorbidities. However, we also demonstrated a lack of evidence from low- and middle-income countries, both on the burden of disease of HZ and on the efficacy and effectiveness of RZV, highlighting the need for improved global surveillance. The global uptake of the vaccine, including in lower resource settings, will depend on additional research as well as on consideration of factors such as the cost-effectiveness, particularly in regions with competing healthcare priorities and limited resources.

Supplementary Materials: The following supporting information can be downloaded at: https://www.mdpi.com/article/10.3390/vaccines13030250/s1, Table S1. Critical appraisal results using the Cochrane Collaboration Risk of Bias 2 Assessment tool. Table S2. Critical appraisal results using the ROBINS-I tool (Risk Of Bias In Non-randomized Studies—of Interventions).

Author Contributions: J.H. and M.M. conceptualized the study and provided supervision for the manuscript. L.R.W. and M.M. performed the formal analysis. L.R.W. performed the data visualization and wrote the original draft. All authors critically reviewed and edited the manuscript and approved the decision to submit for publication. The authors alone are responsible for the views expressed in this article and they do not necessarily represent the views, decisions, or policies of the institutions with which they are affiliated. All authors have read and agreed to the published version of the manuscript.

Funding: This research was funded by the Medical Research Council Doctoral Training Partnership Supplement Fund (to LRW).

Institutional Review Board Statement: Not applicable.

Informed Consent Statement: Not applicable.

Data Availability Statement: Data were retrieved from the articles mentioned in the references.

Acknowledgments: We would like to thank Roodly Archer for her significant support with this project.

Conflicts of Interest: The authors declare no conflict of interest.

References

1. Arvin, A.M. Varicella-zoster virus. *Clin. Microbiol. Rev.* **1996**, *9*, 361–381. [CrossRef] [PubMed]
2. Hope-Simpson, R.E. The nature of herpes zoster: A long-term study and a new hypothesis. *Proc. R. Soc. Med.* **1965**, *58*, 9–20. [CrossRef] [PubMed]
3. Pan, C.X.; Lee, M.S.; Nambudiri, V.E. Global herpes zoster incidence, burden of disease, and vaccine availability: A narrative review. *Ther. Adv. Vaccines Immunother.* **2022**, *10*, 25151355221084535. [CrossRef]
4. Harpaz, R.; Ortega-Sanchez, I.R.; Seward, J.F. Prevention of herpes zoster: Recommendations of the Advisory Committee on Immunization Practices (ACIP). *MMWR Recomm. Rep.* **2008**, *57*, 1–30; quiz CE2–CE4.
5. Schmader, K.E. Epidemiology and impact on quality of life of postherpetic neuralgia and painful diabetic neuropathy. *Clin. J. Pain* **2002**, *18*, 350–354. [CrossRef]
6. Johnson, R.W.; Alvarez-Pasquin, M.J.; Bijl, M.; Franco, E.; Gaillat, J.; Clara, J.G.; Labetoulle, M.; Michel, J.P.; Naldi, L.; Sanmarti, L.S.; et al. Herpes zoster epidemiology, management, and disease and economic burden in Europe: A multidisciplinary perspective. *Ther. Adv. Vaccines* **2015**, *3*, 109–120. [CrossRef]

7. Cohen, J.I. Herpes Zoster. *N. Engl. J. Med.* **2013**, *369*, 255–263. [CrossRef]
8. Brisson, M.; Edmunds, W.J.; Law, B.; Gay, N.J.; Walld, R.; Brownell, M.; Roos, L.L.; De Serres, G. Epidemiology of varicella zoster virus infection in Canada and the United Kingdom. *Epidemiol. Infect.* **2001**, *127*, 305–314. [CrossRef]
9. Insinga, R.P.; Itzler, R.F.; Pellissier, J.M.; Saddier, P.; Nikas, A.A. The incidence of herpes zoster in a United States administrative database. *J. Gen. Intern. Med.* **2005**, *20*, 748–753. [CrossRef]
10. Curran, D.; Callegaro, A.; Fahrbach, K.; Neupane, B.; Vroling, H.; van Oorschot, D.; Yawn, B.P. Meta-Regression of Herpes Zoster Incidence Worldwide. *Infect. Dis. Ther.* **2022**, *11*, 389–403. [CrossRef]
11. Hillebrand, K.; Bricout, H.; Schulze-Rath, R.; Schink, T.; Garbe, E. Incidence of herpes zoster and its complications in Germany, 2005–2009. *J. Infect.* **2015**, *70*, 178–186. [CrossRef] [PubMed]
12. McKay, S.L.; Guo, A.; Pergam, S.A.; Dooling, K. Herpes Zoster Risk in Immunocompromised Adults in the United States: A Systematic Review. *Clin. Infect. Dis.* **2020**, *71*, e125–e134. [CrossRef] [PubMed]
13. Yawn, B.P.; Gilden, D. The global epidemiology of herpes zoster. *Neurology* **2013**, *81*, 928–930. [CrossRef] [PubMed]
14. van Oorschot, D.; Vroling, H.; Bunge, E.; Diaz-Decaro, J.; Curran, D.; Yawn, B. A systematic literature review of herpes zoster incidence worldwide. *Hum. Vaccines Immunother.* **2021**, *17*, 1714–1732. [CrossRef]
15. Bardach, A.E.; Palermo, C.; Alconada, T.; Sandoval, M.; Balan, D.J.; Nieto Guevara, J.; Gómez, J.; Ciapponi, A. Herpes zoster epidemiology in Latin America: A systematic review and meta-analysis. *PLoS ONE* **2021**, *16*, e0255877. [CrossRef]
16. Kawai, K.; Gebremeskel, B.G.; Acosta, C.J. Systematic review of incidence and complications of herpes zoster: Towards a global perspective. *BMJ Open* **2014**, *4*, e004833. [CrossRef]
17. Hussey, H.; Abdullahi, L.; Collins, J.; Muloiwa, R.; Hussey, G.; Kagina, B. Varicella zoster virus-associated morbidity and mortality in Africa—A systematic review. *BMC Infect. Dis.* **2017**, *17*, 717. [CrossRef]
18. Schmader, K.E.; Oxman, M.N.; Levin, M.J.; Johnson, G.; Zhang, J.H.; Betts, R.; Morrison, V.A.; Gelb, L.; Guatelli, J.C.; Harbecke, R.; et al. Persistence of the efficacy of zoster vaccine in the shingles prevention study and the short-term persistence substudy. *Clin. Infect. Dis.* **2012**, *55*, 1320–1328. [CrossRef]
19. Oxman, M.N.; Levin, M.J.; Johnson, G.R.; Schmader, K.E.; Straus, S.E.; Gelb, L.D.; Arbeit, R.D.; Simberkoff, M.S.; Gershon, A.A.; Davis, L.E.; et al. A vaccine to prevent herpes zoster and postherpetic neuralgia in older adults. *N. Engl. J. Med.* **2005**, *352*, 2271–2284. [CrossRef]
20. Baxter, R.; Bartlett, J.; Fireman, B.; Marks, M.; Hansen, J.; Lewis, E.; Aukes, L.; Chen, Y.; Klein, N.P.; Saddier, P. Long-Term Effectiveness of the Live Zoster Vaccine in Preventing Shingles: A Cohort Study. *Am. J. Epidemiol.* **2018**, *187*, 161–169. [CrossRef]
21. Leroux-Roels, I.; Leroux-Roels, G.; Clement, F.; Vandepapelière, P.; Vassilev, V.; Ledent, E.; Heineman, T.C. A phase 1/2 clinical trial evaluating safety and immunogenicity of a varicella zoster glycoprotein e subunit vaccine candidate in young and older adults. *J. Infect. Dis.* **2012**, *206*, 1280–1290. [CrossRef]
22. O'Connor, A.M. Interpretation of Odds and Risk Ratios. *J. Vet. Intern. Med.* **2013**, *27*, 600–603. [CrossRef]
23. Lal, H.; Cunningham, A.L.; Godeaux, O.; Chlibek, R.; Diez-Domingo, J.; Hwang, S.J.; Levin, M.J.; McElhaney, J.E.; Poder, A.; Puig-Barberà, J.; et al. Efficacy of an adjuvanted herpes zoster subunit vaccine in older adults. *N. Engl. J. Med.* **2015**, *372*, 2087–2096. [CrossRef] [PubMed]
24. Cunningham, A.L.; Lal, H.; Kovac, M.; Chlibek, R.; Hwang, S.J.; Díez-Domingo, J.; Godeaux, O.; Levin, M.J.; McElhaney, J.E.; Puig-Barberà, J.; et al. Efficacy of the Herpes Zoster Subunit Vaccine in Adults 70 Years of Age or Older. *N. Engl. J. Med.* **2016**, *375*, 1019–1032. [CrossRef] [PubMed]
25. Kovac, M.; Lal, H.; Cunningham, A.L.; Levin, M.J.; Johnson, R.W.; Campora, L.; Volpi, A.; Heineman, T.C. Complications of herpes zoster in immunocompetent older adults: Incidence in vaccine and placebo groups in two large phase 3 trials. *Vaccine* **2018**, *36*, 1537–1541. [CrossRef]
26. Willer, D.O.; Oostvogels, L.; Cunningham, A.L.; Gervais, P.; Gorfinkel, I.; Hyung Kim, J.; Talarico, C.; Wascotte, V.; Zahaf, T.; Colindres, R.; et al. Efficacy of the adjuvanted recombinant zoster vaccine (RZV) by sex, geographic region, and geographic ancestry/ethnicity: A post-hoc analysis of the ZOE-50 and ZOE-70 randomized trials. *Vaccine* **2019**, *37*, 6262–6267. [CrossRef]
27. Curran, D.; Kim, J.H.; Matthews, S.; Dessart, C.; Levin, M.J.; Oostvogels, L.; Riley, M.E.; Schmader, K.E.; Cunningham, A.L.; McNeil, S.A.; et al. Recombinant Zoster Vaccine Is Efficacious and Safe in Frail Individuals. *J. Am. Geriatr. Soc.* **2021**, *69*, 744–752. [CrossRef]
28. Dagnew, A.F.; Rausch, D.; Hervé, C.; Zahaf, T.; Levin, M.J.; Schuind, A. Efficacy and serious adverse events profile of the adjuvanted recombinant zoster vaccine in adults with pre-existing potential immune-mediated diseases: A pooled post hoc analysis on two parallel randomized trials. *Rheumatology* **2021**, *60*, 1226–1233. [CrossRef]
29. Kim, J.H.; Diaz-Decaro, J.; Jiang, N.; Hwang, S.J.; Choo, E.J.; Co, M.; Hastie, A.; Hui, D.S.C.; Irimajiri, J.; Lee, J.; et al. The adjuvanted recombinant zoster vaccine is efficacious and safe in Asian adults $\geq$50 years of age: A sub-cohort analysis of the ZOE-50 and ZOE-70 randomized trials. *Hum. Vaccines Immunother.* **2021**, *17*, 2050–2057. [CrossRef]

30. Boutry, C.; Hastie, A.; Diez-Domingo, J.; Tinoco, J.C.; Yu, C.J.; Andrews, C.; Beytout, J.; Caso, C.; Cheng, H.S.; Cheong, H.J.; et al. The Adjuvanted Recombinant Zoster Vaccine Confers Long-Term Protection Against Herpes Zoster: Interim Results of an Extension Study of the Pivotal Phase 3 Clinical Trials ZOE-50 and ZOE-70. *Clin. Infect. Dis.* **2022**, *74*, 1459–1467. [CrossRef]
31. Strezova, A.; Diez-Domingo, J.; Al Shawafi, K.; Tinoco, J.C.; Shi, M.; Pirrotta, P.; Mwakingwe-Omari, A. Long-term Protection Against Herpes Zoster by the Adjuvanted Recombinant Zoster Vaccine: Interim Efficacy, Immunogenicity, and Safety Results up to 10 Years After Initial Vaccination. *Open Forum Infect. Dis.* **2022**, *9*, ofac485. [CrossRef] [PubMed]
32. Oostvogels, L.; Heineman, T.C.; Johnson, R.W.; Levin, M.J.; McElhaney, J.E.; Van den Steen, P.; Zahaf, T.; Dagnew, A.F.; Chlibek, R.; Diez-Domingo, J.; et al. Medical conditions at enrollment do not impact efficacy and safety of the adjuvanted recombinant zoster vaccine: A pooled post-hoc analysis of two parallel randomized trials. *Hum. Vaccines Immunother.* **2019**, *15*, 2865–2872. [CrossRef] [PubMed]
33. Bastidas, A.; de la Serna, J.; El Idrissi, M.; Oostvogels, L.; Quittet, P.; López-Jiménez, J.; Vural, F.; Pohlreich, D.; Zuckerman, T.; Issa, N.C.; et al. Effect of Recombinant Zoster Vaccine on Incidence of Herpes Zoster After Autologous Stem Cell Transplantation: A Randomized Clinical Trial. *JAMA* **2019**, *322*, 123–133. [CrossRef] [PubMed]
34. Stadtmauer, E.A.; Sullivan, K.M.; El Idrissi, M.; Salaun, B.; Alonso Alonso, A.; Andreadis, C.; Anttila, V.J.; Bloor, A.J.; Broady, R.; Cellini, C.; et al. Adjuvanted recombinant zoster vaccine in adult autologous stem cell transplant recipients: Polyfunctional immune responses and lessons for clinical practice. *Hum. Vaccines Immunother.* **2021**, *17*, 4144–4154. [CrossRef]
35. Dagnew, A.F.; Ilhan, O.; Lee, W.S.; Woszczyk, D.; Kwak, J.Y.; Bowcock, S.; Sohn, S.K.; Rodriguez Macías, G.; Chiou, T.J.; Quiel, D.; et al. Immunogenicity and safety of the adjuvanted recombinant zoster vaccine in adults with haematological malignancies: A phase 3, randomised, clinical trial and post-hoc efficacy analysis. *Lancet Infect. Dis.* **2019**, *19*, 988–1000. [CrossRef]
36. Sun, Y.; Jackson, K.; Dalmon, C.A.; Shapiro, B.L.; Nie, S.; Wong, C.; Arnold, B.F.; Porco, T.C.; Acharya, N.R. Effectiveness of the recombinant zoster vaccine among Kaiser Permanente Hawaii enrollees aged 50 and older: A retrospective cohort study. *Vaccine* **2021**, *39*, 3974–3982. [CrossRef]
37. Kochhar, G.S.; Desai, A.; Caldera, D.F.; El Hachem, S.; Aoun, E.; Sandhu, D.; Mohan, B.P.; Dulai, P.S.; Farraye, F.A. Effectiveness of recombinant zoster vaccine (RZV) in patients with inflammatory bowel disease. *Vaccine* **2021**, *39*, 4199–4202. [CrossRef]
38. Izurieta, H.S.; Wu, X.; Forshee, R.; Lu, Y.; Sung, H.M.; Agger, P.E.; Chillarige, Y.; Link-Gelles, R.; Lufkin, B.; Wernecke, M.; et al. Recombinant Zoster Vaccine (Shingrix): Real-World Effectiveness in the First 2 Years Post-Licensure. *Clin. Infect. Dis.* **2021**, *73*, 941–948. [CrossRef]
39. Sun, Y.; Kim, E.; Kong, C.L.; Arnold, B.F.; Porco, T.C.; Acharya, N.R. Effectiveness of the Recombinant Zoster Vaccine in Adults Aged 50 and Older in the United States: A Claims-Based Cohort Study. *Clin. Infect. Dis.* **2021**, *73*, 949–956. [CrossRef]
40. Lu, A.; Sun, Y.; Porco, T.C.; Arnold, B.F.; Acharya, N.R. Effectiveness of the Recombinant Zoster Vaccine for Herpes Zoster Ophthalmicus in the United States. *Ophthalmology* **2021**, *128*, 1699–1707. [CrossRef]
41. Bruxvoort, K.J.; Qian, L.; Wu, J.; Florea, A.; Ackerson, B.; Sy, L.S.; Vega Daily, L.; Takhar, H.; Tseng, H.F. Herpes Zoster Following Recombinant Zoster Vaccine with or Without Concomitant Vaccination. *Open Forum Infect. Dis.* **2022**, *9*, ofac011. [CrossRef] [PubMed]
42. Khan, N.; Wang, L.; Trivedi, C.; Pernes, T.; Patel, M.; Xie, D.; Yang, Y.X. Efficacy of Recombinant Zoster Vaccine in Patients with Inflammatory Bowel Disease. *Clin. Gastroenterol. Hepatol.* **2022**, *20*, 1570–1578.e1571. [CrossRef] [PubMed]
43. Parameswaran, G.I.; Drye, A.F.; Wattengel, B.A.; Carter, M.T.; Doyle, K.M.; Mergenhagen, K.A. Increased Myocardial Infarction Risk Following Herpes Zoster Infection. *Open Forum Infect. Dis.* **2023**, *10*, ofad137. [CrossRef]
44. Parameswaran, G.I.; Wattengel, B.A.; Chua, H.C.; Swiderek, J.; Fuchs, T.; Carter, M.T.; Goode, L.; Doyle, K.; Mergenhagen, K.A. Increased Stroke Risk Following Herpes Zoster Infection and Protection with Zoster Vaccine. *Clin. Infect. Dis.* **2023**, *76*, e1335–e1340. [CrossRef]
45. Schwarz, T.F.; Aggarwal, N.; Moeckesch, B.; Schenkenberger, I.; Claeys, C.; Douha, M.; Godeaux, O.; Grupping, K.; Heineman, T.C.; Fauqued, M.L.; et al. Immunogenicity and Safety of an Adjuvanted Herpes Zoster Subunit Vaccine Coadministered with Seasonal Influenza Vaccine in Adults Aged 50 Years or Older. *J. Infect. Dis.* **2017**, *216*, 1352–1361. [CrossRef]
46. Maréchal, C.; Lal, H.; Poder, A.; Ferguson, M.; Enweonye, I.; Heineman, T.C.; Hervé, C.; Rheault, P.; Talli, J.; Wauters, D.; et al. Immunogenicity and safety of the adjuvanted recombinant zoster vaccine co-administered with the 23-valent pneumococcal polysaccharide vaccine in adults ≥50 years of age: A randomized trial. *Vaccine* **2018**, *36*, 4278–4286. [CrossRef]
47. Strezova, A.; Lal, H.; Enweonye, I.; Campora, L.; Beukelaers, P.; Segall, N.; Heineman, T.C.; Schuind, A.E.; Oostvogels, L. The adjuvanted recombinant zoster vaccine co-administered with a tetanus, diphtheria and pertussis vaccine in adults aged ≥50 years: A randomized trial. *Vaccine* **2019**, *37*, 5877–5885. [CrossRef]
48. Min, J.Y.; Mwakingwe-Omari, A.; Riley, M.; Molo, L.Y.; Soni, J.; Girard, G.; Danier, J. The adjuvanted recombinant zoster vaccine co-administered with the 13-valent pneumococcal conjugate vaccine in adults aged ≥50 years: A randomized trial. *J. Infect.* **2022**, *84*, 490–498. [CrossRef]

49. Naficy, A.; Kuxhausen, A.; Pirrotta, P.; Leav, B.; Miller, J.; Anteyi, K.; Danier, J.; Breuer, T.; Mwakingwe-Omari, A. No immunological interference or safety concerns when adjuvanted recombinant zoster vaccine is coadministered with a COVID-19 mRNA-1273 booster vaccine in adults aged 50 years and older: A randomized trial. *Clin. Infect. Dis.* **2023**, *77*, 1238–1246. [CrossRef]
50. Galgani, I.; Põder, A.; Jõgi, R.; Anttila, V.J.; Milleri, S.; Borobia, A.M.; Launay, O.; Testa, M.; Casula, D.; Grassano, L.; et al. Immunogenicity and safety of the non-typable Haemophilus influenzae-Moraxella catarrhalis (NTHi-Mcat) vaccine administered following the recombinant zoster vaccine versus administration alone: Results from a randomized, phase 2a, non-inferiority trial. *Hum. Vaccines Immunother.* **2023**, *19*, 2187194. [CrossRef]
51. Chlibek, R.; Pauksens, K.; Rombo, L.; van Rijckevorsel, G.; Richardus, J.H.; Plassmann, G.; Schwarz, T.F.; Catteau, G.; Lal, H.; Heineman, T.C. Long-term immunogenicity and safety of an investigational herpes zoster subunit vaccine in older adults. *Vaccine* **2016**, *34*, 863–868. [CrossRef] [PubMed]
52. Schwarz, T.F.; Volpe, S.; Catteau, G.; Chlibek, R.; David, M.P.; Richardus, J.H.; Lal, H.; Oostvogels, L.; Pauksens, K.; Ravault, S.; et al. Persistence of immune response to an adjuvanted varicella-zoster virus subunit vaccine for up to year nine in older adults. *Hum. Vaccines Immunother.* **2018**, *14*, 1370–1377. [CrossRef] [PubMed]
53. Hastie, A.; Catteau, G.; Enemuo, A.; Mrkvan, T.; Salaun, B.; Volpe, S.; Smetana, J.; Rombo, L.; Schwarz, T.; Pauksens, K.; et al. Immunogenicity of the Adjuvanted Recombinant Zoster Vaccine: Persistence and Anamnestic Response to Additional Doses Administered 10 Years After Primary Vaccination. *J. Infect. Dis.* **2021**, *224*, 2025–2034. [CrossRef] [PubMed]
54. Johnson, M.J.; Liu, C.; Ghosh, D.; Lang, N.; Levin, M.J.; Weinberg, A. Cell-Mediated Immune Responses After Administration of the Live or the Recombinant Zoster Vaccine: 5-Year Persistence. *J. Infect. Dis.* **2022**, *225*, 1477–1481. [CrossRef] [PubMed]
55. Weinberg, A.; Schmid, D.S.; Leung, J.; Johnson, M.J.; Miao, C.; Levin, M.J. Predictors of Five-Year Persistence of Antibody Responses to Zoster Vaccines. *J. Infect. Dis.* **2023**, *228*, 1367–1374. [CrossRef]
56. Xia, Y.; Zhang, X.; Zhang, L.; Fu, C. Efficacy, effectiveness, and safety of herpes zoster vaccine in the immunocompetent and immunocompromised subjects: A systematic review and network meta-analysis. *Front. Immunol.* **2022**, *13*, 978203. [CrossRef]
57. Racine, É.; Gilca, V.; Amini, R.; Tunis, M.; Ismail, S.; Sauvageau, C. A systematic literature review of the recombinant subunit herpes zoster vaccine use in immunocompromised 18–49 year old patients. *Vaccine* **2020**, *38*, 6205–6214. [CrossRef]
58. Mbinta, J.F.; Nguyen, B.P.; Awuni, P.M.A.; Paynter, J.; Simpson, C.R. Post-licensure zoster vaccine effectiveness against herpes zoster and postherpetic neuralgia in older adults: A systematic review and meta-analysis. *Lancet Healthy Longev.* **2022**, *3*, e263–e275. [CrossRef]
59. Silverii, G.A.; Clerico, A.; Fornengo, R.; Gabutti, G.; Sordi, V.; Peruzzi, O.; Tafuri, S.; Mannucci, E.; Dicembrini, I. Efficacy and effectiveness of Herpes zoster vaccination in adults with diabetes mellitus: A systematic review and meta-analysis of clinical trials and observational studies. *Acta Diabetol.* **2023**, *60*, 1343–1349. [CrossRef]
60. Tricco, A.C.; Zarin, W.; Cardoso, R.; Veroniki, A.A.; Khan, P.A.; Nincic, V.; Ghassemi, M.; Warren, R.; Sharpe, J.P.; Page, A.V.; et al. Efficacy, effectiveness, and safety of herpes zoster vaccines in adults aged 50 and older: Systematic review and network meta-analysis. *BMJ* **2018**, *363*, k4029. [CrossRef]
61. Zeevaert, R.; Thiry, N.; Maertens de Noordhout, C.; Roberfroid, D. Efficacy and safety of the recombinant zoster vaccine: A systematic review and meta-analysis. *Vaccine X* **2023**, *15*, 100397. [CrossRef] [PubMed]
62. de Oliveira Gomes, J.; Gagliardi, A.M.Z.; Andriolo, B.N.G.; Torloni, M.R.; Andriolo, R.B.; Puga, M.E.; Canteiro Cruz, E. Vaccines for preventing herpes zoster in older adults. *Cochrane Database Syst. Rev.* **2023**, *10*, CD008858. [CrossRef] [PubMed]
63. Godeaux, O.; Kovac, M.; Shu, D.; Grupping, K.; Campora, L.; Douha, M.; Heineman, T.C.; Lal, H. Immunogenicity and safety of an adjuvanted herpes zoster subunit candidate vaccine in adults ≥50 years of age with a prior history of herpes zoster: A phase III, non-randomized, open-label clinical trial. *Hum. Vaccines Immunother.* **2017**, *13*, 1051–1058. [CrossRef] [PubMed]
64. Vink, P.; Delgado Mingorance, I.; Maximiano Alonso, C.; Rubio-Viqueira, B.; Jung, K.H.; Rodriguez Moreno, J.F.; Grande, E.; Marrupe Gonzalez, D.; Lowndes, S.; Puente, J.; et al. Immunogenicity and safety of the adjuvanted recombinant zoster vaccine in patients with solid tumors, vaccinated before or during chemotherapy: A randomized trial. *Cancer* **2019**, *125*, 1301–1312. [CrossRef]
65. Vink, P.; Ramon Torrell, J.M.; Sanchez Fructuoso, A.; Kim, S.J.; Kim, S.I.; Zaltzman, J.; Ortiz, F.; Campistol Plana, J.M.; Fernandez Rodriguez, A.M.; Rebollo Rodrigo, H.; et al. Immunogenicity and Safety of the Adjuvanted Recombinant Zoster Vaccine in Chronically Immunosuppressed Adults Following Renal Transplant: A Phase 3, Randomized Clinical Trial. *Clin. Infect. Dis.* **2020**, *70*, 181–190. [CrossRef]
66. López-Fauqued, M.; Campora, L.; Delannois, F.; El Idrissi, M.; Oostvogels, L.; De Looze, F.J.; Diez-Domingo, J.; Heineman, T.C.; Lal, H.; McElhaney, J.E.; et al. Safety profile of the adjuvanted recombinant zoster vaccine: Pooled analysis of two large randomised phase 3 trials. *Vaccine* **2019**, *37*, 2482–2493. [CrossRef]

67. Goud, R.; Lufkin, B.; Duffy, J.; Whitaker, B.; Wong, H.L.; Liao, J.; Lo, A.C.; Parulekar, S.; Agger, P.; Anderson, S.A.; et al. Risk of Guillain-Barré Syndrome Following Recombinant Zoster Vaccine in Medicare Beneficiaries. *JAMA Intern. Med.* **2021**, *181*, 1623–1630. [CrossRef]
68. GlaxoSmithKline. GSK Pricing Information. Available online: https://www.gskforyou.com/gsk-pricing-information/ (accessed on 9 May 2024).

vaccines

MDPI

Systematic Review

Immunogenicity, Efficacy, and Effectiveness of Two-Dose and Shorter Schedules of Hepatitis E Vaccine: A Systematic Review

Bilal Azam [1], Melanie Marti [2], Amit Goel [3] and Rakesh Aggarwal [1,*]

[1] Department of Gastroenterology, Jawaharlal Institute of Postgraduate Medical Education and Research, Puducherry 605006, India; bilalazampgi@gmail.com
[2] Immunization, Vaccines and Biologicals, World Health Organization, 1211 Geneva, Switzerland
[3] Department of Hepatology, Sanjay Gandhi Postgraduate Institute of Medical Sciences, Lucknow 226014, India; agoel.ag@gmail.com
* Correspondence: aggarwal.ra@gmail.com

Abstract: Background: Hepatitis E virus (HEV) is a leading cause of acute viral hepatitis in adults. The schedule for HEV 239, the only approved anti-HEV vaccine, consists of three doses at 0, 1, and 6 months, which is unsuitable for use in emergency and outbreak situations where quick protection is desired. We, therefore, undertook a systematic review of data on immunogenicity, efficacy, and effectiveness of alternative accelerated schedules. **Methods**: Data sources on immunogenicity, efficacy, and effectiveness of the HEV 239 vaccine following accelerated schedules published between 22 January 2005 and February 2024 were identified from five electronic databases, and the relevant data were extracted. **Results**: The search identified seven relevant reports, including one phase II pre-licensure trial, three reports from the phase III licensure trial, and three post-licensure reports. In these studies, following administration of the HEV 239 vaccine in two doses at 0 and 1 month or a three-dose rapid (0, 7, and 21 days) schedule, anti-HEV antibody seroconversion rates were similar to and geometric mean concentrations of anti-HEV antibody were only slightly lower than those following the standard three-dose schedule. In individuals who were seropositive for anti-HEV antibodies at baseline, the antibody response persisted for several years irrespective of the number of vaccine doses, and in those who were seronegative at baseline, administration of two vaccine doses induced antibodies whose level remained substantially high till at least 13 months of follow-up. Administration of two doses was also associated with a high protective efficacy against HEV infection and associated disease. **Conclusions**: The available data indicate that two doses of HEV 239 administered one month apart confer sufficiently high antibody titers and protection for at least 13 months, a duration which should be adequate for its use as an outbreak control measure.

Keywords: hepatitis E; HEV 239; shorter schedule; immunogenicity; efficacy

1. Introduction

Hepatitis E is the most common cause of acute viral hepatitis in adults. It is caused by infection with hepatitis E virus (HEV), which has 27–34 nm diameter virions with a single-stranded RNA [1]. The viral genome has three open reading frames [1]; of these, the ORF1 encodes for the viral non-structural proteins, ORF2 for the capsid protein, and ORF3 for a protein with multiple functions. The virus has eight genotypes, four of which (namely, genotypes 1–4) are most frequently associated with human infections [2,3]. Genotypes 1 and 2 HEV affect only humans; by contrast, genotypes 3 and 4 HEV primarily infect pigs and several other mammalian species and are only occasionally transmitted to humans [2].

Clinical consequences of HEV infection vary from asymptomatic infection to typical acute hepatitis and occasionally acute liver failure, especially in pregnant women [4]. An infrequent presentation is chronic HEV infection, observed with genotypes 3 and 4 viruses, especially among those with immunosuppression [5].

HEV 239 (Hecolin®) is a hepatitis E vaccine that contains a recombinant 239-amino acid protein corresponding to amino acid 368–606 of ORF2 protein of genotype 1 HEV, expressed in *Escherichia coli* [6,7]. It is approved in China (2011) and Pakistan (2021) and has recently received marketing authorization in India. The recommended schedule is three intramuscular doses of 0.5 mL each (containing 30 μg of HEV antigen) at 0, 1, and 6 months among persons aged 16 years or above. This regimen is known to induce a strong antibody response and provides good protection against hepatitis E for at least 10 years [8]. The use of this three-dose (0, 1, 6 months) schedule was based on the results of a phase II study [9], in which this schedule induced a higher antibody titer compared to a two-dose schedule (0, 6 months), though the seroconversion rates with the two schedules were similar [9].

An important use case for this vaccine is for the control of HEV outbreaks [10], as exemplified by its recent use in an internally displaced population in Bentiu, South Sudan [10]. However, the three-dose schedule spread over 6 months is difficult to implement during outbreaks, especially when these occur in areas with mobile populations, conflict situations, and humanitarian emergencies. For instance, in the South Sudan campaign, though 86% of the eligible population took the first dose, the coverage for the second and third doses was only 73% and 58%, respectively [10].

Thus, there is a need for alternative schedules of this vaccine with fewer doses or a more rapid time-course. The regimens with fewer doses, besides being more practical and easier to administer, will also be less costly. Further, the shorter schedules should also be useful for emergency responders and international humanitarian workers, who need to be rapidly deployed.

We, therefore, decided to undertake a systematic review of the available data on immunogenicity, efficacy/effectiveness, safety, and duration of protection following the HEV 239 vaccine when administered in shorter-duration schedules with fewer than three doses or with reduced time intervals between doses.

2. Materials and Methods

Relevant articles were identified through a search of several databases [Medline OvidSP, EMBASE, Cochrane CENTRAL, PubMed, and International Clinical Trials Registry], using the following search terms: 'Hepatitis E vaccin*'; 'HEV 239'; 'Hecolin'; 'Hepatitis E/prevention and control'; and 'Hepatitis E*/immunolog*' on 22 February 2024. Titles and abstracts of the articles so identified were screened using the inclusion and exclusion criteria in Table 1. From the selected studies, data on seroconversion rates and antibody titers at different time points for various schedules were extracted by two reviewers.

Table 1. Inclusion and exclusion criteria applied to the results of the literature search.

Inclusion Criteria
• Contains data on immunogenicity, efficacy, or effectiveness of *Escherichia coli* expressed HEV 239 virus-like particle (VLP) recombinant protein vaccine (Hecolin®), with fewer than 3 doses or a shorter time interval between doses; • Either a clinical trial or observational study; • Populations: All; • Language restriction: None.
Exclusion Criteria
• Not hepatitis E vaccine or Hecolin®; • Non-human studies; • Pre-clinical studies, systematic reviews, and the grey literature.

3. Results

3.1. A Literature Search

The initial search identified a total of 47 records (Figure 1). After two reviewers (BA, RA) screened their titles and abstracts, 14 sources were identified for full-text assessment. Of these, seven papers met the inclusion criteria and were further analyzed; these are summarized in Table 2. A list of data sources that were excluded is available as Supplementary Materials Table S1.

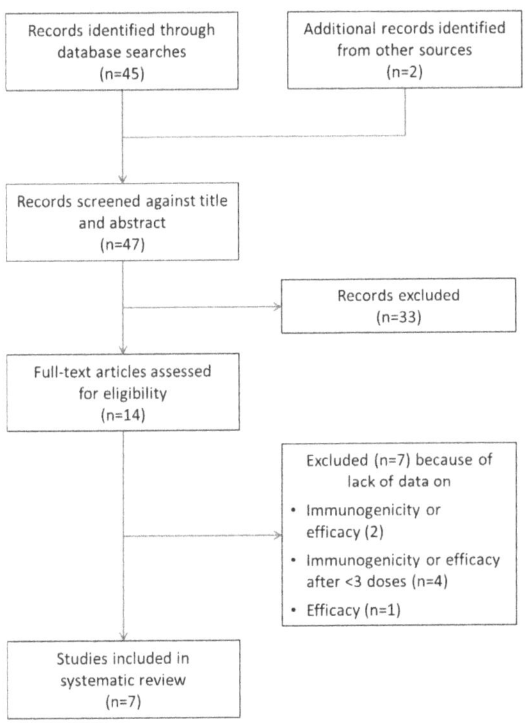

Figure 1. Flow chart showing the process of the literature search and screening for eligibility.

Table 2. List of studies identified for inclusion in the review.

Author, Year (Reference Number); Location	Brief Description	Type of Data Included	Number of Planned Doses/Schedules	Characteristics of Study Subjects	Number of Subjects
During Initial Vaccine Development					
Zhang et al., 2009 [9]; China	Pre-licensure phase II study	Immunogenicity, efficacy	2 doses (0, 6 months) vs. 3 doses (0, 1, and 6 months)	Healthy adults (age 16–55 years); seronegative	457
Zhu et al., 2010 [11]; China Zhang et al., 2015 [12]; China Huang et al., 2024 [6]; China	Phase III (licensure) study Longer term follow-up (4.5 years) of phase III study Longer term follow-up (10 years) of phase III study	Immunogenicity, efficacy	3 doses (0, 1, and 6 months); however, it includes data on immunogenicity and efficacy in some subjects who received fewer doses	Community volunteers aged 16–65 years; irrespective of HEV serostatus (47% seropositive)	112,604
Post-Licensure Studies					
Chen et al., 2019 [13]; China	Clinical trial of a 3-dose accelerated schedule (0, 7, and 21 days)	Immunogenicity	3 doses in accelerated (0, 7, and 21 days) vs. usual (0, 1, and 6 months) schedule	Healthy adults aged 18 years or older; seronegative	126
Øverbø et al., 2023 [14]; Bangladesh	Clinical trial of a 2-dose schedule versus a 3-dose schedule of hepatitis B vaccine	Immunogenicity, efficacy	2 doses (0 and 1 months)	Healthy volunteers aged 16–39 years, irrespective of serostatus (33% seropositive)	100
Kao et al., 2024 [15]; USA	Phase I study for the United States population	Immunogenicity	3 doses (0, 1, and 6 month); includes data on antibody response after 1 or 2 doses.	Healthy adults in the United States; seronegative	25

3.2. Immunogenicity

The data on antibody responses following one or two doses or following rapid three-dose regimens of the HEV 239 vaccine in humans were available from reports on pre-licensure phase II [9] and phase III [6,11,12] trials during vaccine development and from three reports on post-licensure studies [13–15]. Some of these reports were studies using the standard three-dose schedule that also provided data at a timepoint before the third vaccine dose had been administered or on study participants who, for some reason, did not receive all three planned doses.

3.2.1. Pre-Licensure Phase II Trial

This study included healthy persons aged 16–65 years (33% women) in China who were negative for anti-HEV antibodies [9]. It had two parts: a dose-escalation component to determine the optimum amount of antigen in each dose and a dose-scheduling component to determine the optimum number of vaccine doses.

In the dose-scheduling study, 457 persons (mean age: 32.8 s ± 12.5 years) were randomly assigned to receive two doses (20-µg each, at 0 and 6 months) of HEV 239, three doses (20-µg each, at 0, 1 and 6 months) of HEV 239, or three doses of hepatitis B vaccine (5-µg each, at 0, 1 and 6 months; control group) by intramuscular route. Immunogenicity was assessed using seroconversion rates and geometric mean concentrations (GMC) of anti-HEV antibody, using the Wantai anti-HEV assay at months 0 (baseline), 2 (one month after the second dose in the three-dose group), 6 (before the final dose), 7 (one month after the final dose), and 13 (7 months after the final dose).

The seroconversion rates at 7 months with the two-dose and the three-dose schedules were similar (98% vs. 100%) (Table 3). However, the former schedule was associated with significantly lower anti-HEV antibody titers [GMC (95% CI) = 8.6 (6.5–11.3) WU/mL] than the three-dose schedule [15.9 (13.8–18.2); $p < 0.05$], with a GMC ratio (after two doses versus after three doses) of 0.54 (Table 3).

Table 3. Results of seroconversion and antibody titers at 7 months after starting vaccination in phase II trial of HEV 239 vaccine (Zhang et al., 2009) [9].

Vaccine Administered and the Dose Schedule	*n*	Seropositivity (%)	IgG Anti-HEV, WU/mL; Geometric Mean Concentration (95% CI)
HEV 239; 20 µg × 3 doses (0, 1, and 6 months)	128	100	15.9 (13.8–18.2)
HEV 239; 20 µg × 2 doses (0 and 6 months)	109	98	8.6 (6.5–11.3)
HBV vaccine; 5 µg × 3 doses (0, 1, and 6 months)	131	8	-

3.2.2. Phase III (Licensure) Trial

In this large field trial in China [6,11,12], 112,604 healthy adults of either sex aged 16–65 years (mean [standard deviation] age = 44.7 [11.1] years; 56.5% female), irrespective of their HEV serostatus (47% seropositive at baseline), were randomized to receive three intramuscular doses (at 0, 1, and 6 months) of either HEV239 (30-µg each) or a hepatitis B vaccine (5-µg each), and were followed up for safety and efficacy (occurrence of clinical hepatitis E) beginning one month after administration of the third dose. In addition, in a subset of 11,165 subjects ('the immunogenicity subset', including 5567 in the HEV 239 arm and 5598 in the comparator HBV vaccine arm), blood specimens were collected at various time points up to 55 months after the first dose and tested for anti-HEV antibody titers using the Wantai quantitative assay.

Of the 5567 persons in the HEV 239 arm in the immunogenicity subset, some failed to complete the intended three-dose schedule but were, nevertheless, followed up as originally planned. Thus, 184 (3.3%) subjects missed the third dose (receiving two doses at 0 and 1 months, respectively), and 189 (3.4%) missed the second dose (receiving the first and the third doses at 0 and 6 months, respectively). For these participants, antibody titer data at the 43-month follow-up (i.e., 3 years after the completion of one month since the last planned dose) were available for 117 and 125 participants, respectively (data at 55 months were available for very few participants and, hence, were not reported) (Table 4 and Figure 2).

Table 4. Results of seroconversion and antibody titers at 7 and 44 months after starting vaccination in the phase III trial of HEV 239 vaccine (Zhu et al., 2010 [11]; Zhang et al., 2015 [12]).

Number of Doses Received and Time Since the First Dose	Three Doses (0, 1, 6 Month)	Two Doses (0, 1 Month)	Two Doses (0, 6 Month)	One Dose (0 Month)
Seronegative at Baseline				
Seropositivity rate				
7 months	99.9%	98%	100%	98%
13 months	100%	100%	100%	100%
43 months	92%	82%	80%	39%
Anti-HEV antibody titer (WHO Units/mL), Geometric mean concentration (95% confidence interval)				
7 months	14.96 (14.48–15.45)	2.06 (1.68–2.51)	7.03 (5.67–8.72)	0.62 (0.45–0.87)
13 months	4.09 (3.81–4.39)	1.22 (0.61–2.43)	2.13 (1.58–2.87)	0.37 (0.13–1.11)
43 months	0.39 (0.37–0.41)	0.20 (0.14–0.29)	0.21 (0.15–0.29)	0.11 (0.05–0.24)
Seropositive at Baseline				
Seropositivity rate				
7 months	-	-	-	-
43 months	99.8%	100%	100%	100%
Anti-HEV antibody titer (WHO Units/mL), Geometric mean concentration (95% confidence interval)				
7 months	24.74 (14.74–34.74)	15.01 (12.01–17.01)	24.54 (14.54–34.54)	9.01 (7.01–10.01)
43 months	3.77 (2.77–4.77)	2.77 (1.77–3.77)	3.57 (2.57–4.57)	2.00 (1.34–2.77)

In individuals with baseline anti-HEV seropositivity (Figure 2a), GMC for anti-HEV remained high at 43 months of follow-up, irrespective of whether they had received one, two, or three doses of the vaccine.

By contrast, in individuals who were seronegative for anti-HEV at baseline (Figure 2b), the peak anti-HEV antibody concentration at 7 months (i.e., one month after completion of the planned schedule) and 3 years thereafter (i.e., 43 months from the start of vaccination) were somewhat lower in those who received two doses (whether 0–1 month, or 0–6 month) than those following the three-dose schedule, but were higher than those who had received only one dose or the placebo.

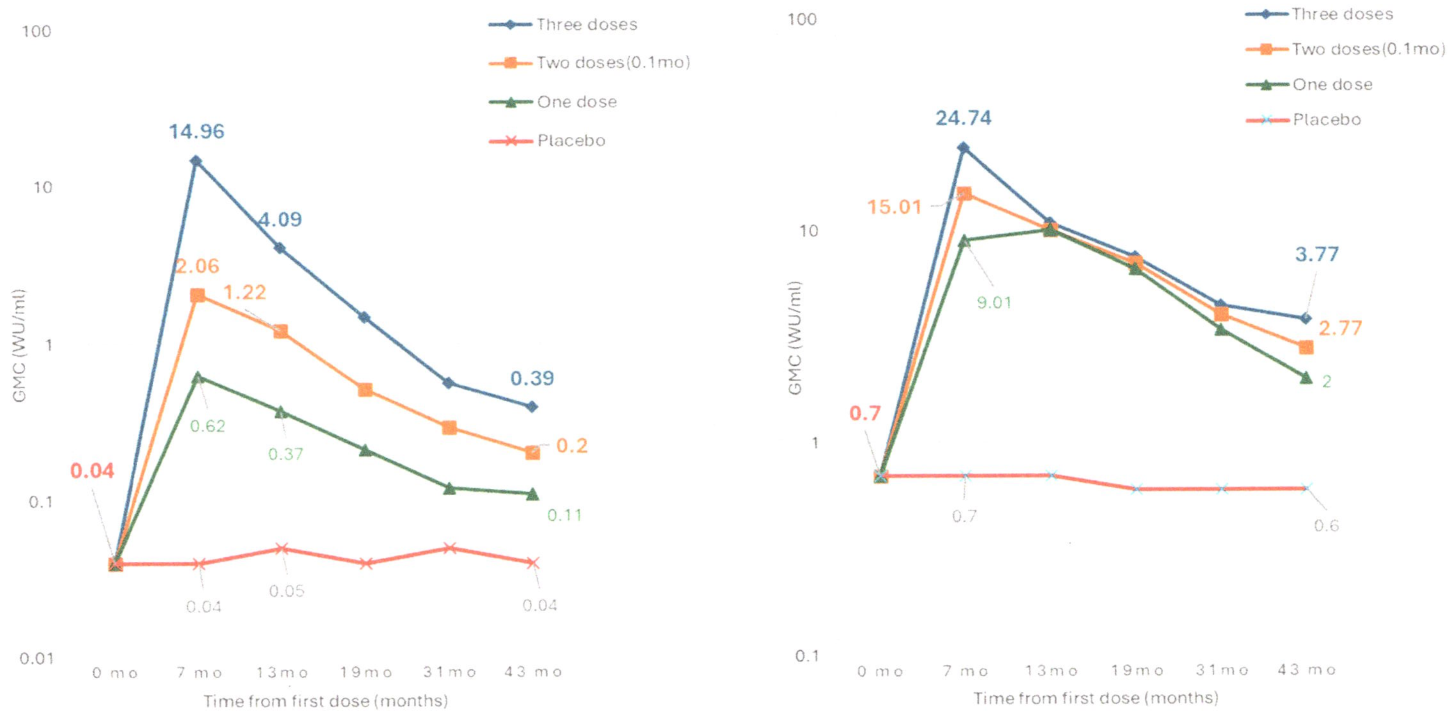

(**a**) Seronegative at baseline

(**b**) Seropositive at baseline

Figure 2. Geometric mean concentration of IgG anti-HEV and seropositivity rates among participants in immunogenicity sub-group. The left panel shows data for those who were seronegative for anti-HEV antibodies at baseline, and the right panel shows data for those who were seropositive at baseline.

3.2.3. Phase I Study in the United States

In a phase I study performed in the United States [15] in 2019, healthy volunteers (n = 25; age: 18–45 years; 19 [76%] women, all seronegative for anti-HEV antibody at baseline) were randomized to receive either HEV 239 vaccine (n = 20) or a placebo (n = 5) by intramuscular route at 0, 1, and 6 months. They were followed up to 6 months after the third dose. The seropositivity rate one month after the second dose was 100%, and GMC was 6.16 (1.68–18.77) WHO Units (WU)/mL. These anti-HEV levels were only somewhat lower than those achieved 1 month after the third dose [11.5 (2.72–33.02)] WU/mL, with a ratio of GMCs after two doses and after three doses being 0.54.

3.2.4. Two-Dose (0–1 Month) Schedule Study

In a randomized, controlled trial in Bangladesh, designed to specifically study a two-dose HEV 239 schedule [14], 100 individuals (mean age = 26.1 ± 9.6 years; 52% males; 33% seropositive for anti-HEV antibody at baseline) were randomized to receive two intramuscular doses (at 0 and 1 month) either of HEV 239 or hepatitis B vaccine and were followed up for 24 months from the first dose. The seropositivity rates following the two-dose schedule of HEV 239 at 2 and 24 months from the first dose were 100% and 98%, respectively, and the GMC for anti-HEV antibody was 49.5 (31.5–77.7) WU/mL and 6.4 (3.6–11.3) WU/mL, respectively (Table 5).

Table 5. Results of seroconversion and antibody titers at 2 and 24 months after starting vaccination in the Bangladesh trial of HEV 239 vaccine (Øverbø et al., Vaccine 2023) [14].

Time Since First Dose	Seropositivity Rate	Antibody Titer (WHO Units/mL), Geometric Mean Concentration (95% Confidence Interval)
		Overall (n = 50)
2 months	100%	49.5 (31.5–77.7)
24 months	98%	6.4 (3.6–11.3)
		Seropositive at baseline (n = 20)
2 months	100%	189.3 (122.3–293.1)
24 months	100%	36.1 (23.2–56.4)
		Seronegative at baseline (n = 30)
2 months	100%	20.2 (12.6–32.5)
24 months	95%	1.6 (1.0–2.5)

3.2.5. Rapid (0–7–21 Day) Three-Dose Accelerated Schedule Study

This randomized trial in China assessed the immunogenicity of an accelerated three-dose HEV 239 schedule administered over three weeks [13]. In this trial, 126 healthy individuals (mean age = 49.83 ± 10.67 years; 48% male), seronegative for anti-HEV, were randomized to receive three doses of HEV 239, in either an accelerated schedule (0, 7, and 21 days; n = 63) or the standard schedule (0, 1, and 6 months; n = 63). At seven months after the first dose, seropositivity rates in both groups were 100%, whereas GMC was somewhat lower with the accelerated schedule [5.0 (4.5–6.5) WU/mL] than the routine schedule [9.5 (8.0–10.1) WU/mL], with a GMC ratio of 0.53. The GMC antibody titer after the second dose of the routine schedule [5.0 (4.0–6.0) WU/mL] was similar to that after the rapid three-dose schedule.

3.3. Vaccine Efficacy

Data on vaccine efficacy were available from the pre-licensure phase II [9] and phase III [6,11,12] trials and from a post-licensure study in Bangladesh [14].

3.3.1. Pre-Licensure Phase II Trial

This trial, though primarily meant to assess vaccine immunogenicity, also assessed the rates of new HEV infections [9]. For this, the HEV-seronegative study participants who had received three-dose schedule of HEV 239 vaccine (0, 1, and 6 months; n = 155), two-dose schedule of HEV 239 (0 and 6 months; n = 151), or three-dose schedule of the control hepatitis B vaccine (0, 1, and 6 months; n = 151) were followed up for evidence of HEV infection for 6 months after the last dose. HEV infection was defined as the occurrence of a greater than three-fold rise in the levels of IgG anti-HEV antibody in paired sera collected at 7 and 13 months, thereby excluding any antibody rise that occurred during the first seven months and could be related to the vaccine itself.

In all, nine instances of HEV infection were recorded in the control group and one each in the two-dose and the three-dose HEV vaccine groups. All these infections were sub-clinical. Thus, the protective efficacy against HEV infection following the two-dose schedule (85%; 95% CI = 10–99%) was comparable to that with the three-dose schedule (89%; 31–100%).

3.3.2. Phase III (Licensure) Trial

This trial is the only study that had an assessment of the clinical efficacy of HEV 239 as the primary objective [6,11,12]. The primary efficacy analysis (per protocol) compared the rate of hepatitis E illness during the period from one month after the third dose till the end of follow-up in the participants who had received three doses of vaccine or placebo. Hepatitis E illness was defined by (i) occurrence of constitutional symptoms lasting at least three days, (ii) serum ALT elevation (at least 2.5-fold the upper limit of normal), and (iii) evidence of recent HEV infection (anti-HEV IgM or HEV RNA; and a $\geq$four-time increase in anti-HEV IgG concentration) [11].

In the most recent report, the trial participants in the per-protocol cohorts were followed up for 113 months beginning one month after the 6-month dose to obtain data on long-term efficacy [6]. In this report, in addition to the participants in the original study, residents in the 11 townships covered by the surveillance system who had not been enrolled in the trial and had been born between 1941 and 1991 (similar to the participant group) were included as an additional external control cohort (n = 178,236) to further evaluate vaccine efficacy.

In the per-protocol analysis, the protective efficacy of HEV 239 against HEV-associated illness was 89% (76–96%) at 102 months and 87% (73–94%) at 120 months of follow-up. Further, in a modified intention-to-treat analysis (those participants who had received any dose of HEV 239 vaccine and were followed up for efficacy up to 120 months from the beginning of vaccination), too, the efficacy was high during the extended follow-up, i.e., 85% (72–93%) at 102 months and 83% (69–91%) at 120 months.

An additional analysis evaluated vaccine efficacy after two doses (at 0 and 1 months) of the vaccine by combining data (i) for the participants who had received only two doses (followed up from 15 days after the second dose up to 120 months) for the entire follow-up period and (ii) for the participants who received three doses during the follow-up period beginning 15 days after the second dose till administration of the third dose. The participants (n = 250) who had received only the first and the third doses (i.e., two doses at 0 and 6 months) were excluded from this analysis. In this analysis, six cases of acute hepatitis E were recorded among placebo recipients (n = 3765 between 6 months to 30 months, and

n = 52,428 till administration of the third dose) and none among the HEV 239 vaccine recipients (n = 3542 between 6 months to 30 months, and n = 52,235 till administration of third dose), indicating efficacy of 100.0%, albeit with broad 95% confidence intervals (15.4–100.0%) [6].

During the follow-up from 30–120 months after the start of vaccination, the number of new hepatitis E cases in the placebo group was too few, leading to inadequate statistical power for the estimation of the long-term efficacy of the two-dose regimen. However, a comparison of the number of cases among two-dose vaccine recipients with those in the post-hoc external control cohort showed a high efficacy (standardized for age and sex) rate (Table 6).

Table 6. Long-term vaccine efficacy in participants administered with two doses (first and second dose) (Huang et al., 2024) [6].

Time Period * (Months from the Start of Vaccination)	Disease Incidence (Per 100,000 Person Years)			Vaccine Efficacy, % (95% Confidence Interval) **	
	HEV 239 Vaccine Group (n = 3542)	Placebo Group (n = 3765)	Post-Hoc External Control Group (n = 178,236)	Vaccine vs. Placebo	Vaccine vs. External Control Cohort *
1.5–30	0.0	2.3	2.0	100 (+15.4 to 100)	100 (31.1 to 100)
1.5–54	0.3	1.8	2.1	83.4 (−36.7 to 99.6)	85.7 (19.1 to 99.6)
1.5–78	0.2	1.5	2.0	83.4 (−36.5 to 99.6)	88.1 (32.8 to 99.7)
1.5–102	0.2	1.5	1.9	85.8 (−10.4 to 99.7)	89.1 (39.0 to 99.7)
1.5–120	0.2	1.3	1.8	85.8 (−10.4 to 99.7)	89.9 (43.4 to 99.7)

* The time periods relate to the time period beginning with the first vaccine dose over which efficacy was assessed. These begin at 1.5 months, i.e., 15 days after the 2nd dose, which was administered one month after the first dose, and continue for variable time after vaccination. ** The vaccine efficacy results are from post-hoc analysis and are standardized for age and sex.

Of the 13 cases of hepatitis E that occurred in the placebo group in this trial in whom virus genotype could be identified, 12 had infection with genotype 4 HEV and one with genotype 1 HEV; hence, the evidence for the protection afforded by the vaccine was primarily for genotype 4 HEV [11].

3.3.3. Two-Dose Schedule Study

In this Bangladesh trial, 100 individuals were randomized into two groups [HEV 239 vs. HBV control] (n = 50 each) and followed up to 23 months after the last dose for episodes of subclinical HEV infection. Five cases of HEV infection were observed in the 45 controls and none in the 43 subjects who received HEV 239, with a protective efficacy against HEV infection of 100% (82–100%).

3.4. *Vaccine Effectiveness*

No data are available on the effectiveness of HEV 239 in real-life settings, whether for a three or two-dose schedule.

3.5. *Vaccine Safety*

Data on the safety of a two-dose schedule of HEV 239 are available only from a pre-licensure study [9] in China with a head-to-head comparison of two-dose (0, 6 months) vs.

threes-dose (0, 1, 6 months) schedules (each dose of 20 μg instead of 30 μg in the marketed product) [9]. In this study, there was no significant difference in the frequencies of all local (5.2 and 8.5 per 100 vaccine doses, respectively) or systemic (4.9 and 7.6 per 100 doses, respectively) adverse events or severe (grade 3 or above) local (0 and 1.6 per 100 doses) or systemic (0 in both) adverse events.

In another study [13], where an accelerated three-dose schedule (0, 7, and 21 days) was compared with the routine three-dose schedule (0, 1, and 6 months) of HEV 239 vaccine, the rates of solicited local (8/62 [12.9%] vs. 8/63 [12.7%]) and systemic (12/62 [19.4%] vs. 11/63 [17.5%]) adverse events were similar. The rates of unsolicited adverse events were 16/62 (25.8%) and 10/63 (15.9%), respectively, with no significant difference. No serious adverse event was observed in either group.

4. Discussion

Our systematic review of immunogenicity data following intramuscular administration of two doses of HEV 239 vaccine showed a high seroconversion rate similar to that following the three-dose schedule and anti-HEV antibody titers, which were somewhat lower than those following the conventionally recommended three-dose schedule. Similar results were also seen following administration of three doses in a rapid 21-day schedule. Further, two vaccine doses were associated with a good protective efficacy rate for at least one year.

There is sufficient evidence to indicate that anti-HEV antibodies are protective against HEV infection [16]. However, the titer defining the protection threshold remains unknown. Despite the lack of data on the protection threshold for antibody concentration, we believe that reasonably robust conclusions are possible from our analysis. Further, the trial data primarily support protection against genotype 4 HEV, a heterologous strain of the genotype 1 protein contained in the vaccine [11]. However, there are in vitro data that anti-HEV antibodies provide cross-protection across HEV genotypes [17,18].

In the pre-licensure phase II study [9], a two-dose schedule showed a seroconversion rate similar to that with the three-dose schedule (98% vs. 100%), albeit with slightly lower anti-HEV antibody titers (GMC = 8.6 vs. 15.9 WU/mL). However, the inter-dose interval in the two-dose schedule in this study was 6 months, and the schedule was no shorter than the conventional three-dose schedule. Further, albeit less importantly, each dose contained a smaller amount (20 μg) of HEV antigen than the marketed preparation (30 μg); it is possible that the results with the latter dose could have been different. These considerations limit the value of these data. However, these data are of importance because these represent the only randomized comparison of two-dose and three-dose schedules. Importantly, in this comparison, the GMC ratio of the titers in the two groups was 0.54. In this context, it is important to consider that in trials comparing different schedules for various vaccines, GMC ratios of above 0.50 are often considered non-inferior [16].

The most relevant data on the value of a shorter-dose schedule are those from the phase III licensure field trial, which have been published as three reports with 19-month, 5-year, and 10-year follow-ups, respectively, from the start of vaccination [6,11,12]. In this trial, some participants did not receive the intended three doses, creating two distinct subsets of participants who had received only two doses, i.e., (i) the planned first and second doses (at 0 and 1 month) or (ii) the planned first and third doses (at 0 and 6 months), which could be compared with those who had received all three planned doses. Of these, the former subset (0, 1 month), being a shorter-duration schedule, is of primary relevance. Though such post-hoc comparisons being non-randomized have limitations, they provide useful information about the response expected following the administration of two doses of the HEV vaccine.

In this trial, in individuals with baseline anti-HEV seropositivity, anti-HEV GMC remained high till 43 months of follow-up, irrespective of the number of doses received, whether one, two, or three. These data suggest that two doses of the HEV 239 vaccine in a 0–1-month schedule are highly likely to provide durable anti-HEV antibody concentration and, hence, protection against HEV infection and disease in HEV-seropositive persons.

By contrast, in individuals who were seronegative for anti-HEV at baseline, the anti-HEV levels reached immediately after vaccination and at all time points thereafter till 43 months were lower after two vaccine doses than after the usual three doses. However, notably, the GMC following the two-dose schedule in the participants who were seronegative at baseline was quite high till at least 13 months of follow-up, being higher at this time point than the GMC observed at 43 months following the usual three-dose schedule. This duration of antibody persistence may be quite sufficient for controlling a disease outbreak, as further discussed below.

In a trial in Bangladesh, which specifically assessed a short two-dose schedule (0–1 months) of HEV 239 [14], seropositivity rates and antibody titers were fairly high, i.e., consistent with the data from the phase III trial. Unfortunately, this study lacked a group with the three-dose schedule, and hence, a head-to-head comparison of the two-dose vs. three-dose schedule of HEV 239 was not available.

Another alternative accelerated schedule with three doses given at 0–7–21 days has also been assessed in one study [13] through comparison with the standard three-dose (0–1–6 month) schedule. This accelerated schedule also led to 100% seropositivity, with antibody GMC only marginally lower than the standard regimen, suggesting that this schedule can be an option in situations necessitating the use of a shorter regimen. However, this schedule, though as quick as the two-dose (0–1 month) schedule, would be costlier and programmatically more challenging. Hence, the two-dose regimen (0–1 month) would appear to score over the 21-day three-dose schedule.

Beyond the immunogenicity data, data on efficacy are also available from three studies [6,9,14]. With regards to protection against sub-clinical infection, the two-dose schedule of HEV 239 in phase II pre-licensure study [9] and the Bangladesh trial [14] showed efficacy rates of 85% and 100%, respectively. However, the interpretation of these studies is limited by the fact that they did not look at clinical disease and instead looked at serological evidence of HEV infection. By comparison, in the phase III licensure trial, efficacy was assessed as protection against clinical disease. In this trial, the protection following two doses was found to be 100%, albeit with wide confidence intervals, and this lasted till at least 30 months after vaccination [6]; after this time point, the low number of cases precluded any reliable conclusion. Even after 30 months, a comparison with a post-hoc general population control group showed that the two-dose schedule was a good protection; however, for this post-hoc comparison, a possibility of bias cannot be excluded. Even if one were to ignore this delayed protection, the 30-month duration of protection is by itself sufficient in situations where a rapid schedule is most required, such as for the control of a hepatitis E outbreak.

In fact, in parts of the world where outbreaks of hepatitis E occur, the background circulation of HEV is higher, and the baseline anti-HEV seropositivity rate is likely to be higher. Given that (i) in seropositive persons, even one dose of HEV 239 leads to a long-duration boosting of anti-HEV antibodies persisting beyond 43 months, and (ii) in seronegative persons, two doses of HEV 239 lead to fairly high anti-HEV GMC at least till 13 months, it appears quite reasonable to use two-dose (0, 1 month) schedule to control hepatitis E outbreaks in disease-endemic areas.

HEV vaccination is expected, in addition to the induction of specific antibody responses, to induce specific cellular immune responses, which are likely to play a complementary role in protection against HEV infection. However, these responses have not been studied in detail in the available studies, either following the usual three-dose schedule or fewer doses.

Further, our analysis shows that the two-dose schedule was as safe as the three-dose schedule. Though these data are based on a small-size study, a schedule with fewer doses would, in any case, not be expected to raise a safety concern.

In conclusion, our systematic review strongly supports the use of a rapid or a shortened two-dose schedule for the HEV 239 vaccine for the control of hepatitis E outbreaks.

Supplementary Materials: The following supporting information can be downloaded at https://www.mdpi.com/article/10.3390/vaccines13010028/s1, Table S1: List of studies excluded from the final review.

Author Contributions: Conceptualization, M.M. and R.A.; methodology, R.A.; formal analysis, B.A., A.G. and R.A.; investigation, B.A., A.G. and R.A.; resources, M.M.; data curation, B.A., A.G. and R.A.; writing—original draft preparation, B.A.; writing—review and editing, M.M., A.G. and R.A.; visualization, B.A. and R.A.; supervision, R.A.; project administration, M.M. and R.A.; funding acquisition, M.M. and A.G. All authors have read and agreed to the published version of the manuscript.

Funding: B.A. was supported by the World Health Organization for this work. WHO reference number: 2024/1453007-0.

Institutional Review Board Statement: Not applicable.

Informed Consent Statement: Not applicable.

Data Availability Statement: Data were retrieved from the articles mentioned in the references.

Conflicts of Interest: B.A. was supported by the World Health Organization for this work. All the other three authors (M.M., A.G. and R.A.) declare that they have no competing financial interests or personal relationships that could have appeared to influence the work reported in this paper.

References

1. Kenney, S.P.; Meng, X.J. Hepatitis E virus genome structure and replication strategy. *Cold Spring Harb. Perspect. Med.* **2019**, *9*, a031724. [CrossRef] [PubMed]
2. Goel, A.; Aggarwal, R. Hepatitis E: Epidemiology, Clinical Course, Prevention, and Treatment. *Gastroenterol. Clin. N. Am.* **2020**, *49*, 315–330. [CrossRef]
3. Nelson, K.E.; Labrique, A.B.; Kmush, B.L. Epidemiology of genotype 1 and 2 hepatitis E virus infections. *Cold Spring Harb. Perspect. Med.* **2019**, *9*, a031732. [CrossRef] [PubMed]
4. Kamar, N.; Izopet, J.; Pavio, N.; Aggarwal, R.; Labrique, A.; Wedemeyer, H.; Dalton, H.R. Hepatitis E virus infection. *Nat. Rev. Dis. Prim.* **2017**, *3*, 17086. [CrossRef] [PubMed]
5. Peron, J.M.; Larrue, H.; Izopet, J.; Buti, M. The pressing need for a global HEV vaccine. *J. Hepatol.* **2023**, *79*, 876–880. [CrossRef] [PubMed]
6. Huang, S.; Zhang, X.; Su, Y.; Zhuang, C.; Tang, Z.; Huang, X.; Chen, Q.; Zhu, K.; Hu, X.; Ying, D.; et al. Long-term efficacy of a recombinant hepatitis E vaccine in adults: 10-year results from a randomised, double-blind, placebo-controlled, phase 3 trial. *Lancet* **2024**, *403*, 813–823. [CrossRef]
7. Innis, B.L.; Lynch, J.A. Immunization against hepatitis E. *Cold Spring Harb. Perspect. Med.* **2018**, *8*, a032573. [CrossRef] [PubMed]
8. Oct2014_Session8_HEV_recommendations.pdf. Available online: https://terrance.who.int/mediacentre/data/sage/SAGE_Docs_Ppt_Oct2014/8_session_hepE/Oct2014_Session8_HEV_recommendations.pdf (accessed on 13 April 2024).
9. Zhang, J.; Liu, C.B.; Li, R.C.; Li, Y.M.; Zheng, Y.J.; Li, Y.P.; Luo, D.; Pan, B.-B.; Nong, Y.; Ge, S.-X.; et al. Randomized-controlled phase II clinical trial of a bacterially expressed recombinant hepatitis E vaccine. *Vaccine* **2009**, *27*, 1869–1874. [CrossRef] [PubMed]
10. Nesbitt, R.C.; Asilaza, V.K.; Gignoux, E.; Koyuncu, A.; Gitahi, P.; Nkemenang, P.; Duncker, J.; Antier, Z.; Haile, M.; Gakima, P.; et al. Vaccination coverage and adverse events following a reactive vaccination campaign against hepatitis E in Bentiu displaced persons camp, South Sudan. *PLoS Negl. Trop. Dis.* **2024**, *18*, e0011661. [CrossRef] [PubMed]
11. Zhu, F.C.; Zhang, J.; Zhang, X.F.; Zhou, C.; Wang, Z.Z.; Huang, S.J.; Wang, H.; Yang, C.-L.; Jiang, H.-M.; Cai, J.-P.; et al. Efficacy and safety of a recombinant hepatitis E vaccine in healthy adults: A large-scale, randomised, double-blind placebo-controlled, phase 3 trial. *Lancet* **2010**, *376*, 895–902. [CrossRef]

12. Zhang, J.; Zhang, X.F.; Huang, S.J.; Wu, T.; Hu, Y.M.; Wang, Z.Z.; Wang, H.; Jiang, H.-M.; Wang, Y.-J.; Yan, Q.; et al. Long-term efficacy of a hepatitis E vaccine. *N. Engl. J. Med.* **2015**, *372*, 914–922. [CrossRef]
13. Chen, Z.; Lin, S.; Duan, J.; Luo, Y.; Wang, S.; Gan, Z.; Yi, H.; Wu, T.; Huang, S.; Zhang, Q.; et al. Immunogenicity and safety of an accelerated hepatitis E vaccination schedule in healthy adults: A randomized, controlled, open-label, phase IV trial. *Clin. Microbiol. Infect.* **2019**, *25*, 1133–1139. [CrossRef]
14. Øverbø, J.; Aziz, A.; Zaman, K.; Clemens, J.; Halle Julin, C.; Qadri, F.; Stene-Johansen, K.; Biswas, R.; Islam, S.; Bhuiyan, T.R.; et al. Immunogenicity and safety of a two-dose regimen with hepatitis E virus vaccine in healthy adults in rural Bangladesh: A randomized, double-blind, controlled, phase 2/pilot trial. *Vaccine* **2023**, *41*, 1059–1066. [CrossRef] [PubMed]
15. Kao, C.M.; Rostad, C.A.; Nolan, L.E.; Peters, E.; Kleinhenz, J.; Sherman, J.D.; Tippett, A.; Shih, J.W.K.; Yildirim, I.; Agbakoba, V.; et al. A phase 1, double-blinded, placebo-controlled clinical trial to evaluate the safety and immunogenicity of HEV-239 (Hecolin®) vaccine in healthy US adults. *J. Infect. Dis.* **2024**, *230*, 1093–1101. [CrossRef] [PubMed]
16. Zhang, J.; Zhang, X.F.; Zhou, C.; Wang, Z.Z.; Huang, S.J.; Yao, X.; Liang, Z.-L.; Wu, T.; Li, J.-X.; Yan, Q.; et al. Protection against hepatitis E virus infection by naturally acquired and vaccine-induced immunity. *Clin. Microbiol. Infect.* **2014**, *20*, O397–O405. [CrossRef] [PubMed]
17. Gu, Y.; Tang, X.; Zhang, X.; Song, C.; Zheng, M.; Wang, K.; Zhang, J.; Ng, M.-H.; Hew, C.-L.; Li, S.; et al. Structural basis for the neutralization of hepatitis E virus by a cross-genotype antibody. *Cell Res.* **2015**, *25*, 604–620. [CrossRef]
18. Zhang, J.; Shih, J.W.; Wu, T.; Li, S.W.; Xia, N.S. Development of the hepatitis E vaccine: From bench to field. *Semin. Liver Dis.* **2013**, *33*, 79–88. [CrossRef]

vaccines

MDPI

Article

Regional Disparities in HPV Vaccination Coverage Among Girls Aged 9 to 14 Years in Togo: Lessons Learned from the Recent Supplementary Immunization Activities

Dadja Essoya Landoh [1,*], Issifou Yaya [2,3,4], Amevegbe Boko [5], Kodjovi Adjeoda [5], Yaovi Temfan Toke [6], Adidja Amani [7], Yerima Mouhoudine [8], Ado Mpia Bwaka [9], Nsiari-Mueyi Joseph Biey [9], Charles Shey Wiysonge [7], Franck Fortune Roland Mboussou [10], Hèzouwè Looky-Djobo [5], Tsidi Agbeko Tamekloe [1], Toyi Nyulelen Mangbassim [6], Tchasso Kenao [6], Amadou Bailo Diallo [1], Fatoumata Binta Tidiane Diallo [1], Benido Impouma [7], Ann Lindstrand [11], Marin Kokou Wotobe [8] and Didier Koumavi Ekouevi [12]

1 World Health Organization, Country Office, Lomé BP 1504, Togo; tamekloet@who.int (T.A.T.); dialloa@who.int (A.B.D.); boussokadi@yahoo.fr (F.B.T.D.)
2 Patient-Reported Outcomes Research (PROQOL), Health Economics Clinical Trial Unit (URC-ECO), Hotel-Dieu Hospital, AP-HP, 75004 Paris, France; iyayad@yahoo.fr
3 CHU-SO, Unité de Recherche en Santé des Populations (URESAP), Épidemiologie des Maladies Infectieuses et Sciences Sociales (Épidé-MISS), Lomé BP 1515, Togo
4 ECEVE, UMR-S 1123, Paris Cité University, Inserm, 75006 Paris, France
5 Division de l'Immunisation, Ministère de la Santé, Lomé BP 386, Togo; amevegbe12@yahoo.fr (A.B.); adjtg@yahoo.fr (K.A.); lookydjobo@yahoo.fr (H.L.-D.)
6 Fonds des Nations Unies pour L'enfance (UNICEF), Bureau Togo, Lomé BP 4042, Togo; yawovitemfan@gmail.com (Y.T.T.); machristian2008@yahoo.fr (T.N.M.); tkenao@unicef.org (T.K.)
7 World Health Organization, Regional Office for Africa, Brazzaville P.O. Box 06, Congo; amaniad@who.int (A.A.); sheyc@who.int (C.S.W.); impoumab@who.int (B.I.)
8 Ministère de la Santé, Lomé BP 386, Togo; dineyerima@yahoo.fr (Y.M.); wotobemarin@yahoo.fr (M.K.W.)
9 World Health Organization, IST West Africa, Ouagadougou P.O. Box 7019, Burkina Faso; bwakaa@who.int (A.M.B.); bieyj@who.int (N.-M.J.B.)
10 World Health Organization, IST Central Africa, Libreville, Gabon; mboussouf@who.int
11 Department of Immunization, Vaccines and Biologicals (IVB), World Health Organization, 1211 Geneva, Switzerland; lindstranda@who.int
12 Centre de Formation et de Recherche en Santé Publique, Université de Lomé, Lomé BP 1515, Togo; didier.ekouevi@gmail.com
* Correspondence: mlandoh@yahoo.fr

Abstract: Background/Objectives: Human papillomavirus (HPV) vaccination is a critical intervention to prevent cervical cancer, especially in settings where screening is limited. In Togo, cervical cancer is the second most common cancer in women. Togo conducted an HPV vaccination campaign for girls aged 9–14 from 27 November to 1 December 2023, followed by introduction of the vaccine into routine immunization. This study aimed to assess regional disparities in vaccination coverage during this campaign. Methods: A cross-sectional study was conducted using data from the nationwide HPV vaccination campaign. The target population included girls aged 9–14, following school and community-based enumeration. The campaign employed school-based, health facility-based, and community-based vaccination strategies. Data were collected via multiple tools, and monitoring was carried out through daily reports and digital tracking. Results: Out of the estimated 654,402 eligible girls, 304,457 (46.5%) were vaccinated. Vaccine coverage varied significantly by region, ranging from 76% in Kara to 15% in Grand Lomé. In-school settings accounted for 91.3% of vaccinations, with the fixed strategy covering 55.4%. In total, 11 districts exceeded 80% vaccine coverage, while 15 districts had <50%. The highest rate of adverse events following immunization was observed in the Maritime region, primarily involving minor symptoms. Conclusion: Although progress was made in HPV vaccination coverage in Togo, regional disparities highlight the need for targeted interventions. Strategies such as expanding vaccine access, enhancing awareness campaigns, and integrating HPV vaccination into routine immunization could improve coverage. Addressing logistical and cultural barriers is also crucial for equitable vaccination, aiming to achieve international benchmarks and reduce HPV-related disease burdens. Further research should explore qualitative factors influencing vaccine acceptance.

Keywords: HPV vaccination; girls; supplementary immunization activities; coverage; disparities; Togo

1. Introduction

Human papillomavirus (HPV) is a common virus that encompasses over 200 distinct types, categorized into five primary genera: Alpha, Beta, Gamma, Mu, and Nu [1]. These HPV types are typically classified as either low-risk (LR—non-carcinogenic) or high-risk (HR—carcinogenic) [2]. Persistent infection with high-risk strains of HPV, particularly types 16 and 18, is strongly associated with the development of cervical cancer. Additionally, HPV infection has been implicated in the development of other cancers, including those of the anus, penis, vagina, vulva, and oropharynx [3].

More than half a million (604,000) new cases of cervical cancer are reported worldwide in 2020, of which 342,000 deaths occurred, and approximately 90% of these deaths occurred in low- and middle-income countries, including Sub-Saharan Africa [4], where the estimated pooled prevalence of HPV among women is 32.3% [5]. This region bears one of the highest global burdens of HPV, which is reflected in high cervical cancer incidence rates [6].

HPV vaccination is crucial in reducing the global cervical cancer burden, especially in developing countries where effective screening and treatment are lacking, making vaccination particularly important [7]. Studies show that widespread vaccination can reduce cervical cancer incidence by nearly 90% among young girls vaccinated before the age of 17 years, with a single dose providing 97.5% protection against persistent infections with HPV types 16 and 18 [8,9]. These findings highlight the critical role of high HPV vaccination coverage, particularly in resource-limited settings, in significantly lowering cervical cancer rates and protecting women's health.

Primary prevention of cervical cancer is essentially based on HPV vaccination and healthy lifestyles [10]. Three vaccine types are currently available and marketed in many countries around the world to prevent HPV related disease: the bivalent vaccines (against genotype 16 and 18), the quadrivalent vaccine (against genotype 6, 11, 16, and 18) and the nonavalent vaccine (against genotypes 6, 11, 16, 18, 31, 33, 45, 52, and 58). All three vaccines include the oncogenic genotypes 16 and 18 that cause most of the cervical cancer [11]. HPV vaccination has been shown to be cost-efficient in low-income countries, including those of Sub-Saharan Africa [12,13].

Overall, raising awareness about HPV and its link to cancer, promoting vaccination, and ensuring access to screening services are essential strategies for reducing the burden of HPV-related cancers [14].

In Togo, cervical cancer ranks as the third most common cancer in terms of incidence (19.1 cases per 100,000 individuals) in both sexes, following prostate cancer (32 cases per 100,000) and breast cancer (30.7 cases per 100,000). Among women, cervical cancer is the second most common cancer (15.7%) after breast cancer (29.4%), based on the GLOBOCAN 2020 global estimates [15]. To mitigate the morbidity and mortality associated with cervical cancer, Togo conducted a nationwide catch-up vaccination campaign with the human papillomavirus (HPV) vaccine for girls aged 9 to 14 years from 27 November to 1 December 2023. Following this, on 4 December 2023, the HPV vaccine was introduced into the routine immunization schedule for 9-year-old girls. Togo conducted a demonstration of the HPV vaccine introduction, covering a cohort of 15,272 girls aged 10 years who received two doses of HPV Vaccine in 2015 and 2016 in two health districts (Tchamba and Golfe) [16].

Since the launch of the Vaccine Alliance (Gavi) program in the country, Togo has consistently achieved over 90% vaccine coverage for most antigens under the Expanded Program on Immunization [17,18], despite the socio-cultural challenges that could have favored vaccination hesitancy in some administrative regions. From the scientific literature review, it appeared that vaccine acceptance can be influenced by several factors, including myths and misconceptions about vaccination and knowledge gaps about immunization. In many low- and middle-income countries, as in Togo, there may be challenges to achieving high vaccination coverage rates, such as limited access to healthcare services, vaccine supply chain issues, and vaccine hesitancy among some communities.

In Togo, disparities in vaccination coverage can exist across regions due to various factors, such as access to healthcare services, socioeconomic status, and cultural beliefs [17, 18]. These regional disparities may be particularly pronounced due to the country's geographical and socio-economic diversity. Factors such as urbanization, infrastructure development, and availability of healthcare facilities can significantly impact vaccination coverage rates in different regions.

This study aimed at analyzing the regional disparities in the HPV vaccination coverage in Togo, during the national vaccination campaign held in November 2023. Understanding these disparities is crucial for designing targeted interventions to improve HPV vaccination coverage and reduce the burden of HPV-related diseases in Togo. Research on regional disparities in HPV vaccination coverage can provide insights into the underlying factors contributing to these disparities and inform strategies to address them effectively.

2. Materials and Methods

2.1. Study Design

This study is a cross-sectional study using data from the recent HPV vaccination campaign targeting girls aged 9 to 14 years. The campaign was implemented nationwide from 27 November to 1 December 2023, aiming to vaccinate at least 90% of the target population with the Cervarix™ bivalent HPV vaccine (GlaxoSmithKline (GSK) in Rixensart, Belgium).

2.2. Target Population and Sampling

The target population for the vaccination campaign was adolescent girls aged 9 to 14 years. Before the campaign, a census was conducted by district teams to enumerate all eligible girls across the country. The enumeration process varied by region. In districts with high net school enrollment rates for girls (above 95%), school-based enumeration was through collaboration with school heads and teachers. In regions like Savanes and Kara, where the net enrollment rate for girls is around 80%, in addition to school-based enumeration, community-based enumeration was carried out by community health workers (CHWs) to ensure that out-of-school girls were also counted.

Given the high school enrollment rate in Togo (93.1% for girls in the 2021–2022 academic year), the majority of the target population was expected to be enrolled in school, with a comprehensive strategy to reach both in-school and out-of-school girls.

2.3. Vaccination Campaign Strategies

The campaign was conducted using three main settings to administer the HPV vaccine:

- School-based vaccination: the vaccination was administered directly in schools to reach most girls who were enrolled in educational institutions, including public, private, and Koranic schools.
- Health facility-based vaccination: out-of-school girls, as well as in-school girls who missed their vaccination at school, were vaccinated at designated health facilities.
- Community-based vaccination: in cases where girls could not be vaccinated at schools or health facilities, mobile vaccination teams were deployed in the communities. This approach involved outreach vaccination strategies to reach out-of-school girls in remote areas and ensure that no one was left behind.

These strategies were supported by a schedule of visits to public and private schools, including Koranic schools. A high school enrollment rate among girls was a crucial factor in the campaign's planning and implementation. Overall, fixed, outreach and mobile strategies were used in the three setting to cover a maximum of the target population.

2.4. Data Collection Tools and Procedures

To ensure systematic data collection during the campaign, a range of tools were developed and deployed, including the following: enumeration and vaccination form (for collecting data on vaccinated girls), out-of-school girls survey form (to identify and record out-of-school girls eligible for vaccination), school survey form (to track in-school girls and vaccination progress), household convenience survey form (for rapid assessment of households), vaccination card (to document each girl's vaccination status), summary of vaccination results form (to consolidate data at the end of each day).

Additionally, several training and guidance documents were prepared for the vaccination teams, such as training manuals for supervisors and vaccinators, and protocols on detecting, reporting, and managing potential adverse events following immunization (AEFI). Training sessions and micro-planning activities were conducted a month prior to the campaign, involving health and education stakeholders at various levels (regional health directors, district health workers, and education staff). Partners such as the WHO, UNICEF, and Gavi consultants also contributed to these preparations' activities.

The bivalent vaccine (Cervarix™ GlaxoSmithKline (GSK) in Rixensart, Belgium)., with 672,200 doses for the campaign and other supplies, were received in July 2023, several months before the start of the campaign, and stored according to standard procedures at the national level. A week before the launch of the campaign, the vaccine (625,522 doses), injection equipment, and other supplies were pre-positioned in the health facilities by the district's teams.

The vaccination teams comprised four members each: two vaccinators (one tasked with collecting the vaccine and the other with its administration) and two recorders (one verifying the age of the recipients, completing vaccination cards and enumeration sheets, and the other filling out tally sheets and ensuring their accuracy). Throughout the vaccination sessions, the vaccinators informed the girls about the targeted disease, vaccination objectives, and common side effects, and advised them to seek medical care in case of adverse reactions. Additionally, each vaccination team conducted awareness sessions on menstrual hygiene and puberty management during school visits.

The Cervarix vaccine was administered intramuscularly in the deltoid region of the left arm. The dose administered per girl aged 9 to 14 was 0.5 mL.

2.5. Monitoring and Quality Control

A robust monitoring system was established to track daily progress at both the operational and national levels. Data were collected through various forms, including enumeration sheets, tally sheets from immunization teams, and waste management sheets. These were submitted to health facility managers, who then reported daily figures to district health authorities. The Division of Immunization compiled these data and produced daily immunization bulletins, with support from partners.

For real-time monitoring, data were entered into the District Health Information System 2 (DHIS2), with technical support from the Health Information Systems Program (HISP). Personal data were not collected, and all variables were configured to facilitate analysis.

At the end of each day, coordination meetings were held at districts and region level to review progress and address any challenges encountered during the vaccination sessions.

2.6. Data Management and Analysis

Once the vaccination campaign was completed, all data collected during the campaign were transferred to EPI-Info 7.2 software for analysis. Descriptive statistical analyses were performed to assess the coverage, identify gaps, and evaluate the overall success of the campaign.

Virtual debriefing meetings were organized with stakeholders from all districts and regions to discuss the campaign's results, identify key findings, and strategize for reaching girls who were missed during the campaign.

2.7. Ethical Considerations

The study followed ethical guidelines by not collecting any personal data during the campaign. The emphasis was placed on maintaining the privacy and confidentiality of the girls involved. All participants, including the girls and their guardians, were fully informed about the purpose of the vaccination, potential side effects, and advised to seek medical assistance in case of adverse reactions. Additionally, awareness-raising sessions on menstrual hygiene and puberty management were integrated into the vaccination visits, further supporting the girls' health and well-being beyond the HPV vaccination. An oral consent was obtained from the parents prior to the vaccination.

The Supplementary Immunization Activities (SIA) using Cervarix was recommended by the National Immunization Technical Advisory Group (NITAG) [19] and approved by the Inter agency Coordination Committee (ICC)

3. Results

According to the census, the number of girls aged 9 to 14 expected to be vaccinated against HPV was estimated at 654,402 (111,787 girls of 9 years and 542,615 aged from 10 to 14 years), including 179,969 in Grand Lomé Region, 104,442 in Maritime, 141,842 in Plateaux, 63,910 in Centrale, 79,655 in Kara, and 84,583 in Savanes Region.

A total of 304,457 girls (62,284 girls aged 9 and 242,173 girls aged 10–14) were vaccinated out of the 654,402 girls expected (Table 1), with overall administrative coverage of 46.5% (56% for girls aged 9 and 45% for girls aged 10–14).

Vaccination coverage for girls aged 9–14 varies from 76% (Kara region) to 15% (Grand Lomé region). Figure 1 shows administrative vaccination coverage by region.

Table 1. Number of girls vaccinated against HPV by region, vaccination campaign for girls aged 9 to 14 to prevent cervical cancer in Togo, December 2023.

Region	Expected Number of 9-Year-Old Girls	Expected Number of Girls Aged 10 to 14	Expected Number of Girls Aged 9 to 14	Number of 9-Year-Old Girls Vaccinated	Number of Girls Aged 10 to 14 Vaccinated	Number of Girls Aged 9 to 14 Vaccinated	Number of HPV Vaccine Doses Used	Number of AEFI Reported	
								Serious AEFI	Minor AEFI
Grand Lomé	30,743	149,226	179,969	5092	21,519	26,611	27,068	0	13
Maritime	17,841	86,601	104,442	6998	30,183	37,181	37,673	0	148
Plateaux	24,230	117,612	141,842	15,900	61,030	76,930	77,356	0	185
Centrale	10,917	52,993	63,910	8772	34,034	42,806	43,061	0	43
Kara	13,607	66,048	79,655	12,679	47,644	60,323	60,740	1	33
Savanes	14,449	70,135	84,583	12,843	47,763	60,606	62,572	0	50
Total	111,787	542,615	654,402	62,284	242,173	304,457	308,470	1	472

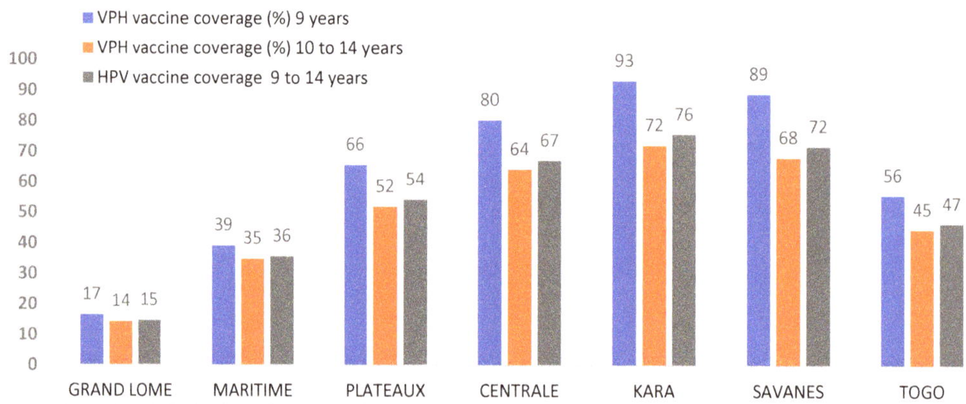

Figure 1. Administrative HPV vaccination coverage by region during SIA for girls aged 9–14 in Togo in December 2023.

The median HPV vaccination coverage was 61.6% (IQR: 40.7–80.2%), with great variability within and between regions. The disaggregated vaccine coverage by district showed that Dankpen district had the highest administrative coverage (100%) and Golfe district the lowest (13%). Moreover, 11 districts out of the 39 (28%) exceeded 80% vaccination coverage: Plateaux region (Anié and Est-Mono); Central region (Blitta and Sotouboua); Kara region (Bassar, Dankpen, and Doufelgou) and Savanes region (Kpendjal, Kpendjal-Ouest, Oti, Oti-Sud). A total of 15 districts out of 39 (38%) did not achieve 50% administrative coverage: Grand Lomé region (all districts: Agoè and Golfe); Maritime region (all districts: Avé, Bas-Mono, Lacs, Vo, Yoto, Zio); Plateaux region (Danyi, Haho, Kloto, Kpélé, Moyen-Mono, Ogou, Wawa); Central region (Tchaoudjo). Figure 2 shows vaccine coverage disaggregated by district, while Figure 3 highlights the performance of the districts. The details are displayed in Appendix A

Apart from the school environment, the target group was found and vaccinated in out-of-school settings. A total of 26,353 girls were vaccinated in out-of-school settings (8.7% of the total vaccinated) and 278,104 in schools (91.3%). In addition, 55.4% of the girls were vaccinated through the fixed strategy, while 4.2% during the mobile strategy (Table 2).

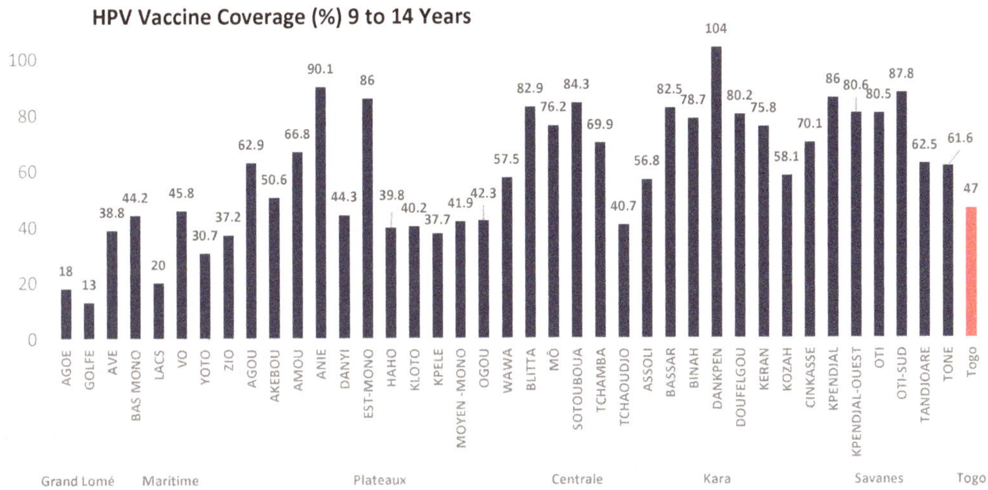

Figure 2. Administrative vaccination coverage by district during the HPV vaccination campaign for girls aged 9–14 in Togo in December 2023.

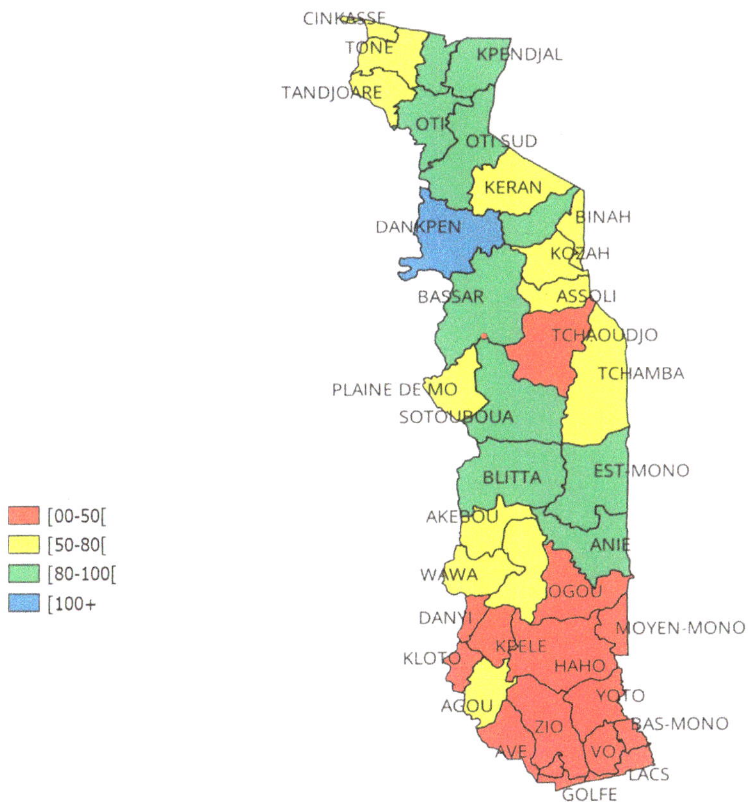

Figure 3. Performance of districts, administrative vaccination coverage during the HPV vaccination campaign for girls aged 9–14 in Togo in December 2023.

Table 2. Vaccination coverage by settings, by strategy, and by region during the cervical cancer vaccination campaign for girls aged 9–14 in Togo in December 2023.

Region (Nb of Girls Vaccinated)	Settings		Strategy		
	In School, n (%)	Out of School, n (%)	Fixed, n (%)	Out Reach, n (%)	Mobile, n (%)
Grand Lomé (26,611)	24,790 (93.2)	1821 (6.8)	7561 (28.4)	17,160 (64.5)	1890 (7.1)
Maritime (37,181)	35,961 (96.7)	1220 (3.3)	20,230 (54.4)	15,172 (40.8)	1779 (4.8)
Plateaux (76,930)	70,401 (91.5)	6529 (8.5)	47,176 (61.3)	27,180 (35.3)	2574 (3.3)
Centrale (42,806)	39,646 (92.6)	3160 (7.4)	25,153 (58.8)	16,589 (38.8)	1064 (2.5)
Kara (60,323)	55,913 (92.7)	4410 (7.3)	33,794 (56.0)	23,912 (39.6)	2617 (4.3)
Savanes (60,606)	51,393 (84.8)	9213 (15.2)	34,786 (57.4)	22,887 (37.8)	2933 (4.8)
Togo (304,457)	278,104 (91.3)	26,353 (8.7)	168,700 (55.4)	122,900 (40.4)	12,857 (4.2)

Vaccination coverage for girls in and out of school is broadly in line with school enrollment rates by region (Grand Lomé = 98.1%; Maritime 96.8%; Plateaux = 95.7%; Centrale 93.0%; Kara = 91.6%, Savanes = 80.4%), although there are some regions having low coverage rates recorded.

Concerning the AEFI, the highest rate of notification (145.5/100,000 doses) was recorded in the Maritime region. For minor AEFI, the most frequently reported signs were injection site reaction (pain, redness, swelling, which accounted for 86.8%); fever (19.3%) and headache (17.6%). A total of seven serious AEFI cases were recorded throughout the country, including three in the Kara region, and were investigated, with positive outcomes.

4. Discussion

This research focused on assessing HPV vaccination coverage in Togo, following a nationwide campaign that targeted girls aged 9 to 14 years old. We sought to identify discrepancies in vaccine uptake among vulnerable population groups. The quantitative analysis revealed that approximately half of the target population received the HPV vaccine, with a similar coverage for both in-school and out-of-school girls. This level of coverage, though significant, highlights gaps when compared to global standards, such as those found in high-income countries. Additionally, regional disparities were observed, particularly a south–north gradient, with socioeconomic factors potentially influencing access to vaccines.

Prior to the implementation of the campaign, the readiness assessment tool was used to assess key components of campaign preparedness, including cold chain management, staff training, vaccine supply, AEFI monitoring, community awareness, coordination, and resource mobilization. This systematic approach helps identify gaps early and implement corrective actions in all districts. All the districts received similar support during preparation and implementation of the campaign.

The HPV vaccination coverage observed in Togo is comparable to findings from a similar study in Tanzania, which reported a 49% coverage rate [20]. However, these results contrast sharply with a systematic review and meta-analysis of school-aged adolescent girls in sub-Saharan Africa, which indicated a significantly lower uptake rate of 28.53% [21]. When compared to high-income countries like the USA (62.8%), Australia (83%) [22], and Scotland (94.4%) [23], Togo's HPV vaccination coverage lags substantially. This discrepancy likely stems from differences in healthcare infrastructure, vaccine availability, and routine immunization practices between low-resource and developed countries.

The study showed notable regional variations in HPV vaccination coverage within Togo, with a clear south-to-north gradient. Surprisingly, the southern regions, including Lomé, which have higher literacy rates and socioeconomic status, showed lower vaccination coverage compared to some northern regions. This suggests that factors beyond education and economic status may play a significant role in vaccine uptake. Such factors may include awareness, effectiveness, and involvement of local communities during the vaccination campaign. Also, within a region, there are vaccine coverage variations between districts. Most districts with low vaccine coverage are urban, with high impact from misinformation circulating in social medias. The observed disparities highlight the need for region-specific interventions to ensure equitable uptake of the HPV vaccine across the country. We found that the HPV vaccine coverage was 104% in Dankpen district. This discrepancy could be explained by possible inaccuracy in estimating the target population during enumeration process, and data recording errors during the implementation of the supplementary immunization activities. The HPV vaccine coverage rates were consistently higher among 9-year-old girls compared to those aged 10–14 across all regions. This could be attributed to a higher refusal rate among the older age group. Nine-year-old girls, who are most often in primary school, encountered less resistance than their older counterparts in secondary school. Additionally, girls aged 10–14 may have greater exposure to rumors on social media, which could contribute to higher refusal rates.

Several barriers may contribute to the low HPV vaccination rate in Togo [17,18]. Firstly, this campaign was implemented in a context where rumors about the HPV vaccine were widespread on social media, particularly in the southern regions. This led to significant cases of vaccine refusal, especially in these southern regions. Secondly, concerns about side effects, fueled by misinformation, continue to affect vaccine acceptance in Togo. Misconceptions such as the false belief that the HPV vaccine causes infertility or promotes promiscuity are prevalent in some communities, undermining trust in the vaccination. Thirdly, low awareness may also have played a role in the low coverage. In fact, a lack of public understanding of HPV, its risks, and the benefit of vaccination is a major barrier in Togo. This could be explained partly by the limited education and awareness campaigns on the importance of HPV. The absence of comprehensive information prevents individuals from recognizing the importance of vaccination in preventing cervical cancer.

To address these barriers and increase HPV vaccination coverage across Togo, a multi-pronged approach is necessary. Key strategies include vaccine access expansion, by improving healthcare infrastructure and logistics to ensure broader availability of vaccines, particularly in underserved regions. Awareness raising by implementing targeted education campaigns and community dialogues to dispel myths about the vaccine and provide accurate information about the safety of HPV vaccine and its efficacy could also improve coverage. These campaigns should focus on promoting the benefits of vaccination for preventing HPV-related diseases. In addition, healthcare providers and community leaders should use evidence-based communication strategies to counter misinformation and build trust in vaccination programs. Furthermore, HPV vaccination should be incorporated into routine immunization schedules and financial barriers reduced through free vaccination programs. Finally, government agencies, healthcare providers, community organizations, and international partners should work together to overcome logistical, financial, and cultural barriers to vaccination.

Limitations

While this study provides valuable insights into HPV vaccination coverage in Togo, there are several limitations. First, the study focused primarily on quantitative data, with limited assessment of the qualitative factors that influence vaccine uptake, such as cultural beliefs and community engagement. Furthermore, the study did not account for potential biases in self-reported vaccination data, which could influence the accuracy of the reported coverage rates.

Future research should explore the qualitative aspects of HPV vaccination uptake, including the role of cultural, social, and religious factors in shaping attitudes toward vaccination. Studies that investigate the effectiveness of targeted educational campaigns and intervention strategies in different regions could provide valuable insights for improving vaccine acceptance. Additionally, longitudinal studies tracking vaccination coverage and its impact on cervical cancer incidence would contribute to understanding the long-term outcomes of HPV vaccination programs in low-resource settings.

The findings of this study have important policy implications for improving HPV vaccination coverage in Togo. Policymakers should prioritize efforts to strengthen healthcare infrastructure, particularly in rural and difficult to access areas, to ensure equitable access to vaccination services. Offering free HPV vaccinations could reduce financial barriers and improve uptake among vulnerable populations. Moreover, launching national awareness campaigns that address common misconceptions and promote the benefits of vaccination is critical for increasing public acceptance. Finally, integrating HPV vaccination into the broader national immunization program would ensure its sustainability and long-term success in reducing HPV-related disease burdens. By addressing these policy priorities, Togo can move closer to achieving international benchmarks for HPV vaccination and improving public health outcomes.

5. Conclusions

Significant progress has been made in HPV vaccination coverage among girls aged 9 to 14 in Togo; however, disparities persist compared to high-income countries, but also between the different regions. Further interventions and investigations are needed to identify and address barriers to vaccine acceptance, to implement targeted interventions, and to strengthen healthcare systems. Toward these strategies, stakeholders can enhance HPV vaccination coverage, improve equity, and mitigate the impact of HPV-related diseases in vulnerable populations.

Author Contributions: Conceptualization: D.E.L., I.Y., A.B., K.A., Y.T.T. and D.K.E.; Methodology: D.E.L., I.Y., A.B., K.A., Y.T.T., A.A., Y.M., A.M.B., N.-M.J.B., C.S.W., F.F.R.M., H.L.-D., T.A.T., T.N.M., T.K., A.B.D., F.B.T.D., B.I., A.L., M.K.W. and D.K.E.; Formal analysis: D.E.L., I.Y., A.B., K.A., Y.T.T. and D.K.E.; Writing—original draft: D.E.L., I.Y., A.B., K.A., Y.T.T., Y.M., A.M.B., T.A.T., T.N.M., T.K., A.B.D., F.B.T.D., A.L., M.K.W. and D.K.E.; Writing—review & editing: D.E.L., I.Y., A.B., K.A., Y.T.T., A.A., Y.M., A.M.B., N.-M.J.B., C.S.W., F.F.R.M., H.L.-D., T.A.T., T.N.M., T.K., A.B.D., F.B.T.D., B.I., A.L., M.K.W. and D.K.E.; Supervision: D.E.L., I.Y., A.B., K.A., Y.T.T., A.A., Y.M., A.M.B., N.-M.J.B., C.S.W., F.F.R.M., H.L.-D., T.A.T., T.N.M., T.K., A.B.D., F.B.T.D., B.I., A.L., M.K.W. and D.K.E.; D.K.E. was responsible of the scientific coordination of the study. All authors have read and agreed to the published version of the manuscript.

Funding: This research received no external funding. However, the HPV vaccine costs and the SIA operational costs were financed by the Togolese Government and Gavi, the Vaccine Alliance.

Institutional Review Board Statement: Ethics approval was not required. However, the National Immunization Technical Advisory Group (NITAG) recommended the introduction of the HPV vaccine in Togo. For this study, secondary data were obtained from the Division of Immunization at the Ministry of Health of Togo after clearance from the department. The Division of Immunization authorized the use of data.

Informed Consent Statement: Patient consent was waived due to the fact that the NITAG recommended the introduction of the HPV vaccine in the country.

Data Availability Statement: Extracted data are with the authors and at the Ministry of Health and available for sharing on request.

Acknowledgments: We are thankful to the Ministry of Health of Togo through the Secretary-General for approving the publication of these results.

Conflicts of Interest: The authors declare that they have no competing interests. D.E.L., A.A., A.B., N.-M.J.B., C.S.W., F.F.R.M., A.B.D., F.B.T.D., A.L. are working for the World Health Organization. Y.T.T., T.N.M., and T.K. work for Unicef Togo country office. The authors are solely responsible for the opinions expressed in this publication and do not necessarily represent the decisions, policies, or views of the World Health Organization and UNICEF.

Abbreviations

The following abbreviations are used in this manuscript:

AEFI	Adverse Events Following Immunization
DHIS2	District Health Information System 2
Gavi	Gavi, the Vaccine Alliance
GLOBOCAN	Global Cancer Observatory
HISP	Health Information Systems Program
HPV	Human Papillomavirus
ICC	Inter-Agency Coordination Committee
NITAG	National Immunization Technical Advisory Group
SIA	Supplementary Immunization Activities
UNICEF	United Nations International Children's Emergency Fund
WHO	World Health Organization

Appendix A

Table A1. Target populations and administrative HPV vaccine coverage by district and region, vaccination campaign among girls of 9 to 14 years old in Togo, December 2023.

Region/ District	Total Population 2022 by, District	Target Population 9-Year-Old Girls	Target Population 9-Year-Old Girls	Target Population 9-Year-Old Girls	Number of 9-Year-Old Girls Vaccinated	Number of 10- to 14-Year-Old Girls Vaccinated	Total Number of 9- to 14-Year-Old Girls Vaccinated	Number of HPV Vaccine Doses Used	HPV Vaccine Coverage (%) 9 Years	HPV Vaccine Coverage (%) 10 to 14 Years	HPV Vaccine Coverage (%) 9 to 14 Years
AGOE	902,997	12,371	60,049	72,420	2413	10,581	12,994	13,056	20	18	18
GOLFE	1,341,003	18,372	89,177	107,548	2679	10,938	13,617	14,012	15	12	13
REGION GRAND LOME	2,244,000	30,743	149,226	179,969	5092	21,519	26,611	27,068	16.6	14.4	14.8
AVE	121,640	1666	8089	9756	779	3008	3787	3852	46.7	37.2	38.8
BAS MONO	111,212	1524	7396	8919	617	3325	3942	4000	40.5	45.0	44.2
LACS	232,255	3182	15,445	18,627	849	2875	3724	3785	26.7	18.6	20.0
VO	267,980	3671	17,821	21,492	1736	8100	9836	9938	47.3	45.5	45.8
YOTO	210,264	2881	13,983	16,863	1018	4160	5178	5240	35.3	29.8	30.7
ZIO	358,920	4917	23,868	28,785	1999	8715	10,714	10,858	40.7	36.5	37.2
REGION MARITIME	1,302,271	17,841	86,601	104,442	6998	30,183	37,181	37,673	39.2	34.9	35.6
AGOU	110,370	1512	7340	8852	989	4577	5566	5624	65.4	62.4	62.9
AKEBOU	79,469	1089	5285	6373	867	2356	3223	3264	79.6	44.6	50.6
AMOU	136,200	1866	9057	10,923	1370	5928	7298	7368	73.4	65.4	66.8
ANIE	159,739	2188	10,623	12,811	2550	8999	11,549	11,573	116.5	84.7	90.1
DANYI	50,424	691	3353	4044	355	1437	1792	1754	51.4	42.9	44.3
EST-MONO	155,185	2126	10,320	12,446	2493	8216	10,709	10,760	117.3	79.6	86.0
HAHO	315,921	4328	21,009	25,337	1980	8106	10,086	10,122	45.7	38.6	39.8
KLOTO	182,030	2494	12,105	14,599	1092	4773	5865	5934	43.8	39.4	40.2
KPELE	97,726	1339	6499	7838	611	2341	2952	3012	45.6	36.0	37.7
MOYEN-MONO	97,946	1342	6513	7855	615	2680	3295	3328	45.8	41.1	41.9

Table A1. *Cont.*

Region/ District	Total Population 2022 by, District	Target Population 9-Year-Old Girls	Target Population 9-Year-Old Girls	Target Population 9-Year-Old Girls	Number of 9-Year-Old Girls Vaccinated	Number of 10- to 14-Year-Old Girls Vaccinated	Total Number of 9- to 14-Year-Old Girls Vaccinated	Number of HPV Vaccine Doses Used	HPV Vaccine Coverage (%) 9 Years	HPV Vaccine Coverage (%) 10 to 14 Years	HPV Vaccine Coverage (%) 9 to 14 Years
OGOU	252,973	3466	16,823	20,288	1836	6740	8576	8625	53.0	40.1	42.3
WAWA	130,622	1790	8686	10,476	1142	4877	6019	5992	63.8	56.1	57.5
REGION PLATEAUX	1,768,605	24,230	117,612	141,842	15,900	61,030	76,930	77,356	65.6	51.9	54.2
BLITTA	177,072	2426	11,775	14,201	2496	9281	11,777	11,793	102.9	78.8	82.9
MÔ	47,615	652	3166	3819	541	2342	2883	2898	83%	74%	75.5%
SOTOUBOUA	157,067	2152	10,445	12,597	2004	8614	10,618	10,676	93.1	82.5	84.3
TCHAMBA	168,352	2306	11,195	13,502	1935	7502	9437	9526	83.9	67.0	69.9
TCHAOUDJO	246,780	3381	16,411	19,792	1796	6269	8065	8168	53.1	38.2	40.7
REGION CENTRALE	796 886	10 917	52 993	63 910	8 772	34 008	42,780	43,061	80%	64%	66.9%
ASSOLI	66,598	912	4429	5341	534	2502	3036	3105	58.5	56.5	56.8
BASSAR	153,927	2109	10,236	12,345	2065	8118	10,183	10,259	97.9	79.3	82.5
BINAH	90,864	1245	6042	7287	1114	4618	5732	5770	89.5	76.4	78.7
DANKPEN	165,417	2266	11,000	13,266	3708	10,088	13,796	13,818	163.6	91.7	104.0
DOUFELGOU	102,245	1401	6799	8200	1342	5234	6576	6614	95.8	77.0	80.2
KERAN	119,892	1643	7973	9615	1626	5667	7293	7394	99.0	71.1	75.8
KOZAH	294,260	4031	19,568	23,600	2290	11,417	13,707	13,780	56.8	58.3	58.1
REGION KARA	993,203	13,607	66,048	79,655	12,679	47,644	60,323	60,740	93.2	72.1	75.7
CINKASSE	100,491	1377	6683	8059	1125	4524	5649	5680	81.7	67.7	70.1
KPENDJAL	77,679	1064	5166	6230	1123	4234	5357	5374	105.5	82.0	86.0
KPENDJAL-OUEST	118,212	1620	7861	9481	1816	5822	7638	7656	112.1	74.1	80.6
OTI	119,152	1632	7924	9556	1336	6356	7692	7710	81.8	80.2	80.5
OTI-SUD	122,891	1684	8172	9856	2071	6580	8651	8692	123.0	80.5	87.8
TANDJOARE	150,993	2069	10,041	12,110	1420	6152	7572	7614	68.6	61.3	62.5
TONE	365,237	5004	24,288	29,292	3952	14,095	18,047	19,846	79.0	58.0	61.6
REGION SAVANES	1,054,655	14,449	70,135	84,583	12,843	47,763	60,606	62,572	88.9	68.1	71.7
TOTAL PAYS	8,159,620	111,787	542,615	654,402	62,284	242,173	304,457	308,470	55.7	44.6	46.5

References

1. De Villiers, E.-M.; Fauquet, C.; Broker, T.R.; Bernard, H.-U.; zur Hausen, H. Classification of papillomaviruses. *Virology* **2004**, *324*, 17–27. [PubMed]
2. Gheit, T. Mucosal and Cutaneous Human Papillomavirus Infections and Cancer Biology. *Front. Oncol.* **2019**, *9*, 355. [CrossRef] [PubMed]
3. de Martel, C.; Plummer, M.; Vignat, J.; Franceschi, S. Worldwide burden of cancer attributable to HPV by site, country and HPV type. *Int. J. Cancer.* **2017**, *141*, 664–670. [PubMed]
4. World Health Organization (WHO). Cervical Cancer. 2024. Available online: https://www.who.int/news-room/fact-sheets/detail/cervical-cancer (accessed on 14 August 2024).
5. Seyoum, A.; Assefa, N.; Gure, T.; Seyoum, B.; Mulu, A.; Mihret, A. Prevalence and Genotype Distribution of High-Risk Human Papillomavirus Infection Among Sub-Saharan African Women: A Systematic Review and Meta-Analysis. *Front. Public Health* **2022**, *10*, 890880.
6. De Vuyst, H.; Alemany, L.; Lacey, C.; Chibwesha, C.J.; Sahasrabuddhe, V.; Banura, C.; Denny, L.; Parham, G.P. The burden of human papillomavirus infections and related diseases in sub-saharan Africa. *Vaccine* **2013**, *31* (Suppl. S5), F32–F46. [PubMed]
7. World Health Organization (WHO). Cervical Cancer Action–Strategies for HPV Vaccination in the Developing World–PAHO/WHO | Pan American Health Organization. 2009. Available online: https://www.paho.org/en/documents/cervical-cancer-action-strategies-hpv-vaccination-developing-world (accessed on 14 August 2024).

8. Lei, J.; Ploner, A.; Elfström, K.M.; Wang, J.; Roth, A.; Fang, F.; Sparén, P. HPV Vaccination and the Risk of Invasive Cervical Cancer. *N. Engl. J. Med.* **2020**, *383*, 1340–1348. [PubMed]
9. Barnabas, R.V.; Brown, E.R.; Onono, M.A.; Bukusi, E.A.; Njoroge, B.; Winer, R.L.; Galloway, D.A.; Pinder, L.P.; Donnell, D.; Wakhungu, I.; et al. Efficacy of single-dose HPV vaccination among young African women. *NEJM Evid.* **2022**, *1*, EVIDoa2100056. [PubMed]
10. Pathak, P.; Pajai, S.; Kesharwani, H. A Review on the Use of the HPV Vaccine in the Prevention of Cervical Cancer. *Cureus* **2022**, *14*, e28710. [CrossRef] [PubMed]
11. Pinto, L.A.; Dillner, J.; Beddows, S.; Unger, E.R. Immunogenicity of HPV prophylactic vaccines: Serology assays and their use in HPV vaccine evaluation and development. *Vaccine* **2018**, *36*, 4792–4799. [CrossRef] [PubMed]
12. Murewanhema, G.; Moyo, E.; Dzobo, M.; Mandishora-Dube, R.S.; Dzinamarira, T. Human papilloma virus vaccination in the resource-limited settings of sub-Saharan Africa: Challenges and recommendations. *Vaccine X* **2024**, *20*, 100549. [PubMed]
13. Black, E.; Richmond, R. Prevention of Cervical Cancer in Sub-Saharan Africa: The Advantages and Challenges of HPV Vaccination. *Vaccines* **2018**, *6*, 61. [CrossRef]
14. Rathod, S.; Potdar, J.; Gupta, A.; Sethi, N.; Dande, A. Empowering Women's Health: Insights Into HPV Vaccination and the Prevention of Invasive Cervical Cancer. *Cureus* **2023**, *15*, e49523. [CrossRef]
15. Gavi, the Vaccine Alliance. Togo Introduces Human Papillomavirus Vaccine to Protect Adolescent Girls from the Leading Cause of Cervical Cancer. 2024. Available online: https://www.gavi.org/news/media-room/togo-introduces-human-papillomavirus-vaccine-protect-adolescent-girls-leading (accessed on 15 August 2024).
16. Ministère de la Santé du Togo: Rapport Global. Projet de Démonstration de la Vaccination Contre le Virus du Papillome Humain Pour la Prévention et le Contre le du Cancer du Col de L'utérus; Togo—2015 a 2017. Available online: https://www.google.com/url?sa=t&source=web&rct=j&opi=89978449&url=https://www.pev.tg/download/rapport-global-2ans-projet-demo-vaccin-vph-cancer-col-togo-vf/&ved=2ahUKEwj4lJDPuJiMAxXWBfsDHeYCDDQQFnoECCwQAQ&usg=AOvVaw06EGIMdQvNgpM6XPgHe6aj (accessed on 19 March 2025).
17. Landoh, D.E.; Ouro-Kavalah, F.; Yaya, I.; Kahn, A.-L.; Wasswa, P.; Lacle, A.; Gitta, S.N.; Soura, A.B. Predictors of incomplete immunization coverage among one to five years old children in Togo. *BMC Public Health* **2016**, *16*, 968. [CrossRef] [PubMed]
18. Ekouevi, D.K.; Gbeasor-Komlanvi, F.A.; Yaya, I.; Zida-Compaore, W.I.; Boko, A.; Sewu, E.; Lacle, A.; Ndibu, N.; Toke, T.; Landoh, D.E.; et al. Incomplete immunization among children aged 12–23 months in Togo: A multilevel analysis of individual and contextual factors. *BMC Public Health* **2018**, *18*, 952.
19. Ministère de la Santé, de l'Hygiène Publique République Togolaise. *Avis sur l'introduction du Schéma Vaccinal Simplifié Monodose du Vaccin Contre le Papillomavirus Humain dans la Vaccination de Routine au Togo GTCV–Togo*; Ministère de la Santé, de l'Hygiène Publique République Togolaise: Lomé, Togo, 2023.
20. Mendes Lobão, W.; Duarte, F.G.; Burns, J.D.; de Souza Teles Santos, C.A.; Chagas de Almeida, M.C.; Reingold, A.; Duarte Moreira, E. Low coverage of HPV vaccination in the national immunization programme in Brazil: Parental vaccine refusal or barriers in health-service based vaccine delivery? *PLoS ONE* **2018**, *13*, e0206726. [CrossRef] [PubMed]
21. Asgedom, Y.S.; Kebede, T.M.; Seifu, B.L.; Mare, K.U.; Asmare, Z.A.; Asebe, H.A.; Kase, B.F.; Shibeshi, A.H.; Tebeje, T.M.; Sabo, K.G.; et al. Human papillomavirus vaccination uptake and determinant factors among adolescent schoolgirls in sub-Saharan Africa: A systematic review and meta-analysis. *Hum. Vaccines Immunother.* **2024**, *20*, 2326295. [CrossRef] [PubMed]
22. Brotherton, J.M.L.; Murray, S.L.; Hall, M.A.; Andrewartha, L.K.; Banks, C.A.; Meijer, D.; Pitcher, H.C.; Scully, M.M.; Molchanoff, L. Human papillomavirus vaccine coverage among female Australian adolescents: Success of the school-based approach. *Med. J. Aust.* **2013**, *199*, 614–617. [PubMed]
23. Loke, A.Y.; Kwan, M.L.; Wong, Y.-T.; Wong, A.K.Y. The Uptake of Human Papillomavirus Vaccination and Its Associated Factors Among Adolescents: A Systematic Review. *J. Prim. Care Community Health* **2017**, *8*, 349–362. [CrossRef] [PubMed]

vaccines

MDPI

Conference Report

The 2024 Annual Meeting of the Essential Programmes on Immunization Managers in Central Africa: A Peer Learning Platform

Franck Mboussou [1,*], Audry Mulumba [2], Celestin Traore [3], Florence Conteh-Nordman [4], Shalom Tchokfe Ndoula [5], Antoinette Demian Mbailamen [6], Jean Claude Bizimana [7], Christian Akani [1], Yolande Vuo-Masembe [1], Bridget Farham [1], Marcelin Menguo Nimpa [8], Thomas Noel Gaha [9], Martin Morand [4], Lynda Rey [4], Maria Carolina Danovaro-Holliday [10], Charles Shey Wiysonge [1] and Benido Impouma [1]

1 World Health Organization Regional Office for Africa, Brazzaville P.O. Box 06, Congo; sheyc@who.int (C.S.W.)
2 Essential Immunization Programme, Ministry of Health, 30 Avenue de la Justice, Kinshasa M7MG+2X8, Democratic Republic of the Congo
3 UNICEF Regional Office for West and Central Africa, Dakar P.O. Box 29720, Senegal
4 Gavi Secretariat, 1218 Le Grand-Saconnex, Switzerland; lrey@gavi.org (L.R.)
5 Essential Immunization Programme, Ministry of Health, 8 Rue 3038 Quartier du Lac, Yaoundé P.O. Box 1937, Cameroon
6 Essential Immunization Programme, Ministry of Health, Ndjamena P.O. Box 548, Chad
7 Essential Immunization Programme, Ministry of Health, Rue Pierre Ngendandumwe, Bujumbura J968+H3J, Burundi
8 World Health Organization, Democratic Republic of Congo Country Office, 42 Avenue des Cliniques, Kinshasa 01206, Democratic Republic of the Congo
9 UNICEF, Democratic Republic of Congo Country Office, 372 Concession Immotex, Kinshasa M7H9+HQW, Democratic Republic of the Congo
10 World Health Organization Headquarters, 1211 Geneva, Switzerland
* Correspondence: mboussouf@who.int

Abstract: Background: Since 1974, Essential Programme on Immunisation managers from ten Central African countries meet yearly with partners to review progress made and share experiences and lessons learned from the implementation of immunization programmes. The 2024 meeting occurred in Kinshasa, Democratic Republic of Congo, in September 2024. This conference report summarizes the key takeaways from discussions on using immunization data for decision-making, the implementation of the Big Catch-Up (BCU) initiative to reduce the burden of zero-dose children, and progress and challenges in introducing selected new vaccines. Conference Takeaways: Inaccurate administrative data on routine immunization observed in most countries, compared to WHO/UNICEF Estimates of National Immunization Coverage and national survey estimates, affect timely decisions to improve the Expanded Programme on Immunization (EPI) performance. Five countries in Central Africa are among the priority countries of the BCU initiative but, as of the end of August 2024, are yet to formally start its implementation. Cameroon and Central African Republic introduced the malaria vaccine in January 2024 and August 2024, respectively, while the Democratic Republic of Congo, Chad, and Burundi have planned to do so by 2025. Conclusions and Recommendations: Meeting participants put forward several recommendations for countries and immunization partners, including but not limited to (i) investing more in routine immunization data quality assurance to better use data to inform decisions, (ii) accelerating the implementation of the BCU initiative to close the immunity gap resulting from routine immunization disruptions due to the COVID-19 pandemic, (iii) updating malaria vaccine introduction plans to invest more in demand generation and community engagement, and (iv) learning from Cameroon's experience in tackling hesitancy to human papilloma virus vaccine. It is critical to set up an appropriate mechanism for monitoring the implementation of these recommendations.

Keywords: immunization; Central Africa; big catch-up; peer learning

1. Introduction

In 1974, the World Health Organization (WHO) established the Expanded Programme on Immunization to ensure equitable access to life-saving vaccines for every child, regardless of geographic location or socioeconomic status [1]. Later, this programme evolved into the Essential Programme on Immunization (EPI), seeking to safeguard individuals of all ages through comprehensive immunization efforts [1]. Countries across the world gradually set up the EPI at the national level. In the Central Africa subregion made up of 10 countries (Angola, Burundi, Cameroon, Central African Republic (CAR), Chad, Congo, Democratic Republic of the Congo, Equatorial Guinea, Gabon, and São Tomé and Príncipe), the EPI was operational in all countries by 1984. As a result of the implementation of the EPI in Central Africa, (i) the number of antigens provided to children and adolescents increased from 6 in 1984 to 13 in 2024; (ii) the number of children vaccinated yearly with the first dose of the pentavalent vaccine—Diphtheria, Tetanus, Pertussis, *Haemophilus influenzae* type b, and Hepatitis B—(Penta 1) increased from 1.6 million in 2000 to 7.9 million in 2023; and (iii) the median coverage with the third dose of the pentavalent vaccine (Penta 3) increased from 38.5% [range: 31%;82%] in 2000 to 72% [range: 42%;89%] in 2023, as per the 2024 revision of the WHO and UNICEF Estimates of National Immunization Coverage (WUENIC) [2]. Despite this significant and commendable progress, most countries in Central Africa are still off-track towards achieving global immunization agenda 2030 (IA2030) targets [3]. Since 1974, EPI managers from Central African countries meet every year with partners and other stakeholders to review progress made and share experiences and lessons learned from implementing national immunization programmes in line with global and regional goals. Organized jointly by the WHO Regional Office for Africa and UNICEF Regional Office for West and Central Africa, the 2024 annual EPI managers' meeting took place in Kinshasa, Democratic Republic of Congo, from 9 to 12 September 2024 and attracted 157 participants from 10 countries of the subregion and immunization partners. The meeting's methods included oral presentations from subject matter experts, panel discussions on selected topics, and country posters on EPI progress. This report summarizes the key takeaways from discussions on three key topics: use of immunization data for decision-making, implementation of the big catch-up (BCU) initiative aiming at reducing the burden of zero-dose and under immunized children [3], and progress and challenges in the introduction of selected new vaccines (Malaria vaccines and Human Papillomavirus vaccines).

2. Conference Section

2.1. Routine Immunization Data Use to Inform Decisions

Discussion surrounding the use of routine vaccination coverage data to inform decision-making showed that all countries in Central Africa have set up a system for collecting data on vaccine uptake and computing immunization coverage to monitor EPI progress. At health facility level, the system involves paper-based data collection/reporting tools, which include registers, tally sheets, coverage wall charst, monthly reporting forms, etc. In 6 of the 10 countries (Angola, Burundi, Cameroon, Chad, Congo, and Democratic Republic of Congo), monthly reports from health facilities are submitted to the regional and national level through an electronic tool for aggregated data reporting, i.e., District Health Information Software 2 (DHIS2). The remaining four countries use a Microsoft Excel-based tool for data transmission from the district level to the national level: the district vaccination management data tool (DVMDT) and are in the process of transitioning to DHIS 2. In all countries, target populations for EPI are derived from census projections. Suboptimal data quality assurance processes and inaccurate estimates of target populations, including outdated censuses or incomplete civil registration and vital statistics (CRVSs), have led to overestimating immunization coverage in some countries. Of the 10 countries in Central Africa, administrative coverage with Penta 3 in 2023 was similar to WUENIC estimates in 5 countries (Burundi, Congo, Equatorial Guinea, Gabon, and São Tomé and Príncipe). In Angola, Cameroon, Central African Republic, Chad, and the Democratic Republic of Congo, the administrative penta 3 coverage in 2023 was more significant than WUENIC, suggesting the underestimation of target populations, the overreporting of children vaccinated, or a combination of both (Figure 1). In these countries, the proportion of districts with administrative penta 3 coverage in 2023 of at least 80% was 51% in Angola, 54% in Cameroon, 80% in Central African Republic and Chad, and 85% in the Democratic Republic of Congo, suggesting disparities in the EPI performance between districts.

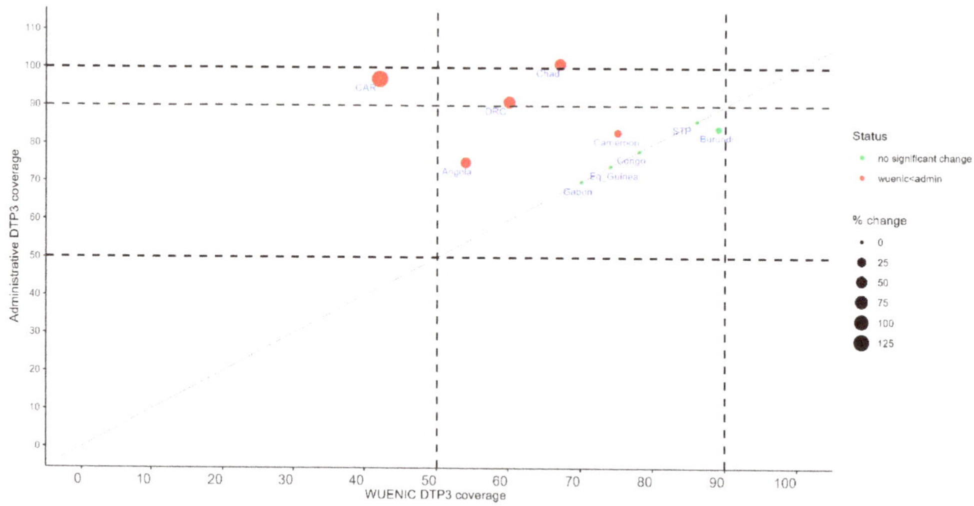

Figure 1. WUENIC and administrative coverage with the third dose of pentavalent vaccine in 2023 in Central Africa. Dashed lines earmark 50%, 80%, and 90% coverage; the solid line represents the diagonal.

Based on WUENIC estimates, the median Penta 1 to Penta 3 dropout rate in 2023 was 6%, with four countries recording over 10% (Democratic Republic of Congo (20%), Chad (17%), Angola (15%) and Central African Republic (12%)) and three countries recording less than 5% (Burundi (0%), Gabon (3%) and Congo (4%)).

While WUENIC data are used to monitor and compare the performance of immunization programmes at the national and international levels in a standardized way [4], microplanning and actions aiming to improve the routine immunization performance are undertaken using administrative coverage data. Immunization coverage surveys (ICSs) are among the data sources used to generate WUENIC estimates in addition to administrative data and other programmatic and operational considerations. In 2023–2024, seven countries conducted an ICS: Cameroon, Central African Republic, Chad, Congo, the Democratic Republic of Congo, Equatorial Guinea, and São Tomé and Príncipe. The Democratic Republic of Congo also employed a Demographic and Health Survey (DHS) in 2023–2024, as did Angola. Limited technical capacities, financial resources (especially when a sample representative of districts is required), and low vaccination card availability were identified as the main challenges of ICSs in Central Africa. None of the Central African countries have managed to deploy an electronic immunization registry nationwide, failing to leverage the COVID-19 vaccination individual data systems to strengthen routine immunization data management and use for decision-making [5].

Inaccurate administrative data, especially the overestimation of immunization coverage, affects timely and well-informed decision-making aiming to improve EPI performance. The following recommendations were adopted to enhance effective use of quality data for decision-making: (i) conduct data triangulation exercises annually to adjust population size estimates using WHO methods for Assessing and Improving the Accuracy of Target Population Estimates for Immunization Coverage [6]; (ii) invest more in data quality self-assessments and audits to improve routine immunization data accuracy; (iii) consider deploying electronic immunization registries, including digital vaccination cards learning from the experience of countries in other regions, and leveraging COVID-19 vaccination experience; and (iv) conduct immunization coverage surveys representative of the district level more frequently.

2.2. Efforts to Reduce the Burden of Zero-Dose Children

During the meeting, a discussion panel was dedicated to countries' efforts in reducing the burden of zero-dose and under-immunized children. Zero-dose refers to children who have failed to receive any routine vaccination, while under-immunized refers to children who have received some, but not all, of their recommended scheduled vaccinations. In all Central African countries, COVID-19 disruptions have led to a dramatic increase in the number of zero-dose and under-immunized children. From 2019 to 2023, based on WUENIC (2023 revision) and the United Nations Population Division (UNPD) estimates (2024 revision), Central Africa recorded an estimated 13.9 million of zero-dose and under-immunized children (8.9 million zero-dose children and 5.0 million under-immunized children). Table 1 presents the distribution of the estimated number of zero-dose and under-immunized children by country in Central Africa from 2019 to 2023.

Table 1. Distribution of zero-dose and under-immunized children in Central Africa (2019–2023).

Country	Surviving Infants (2019–2023 Cohorts)	# Zero-Dose Children	# Under-Immunized Children	# Zero-Dose and Under-Immunized Children	% of All Zero-Dose and Under-Immunized Children in Central Africa
Angola	6,389,000	2,468,000	744,000	3,212,000	23
Burundi	2,200,000	119,000	57,000	176,000	1
Cameroon	4,503,000	1,088,000	243,000	1,331,000	10
Central African Republic	1,054,000	485,000	127,000	612,000	4
Chad	3,683,000	818,000	743,000	1,561,000	11
Congo	899,000	172,000	34,000	206,000	1
Democratic Republic of Congo	19,920,000	3,636,000	3,050,000	6,686,000	48
Equatorial Guinea	258,000	59,000	25,000	84,000	1
Gabon	334,000	93,000	15,000	108,000	1
São Tomé and Príncipe	31,000	2000	-	2000	0
Total	**39,271,000**	**8,940,000**	**5,038,000**	**13,978,000**	**100**

#: Number.

Angola, Chad, Cameroon, and the Democratic Republic of Congo account for 91% of zero-dose and under-immunized children in the subregion.

To close the immunity gaps caused by the backsliding of immunization coverage during the COVID-19 pandemic and catch up on vaccination of 90% of zero-dose children by the end of 2025, WHO, UNICEF, Gavi Secretariat and Gates Foundation set up the BCU initiative in 2023 [7]. Five Central African countries are among the priority countries for this initiative: Burundi, Cameroon, Chad, Central African Republic, and Democratic

Republic of Congo. Having transitioned out of Gavi support in 2024, Angola is not part of the priority countries but has engaged in BCU activities. As of the end of August 2024, as part of the BCU initiative preparedness, the priority five countries had revised their immunization schedules to extend vaccination targets to children aged 24–59 months and allow delayed vaccination. However, at the time of this meeting, the revised schedules were yet to be officially validated and disseminated within the health system in Burundi and Central African Republic. In addition, vaccination data collection tools were revised and deployed to capture vaccine doses given to children aged 24–59 months in three countries: Cameroon, Chad, and the Democratic Republic of Congo. In Burundi and the Central African Republic, the tools have been revised but not yet distributed in health facilities. As of the end of August 2024, Gavi had approved a total of 21 million vaccine doses for the five BCU priority countries , including 10.3 million doses already shipped in four countries (49%), with Burundi yet to receive the first shipment.

As of the end of August 2024, none of the five countries have started to formally implement BCU activities, particularly the periodic intensification of routine immunization (PIRI) campaigns to catch up on vaccination of children missed since 2020. Cameron has scheduled three rounds of BCU PIRI in September and December 2024 and January 2025. In Chad, the first round of the BCU PIRI was scheduled for December 2024 in the 23 regions that make up the country. Burundi had planned four rounds of BCU PIRIs separated by four weeks, with the first round scheduled in late December 2024. In Central African Republic and the Democratic Republic of Congo, BCU PIRIs are planned for the first quarter of 2025. Angola, a country that transitioned out of Gavi support in 2024, benefited from Gavi funding through the Middle-Income Countries Approach (MICs) to catch up on the vaccination of zero-dose children. With USD 9.1 million received out of USD 43 million required, MIC funding had already contributed to reducing the zero-dose burden by 21% at the time of the meeting. The funding gap for BCU in Angola was yet to be covered. Wrapping up this discussion, participants adopted the following recommendations: (i) Burundi and Central African Republic are to ensure that revised schedules and tools to accommodate delayed vaccination are distributed to all health facilities, (ii) the five BCU priority countries are to make all necessary arrangements to conduct the first PIRI rounds by end January 2025, and (iii) international partners are to support the Government of Angola to raise funds through public–private partnership to cover the BCU funding gap.

2.3. *Introduction of New Vaccines*

Discussion on progress in new vaccine introduction focused on the rollout of malaria vaccines and progress in revitalization of HPV vaccination.

Vaccination has been recently added to the malaria prevention package, following prequalification by the World Health Organization (WHO) of two vaccines: RTS/AS01, approved in 2022 [8], and R21/Matrix-M, approved in 2023 [9]. As of the end of August 2024, two countries have started to roll out malaria vaccines in Central Africa: Cameroon and Central African Republic. Cameroon started to administer RTS/AS01 vaccine on 22 January 2024 in 42 districts at most risk of malaria of the 200 health districts in the country [10]. The recommended schedule in Cameroon comprises four doses that are administered to children at 6, 7, 9, and 24 months of age. By end July 2024, i.e., six months into the vaccine rollout, 74 401 children were vaccinated with the first malaria vaccine dose, providing 50% coverage, against 26% for the second dose and 7% for the third dose. Cameroon conducted a mini post-introduction evaluation of malaria vaccine in May–June 2024. The following causes of low vaccination coverage and high dropout rate were identified: (i) the fact that vaccination schedules for the first and second doses do not match existing contacts with immunization services as per the official schedule, (ii) insufficient investment in demand generation, outreach and mobile vaccination sessions, and a robust defaulters' tracking system, and (iii) suboptimal use of the missed opportunities for vaccination approach. Central African Republic started to roll out R21/Matrix-M vaccine on 22 August 2025 in all the 35 districts of the country. The recommended schedule in Central African Republic comprises four doses administered to children at 6, 7, 9, and 16 months of age. The initial results of malaria vaccine rollout in Central African Republic were not available at the time of the EPI managers meeting. Three other countries had planned to roll out malaria vaccine in the last quarter of 2024 or the first quarter of 2025: Burundi (first quarter 2025), Chad (October 2024), and Democratic Republic of Congo (October 2024).

In December 2022, the Gavi Board approved the revitalization of the Alliance's Human Papillomavirus (HPV) vaccine programme with the aim of reaching over 86 million girls with HPV vaccine by 2025 to avert over 1.4 million future deaths from cervical cancer [11]. In Central Africa, apart from Cameroon and São Tomé and Príncipe, who pioneered the introduction of HPV vaccine in Central Africa in 2020 and 2021, respectively, no other Gavi eligible country has started to roll out these vaccines.

Cameroon started to administer HPV vaccines to girls aged 9–13 years using a school-based implementation strategy while dealing with COVID-19 vaccination, resulting in low uptake. The coverage in girls was 18.2% in 2021 and 20.3% in 2022. Concerns about vaccine safety, fear of infertility and the negative influence of social media exacerbated by the COVID-19 pandemic are known to be the main reasons for HPV vaccine hesitancy in Cameroon [12]. In 2022, WHO updated recommendations on HPV vaccine, adding an alternative single dose schedule. As a follow-up, Cameroon switched to a single-dose schedule and extended the target population to boys from the same age group in 2023. As a result, the HPV vaccine coverage in girls increased to 56.8% in 2023 compared to 20.3% in 2022. The coverage in boys in 2023 was 26%. Lessons learned from Cameroon underline the need for innovative communication, political commitment, and advocacy targeting faith leaders to sustain and expand vaccination efforts.

São Tomé and Príncipe has been less impacted by HPV vaccine hesitancy, despite the context of the COVID-19 pandemic, using a two-dose schedule. In 2022, the HPV coverage in girls aged 9–14 years was 74% with the first dose and 55% with the second dose, compared to 80% with the first dose and 58% with the second dose in 2023.

In addition to Cameroon and São Tomé and Príncipe, two other Gavi-eligible countries have planned to introduce HPV vaccine: Burundi in 2025 and the Democratic Republic of Congo in 2026.

Among the three Gavi non-eligible countries in Central Africa, Equatorial Guinea implemented an HPV vaccine demonstration project in 2024 in one district, achieving 80.3% coverage of girls aged 9–13. Leveraging lessons from the demonstration project, the Equatorial Guinea Government has planned a nationwide rollout by 2026. Angola has planned to introduce the HPV vaccine to girls aged 9–12 in 2025, as 1.4 million vaccine doses out of 2.2 million needed to reach 2.13 million girls have already been delivered. Gabon is contemplating starting a demonstration project in the coming years. It is critical for Burundi, Democratic Republic of Congo, Equatorial Guinea, and Angola to learn from Cameroon and São Tomé and Príncipe's experience on schedules, primary and secondary target groups, and response to vaccine hesitancy to ensure successful introduction of HPV vaccine.

Table 2 summarizes the status of malaria and HPV vaccines in Central African countries as of the end of August 2025.

Table 2. Status of introduction of malaria and human papilloma virus vaccines in Central African countries as of the end of August 2024.

Country	Malaria Vaccine Introduction	HPV Vaccine Introduction
Angola	Not yet planned	Planned in 2025
Burundi	Planned in 2025	Planned in 2025
Cameroon	Introduced in January 2024	Introduced in 2020
Chad	Planned in October 2024	Not yet planned
Central African Republic	Planned in September 2025	Not yet Planned
Congo	Not yet planned	Not yet planned
Democratic Republic of Congo	Planned in October 2024	Planned in 2026
Equatorial Guinea	Demonstration in 2024; introduction planned in 2026	Not yet planned
Gabon	Not yet planned	Not yet planned
São Tomé and Príncipe	Not yet planned	Introduced in 2021

3. Conclusions

The 2024 EPI managers meeting in Central Africa offered an opportunity to share experiences and devise solutions. It allowed for the exploration of ways to deal better with the common issue of data quality in routine immunization to inform timely decisions. The meeting was also a successful peer learning platform for EPI managers and other stakeholders in immunization programmes on the topics of data use for decision-making, BCU readiness and implementation and introduction of malaria and HPV vaccines, among other topics not covered in this report.

The discussions during the meeting highlighted immunization data quality issues in most countries, leading to overestimation of immunization coverage and preventing timely decision-making. Participants recommended that countries invest more in routine immunization data quality assurance for a better use of data to inform decisions.

The high burden of zero-dose children resulting from routine immunization disruptions during the emergency phase of the COVID-19 pandemic was discussed. The implementation of the BCU Initiative sponsored by Gavi in five priority countries, among those with the highest number of zero-dose children, has been delayed mainly due to competing priorities. In Angola, a country that transitioned out of Gavi support in 2024, the implementation of catch-up vaccination activities was slowed down for financial reasons. Given the urgent need for reducing immunity gaps to prevent resurgence of long-forgotten vaccine preventable diseases, it is critical to accelerate the implementation of the BCU initiative in Gavi eligible countries and to support Angola's efforts in raising local funding for catch-up vaccinations through public–private partnership.

The first six months of the malaria vaccine rollout in Cameroon have shown suboptimal coverage for the first dose and a high dropout rate for the second and the third doses. A mini PIE conducted four months into the introduction showed that the vaccination schedule with appointments for the first and second doses not matching existing contacts with health facilities for vaccination, and that insufficient investment in demand generation and outreach/mobile vaccination sessions, are the main drivers of low coverage and children's retention rate. Central African Republic and the three other countries that will introduce malaria vaccines in the fourth quarter of 2024 or the first quarter of 2025 were urged to update their introduction plan to ensure enough investment in demand generation and community engagement to allow time for mothers to become familiar with new appointments related to malaria vaccines.

HPV vaccine introduction in Cameroon was hampered by high vaccine hesitancy, contributing to low acceptance. Switching from a two-dose to a single-dose schedule and extending the target population to boys contributed to improved coverage in girls.

It is critical for countries planning to introduce HPV vaccine to learn from Cameroon's experience in tackling vaccine hesitancy and contemplate a single dose schedule.

Lessons learned and recommendations from the meeting, if implemented, will ultimately contribute to improving EPI's performance in these programme areas. Indeed, peer learning has been shown to play an important role in rapidly advancing technical capacities to drive policy change and address issues that affect vaccination [13].

It is critically important and urgent that the meeting organizers set up an appropriate mechanism for monitoring the implementation of the meeting's recommendations and document best practices. Adding a page on the meeting website, displaying the action points for EPIs by country and for partners, and allowing online monthly updates, coupled with regular meetings to monitor progress in implementing action points, would increase the chance of turning the meeting recommendations into concrete actions. EPI managers are expected to lead the required changes for more efficient and effective immunization programmes. To this end, international partners are urged to set up a training programme on transformational leadership for EPI managers and key EPI staff. The participants agreed that the 2025 EPI managers' meeting will occur in São Tomé and Príncipe.

Limitations

This paper is a meeting report. The content was developed using oral presentations and panel discussion summaries. The situation may have evolved since the meeting's conclusion, so the interpretation of the results presented here should take into account these limitations.

Author Contributions: Conceptualization, F.M., C.T., B.I. and F.C.-N.; methodology, F.M., S.T.N., A.D.M., A.M., J.C.B. and T.N.G.; formal analysis, F.M., M.C.D.-H., Y.V.-M., C.A., L.R., M.M. and B.F.; data curation, C.A., M.M.N. and F.M.; writing—original draft preparation, F.M. and C.A.; writing—review and editing, C.S.W., B.F., B.I., A.M., S.T.N., A.D.M., M.M., L.R., M.C.D.-H., Y.V.-M., C.T. and J.C.B.; supervision, B.I. and C.S.W.; project administration, F.M., B.F., T.N.G., M.M.N. and F.C.-N. All authors have read and agreed to the published version of the manuscript.

Funding: This research received no external funding.

Institutional Review Board Statement: Not applicable.

Informed Consent Statement: Not applicable.

Data Availability Statement: All the presentations and materials from the 2024 EPI Managers meeting in Central Africa are available and downloadable at the following link: https://who-ist-ca.github.io/Reunion-Annuelle-PEV/epi/agenda.html (accessed on 7 March 2025).

Acknowledgments: The authors would like to express their gratitude to Ministries of Health in Central Africa for attending the meeting and sharing their experience on the implementation of Essential Programmes on Immunization.

Conflicts of Interest: The authors declare no conflicts of interest.

References

1. World Health Organization. 50th Anniversary of the Expanded Programme on Immunization (EPI). Available online: https://www.who.int/news-room/events/detail/2024/01/01/default-calendar/50th-anniversary-of-the-expanded-programme-on-immunization-(epi) (accessed on 11 January 2025).
2. World Health Organization. Immunization Data. Available online: https://immunizationdata.who.int/global?topic=&location= (accessed on 11 January 2025).
3. World Health Organization. The Big Catch-Up: An Essential Immunization Recovery Plan for 2023 and Beyond. Available online: https://www.who.int/publications/i/item/9789240075511 (accessed on 11 January 2025).

4. World Health Organization. WHO/UNICEF Estimates of National Immunization Coverage. Available online: https://www.who.int/teams/immunization-vaccines-and-biologicals/immunization-analysis-and-insights/global-monitoring/immunization-coverage/who-unicef-estimates-of-national-immunization-coverage (accessed on 4 March 2025).
5. Mboussou, F.; Nkamedjie, P.; Oyaole, D.; Farham, B.; Atagbaza, A.; Nsasiirwe, S.; Costache, A.; Brooks, D.; Wiysonge, C.S.; Impouma, B. Rapid assessment of data systems for COVID-19 vaccination in the WHO African Region. *Epidemiol. Infect.* **2024**, *152*, e50. [CrossRef] [PubMed]
6. World Health Organization. Assessing and Improving the Accuracy of Target Population Estimates for Immunization Coverage. Available online: https://www.who.int/publications/m/item/assessing-and-improving-the-accuracy-of-target-population-estimates-for-immunization-coverage (accessed on 18 January 2025).
7. World Health Organization. WHO Recommends Groundbreaking Malaria Vaccine for Children at Risk. Available online: https://www.who.int/news/item/06-10-2021-who-recommends-groundbreaking-malaria-vaccine-for-children-at-risk (accessed on 2 February 2025).
8. World Health Organization. WHO Recommends R21/Matrix-M Vaccine for Malaria Prevention in Updated Advice on Immunization. Available online: https://www.who.int/news/item/02-10-2023-who-recommends-r21-matrix-m-vaccine-for-malaria-prevention-in-updated-advice-on-immunization (accessed on 2 February 2025).
9. O'Brien, K.L.; Lemango, E. The big catch-up in immunisation coverage after the COVID-19 pandemic: Progress and challenges to achieving equitable recovery. *Lancet* **2023**, *402*, 510–512. [CrossRef] [PubMed]
10. Gavi, the Vaccine Alliance. Cameroon's Historic Malaria Vaccine Introduction Shows Signs of Success, on Year on. Available online: https://www.gavi.org/vaccineswork/cameroons-historic-malaria-vaccine-introduction-shows-signs-success-one-year (accessed on 5 March 2025).
11. Gavi, the Vaccine Alliance. Human Papillomavirus Vaccine Support. Available online: https://www.gavi.org/types-support/vaccine-support/human-papillomavirus (accessed on 18 January 2025).
12. Haddison, E.; Tambasho, A.; Kouamen, G.; Ngwafor, R. Vaccinators' Perception of HPV Vaccination in the Saa Health District of Cameroon. *Front. Public Health* **2022**, *9*, 748910. [CrossRef] [PubMed]
13. Adamu, A.A.; Ndwandwe, D.; Jalo, R.I.; Ndoutabe, M.; Wiysonge, C.S. Peer learning in immunisation programmes. *Lancet* **2024**, *404*, 334–335. [CrossRef] [PubMed]

vaccines

MDPI

Conference Report

WHO Workshop Report: Regulatory Science to Inform Clinical Pathways for Shigella Vaccines Intended for Use in Children in Low- and Middle-Income Countries

Robert W. Kaminski [1,*], Patricia B. Pavlinac [2], James A. Platts-Mills [3], Elizabeth T. Rogawski McQuade [4], William P. Hausdorff [5,6], Richard A. Isbrucker [7], Kirsten S. Vannice [8], Marco Cavaleri [9], Sonali Kochhar [2,10], Kirsty Mehring-LeDoare [1], Godwin Enwere [11], Annelies Wilder-Smith [1], Karen L. Kotloff [12], Samba Sow [12,13] and Birgitte K. Giersing [1]

1 Department of Immunization, Vaccines and Biologicals, World Health Organization, 1211 Geneva, Switzerland; mehringlek@who.int (K.M.-L.); wildersmitha@who.int (A.W.-S.); giersingb@who.int (B.K.G.)
2 Department of Global Health, University of Washington, Seattle, WA 98105, USA; ppav@uw.edu (P.B.P.); sonalikochhar@yahoo.co.in (S.K.)
3 Department of Medicine, Infectious Diseases and International Health, University of Virginia, Charlottesville, VA 22908, USA; jp5t@uvahealth.org
4 Department of Epidemiology, Emory University, Atlanta, GA 30322, USA; erogaws@emory.edu
5 Center for Vaccine Innovation and Access, PATH, Washington, DC 20001, USA; whausdorff@path.org
6 Faculty of Medicine, Université Libre de Bruxelles, 1050 Brussels, Belgium
7 Health Canada, Ottawa, ON K1A 0K9, Canada; richard.isbrucker@hc-sc.gc.ca
8 Bill & Melinda Gates Foundation, 440 5th Ave. N, Seattle, WA 98109, USA; kirsten.vannice@gatesfoundation.org
9 European Medicines Agency, 1083 HS Amsterdam, The Netherlands; marco.cavaleri@ema.europa.eu
10 Global Healthcare Consulting, Gurgaon 122503, India
11 Vaccine Assessment Team Pre-Qualification, World Health Organization, 1211 Geneva, Switzerland; enwereg@who.int
12 Center for Vaccine Development and Global Health, University of Maryland, Baltimore, MD 21201, USA; kkotloff@som.umaryland.edu (K.L.K.); ssow@cvd-mali.org (S.S.)
13 Centre pour le Développement des Vaccins, Bamako P.O. Box 251, Mali
* Correspondence: kaminskir@who.int

Abstract: Infectious diarrhea caused by *Shigella* remains a significant global health concern, and several vaccine candidates are approaching phase III clinical studies in the target population of young children in low- and middle-income countries. The World Health Organization (WHO) has published preferred product characteristics (PPCs) for *Shigella* vaccines to provide strategic guidance that aids in advancing product development and highlights policy considerations for use in LMIC settings where the vaccine is most needed. However, the selection of appropriate clinical endpoints was not clearly defined within the PPCs and remains an important issue for phase III study design. Previously, an expert panel identified areas of alignment and consensus on many clinical study design components while also recognizing that further discussions and data were required to solidify recommendations on key study design aspects. Therefore, WHO convened a diverse range of stakeholders, including manufacturers, regulators, and policymakers across national, regional, and global levels, with the aim of achieving consensus and soliciting inputs from the regulatory community surrounding vaccine phase III study design considerations. The intent of this report is to outline the key points from those discussions to inform the phase III design strategies and investment decisions of product developers and donors and to share recommendations for next steps.

Keywords: *Shigella*; vaccines; children; phase III study; endpoints; safety; low- and middle-income countries

1. Introduction/Background

Diarrheal disease remains a significant global health threat, with an estimated 1.1 million diarrheal-related deaths in 2021, affecting all age groups across diverse geographical regions [1,2]. However, the most significant impact is among children under 5 years old in low- and middle-income countries (LMICs). *Shigella* remains a leading cause of diarrheal disease worldwide leading to an estimated 94,000 deaths in 2019, with the greatest burden of morbidity and mortality seen in children between 6 months and two years of age [3]. Both symptomatic and asymptomatic *Shigella* infections in young children can also lead to growth faltering and stunting [4,5], with long-lasting detrimental effects on physical and cognitive development [6], increasing susceptibility to other infectious diseases. Thus, preventing *Shigella* infections through improved sanitation, vaccination, and ready access to healthcare and antibiotic treatment is essential for reducing the risk of stunting, promoting healthy growth in children, and allowing populations to reach their fullest economic and productivity levels. However, the overuse and misuse of antibiotics contribute to the emergence and spread of antibiotic-resistant strains of *Shigella*, posing a serious public health threat [7,8] recognized by WHO and the US Centers for Disease Control. The WHO Global Antimicrobial Resistance Surveillance System [9] identified *Shigella* as a priority pathogen for the development of new interventions. This underscores the importance of addressing antimicrobial resistance (AMR) through appropriate antibiotic stewardship practices, improved sanitation and hygiene measures, and the development of effective vaccines against *Shigella*.

Several multi-valent *Shigella* vaccines are currently in development [10] designed to target *S. sonnei*, *S. flexneri* 2a, 3a, and *S. flexneri* 6 or 1b, with phase II studies in infant target populations underway or recently completed in Africa and Asia. To further support vaccine introduction, WHO has prioritized defining pathways and evidence requirements for developing safe, effective, and affordable vaccines to combat *Shigella*-induced dysentery and diarrhea in children under 5 years old in LMICs. This strategy aims not only to expedite regulatory approval for the target group but also to ensure the availability of evidence to support efficient policy recommendations and timely implementation. Consequently, WHO has developed preferred product characteristics (PPCs) for *Shigella* vaccines [11], outlining the desirable product attributes for their utilization in LMIC settings and contributing to better health outcomes in vulnerable populations. The WHO PPCs emphasize the need for vaccines that are safe, affordable, and provide long-lasting protection, particularly for infants and young children in LMICs. Key product characteristics outlined in the PPCs include an acceptable safety and reactogenicity profile, efficacy in preventing moderate to severe *Shigella* diarrhea in children from 6–36 months, ease of administration, and stability in varying storage conditions. The PPCs also stress the importance of vaccines that can be integrated into existing immunization programs to maximize coverage and impact.

The clinical pathway to marketing authorization for *Shigella* vaccine developers and funders has been a critical question during the early phases of the product development [12]. A previous WHO-led consultation of experts, policymakers, and regulators determined that an efficacy trial would be on the critical path for licensure for infants in LMICs given the feasibility of the trial, the lack of an established correlate of protection, and the concern of generalizability of the adult controlled human infection model (CHIM) to children living in LMICs [13]. A phase III study of a bivalent (*S. flexneri* 2a and *S. sonnei*) conjugate vaccine is underway (NCT05156528), with other trials likely to follow in the coming years. Additionally, a large multi-country observational study is underway to identify potential trial sites and characterize baseline incidence [14–16]. The Enterics for Global Health (EFGH) *Shigella* surveillance study [16,17] employs cross-sectional and longitudinal study designs to establish incidence and consequences of medically attended *Shigella* diarrhea in children 6–35 months of age in Bangladesh [14], Gambia [18], Kenya [19], Malawi [20], Mali [21], Pakistan [22], and Peru [15].

The selection of appropriate clinical and microbiologic parameters for a phase III study remains an important issue since they can significantly impact study power and efficacy estimates due to the relative sensitivity and specificity of the options for microbiologic confirmation and because the vaccine may preferentially prevent a more severe phenotype rather than all disease. Therefore, an ad hoc expert panel was convened to outline phase III study design considerations for a *Shigella* clinical study in infants from LMICs [23]. The panel identified areas of alignment and consensus on many aspects of study design consideration for a phase III vaccine trial while recognizing that further discussions, data, and regulatory input were needed to solidify recommendations on key aspects. To achieve this goal, WHO convened a diverse range of stakeholders, including vaccine manufacturers, regulators, researchers, and policymakers across national, regional, and global levels, to facilitate discussions aimed at building consensus on *Shigella* vaccine phase III study design considerations.

2. WHO Regulatory Science Workshop

The Regulatory Science Workshop held in Nairobi, Kenya, in 2024 was designed around four discussion domains (see Table 1): (1) vaccine safety considerations, (2) primary clinical endpoints including case definitions and case ascertainment methods, (3) secondary clinical endpoints, and (4) exploratory or descriptive endpoints that could positively impact policy-making decisions. The two-day participatory and interactive workshop had the overarching goal of gaining consensus and informing potential clinical endpoints, case definitions, and case ascertainment methods to better navigate regulatory approval and policy framework. Over 35 regulators from the AFRO, AMRO, EMRO, EURO, and SEARO WHO regions participated in the workshop, particularly those from countries in which the phase III field efficacy study may be conducted. Input from the regulatory community was sought through a series of round table, guided discussions to align clinical endpoints, clinical case definition, and case ascertainment method(s) with regulatory expectations. The intent of this report is to outline the key points from those discussions and further inform the phase III design strategies and investment decisions of product developers and donors.

Table 1. Major discussion domains, complexities, and feedback to inform next steps.

Discussion Domains	Issues/Complexities	Input/Next Steps
Safety Considerations	• Are the safety assessments conducted in phase IIa Shigella vaccine studies sufficient for phase III studies, or are there any recommended additions? • Can the regulatory community expound on adverse events that would be important to capture in the context of a phase III *Shigella* vaccine study?	• Consensus that the safety assessments from phase IIa Shigella vaccine studies are sufficient for phase III studies. • Regulatory bodies require assessing vaccine safety in a minimum of 3000 study participants. • Unexpected AEs (due to new adjuvant introduction, immune-mediated diseases, and gender-specific issues) should be captured.

Table 1. *Cont.*

Discussion Domains	Issues/Complexities	Input/Next Steps
Clinical case definitions	• Two clinical case definitions were considered for a phase III *Shigella* vaccine study (MSD-GEMS and MSD by mVesikari ± dysentery). • MSD-GEMS does not easily account for various disease severities; some parameters are considered subjective. • mVesikari ± dysentery allows post hoc analysis of vaccine impact across a range of disease severities; it is not specifically tailored to Shigella disease.	• Evaluate the use of MSD-GEMS and mVesikari scoring systems using EFGH data sets. • Refine definition(s) to remove subjective measures and ensure robust alignment with Shigella disease. • Convene stakeholders, particularly regulators, to review recommended and refined case definitions.
Laboratory confirmation of *Shigella* infection	• Culture and qPCR considered for Shigella case detection. • Culture allows AST and investigations into vaccine impact on AMR. • qPCR is more sensitive, facilitating lower phase III study sample sizes. • qPCR capable of serotyping but limited to *S. sonnei* and *S. flexneri* serotypes.	• Regulators are open to either culture or PCR as case detection methodology. • PCR will require submission of a data package to support phase III usage. • Efforts are underway to develop a data package; comparisons in the context of the EFGH study. • Both should be performed in a trial regardless of what is used for the primary endpoint.
Secondary endpoints	• Primary endpoint focused on vaccine impact on first Shigella infection with a serotype targeted by the vaccine. • What would be the recommendation(s) for secondary endpoints in a phase III *Shigella* vaccine study? • Provide insights towards modifications or clarifications that would align these endpoints more thoroughly with regulatory expectations. • If qPCR was used for case detection, vaccine impact on infection with serotypes other than *S. sonnei* and *S. flexneri* would be limited.	• Vaccine efficacy against a broad range of disease severities. • Vaccine efficacy across *Shigella* flexneri serotypes not targeted by the vaccine. • The duration, longevity, and durability of vaccine efficacy. • Vaccine efficacy in the target age group for routine immunization, if a broader age range is evaluated.
Vaccine impact on growth faltering/stunting	• *Shigella* is one of many causes of growth-faltering and a trial will not be able to pre-specify Shigella-attributed growth faltering; therefore, it will be underpowered. • Strong adherence to effective treatment in a clinical trial may modify vaccine impact on growth faltering. • The feasibility to measure growth measurements in infant and young child populations using the WHO Growth Measuring and Standards has been accomplished at LMIC sites in a variety of epidemiology studies (e.g., GEMS, VIDA, ABCD, EFGH). • Can the regulatory community comment on the feasibility of collecting sufficient data during a phase III study, over an anticipated follow-up of 2–3 years, to measure vaccine impact on growth faltering?	• Nutritional studies have successfully incorporated impact on growth faltering, suggesting feasibility in a Phase III vaccine study. • However, study design and sample size may be significantly impacted. • Likely more feasible to treat as an exploratory (descriptive) endpoint. • Potential to include in post-marketing surveillance and impact studies.

Table 1. *Cont.*

Discussion Domains	Issues/Complexities	Input/Next Steps
Vaccine impact on antibiotic usage as a proxy for AMR reduction	• Measuring reductions in antibiotic usage may be feasible in a Phase III study. • Would a reduction of total antibiotic use/burden be sufficient, or does the regulatory community suggest more granular data collection (for example, antibiotic dose utilized, duration of antibiotic usage)? • Would a reduction in WHO-recommended antibiotic treatment protocols be sufficient, or should the data sets also focus more widely on classes of antibiotics utilized?	• Estimating the impact of a *Shigella* vaccine on antibiotic usage was recommended even if it would not be included in the vaccine indication since it would be valuable data for policy decisions. • Consensus that if the additional benefit of reduced antibiotic usage was not substantially demonstrated, it would signify the absence of an extra benefit rather than posing a definitive risk. • Convene a WHO Policy Workshop with LMIC stakeholders to further discuss.

3. Vaccine Safety Considerations

Several *Shigella* vaccines have progressed through Phase I and Phase II studies in adult, child, and infant populations, with vaccine safety being a key endpoint of those evaluations. The safety endpoints being assessed in those Phase IIa *Shigella* vaccine studies (NCT04056117, NCT04602975, NCT05073003) include solicited adverse events (AEs) for 7 days, unsolicited AEs for 28 days, and serious AEs (SAEs) and adverse events of special interest (AESIs) for the trial's duration.

There was consensus among the workshop participants that the safety data collected from the previous Phase IIa studies were also appropriate for Phase III studies and should continue to be reported as per standard regulatory guidelines by relatedness, grade, and frequency, with Data and Safety Monitoring Boards (DSMBs) in place for a thorough oversight. Regulatory guidelines, such as those from the FDA and EMA, typically require assessing vaccine safety in a minimum of 3000 study participants. A robust follow-up and monitoring system is crucial to ensure adequate reporting of AESIs. In the context of a Phase III *Shigella* vaccine study, unexpected AEs and immune-mediated diseases should be captured and reported. Additionally, post-marketing commitments such as pharmacovigilance/surveillance and a Risk Management Plan may be required, along with consideration of regional factors. No additional safety endpoints were specifically outlined, but long-term follow-up if co-administration with other vaccines occurs and investigations into comorbidities, such as HIV-exposed subjects and HLA-related autoimmunity, may be anticipated.

4. Primary Vaccine Efficacy Endpoint

There was broad consensus that the primary endpoint for a phase III *Shigella* vaccine study in infant and toddler populations from LMICs should demonstrate vaccine efficacy against only those *Shigella* serotypes targeted by the vaccine (e.g., *S. flexneri* 2a, 3a, and 6 and *S. sonnei*). Furthermore, it was considered important that efficacy should be associated with the first episode of *Shigella*—attributed diarrhea in the trial—as repeat Shigella exposures may be a confounder. It was recommended that a phase III primary endpoint should be vaccine efficacy against the first episode of moderate or severe diarrhea caused by *Shigella* serotypes targeted by the vaccine, aligned with the WHO PPCs and past phase III trials of rotavirus vaccines, to demonstrate a strong public health value. Discussions also identified topics related to the primary endpoint that required additional alignment with regulatory expectations, including clinical case definition(s) and case detection methodologies.

4.1. Clinical Case Definition

Prior to the meeting, there was agreement that more severe diarrhea (as opposed to all diarrhea) would be required as the primary clinical case definition based on the PPCs. Therefore, several clinical case definitions of moderate-or-severe disease (MSD) were discussed with regulators to identify the most suitable definition to serve as a framework for a Shigella Phase III vaccine study. A dichotomous definition [24] was developed for the Global Enteric Multicenter Study (GEMS). The GEMS-MSD definition utilizes diarrhea (≥three abnormally loose stools in 24 h) accompanied by dehydration and/or dysentery (at least one stool containing visible blood according to either the caretaker or the clinician) as criteria.

The modified Vesikari (mVesikari) scoring system, which has been utilized in several enteric vaccine studies, including rotavirus [25], assigns a score across a wide range of signs and symptoms, including duration and maximum number of stools, maximum number and duration of vomiting, temperature, dehydration, and treatment. The scores have been used to rank diarrhea severity into mild (0–6 points), moderate (7–10 points), or severe (≥11 points) illness categories.

Several key attributes of the mVesikari and GEMS-MSD definitions were discussed to ensure the ability to accurately and robustly identify cases that aligned with the trial clinical endpoints of measuring vaccine impact on MSD. The mVesikari score emerged as a potential case definition, yet concerns were raised regarding its applicability to *Shigella*, notably the emphasis of the scoring system on vomiting, which is not as predominant with *Shigella* infections as with rotavirus. It was also noted that the severity definition does not need to distinguish *Shigella* from other etiologies since etiology in a phase III Shigella vaccine study will be determined through culture and/or qPCR methods. Additionally, the score's interpretation and complexity were noted. As an alternative, a refined case definition based on GEMS-MSD criteria was proposed, aiming for simplicity and relevance to *Shigella*, with some experts suggesting an amended GEMS-MSD definition should include diarrhea duration and fever. The discussion also touched upon the importance of clinical case definitions in the context of secondary endpoints and post hoc analyses, particularly in evaluating the vaccine's impact across multiple disease severity subsets. Therefore, a recommendation from the workshop included establishing an expert working group to optimize a case definition modeled after the mVesikari and GEMS-MSD definitions, which would include an objective, simple composite case definition that easily explains the clinical syndrome of more severe shigellosis while also adding additional details than are currently captured in the GEMS-MSD definition. Importantly, the case definition should also be able to disaggregate moderate from severe cases and be more fully aligned with characteristics of *Shigella* disease. The recommended case definition would then be reviewed during a future WHO expert consultation for broader input and alignment prior to generating a meeting report to disseminate finalized recommendations to the global community.

4.2. Microbiological Confirmation Methodology

Classical microbiological culture methods and quantitative polymerase chain reaction (qPCR) are two prevalent techniques for detecting *Shigella* in stool samples and have been utilized in numerous epidemiological studies [26,27]. Both have distinct advantages and disadvantages in terms of sensitivity, specificity, time efficiency, and practical application in clinical settings. As the detection methods have implications for trial size, cost, and feasibility, as well as the ability to compare trial results, it would thus be ideal to formulate a clear recommendation as part of the case definition.

One significant advantage of qPCR is high sensitivity. qPCR can detect low levels of *Shigella* DNA, making it highly effective, even in cases with low bacterial loads or after antibiotic treatment that may not be detected by culture methods [28,29]. Additionally, qPCR allows for (1) rapid processing and results, often within a few hours, which is crucial for timely diagnosis and treatment in clinical settings, or alternatively (2) sample batching to allow simultaneous analysis across multiple samples or centralizing the qPCR analysis during a multisite study, which can positively impact reproducibility. *Shigella* detection by qPCR is accomplished by amplifying the *ipaH* gene, which is also found in enteroinvasive *E. coli* (EIEC). Moreover, qPCR can sometimes detect non-viable bacteria, leading to lower clinical specificity since it amplifies DNA regardless of the bacteria's viability. Recent advances, such as setting cycle threshold cut-offs that optimize specificity, as well as adding serotype specific targets for *Shigella* may overcome these concerns. Also, combining qPCR with a clinical case definition that captures more severe disease will decrease likelihood of asymptomatic detection of *Shigella*.

Culture methods have the advantage of confirming the presence of viable *Shigella* organisms and allow for antibiotic susceptibility testing, which is crucial for selecting appropriate treatments and informing potential exploratory clinical study endpoints. Culturing is generally more cost-effective compared to qPCR and does not require sophisticated equipment. technical training. Despite these benefits, culture methods have notable disadvantages, including being time-consuming, typically requiring 24–48 h or longer to yield results, which delays diagnosis and treatment, and requiring extensive training. Additionally, culture methods are difficult to standardize across laboratories and have lower sensitivity compared to qPCR [28], particularly if the bacterial load in the sample is low or if the bacteria are in a viable but non-culturable state due to prior antibiotic use or sample handling conditions, as *Shigella* can be sensitive to temperature, pH, and oxygen levels during transport. This can result in false-negative results and potentially undetected *Shigella* cases, especially among younger children who are less likely to be culture positive. Moreover, the lower sensitivity substantially impacts clinical trial sample size calculations and therefore may affect the feasibility of successfully conducting a phase III study.

There is an inherent relationship between microbiological methods for confirmation of cases and sample size required to power a phase III pediatric efficacy trial to detect the target vaccine efficacy of at least 60% against vaccine-preventable *Shigella* strains, as outlined in the WHO PPCs. For example, using qPCR for confirmation of *Shigella* infection increases the trial's power compared to traditional culture methods. The calculations show that for a primary endpoint of mVesikari $\geq$9 and/or dysentery with qPCR confirmation for vaccine-preventable strains, a one-year follow-up trial could require ~6000 participants, based on incidence estimated at some EFGH sites. In contrast, using less sensitive culture confirmation would require >15,000 participants to sufficiently power the study. Therefore, qPCR for *Shigella* detection has emerged as an attractive alternative to classic culture methods. Furthermore, advancements and refinements over the past several years have also facilitated the use of qPCR as a means of determining *Shigella* species and serotype directly from stool samples [30,31], further increasing the practicality of the assay with the current PCR serotyping methodology capable of detecting vaccine-preventable serotypes proposed in a phase III study, which include *S. sonnei* and *S. flexneri* 2a, 3a, 6, and 1b [31].

When discussed with the regulatory community, it was noted that while some regulators may prefer culture-based methods due to their ability to definitively detect *Shigella*-attributed diarrhea, regulators are open to considering PCR if appropriate data are generated to demonstrate that it is fit-for-purpose and possible to validate, which could support regulatory acceptance. It was emphasized that clarity on the diagnostic's intended use and interpretation of discordant results between culture and PCR is crucial, with pre-specification in protocols and analysis plans recommended. In particular, justification of the PCR cycle threshold (ct) for selection of actual cases needs to be discussed with regulators before starting the clinical trial. There was a suggestion that the ICH Q2(R2) guideline, which focuses on standard analytical metrics (sensitivity/specificity, range, linearity, limit of detection, accuracy (via spiking known quantities of analyte into a test sample), precision (via reproducibility), and reproducibility (between labs)), is a good resource for understanding data required for licensure submission [32,33]. Much of these data are available or published for the TaqMan Array Card [34,35].

The importance of engaging with regulatory bodies to design the appropriate data package early in the process was underscored. For example, the data package would be different if the qPCR assay was being used as a clinical diagnostic test versus as a biomarker to support clinical endpoints, with the latter not typically requiring formal licensure. It was suggested that a "Type C meeting" with the FDA could be one mechanism to provide guidance once clarity on the intended use and limitations of the assay were established and that engagement with the FDA or EMA, in collaboration with LMIC regulators from countries in which the vaccine is intended to be used, could help pave the way for rapid regulatory approval in LMICs.

Other points of discussion indicated that derivation and validation of a quantitative cutoff could possibly face more scrutiny, and data supporting the clinical specificity of *Shigella* detection at that cutoff would be crucial. Similarly, data would be needed to support the use of a quantitative algorithm to serotype *Shigella*-attributable diarrhea using O-antigen synthesis and modification genes. A semi-quantitative assay would be acceptable, but converting cycle thresholds to copy numbers was advised. Finally, a centralized lab could be used for a multisite study, but if not, data will have to be presented demonstrating the consistency of test performance between sites. Additionally, lessons could be drawn from the use of PCR in malaria vaccine trials [36,37]. Overall, the discussion underscored the importance of robust data, clear regulatory engagement, and contextual clarity in utilizing PCR for *Shigella* detection. Furthermore, regardless of which laboratory method is used for the primary endpoint and determining sample size, both qPCR and culture methods should be employed.

5. Secondary Endpoints

For a phase III Shigella vaccine clinical trial, primary endpoints will focus on key measures to determine vaccine efficacy, such as the prevention of laboratory-confirmed Shigella infections or a significant reduction in severe gastrointestinal symptoms among vaccinated individuals compared to a control group. These endpoints are the trial's main outcomes, guiding regulatory and clinical approval decisions. Secondary endpoints explore additional aspects of vaccine performance, like reduction in all-cause diarrheal disease, duration of illness, or immune response levels, offering further insights into the vaccine's broader effects. Exploratory endpoints investigate less established or long-term outcomes, such as identifying biomarkers of immunity, evaluating vaccine impact across different age groups or geographic regions, or monitoring potential off-target benefits. These endpoints are primarily hypothesis-generating, potentially guiding future vaccine development and public health strategies.

Potential secondary clinical endpoints were also discussed, priority ranked, and, in some cases, modifications were suggested. The highest priority endpoints were largely focused on (i) vaccine efficacy against a broad range of disease severities, including less-severe disease, followed by (ii) vaccine efficacy irrespective of *Shigella* serotype, and (iii) evaluating the longevity of the protective immune response induced through vaccination (Table 2). A secondary endpoint that provides flexibility surrounding which clinical syndrome is vaccine-preventable was an important attribute considered. Using a case definition scoring system, such as mVesikari and/or dysentery, allows us to identify protection against a variety of severity subsets to be evaluated as secondary endpoints in a transparent and feasible manner, whereas there was less clarity on how the GEMS-MSD definition could be categorized into severity subsets. If a new, non-scoring system is developed, it was agreed that it should at least separate mild, moderate, and severe to provide dimensions for endpoint disaggregation. Additionally, if a phase III Shigella vaccine study were to enroll a wide age range (e.g., 6–60 months), establishing efficacy by age cohort would be an important aspect for consideration as a secondary endpoint since these data would be critical to understanding the impact of different vaccination schedule options and have important implications surrounding the role of pre-existing immunity or boosting through pathogen exposure in endemic settings.

Table 2. Recommended prioritization and categorization of secondary endpoints.

Priority	Category	Proposed Secondary Endpoint
1	Vaccine efficacy against broad range of disease severities	Vaccine-preventable subset of *Shigella*-associated disease across a broad range of severities utilizing alternative definitions of disease severity, such as very severe diarrhea and diarrhea of any severity, as determined by mVesikari, as well as dysentery alone.
2	Vaccine efficacy across *Shigella* serotypes not targeted by the vaccine	All *Shigella* moderate or severe diarrhea and/or dysentery episodes, irrespective of serotype
		Shigella moderate or severe diarrhea and/or dysentery due to molecularly confirmed *Shigella flexneri* or *Shigella sonnei*
3	The duration, longevity, and durability of vaccine efficacy	Evaluations of protection longevity afforded by vaccination through evaluation of not only first but also subsequent diarrheal episodes
		Efficacy between first and second vaccination (disease between 6 months and 9 months)
No priority	Not recommended	Vaccine-preventable subset of *Shigella*-associated disease using GEMS-MSD and GEMS-LSD definitions
		Vaccine-preventable subset of *Shigella*-associated disease using hospitalization as a severity indicator

The second highest priority was to evaluate vaccine efficacy against more *Shigella* serotypes than those specifically targeted within the vaccine or to assess vaccine-induced cross-protection. There was a recognition during the discussion of challenges that may be presented depending on the choice of case detection methodologies, specifically culture versus PCR, largely based upon the limitations of qPCR to distinguish beyond *S. sonnei* and *S. flexneri* serotypes. However, there were strategies discussed that could partially mitigate these challenges, such as limiting the secondary endpoint to all *Shigella flexneri* serotypes and *S. sonnei* if PCR was utilized as the case detection method employed in the phase III study. Alternatively, both culture and PCR-based detection methods could be employed if protection against less prominent Shigella serotypes (e.g., *S. boydii*) were to be assessed.

The third priority tier for secondary endpoints included measures of vaccine efficacy duration by capturing not only the first episode of *Shigella* diarrhea after vaccination but throughout the course of the study, which was shown to be valuable to policy decisions in the malaria vaccine field [38]. However, it may be difficult to substantially power the study and may require alternative statistical methods, such as survival analysis, to effectively capture vaccine impact. Several other clinical endpoints were also suggested for consideration, including determining vaccine efficacy (1) stratified by follow-up time, (2) against all-cause diarrhea meeting primary case definition, (3) against caregiver-reported diarrhea, including episodes that did not lead to care-seeking, and (4) stratified by baseline antibody levels. Two additional suggestions were to include subgroup analyses considering country/site, sex, and age and, if budget allows, to evaluate inflammatory markers [39] for vaccine breakthroughs versus unvaccinated cases.

6. Exploratory Endpoints

As the discussions turned to exploratory endpoints, an emphasis was placed on distinguishing between hypothesis-driven and descriptive endpoints. Hypothesized (regulatory) endpoints are pre-specified primary and secondary outcomes used to assess the efficacy and safety of an intervention. The primary endpoints are statistically powered and critical for gaining regulatory approval from bodies like the FDA or EMA. Conversely, descriptive endpoints are exploratory outcomes that provide broader insights into the intervention's real-world impact that may be informative for policy decisions, including long-term safety and effectiveness. All types of endpoints are essential for a comprehensive evaluation of the vaccine's benefits and implications. In the context of a phase III *Shigella* vaccine study, exploratory endpoints associated with the vaccine's impact on AMR/antibiotic usage and growth faltering/stunting were discussed by the convening.

With respect to vaccine impact on growth faltering, the regulatory community asserted that assessing growth is feasible and utilized in nutritional studies, although there was speculation about its relevance at this stage of clinical vaccine development. Concerns were expressed regarding the interpretation of individual z-scores, misclassification of infection, and impact of environmental enteric dysfunction, collectively affecting growth impact. Furthermore, treatment with antibiotics, which would likely be included as standard of care in a phase III Shigella vaccine trial, has been shown to ameliorate impacts of infection on growth [4]. While not crucial for regulatory approval, there was broad agreement that demonstration of vaccine impact on growth faltering would likely be well-received by policymakers and facilitate vaccine introduction decisions. However, large-scale anthropometric data collection requires significant resources, and the expected effects of the vaccine on growth are likely to be very small (<0.1 z-scores for individuals with shigella and <0.01 z-scores on average for the whole trial population). Attempting to observe vaccine effects on overall growth was compared to observing vaccine impacts on all-cause mortality, which is typically beyond study power. Underpowered studies pose high risks; a lack of demonstrated growth effects could dampen vaccine enthusiasm, and caution was expressed to avoid negative results and opportunity costs. Therefore, there was the suggestion that endpoints related to growth faltering may better align with a descriptive exploratory endpoint at this stage of clinical development. Such descriptive endpoints could include changes in anthropometric measures by vaccination status, for example. Length for age (LAZ) at regular intervals (6, 12, 18, and 24 months) in the trial or other pragmatic times based on the regularly scheduled visits can be collected in the trial, but there remains a likelihood post-licensure study data would be needed to fully inform these descriptive exploratory endpoints.

The tremendous impact of antimicrobial resistance (AMR) on communities was well-recognized across various stakeholders, highlighting the importance of strategic national control and policy formulation. There was a suggestion that in phase III trials, an opportunity exists to compare antibiotic usage between vaccinated and unvaccinated groups, with routine data collection on concomitant medications during both scheduled and unscheduled visits. Health books or diaries could be used to cover gaps between visits, supported by additional phone calls or decision support systems (DDS) for comprehensive data collection. Therefore, including a descriptive exploratory endpoint to document the impact of a *Shigella* vaccine on antibiotic usage was recommended even if it would not be included in the vaccine indication since it would be valuable data for policy decisions. It was suggested that a statistically significant difference in antibiotic use between vaccine and placebo groups could positively influence policymakers, especially in LMICs, by demonstrating potential cost and budget impacts, as well as contributing to global AMR reduction efforts. It was noted that training healthcare providers on the vaccine's impact on AMR is also beneficial. Interestingly, there was consensus that if the additional benefit of reduced antibiotic usage was not substantially demonstrated, it would signify the absence of an extra benefit rather than posing a definitive risk. It was also noted as a relevant consideration that if the phase III study was powered for a primary outcome based on PCR, AMR endpoints would be underpowered because they can only be assessed in culture-positive cases. Therefore, meeting participants recommended convening a WHO Policy Workshop with LMIC stakeholders to further discuss how descriptive exploratory endpoints such as reductions in stunting/growth faltering and AMR/antimicrobial usage from a phase III *Shigella* vaccine study can support policy decisions, vaccine implementation, and uptake in LMICs.

7. Correlate Generation and Facilitation of Clinical Studies

In addition to clinical objectives and endpoints, there were also discussions at the workshop surrounding opportunities for correlates of protection (CoP) to be generated as part of the phase III trial. CoPs may empower immunobridging from demonstrated vaccine effectiveness in a phase III efficacy trial conducted under one set of conditions to infer vaccine effectiveness under another set of conditions, such as in a different age group or demographic group, concomitant administration with other vaccines, or with different Shigella vaccine platforms. Immunobridging could be facilitated in a phase III study through nested immunology cohorts (500–1000 subjects). Several efforts underway to support immunobridging were discussed, including the harmonization of antibody binding assays (LPS-ELISA), functional assays (serum bactericidal assays), and the establishment of a WHO International Reference Serum to support phase III vaccine evaluations.

The workshop convening also discussed opportunities to facilitate clinical studies. For Phase III studies conducted at multiple sites across several LMICs, facilitating joint review by multiple national regulatory authorities or ethics committees, especially in the intended countries of use, can foster consensus on aspects such as optimal case definitions and endpoints, ethical and regulatory matters, and common data requirements. The African Vaccine Regulatory Forum (AVAREF) is an example, aiming to harmonize regulatory and ethics practices across the African continent to support product development. Under the African Medicines Regulatory Harmonization (AMRH) program, AVAREF serves as the technical committee for clinical trials, aligning its tools and processes with the African Medicines Agency (AMA) to support regulatory reliance implementation.

Additionally, the EMA (European Medicines Agency) M4ALL (Medicines for All) program is a strategic initiative aimed at enhancing global access to high-quality medicines. This program focuses on fostering international collaboration and harmonizing regulatory standards to ensure that safe, effective, and affordable medicines are available to all populations, particularly in LMICs. M4ALL provides a mechanism for seeking scientific opinions on high-priority vaccines intended for markets outside the EU, in collaboration with the WHO. This process leverages local epidemiology and disease expertise to provide a unified development and assessment pathway, aiming to expedite WHO prequalification and registration in target countries. By working with various stakeholders, including other regulatory agencies, pharmaceutical companies, and international organizations, M4ALL seeks to streamline the development, approval, and distribution processes for essential medicines, addressing critical public health needs worldwide. Key components of the M4ALL program include capacity-building initiatives, technical support, and the promotion of best practices in regulatory science. The program also emphasizes the importance of innovation and the use of modern technologies to overcome barriers in medicine accessibility. By creating a more efficient and unified regulatory environment, M4ALL aims to reduce the time and cost associated with bringing new medicines to market, ultimately improving health outcomes and reducing disparities in healthcare access across different regions.

8. Recommended Efforts to Further Support Clinical, Regulatory, and Policy-Related Strategic Planning

Several workstreams (Table 3) have been identified during the Regulatory Science Workshop to prepare for and inform phase III clinical studies and further support *Shigella* vaccine approval for use in young children living in LMICs. Many of these recommended workstreams could be conducted in parallel to ensure the most expeditious support.

Table 3. Recommended future actions to support phase III study design.

Expert consultation/SME Working Group to Finalize a Case Definition/Scoring System
• Convening of an expert consultation/SME working group to draft a case definition/scoring system for use in a primary endpoint for a *Shigella* phase III study conducted in an LMIC setting. • Present the recommended clinical case definition to vaccine developers, donors, and LMIC stakeholders to gain broad input and consensus prior to finalization. • Publish recommendations and learnings from the expert panel and stakeholder consultations.
qPCR Methodology Qualification and Validation to Support Phase III Studies
• Convene an expert group to review existing data sets and identify gaps to be considered to ensure the *Shigella* qPCR assay is "fit for purpose" in support of a Phase III clinical endpoint. • Utilize data sets generated in the EFGH study to effectively bridge between culture and qPCR methods. • Potentially conduct a "Type C" meeting with the FDA (or similar regulatory body) to present validation and bridging data sets and gain early input.
Convene a WHO Policy Workshop
• Convening of a WHO Policy Workshop/LMIC stakeholder meeting to discuss how outcomes from a phase III *Shigella* vaccine study (such as reductions in stunting/growth faltering and AMR/antimicrobial usage) can further support vaccine implementation and uptake in LMICs. • Publish recommendations and learnings from the WHO Policy Workshop.
Revise WHO Preferred Product Characteristics
• Address any recommended modifications to the WHO PPCs based on inputs from the Regulatory Science Workshop and the WHO Policy Workshop. • Present modified PPCs to the PDVAC for additional input and recommendations.
Explore Potential *Shigella* Combination Vaccines
• Develop a strategic framework to identify and structure considerations for combination vaccines, and once developed, apply the framework to vaccines in the current pipeline. • In parallel, develop combination vaccine value assessments. • Consult extensively with immunization stakeholders and programs at the national and regional levels, including civil society organizations, on potential public health benefits, priority of, and demand for the provisionally preferred combinations identified. • Consult with vaccine manufacturers and developers to assess the probability of technical and regulatory success for. • Where appropriate, signal potential combinations that could be of interest through WHO PPCs.

It was recommended that an expert consultation should be convened to establish a viable clinical case definition for use in the phase III primary and secondary endpoints. A clinical case definition that fully addresses moderate and severe *Shigella* infections in young children in an objective and reproducible manner while allowing differentiation of disease severity could facilitate critical secondary endpoints that will support regulatory approval and market authorization while providing critical input needed for policy and vaccine implementation pathways.

Similarly, it was recommended that experts should engage in the qualification and validation of a qPCR methodology to be used for clinical case detection. Data sets from the EFGH *Shigella* surveillance study could be utilized to compare and bridge between the microbiological culture [40] and qPCR methods [34]. These efforts may culminate in a type-C meeting with the US FDA (or equivalent interaction with a regulatory body in LMICs) to facilitate early consultations on the use of the PCR assay to support the primary endpoint in a future Phase III study.

It was also recommended that WHO should convene a policy workshop with LMIC stakeholders, donors, and policymakers to explore how secondary and exploratory endpoints in a phase III study focused on measuring the ability of a *Shigella* vaccine to diminish antibiotic usage and reduce growth faltering/stunting could support vaccine implementation and country uptake. A meeting report from the Policy Workshop should be crafted and published to disseminate outputs, discussions, and recommendations. It is anticipated that the results of the recommended efforts outlined above may necessitate revisions to the WHO preferred product characteristics guidance document, which will be considered and presented to the Product Development for Vaccines Advisory Committee (PDVAC; https://www.who.int/groups/product-development-for-vaccines-advisory-committee (accessed on 20 April 2025)) for external advice and concurrence.

Recognizing that immunization programs around the world are struggling to accommodate the increasing number of vaccines, the logistics of vaccine delivery, financial constraints, and a limited number of medical visits for vaccination, especially in young children, there is an increased urgency to develop combination vaccines [41]. As *Shigella* vaccines enter phase III studies, considerations need to be taken to promote and advocate for vaccine implementation, which may be more successful if a *Shigella* vaccine were combined with another near-licensure or licensed vaccine. Potential *Shigella* combination vaccines have been explored [42] with an emphasis on manufacturing and compatibility, epidemiological and clinical presentations, and strategy, policy, and regulatory considerations. However, there is a need for a strategic framework that can be applied to identify and structure considerations across public health and economic values to better inform and create demand from stakeholders and de-risk investments. Questions regarding the accessibility and finance of approved Shigella vaccines were not considered in the Regulatory Science Workshop, although they can be important as vaccines move closer to market authorization. Although not a workstream directly linked to the Regulatory Science Workshop, efforts are underway to develop the framework needed to evaluate potential combination vaccines, which may help ensure uptake of a *Shigella* vaccine across LMICs with the greatest need.

There is a significant global health burden posed by *Shigella* infections coupled with increasing antibiotic resistance, underscoring the urgent need for an effective vaccine and driving the strategic priority for WHO. However, the demand for a *Shigella* vaccine may not be sufficient, as global awareness of disease burden is lacking, and countries are facing a multitude of competing interventions, including multiple other vaccines, all of which pose huge economic and logistical challenges requiring prioritization. Therefore, significant investment in vaccine demand mobilization through effective communications and community engagement is needed to ensure vaccines become vaccinations.

Author Contributions: All authors provided substantial contributions to the conception or design of the work; the acquisition, analysis, or interpretation of data for the work; the drafting of the work or revising it critically for important intellectual content; provided final approval of the version to be published; and are in agreement to be accountable for all aspects of the work in ensuring that questions related to the accuracy or integrity of any part of the work are appropriately investigated and resolved. All authors have read and agreed to the published version of the manuscript.

Funding: This meeting report was developed and produced with funding from the Bill and Melinda Gates Foundation (grant number INV 005318). The authors alone are responsible for the views expressed in this manuscript, and they do not necessarily represent the views, decisions, or policies of the institutions with which we are affiliated.

Institutional Review Board Statement: Not applicable.

Informed Consent Statement: Not applicable.

Data Availability Statement: The data presented in this study are available in this article.

Acknowledgments: The authors would like to acknowledge the contributions of Ashwani Arora, Francesca Micoli, Kawsar Talaat, Frederick Sawe, Debbie Spindelman, Chloe Puett, Christine McGrath, Jessica Long, Michelo Simuyandi, Farah Qamar, and Mateusz Hasso-Agopsowicz for tremendous contributions during the virtual consultations that informed discussion topics as well as the presenters and attendees who contributed vital information and insights during the Workshop.

Conflicts of Interest: The authors report no potential conflicts of interest. All authors have submitted the ICMJE Form for Disclosure of Potential Conflicts of Interest. Conflicts that the Editors consider relevant to the content of the manuscript have been disclosed.

References

1. Global Burden of Disease Network. Global Burden of Disease Study 2021 (GBD 2021) Results. Available online: https://vizhub.healthdata.org/gbd-results (accessed on 6 July 2024).
2. Muzembo, B.A.; Kitahara, K.; Mitra, D.; Ohno, A.; Khatiwada, J.; Dutta, S.; Miyoshi, S.-I. Burden of Shigella in South Asia: A Systematic Review and Meta-Analysis. *J. Travel. Med.* **2023**, *30*, taac132. [CrossRef]
3. Perin, J.; Mulick, A.; Yeung, D.; Villavicencio, F.; Lopez, G.; Strong, K.L.; Prieto-Merino, D.; Cousens, S.; Black, R.E.; Liu, L. Global, Regional, and National Causes of under-5 Mortality in 2000-19: An Updated Systematic Analysis with Implications for the Sustainable Development Goals. *Lancet Child. Adolesc. Health* **2022**, *6*, 106–115. [CrossRef] [PubMed]
4. Nasrin, D.; Blackwelder, W.C.; Sommerfelt, H.; Wu, Y.; Farag, T.H.; Panchalingam, S.; Biswas, K.; Saha, D.; Jahangir Hossain, M.; Sow, S.O.; et al. Pathogens Associated with Linear Growth Faltering in Children with Diarrhea and Impact of Antibiotic Treatment: The Global Enteric Multicenter Study. *J. Infect. Dis.* **2021**, *224*, S848–S855. [CrossRef] [PubMed]
5. Rogawski, E.T.; Liu, J.; Platts-Mills, J.A.; Kabir, F.; Lertsethtakarn, P.; Siguas, M.; Khan, S.S.; Praharaj, I.; Murei, A.; Nshama, R.; et al. Use of Quantitative Molecular Diagnostic Methods to Investigate the Effect of Enteropathogen Infections on Linear Growth in Children in Low-Resource Settings: Longitudinal Analysis of Results from the MAL-ED Cohort Study. *Lancet Glob. Health* **2018**, *6*, e1319–e1328. [CrossRef]
6. Prado, E.L.; Dewey, K.G. Nutrition and Brain Development in Early Life. *Nutr. Rev.* **2014**, *72*, 267–284. [CrossRef]
7. Neupane, R.; Bhathena, M.; Das, G.; Long, E.; Beard, J.; Solomon, H.; Simon, J.L.; Nisar, Y.B.; MacLeod, W.B.; Hamer, D.H. Antibiotic Resistance Trends for Common Bacterial Aetiologies of Childhood Diarrhoea in Low- and Middle-Income Countries: A Systematic Review. *J. Glob. Health* **2023**, *13*, 04060. [CrossRef]
8. Awuor, A.O.; Ogwel, B.; Powell, H.; Verani, J.R.; Sow, S.O.; Hossain, M.J.; Ochieng, J.B.; Juma, J.; Jamka, L.P.; Roose, A.; et al. Antibiotic-Prescribing Practices for Management of Childhood Diarrhea in 3 Sub-Saharan African Countries: Findings from the Vaccine Impact on Diarrhea in Africa (VIDA) Study, 2015–2018. *Clin. Infect. Dis.* **2023**, *76*, S32–S40. [CrossRef] [PubMed]
9. Global Antimicrobial Resistance and Use Surveillance System (GLASS) Report: 2022. Available online: https://www.who.int/publications/i/item/9789240062702 (accessed on 12 July 2024).
10. MacLennan, C.A.; Grow, S.; Ma, L.; Steele, A.D. The Shigella Vaccines Pipeline. *Vaccines* **2022**, *10*, 1376. [CrossRef]
11. WHO Preferred Product Characteristics for Vaccines Against Shigella. Available online: https://www.who.int/publications/i/item/9789240036741 (accessed on 6 July 2024).
12. MacLennan, C.A.; Talaat, K.R.; Kaminski, R.W.; Cohen, D.; Riddle, M.S.; Giersing, B.K. Critical Needs in Advancing Shigella Vaccines for Global Health. *J. Infect. Dis.* **2022**, *225*, 1500–1503. [CrossRef]

13. Giersing, B.K.; Isbrucker, R.; Kaslow, D.C.; Cavaleri, M.; Baylor, N.; Maiga, D.; Pavlinac, P.B.; Riddle, M.S.; Kang, G.; MacLennan, C.A. Clinical and Regulatory Development Strategies for Shigella Vaccines Intended for Children Younger than 5 Years in Low-Income and Middle-Income Countries. *Lancet Glob. Health* **2023**, *11*, e1819–e1826. [CrossRef]
14. Khanam, F.; Islam, M.T.; Bhuiyan, T.R.; Hossen, M.I.; Rajib, M.N.H.; Haque, S.; Ireen, M.; Qudrat-E-Khuda, S.; Biswas, P.K.; Bhuiyan, M.A.I.; et al. The Enterics for Global Health (EFGH) *Shigella* Surveillance Study in Bangladesh. *Open Forum Infect. Dis.* **2024**, *11*, S76–S83. [CrossRef] [PubMed]
15. Manzanares Villanueva, K.; Pinedo Vasquez, T.; Peñataro Yori, P.; Romaina Cacique, L.; Garcia Bardales, P.F.; Shapiama Lopez, W.V.; Zegarra Paredes, F.; Perez, K.F.; Rengifo Pinedo, S.; Silva Delgado, H.; et al. The Enterics for Global Health (EFGH) *Shigella* Surveillance Study in Peru. *Open Forum Infect. Dis.* **2024**, *11*, S121–S128. [CrossRef]
16. Atlas, H.E.; Conteh, B.; Islam, M.T.; Jere, K.C.; Omore, R.; Sanogo, D.; Schiaffino, F.; Yousafzai, M.T.; Ahmed, N.; Awuor, A.O.; et al. Diarrhea Case Surveillance in the Enterics for Global Health *Shigella* Surveillance Study: Epidemiologic Methods. *Open Forum Infect. Dis.* **2024**, *11*, S6–S16. [CrossRef] [PubMed]
17. Vannice, K.; MacLennan, C.A.; Long, J.; Steele, A.D. Optimizing Vaccine Trials for Enteric Diseases: The Enterics for Global Health (EFGH) Shigella Surveillance Study. *Open Forum Infect. Dis.* **2024**, *11*, S1–S5. [CrossRef] [PubMed]
18. Conteh, B.; Badji, H.; Jallow, A.F.; Karim, M.; Manneh, A.; Keita, B.; Sarwar, G.; Ceesay, B.E.; Jarju, S.; Jabang, A.M.J.; et al. The Enterics for Global Health (EFGH) Shigella Surveillance Study in The Gambia. *Open Forum Infect. Dis.* **2024**, *11*, S84–S90. [CrossRef]
19. Omore, R.; Awuor, A.O.; Ogwel, B.; Okonji, C.; Sonye, C.; Oreso, C.; Akelo, V.; Amollo, M.; Ogudi, I.; Anyango, R.O.; et al. The Enterics for Global Health (EFGH) Shigella Surveillance Study in Kenya. *Open Forum Infect. Dis.* **2024**, *11*, S91–S100. [CrossRef]
20. Mategula, D.; Ndalama, M.; Lefu, C.; Chinkhumba, J.; Ndeketa, L.; Munthali, V.; Chitala, C.; Malemia, T.; Million, G.; Mbutuka, I.; et al. The Enterics for Global Health (EFGH) Shigella Surveillance Study in Malawi. *Open Forum Infect. Dis.* **2024**, *11*, S101–S106. [CrossRef]
21. Keita, A.M.; Doh, S.; Juma, J.; Nasrin, D.; Traoré, A.; Onwuchekwa, U.; Maguire, R.; Haidara, F.C.; Sow, S.O.; Kotloff, K.L.; et al. The Enterics for Global Health (EFGH) Shigella Surveillance Study in Mali. *Open Forum Infect. Dis.* **2024**, *11*, S107–S112. [CrossRef]
22. Ahmed, N.; Yousafzai, M.T.; Naz Qamar, F. The Enterics for Global Health (EFGH) Shigella Surveillance Study in Pakistan. *Open Forum Infect. Dis.* **2024**, *11*, S113–S120. [CrossRef]
23. Pavlinac, P.B.; Rogawski McQuade, E.T.; Platts-Mills, J.A.; Kotloff, K.L.; Deal, C.; Giersing, B.K.; Isbrucker, R.A.; Kang, G.; Ma, L.-F.; MacLennan, C.A.; et al. Pivotal Shigella Vaccine Efficacy Trials—Study Design Considerations from a Shigella Vaccine Trial Design Working Group. *Vaccines* **2022**, *10*, 489. [CrossRef]
24. Levine, M.M.; Kotloff, K.L.; Nataro, J.P.; Muhsen, K. The Global Enteric Multicenter Study (GEMS): Impetus, Rationale, and Genesis. *Clin. Infect. Dis.* **2012**, *55* (Suppl. S4), S215–S224. [CrossRef]
25. Zaman, K.; Dang, D.A.; Victor, J.C.; Shin, S.; Yunus, M.; Dallas, M.J.; Podder, G.; Vu, D.T.; Le, T.P.M.; Luby, S.P.; et al. Efficacy of Pentavalent Rotavirus Vaccine against Severe Rotavirus Gastroenteritis in Infants in Developing Countries in Asia: A Randomised, Double-Blind, Placebo-Controlled Trial. *Lancet* **2010**, *376*, 615–623. [CrossRef]
26. The MAL-ED Network Investigators The MAL-ED Study: A Multinational and Multidisciplinary Approach to Understand the Relationship Between Enteric Pathogens, Malnutrition, Gut Physiology, Physical Growth, Cognitive Development, and Immune Responses in Infants and Children Up to 2 Years of Age in Resource-Poor Environments. *Clin. Infect. Dis.* **2014**, *59*, S193–S206. [CrossRef]
27. Pavlinac, P.B.; Platts-Mills, J.A.; Tickell, K.D.; Liu, J.; Juma, J.; Kabir, F.; Nkeze, J.; Okoi, C.; Operario, D.J.; Uddin, J.; et al. The Clinical Presentation of Culture-Positive and Culture-Negative, Quantitative Polymerase Chain Reaction (qPCR)-Attributable Shigellosis in the Global Enteric Multicenter Study and Derivation of a Shigella Severity Score: Implications for Pediatric Shigella Vaccine Trials. *Clin. Infect. Dis.* **2021**, *73*, e569–e579. [CrossRef]
28. Liu, J.; Platts-Mills, J.A.; Juma, J.; Kabir, F.; Nkeze, J.; Okoi, C.; Operario, D.J.; Uddin, J.; Ahmed, S.; Alonso, P.L.; et al. Use of Quantitative Molecular Diagnostic Methods to Identify Causes of Diarrhoea in Children: A Reanalysis of the GEMS Case-Control Study. *Lancet* **2016**, *388*, 1291–1301. [CrossRef]
29. Pholwat, S.; Liu, J.; Taniuchi, M.; Haque, R.; Alam, M.M.; Faruque, A.S.G.; Ferdous, T.; Ara, R.; Platts-Mills, J.A.; Houpt, E.R. Use of Molecular Methods to Detect Shigella and Infer Phenotypic Resistance in a Shigella Treatment Study. *J. Clin. Microbiol.* **2022**, *60*, e0177421. [CrossRef] [PubMed]
30. Sun, Q.; Lan, R.; Wang, Y.; Zhao, A.; Zhang, S.; Wang, J.; Wang, Y.; Xia, S.; Jin, D.; Cui, Z.; et al. Development of a Multiplex PCR Assay Targeting O-Antigen Modification Genes for Molecular Serotyping of Shigella Flexneri. *J. Clin. Microbiol.* **2011**, *49*, 3766–3770. [CrossRef] [PubMed]
31. Liu, J.; Pholwat, S.; Zhang, J.; Taniuchi, M.; Haque, R.; Alam, M.; Ochieng, J.B.; Jones, J.A.; Platts-Mills, J.A.; Tennant, S.M.; et al. Evaluation of Molecular Serotyping Assays for Shigella Flexneri Directly on Stool Samples. *J. Clin. Microbiol.* **2021**, *59*, e02455-20. [CrossRef]

32. ICH Q2(R2) Validation of Analytical Procedures—Scientific Guideline | European Medicines Agency. Available online: https://www.ema.europa.eu/en/ich-q2r2-validation-analytical-procedures-scientific-guideline (accessed on 7 July 2024).
33. Center for Drug Evaluation and Research; Office of Regulatory Policy. Q2(R2) Validation of Analytical Procedures. Available online: https://www.fda.gov/regulatory-information/search-fda-guidance-documents/q2r2-validation-analytical-procedures (accessed on 7 July 2024).
34. Liu, J.; Garcia Bardales, P.F.; Islam, K.; Jarju, S.; Juma, J.; Mhango, C.; Naumanga, Q.; Qureshi, S.; Sonye, C.; Ahmed, N.; et al. *Shigella* Detection and Molecular Serotyping with a Customized TaqMan Array Card in the Enterics for Global Health (EFGH): *Shigella* Surveillance Study. *Open Forum Infect. Dis.* **2024**, *11*, S34–S40. [CrossRef]
35. Liu, J.; Kabir, F.; Manneh, J.; Lertsethtakarn, P.; Begum, S.; Gratz, J.; Becker, S.M.; Operario, D.J.; Taniuchi, M.; Janaki, L.; et al. Development and Assessment of Molecular Diagnostic Tests for 15 Enteropathogens Causing Childhood Diarrhoea: A Multicentre Study. *Lancet Infect. Dis.* **2014**, *14*, 716–724. [CrossRef]
36. Kamau, E.; Alemayehu, S.; Feghali, K.C.; Saunders, D.; Ockenhouse, C.F. Multiplex qPCR for Detection and Absolute Quantification of Malaria. *PLoS ONE* **2013**, *8*, e71539. [CrossRef] [PubMed]
37. Walk, J.; Schats, R.; Langenberg, M.C.C.; Reuling, I.J.; Teelen, K.; Roestenberg, M.; Hermsen, C.C.; Visser, L.G.; Sauerwein, R.W. Diagnosis and Treatment Based on Quantitative PCR after Controlled Human Malaria Infection. *Malar. J.* **2016**, *15*, 398. [CrossRef] [PubMed]
38. Global Technical Strategy for Malaria 2016–2030, 2021 Update. Available online: https://www.who.int/publications/i/item/9789240031357 (accessed on 8 November 2024).
39. Babb, C.; Badji, H.; Bhuiyan, M.T.R.; Cornick, J.; Qureshi, S.; Sonye, C.; Shapiama Lopez, W.V.; Adnan, M.; Atlas, H.E.; Begum, K.; et al. Evaluation of Fecal Inflammatory Biomarkers to Identify Bacterial Diarrhea Episodes: Systematic Review and Protocol for the Enterics for Global Health Shigella Surveillance Study. *Open Forum Infect. Dis.* **2024**, *11*, S65–S75. [CrossRef] [PubMed]
40. Horne, B.; Badji, H.; Bhuiyan, M.T.R.; Romaina Cachique, L.; Cornick, J.; Hotwani, A.; Juma, J.; Ochieng, J.B.; Abdou, M.; Apondi, E.; et al. Microbiological Methods Used in the Enterics for Global Health Shigella Surveillance Study. *Open Forum Infect. Dis.* **2024**, *11*, S25–S33. [CrossRef]
41. Hausdorff, W.P.; Madhi, S.A.; Kang, G.; Kaboré, L.; Tufet Bayona, M.; Giersing, B.K. Facilitating the Development of Urgently Required Combination Vaccines. *Lancet Glob. Health* **2024**, *12*, e1059–e1067. [CrossRef]
42. Riddle, M.S.; Louis Bourgeois, A.; Clifford, A.; Jeon, S.; Giersing, B.K.; Jit, M.; Tufet Bayona, M.; Ovitt, J.; Hausdorff, W.P. Challenges and Opportunities in Developing a Shigella-Containing Combination Vaccine for Children in Low- and Middle-Income Countries: Report of an Expert Convening. *Vaccine* **2023**, *41*, 2634–2644. [CrossRef]

vaccines

MDPI

Article

COVID-19 Vaccine Hesitancy Among Pediatric Oncology and Bone Marrow Transplant Patients

Sarah A. O'Neill [1], Son Tran [2], Cora Constantinescu [3] and Tony H. Truong [4,*]

[1] Department of Pediatrics, Alberta Children's Hospital, University of Calgary, Calgary, AB T2N 1N4, Canada; sarah.oneill@ucalgary.ca
[2] Dalla Lana School of Public Health, University of Toronto, Toronto, ON M5S 1A1, Canada
[3] Section of Pediatric Infectious Diseases, Department of Pediatrics, Alberta Children's Hospital, University of Calgary, Calgary, AB T2N 1N4, Canada; cora.constantinescu@albertahealthservices.ca
[4] Section of Pediatric Oncology and Cellular Therapy, Department of Pediatrics, Alberta Children's Hospital, University of Calgary, Calgary, AB T2N 1N4, Canada
* Correspondence: tony.truong@ahs.ca

Abstract: Background/Objectives: Vaccine hesitancy among immunocompromised patients is complex and not well understood. This study aimed to determine the rate of COVID-19 vaccine hesitancy among pediatric oncology and bone marrow transplant (BMT) patients and to understand associated factors. **Methods**: Parents of patients (≤18 years) with cancer or post-BMT completed the Parent Attitudes about Childhood Vaccines Survey. A COVID-19 vaccine hesitancy score (VHS-COVID) was calculated from 0 to 100 (higher scores indicating increasing hesitancy). A small group of patients (patients older than 15 years) were also surveyed directly. **Results**: Among 113 parent respondents, the majority were female (58%) and at least college/university educated (78%). The majority (73%) of patients had cancer (61% leukemia/lymphoma, 37% solid/CNS tumors), while 27% had received BMT for malignant and non-malignant conditions. Only 48% of patients had been vaccinated against COVID-19, compared to 88% of parents. Ineligibility due to phase of cancer/BMT treatment (27%), vaccine hesitancy (24%), and age (24%) were the top three reasons for not vaccinating against COVID-19. Only 13% of parents said they would "definitely vaccinate" if their child became eligible. VHS-COVID scores were higher for parents of patients in surveillance versus active therapy (mean 61 vs. 48; $p = 0.03$). Parents who had received fewer COVID-19 vaccine doses (0–1 vs. ≥2) were more hesitant toward all vaccines ($p = 0.0002$), COVID-19 vaccines ($p = 0.0003$), and influenza vaccines ($p = 0.005$). **Conclusions:** Vaccine hesitancy is common among this population and was demonstrated through beliefs (hesitancy scores) as well as vaccine uptake. Future work should focus on education targeting vaccine eligibility and engaging with vaccine hesitant families in the immunocompromised community.

Keywords: vaccine hesitancy; vaccination; immunization; cancer; pediatric; immunocompromised; public health

1. Introduction

The World Health Organization (WHO) has defined vaccine hesitancy as a 'delay in acceptance of the vaccine despite the availability of vaccination services' [1]. Addressing vaccine hesitancy becomes increasingly complex as we consider unique populations such as pediatric oncology and bone marrow transplant (BMT) patients, who have different vaccine-preventable disease risks and vaccine recommendations compared to the general population [2,3]. Vaccines are generally not provided to pediatric oncology patients during active chemotherapy or to BMT patients until 6 months post-transplant. Cytotoxic and myelosuppressive drugs limit the body's ability to mount a robust immune response, thereby making routine vaccinations less effective in the immunocompromised host. Further, vaccination with live attenuated vaccines (e.g., measles, mumps, rubella, and varicella (MMRV) vaccine) are contraindicated due to the rare chance of developing an illness because of the vaccine [4].

In contrast, the pediatric and adult mRNA-based COVID-19 vaccines are not live vaccines, and although immunocompromised patients may not be able to mount a robust antibody response, possible anti-viral protection and desire to achieve greater herd immunity are desired benefits [5,6]. As such, COVID-19 vaccines are strongly recommended by national advisory committees on immunizations for immunocompromised patients such as cancer and bone marrow transplant patients [7].

Caregivers of childhood cancer survivors have expressed concerns about the COVID-19 vaccine due to the fragile health of their child, the risk of severe complications, inadequate safety information, and unclear necessity [8,9]. Parents have also reported greater hesitancy toward COVID-19 vaccines than routine childhood vaccinations, suggesting that using terms like "vaccine hesitant" may be more precise when referring to a specific vaccine [8].

We are beginning to understand COVID-19 vaccine hesitancy in survivor communities and the general public. However, the literature has yet to explore factors relating to vaccine hesitancy to COVID-19 among pediatric oncology patients undergoing active anti-cancer therapy, a time when they might be at increased severity risk from this disease [10–12]. Vaccine uptake rates have dropped across all childhood immunizations since the pandemic, with many sources citing a loss of confidence associated with the COVID-19 vaccine and COVID restrictions [13,14]. Understanding the hesitancy behind the COVID-19 vaccine may help guide us in understanding how to prevent the loss of confidence around other vaccines as well. For this study, we explored attitudes related to COVID-19 and influenza vaccines, with a brief inquiry into views around routine vaccinations in childhood. To compare parental views with patients, a small group of patients older than 15 years were also surveyed. By evaluating the factors affecting current (COVID-19) and annual respiratory seasonal (influenza) vaccinations, we can provide better information about perceived disease threat, vaccination effectiveness, and safety in our patients and develop strategies to increase vaccine uptake.

2. Materials and Methods

Pediatric oncology and bone marrow transplant patients and their parents were recruited from both the outpatient oncology/BMT clinic and the inpatient ward at the Alberta Children's Hospital (ACH) in Calgary, Alberta, from February 2023 to September 2023. Parents were eligible to complete the survey if their child was under 18 years old, had a current or previous diagnosis of cancer, was in any stage of treatment/remission/follow-up, or had received a bone marrow transplant for any indication (malignant or non-malignant). Participants were excluded if they were unable to read/understand the English survey. Patients who had received the COVID-19 vaccine or had a previous confirmed diagnosis of COVID-19 were not excluded from the study. Patients older than 15 years were also allowed to complete the study to express their individual views. Informed consent was obtained at the start of the study questionnaire. The study was approved by the Health Research Ethics Board of Alberta: Cancer Committee.

Vaccine hesitancy was measured using an adapted version of the Parent Attitudes about Childhood Vaccines survey (PACV) by Opel et al. (2011) [15]. Survey questions maintained the same wording as the original instrument; however, participants were asked to answer the questions as they pertained to their views on a particular vaccine (i.e., routine childhood vaccinations, COVID-19, or influenza). Additionally, the word "shot" in the question stem was replaced by "vaccine", as it is a more familiar term used in Canada. Survey responses were collapsed into three categories: hesitant, neutral/not sure, and non-hesitant. A vaccine hesitancy score was calculated by assigning a numeric score to each response: 2 points for each hesitant response, 1 for neutral/not sure, and 0 for each non-hesitant response. The responses of agree and strongly agree were combined together (Agree); disagree and strongly disagree were combined (Disagree). Hesitant reflects the combined responses of very and somewhat hesitant; not hesitant reflects the combined responses of not hesitant at all and not too hesitant. Concerned reflects the combined responses of very and somewhat concerned; not concerned reflects the combined responses of not concerned at all and not too concerned. For sliding scale questions (e.g., "From 0–10, how sure are you that following the recommended vaccine schedule is a good idea for your child?"), answers were collapsed into hesitant (0–3), not sure (4–7) and non-hesitant (8–10) categories. A raw total vaccine hesitancy score (VHS-Total) was calculated from the sum of each question score and transformed into a 0–100 scale, with higher scores indicating increased hesitancy. Separate scores were also tallied specifically for the COVID-19 and influenza vaccines and are referred to as "VHS-COVID" and "VHS-Flu", respectively.

Potential associations with vaccine hesitancy scores (e.g., COVID vaccination status, treatment status, demographics) were assessed in bivariate analyses using *t*-tests, ANOVA, or Wilcoxon tests as appropriate to the data. Linear regressions were used to evaluate which demographic factors are associated with vaccine hesitancy scores. Predictors that met a significance threshold of $p < 0.1$ (two-tailed) were jointly evaluated in a multiple linear regression model. A manual stepwise backward elimination approach was used to identify significant covariates at a $p < 0.05$ (two-tailed) as required. Statistical analyses were conducted using the SAS statistical program (SAS-PC, version 9.4; SAS Institute Inc., Cary, NC, USA).

3. Results

3.1. Parent Respondents

Overall, 159 responses were received. Surveys were discarded due to respondents not consenting to the study (n = 4) or for not completing at least 2 sections of the survey (Routine Immunizations and Influenza; n = 22). Of the 133 remaining surveys, 113 were completed by parents. The remaining 20 surveys were completed by patients and analyzed separately. Two parents and one patient participant did not complete the final section on COVID-19, and statistics were adjusted accordingly. Among 113 parents, the majority were female (58%) and at least college/university educated (78%) (Table 1). Regarding their children, the majority (73%) were patients with cancer (61% leukemia/lymphoma, 37% solid/CNS tumors), while 27% had received BMT for malignant and non-malignant conditions. Most patients were undergoing active treatment (73%), with the remainder in surveillance/follow-up (27%).

Table 1. Participant demographics and details about the patient's treatment.

	Number (%) of Parent Participants (n = 113)	Number (%) of Patient Participants (n = 20)
Respondent Gender		
Male	43 (39)	8 (42)
Female	64 (58)	10 (53)
Prefer not to disclose	3 (3)	1 (5)
Parental Education		
Master's, Ph.D., professional degree	11 (10)	4 (21)
University degree	33 (30)	2 (11)
College diploma	42 (38)	3 (16)
High school	17 (15)	5 (26)
Below high school	2 (2)	5 (26)
Prefer not to disclose	5 (5)	
Type of Treatment Received		
Cancer	82 (73)	16 (80)
BMT (total)	31 (27) (18 malignant; 13 non-malignant)	4 (20) (all 4 non-malignant)

Table 1. *Cont.*

	Number (%) of Parent Participants (n = 113)	Number (%) of Patient Participants (n = 20)
Treatment Status		
Active	83 (73)	9 (45)
Surveillance	30 (27)	11 (55)
Cancer Type		
Leukemia	36 (36)	4 (25)
Lymphoma	25 (25)	4 (25)
Brain tumor	9 (9)	1 (6)
Solid tumor	28 (28)	7 (44)
Other	2 (2)	0
Relapse status		
Yes	47 (47)	3 (18)
No	49 (49)	14 (82)
Unsure	4 (4)	
Patient's School		
Private school	13 (12)	2 (11)
Public school	78 (71)	16 (84)
Homeschool	4 (4)	1 (5)
Not school age	10 (9)	n/a
Other	5 (5)	
Household Income		
>$100,000	35 (32)	11 (58)
$50,000–100,000	20 (18)	3 (16)
<$50,000	45 (41)	2 (11)
Prefer not to disclose	10 (9)	3 (16)
Patient COVID Vaccine status		
0 doses	59 (52)	3 (15)
1 dose	16 (14)	0 (0)
2 doses	29 (26)	7 (35)
3 or more doses	9 (8)	10 (50)
Parent COVID Vaccine status		
0 doses	14 (12)	n/a
1 dose	19 (17)	n/a
2 doses	48 (42)	n/a
3 or more doses	31 (27)	n/a
Unsure	1 (1)	n/a
Influenza Vaccine status	Parent	Patient
3–5 times in the last 5 years	57 (50)	10 (50)
Never/0–2 times in the last 5 years	56 (49)	10 (50)

Percentages may not total 100% due to rounding.

Despite 56% of all parents reporting that they were at least somewhat hesitant about the COVID-19 vaccine, 88% of parents had received at least one dose (Table 2). In contrast, only 48% of their children had received at least one dose of the COVID-19 vaccine. Ineligibility due to stage of cancer/BMT treatment (27%), vaccine hesitancy (24%), and age (24%) were the top three reasons for not vaccinating their children against COVID-19. Only 13% of parents said they would "definitely vaccinate" their child if they became eligible. Overall, one-quarter of parents were unsure if they can trust the information they receive about COVID-19 vaccines, but the majority (66%) felt they could openly discuss these concerns with their child's doctor.

Table 2. Modified PACV survey questions and parent and patient responses.

Question	Response	Parents (n = 113) N (%)	Patients (n = 20) N (%)
Part 1: Views on Vaccines in General			
1. If you had another infant today, would you want him/her to get all the recommended vaccines?	Yes	81 (72)	n/a
	Not sure	23 (20)	n/a
	No	**9 (8)**	**n/a**
2. Children get more vaccines than are good for them	Disagree	40 (35)	17 (85)
	Not sure	19 (17)	2 (10)
	Agree	**54 (48)**	**1 (5)**
3. It is better for my child to develop immunity by getting sick than to get a vaccine	Disagree	40 (35)	15 (75)
	Not sure	19 (17)	0
	Agree	**54 (48)**	**5 (25)**
4. Overall, how hesitant about childhood vaccines would you consider yourself to be?	**Hesitant**	**37 (33)**	**4 (15)**
	Not sure	11 (10)	1 (5)
	Not hesitant	65 (58)	15 (75)
5. How sure are you that following the recommended vaccine schedule is a good idea for your child?	**0–3 (Not sure)**	**14 (12)**	**2 (10)**
	4–7 (Neutral)	50 (44)	8 (40)
	8–10 (Extremely sure)	49 (43)	10 (50)
Part 2: Views on Annual Influenza Vaccine			
1. Have you ever delayed your child getting *the annual influenza* vaccine for reasons other than illness, allergy, or your child's cancer diagnosis?	**Yes**	**58 (51)**	**10 (50)**
	Not sure	5 (4)	2 (10)
	No	50 (44)	8 (40)
2. Have you ever decided not to get *the annual influenza* vaccine for your child for reasons other than illness, allergy, or your child's cancer diagnosis?	**Yes**	**64 (57)**	**12 (60)**
	Not sure	4 (4)	2 (10)
	No	45 (40)	6 (30)
3. Overall, how hesitant about the influenza vaccine would you consider yourself to be?	**Hesitant**	**50 (44)**	**4 (20)**
	Not sure	13 (12)	3 (15)
	Not hesitant	50 (44)	13 (65)
4. I believe that the illness that the influenza vaccine prevents is severe	**Disagree**	**28 (25)**	**6 (30)**
	Not sure	22 (19)	4 (20)
	Agree	63 (56)	10 (50)
5. It is better for my child to develop immunity by getting sick with influenza than to get a vaccine	Disagree	39 (35)	14 (70)
	Not sure	20 (18)	3 (15)
	Agree	**54 (48)**	**3 (15)**
6. I trust the information I receive about the influenza vaccines	**Disagree**	**17 (15)**	**5 (25)**
	Not sure	36 (32)	2 (10)
	Agree	60 (53)	13 (65)
7. I am able to openly discuss my concerns about influenza vaccines with my child's doctor	**Disagree**	**14 (12)**	**1 (5)**
	Not sure	22 (19)	3 (15)
	Agree	77 (68)	16 (80)

Table 2. *Cont.*

Question	Response	Parents (n = 113) N (%)	Patients (n = 20) N (%)
8. How concerned are you that your child might have a serious side effect from the influenza vaccine?	**Concerned**	**56 (50)**	**6 (30)**
	Not sure	14 (12)	4 (20)
	Not concerned	43 (38)	10 (50)
9. How concerned are you that the influenza vaccine might not prevent the disease?	**Concerned**	**55 (49)**	**4 (20)**
	Not sure	21 (19)	3 (15)
	Not concerned	37 (33)	13 (65)
Part 3: Views on COVID-19 mRNA vaccine			
1. Have you ever delayed your child getting the *COVID-19* vaccine for reasons other than illness, allergy, or your child's cancer diagnosis?	**Yes**	**61 (55)**	**7 (37)**
	Not sure	3 (3)	2 (11)
	No	47 (42)	10 (53)
2. Have you ever decided not to get the *COVID-19* vaccine for your child for reasons other than illness, allergy, or your child's cancer diagnosis?	**Yes**	**59 (53)**	**3 (16)**
	Not sure	3 (3)	1 (5)
	No	49 (44)	15 (79)
3. Overall, how hesitant about the COVID vaccine would you consider yourself to be?	**Hesitant**	**62 (56)**	**4 (21)**
	Not sure	9 (8)	0
	Not hesitant	40 (36)	15 (79)
4. I believe that the illness that the COVID vaccine prevents is severe	**Disagree**	**29 (26)**	**2 (11)**
	Not sure	18 (16)	2 (11)
	Agree	64 (58)	15 (79)
5. It is better for my child to develop immunity by getting sick than to get a COVID vaccine	Disagree	40 (36)	16 (84)
	Not sure	21 (19)	1 (5)
	Agree	**50 (45)**	**2 (10)**
6. I trust the information I receive about COVID vaccines	**Disagree**	**31 (28)**	**3 (16)**
	Not sure	28 (25)	2 (11)
	Agree	52 (47)	14 (74)
7. I am able to openly discuss my concerns about the COVID vaccine with my child's doctor	**Disagree**	**21 (19)**	**1 (5)**
	Not sure	17 (15)	5 (26)
	Agree	73 (66)	13 (68)
8. How concerned are you that your child might have a serious side effect from a COVID vaccine?	**Concerned**	**72 (65)**	**5 (26)**
	Not sure	11 (10)	2 (11)
	Not concerned	28 (25)	12 (63)
9. How concerned are you that a COVID vaccine might not prevent the disease?	**Concerned**	**67 (60)**	**8 (42)**
	Not sure	13 (12)	0
	Not concerned	31 (28)	11 (58)

Hesitant responses are bolded. Survey questions for patients were modified to be directed to them instead of their child. Agree reflects the combined responses of strongly agree and agree; disagree reflects the combined responses of strongly disagree and disagree. Hesitant reflects the combined responses of very and somewhat hesitant; not hesitant reflects the combined responses of not hesitant at all and not too hesitant. Response category on a 0–10 scale, with 0 being 'not at all sure' and 10 being 'extremely sure'. Concerned reflects the combined responses of very and somewhat concerned; not concerned reflects the combined responses of not concerned at all and not too concerned. Percentages may not total 100% due to rounding.

Hesitant views were unique for some participant subgroups and, at times, only expressed toward certain vaccines. Families in the surveillance/follow-up subgroup were more hesitant toward the COVID-19 vaccine compared to those still in the in active treatment subgroup (VHS-COVID, 61 vs. 48; $p = 0.03$), but this difference was not significant for VHS-Total ($p = 0.1$) or VHS-Flu ($p = 0.13$; Table 3). Lower household income (<$50,000) was associated with increased hesitancy toward routine immunizations ($p = 0.04$) as well as flu vaccines ($p = 0.04$), but not for hesitancy toward the COVID-19 vaccine ($p = 0.57$).

Table 3. Hesitancy outcomes for parent respondents based on demographics.

	VHS-Total		VHS-COVID		VHS-Influenza	
	Score, Mean (Median)	p-Value	Score, Mean (Median)	p-Value	Score, Mean (Median)	p-Value
Parental Gender						
Male	48 (54)	0.99	50 (61)	0.61	48 (56)	0.63
Female	47 (52)		53 (64)		45 (50)	
Parental Education						
High	47 (53)	0.56	52 (61)	0.68	46 (56)	0.35
Low	45 (52)		50 (56)		43 (56)	
Type of Treatment Received						
Cancer	47 (52)	0.91	51 (61)	0.94	46 (50)	0.78
BMT	47 (50)		52 (67)		46 (56)	
Treatment Phase						
Active	44 (43)	0.10	48 (56)	0.03	43 (39)	0.13
Surveillance	54 (58)		61 (69)		54 (61)	
Cancer Type						
Leukemia/lymph	51 (61)	0.3	56 (67)	0.2	51 (61)	0.18
Brain/solid	42 (37)		47 (50)		40 (33)	
Relapse status						
Yes	47 (59)	0.6	48 (61)	0.08	45 (56)	0.45
No	49 (52)		57 (67)		48 (50)	
Patient's School						
Public school	49 (59)	0.17	54 (67)	0.07	41 (36)	0.26
Other	41 (40)		44 (44)		48 (61)	
Household Income						
High	42 (43)	0.04	49 (61)	0.57	40 (39)	0.04
Low	53 (63)		55 (67)		53 (61)	
COVID Vaccine status (self)						
0 or 1 dose	62 (65)	0.0002	67 (72)	0.0003	59 (61)	0.005
≥2 doses	41 (42)		45 (50)		41 (30)	
Influenza Vaccine status (self)						
≤2 doses in the last 5 years	51 (50)	0.14	55 (61)	0.15	51 (56)	0.09
3–5 doses in the last 5 years	43 (54)		48 (61)		42 (44)	

Numbers do not total 100% due to partial survey completion or rounding. Parental education level collapsed into high (college diploma, university degree, master's, Ph.D. or professional degree) and low (high school diploma or below). Patient school collapsed into public and other (private, homeschool, not school age, other). Household income collapsed into high (>$50,000/year) and low (<$50,000/year).

Parents who were not regular recipients of the annual influenza vaccine (i.e., received two or fewer in the last 5 years) were generally more hesitant (though not significantly) toward all vaccine categories (VHS-Total, $p = 0.14$; VHS-COVID, $p = 0.15$; and Influenza-VHS, $p = 0.09$), compared to those who received three or more annual influenza vaccines. The following variables were not significantly associated with vaccine hesitancy (VHS-COVID,

VHS-Flu, or VHS-Total) for parent participants: treatment type (cancer vs. BMT), cancer type, relapse status, or additional parental demographic factors (gender, parental education, child's school).

In the multivariable linear regression, only COVID-19 vaccination status was a significant predictor of VHS-Total scores (parents who had one or fewer doses were more hesitant than those with two or more doses, beta 17.44, $p = 0.0086$). For VHS-COVID scores, parents whose children were in surveillance/follow-up were more hesitant compared to those in active therapy (beta 16.24, $p = 0.047$), and those having received one or fewer doses of COVID-19 vaccine (beta 19.33, $p = 0.01$). For the VHS-Flu scores, those with lower household incomes were more hesitant than those with higher incomes (beta 15.88, $p = 0.04$).

3.2. *Patient Respondents (Older than 15 Years)*

Patients older than 15 years had an opportunity to respond to the survey on their own (n = 20). Patient respondents were more balanced in gender split (53% female, 42% male) compared to parent respondents. Similar to the parent population, the majority of respondents were diagnosed with cancer (80%), though over half of the patient group (55%) were in surveillance/follow-up rather than active treatment (45%) (Table 1). Patients self-reported better COVID-19 vaccine uptake (85% had ≥2 doses) compared to parent respondents (69% of parents and 34% of their children had ≥2 doses). This was also reflected in patients having significantly lower vaccine hesitancy scores than parents for VHS-Total (29 vs. 47; $p = 0.0036$) and VHS-COVID (24 vs. 51; $p = 0.0005$) (Table 4).

Table 4. Vaccine hesitancy scores for parent vs. patient respondents.

Hesitancy Outcome	Parent, Mean (Median)	Patient, Mean (Median)	*p*-Value
VHS-Total	47 (52)	29 (17)	0.0036
VHS-COVID	51 (61)	24 (11)	0.0005
VHS-Flu	46 (56)	34 (31)	0.09

Personal uptake of the influenza vaccine was similar between parent and patient respondents (50% were vaccinated in ≥3 of the last 5 years); however, their views about the vaccine differed. Parents were more hesitant than patients about the influenza vaccine (44% vs. 20% at least somewhat hesitant, respectively), despite both groups agreeing that the vaccine prevents serious illness. Further, many parents agreed it was better for their children to gain immunity by being sick with influenza rather than getting the vaccine (48% vs. 15% of patients). Overall, parents were more hesitant toward the influenza vaccine (VHS-Flu, 46 vs. 34 for patients); however, this was not significant ($p = 0.09$).

Among the patient respondents, the type of treatment received and COVID-19 vaccination status significantly affected hesitancy toward all vaccine categories (Table 5). Patients who received ≥2 doses of the COVID vaccine were significantly less hesitant toward all vaccine types ($p = 0.02$), COVID-19 vaccines ($p = 0.02$), and influenza vaccines ($p = 0.03$) than those who were unvaccinated against COVID-19 or had only received one dose. Individuals treated for cancer (n = 16) were less hesitant than patients who received BMT (n = 4); however, these data should be interpreted with caution given small numbers ($p = 0.005$, $p = 0.02$, $p = 0.003$ for VHS-Total, VHS-COVID, and VHS-Flu, respectively). The following variables were not significantly associated with vaccine hesitancy (VHS-COVID, VHS-Flu, or VHS-Total) for patient respondents: treatment phase, cancer type, relapse status, influenza vaccine status, or additional demographic factors (gender, parental education, school, household income).

Table 5. Hesitancy outcomes for patient respondents based on demographics.

	VHS-Total		VHS-COVID		VHS-Influenza	
	Score, Mean (Median)	*p*-Value	Score, Mean (Median)	*p*-Value	Score, Mean (Median)	*p*-Value
Patient Gender						
Male	37 (31)	0.15	35 (31)	0.24	40 (36)	0.24
Female	20 (16)		17 (11)		27 (25)	
Parental Education						
High	22 (16)	0.8	20 (11)	0.65	28 (28)	0.62
Low	31 (17)		11 (11)		36 (33)	
Type of Treatment Received						
Cancer	20 (16)	0.005	16 (11)	0.016	25 (11)	0.003
BMT	64 (59)		67 (72)		74 (72)	
Treatment Phase						
Active	30 (20)	0.4	16 (8)	0.38	42 (33)	0.15
Surveillance	28 (16)		30 (11)		28 (28)	
Cancer Type						
Leukemia/lymph	17 (16)	0.83	13 (11)	0.74	20 (19)	0.49
Brain/solid	23 (16)		19 (11)		29 (28)	
Relapse status						
Yes	23 (16)	0.9	19 (6)	0.52	35 (33)	0.25
No	22 (16)		19 (11)		25 (25)	
School						
Public school	22 (16)	0.09	18 (11)	0.10	28 (28)	0.08
Other	51 (43)		54 (50)		56 (44)	
Household Income						
High	25 (16)	0.52	21 (11)	0.81	28 (28)	0.20
Low	30 (30)		28 (28)		39 (39)	
COVID Vaccine status (self)						
0 or 1 dose	66 (64)	0.02	67 (50)	0.02	67 (67)	0.03
≥2 doses	22 (16)		16 (11)		29 (28)	
Influenza Vaccine status (self)						
≤2 doses in the last 5 years	28 (17)	1.0	25 (11)	0.77	33 (33)	0.88
3–5 doses in the last 5 years	29 (18)		23 (11)		36 (28)	

Numbers do not total 100% due to partial survey completion or rounding. Parental education level collapsed into high (college diploma, university degree, master's, Ph.D. or professional degree) and low (high school diploma or below). Patient school collapsed into public and other (private, homeschool, not school age, other). Household income collapsed into high (>$50,000/year) and low (<$50,000/year).

4. Discussion

Parents of children with cancer and recipients of BMT exhibit hesitancy toward the COVID-19 vaccine despite the best evidence and guidelines supporting their use in this population. The strongest predictor of vaccine hesitancy was the number of COVID-19 vaccine doses received by the parent themselves. Overall, COVID-19 vaccination status, household income, and phase of cancer/BMT treatment were significantly associated with hesitancy scores in Total-VHS, VHS-COVID, and VHS-Flu. Patient respondents displayed less hesitancy than parent respondents for VHS and VHS-COVID.

This study builds on previous work in the survivorship community by including patients undergoing active treatment and was conducted three years into the pandemic to gain insight into belief systems as they have evolved over time. Supporting the work of Wimberley et al., parents surveyed had received more vaccines than their children [9]. Specifically, Wimberly et al. found that 29% of parents were hesitant to vaccinate their childhood cancer survivors against COVID-19, including 11% who would "definitely not" vaccinate. In contrast, only 20% of caregivers were hesitant to vaccinate themselves, and 12% of caregivers would vaccinate their other children differently than the childhood cancer survivor [9]. Contradictory to this, however, our study reports that patients themselves expressed less vaccine hesitancy than their parents toward all vaccine categories. This presents an interesting opportunity for targeting vaccine education toward patients aged 15 years and older, as they begin to express interest in their healthcare decisions and as in some places, such as Alberta, can make autonomous decisions regarding this.

Several studies in adult oncology have demonstrated the prevalence of COVID-19 vaccine hesitancy, up to 42% in a large French survey [16–18]. One study on adolescent and young adult cancer survivors reported that 24% of patients were hesitant about the COVID-19 vaccine, citing lower perceived disease vulnerability and concerns about vaccine safety [19].

Vaccines differ in their history (i.e., well-established, novel, or experimental), how they are perceived (i.e., effectiveness, necessity, and severity of side effects), and who they are offered to (i.e., population-wide or targeted toward specific subgroups). In this study, COVID-19 vaccination status was the strongest predictor of parental vaccine hesitancy (routine and COVID-19 vaccines), suggesting that beliefs and actions around COVID-19 vaccines are closely correlated. However, the same was not true for influenza vaccination status and hesitancy toward influenza vaccines. In addition to concerns about the vaccine itself, the threat of disease perceived by an individual is another important factor to consider. In our study, most parents agreed that influenza posed a serious disease threat (56%); however, many (48%) felt their child would be better off getting sick with the flu than vaccinating against it. There is a higher prevalence of the latter parental belief in our current study (48%) than what was observed from the knowledge, attitudes, and beliefs (KAB) study from the 2017 childhood National Immunization Coverage Survey (cNICS) in Canada. The cNICS, which surveyed Canadian parents about general childhood vaccines, reported that 31% of parents agreed that it is better for children to develop their immunity from natural infections rather than from vaccines [20]. Health care providers should recognize that complacency can often play a role in vaccination status and highlight the risk of disease in their discussions with families.

Parents of children in surveillance were more hesitant toward the COVID-19 vaccine than those in active treatment, but the same was not true toward the influenza vaccine. This supports the work of Temsah et al., who reported that individuals may express increased hesitancy toward some vaccinations and not others [8]. As such, vaccine hesitancy cannot be a blanket term applied to an individual's views on all vaccinations, but factors related to hesitancy and complacency must be explored as they relate to each specific vaccine.

This study was limited by recruiting participants from only one center in Canada. This study took place at the Alberta Children's Hospital, which serves a diverse patient population and is the only pediatric bone marrow transplant center in the province (and one of six in Canada). The survey was only available in English; thus, the data do not include the views of non-English speaking families. Due to the small sample size in our study and lack of statistical power, we may not have been able to detect true differences in both the parent and patient respondents. Additional patient recruitment would allow for a more robust comparison of vaccine hesitancy among patients and parents. The strengths of this study include the opportunity to explore COVID-19 vaccine hesitancy and compare it with routine childhood vaccines and the annual influenza vaccine. We were also able to survey a small group of patient respondents who had unique views regarding vaccine hesitancy compared to parent respondents.

Finally, this study has provided insight into opportunities for specific education with families around vaccine eligibility. The top three reasons parents selected for not vaccinating their child against COVID-19 were vaccine hesitancy and ineligibility due to age or stage of treatment. The COVID-19 vaccine is widely recommended to all immunocompromised patients, and only Canadians less than 6 months old are ineligible for the vaccine due to age. Most parents felt comfortable discussing vaccines with their doctor, which provides an excellent opportunity to address this type of vaccine misinformation and discuss hesitancy.

COVID-19 vaccines were introduced to Canadian adults in December 2020, shortly after the pandemic was declared in March 2020. For pediatric patients, it was not until November 2021 that children 5 years and older became eligible for mRNA vaccines. Lastly, children aged 6 months to 5 years old became eligible in July 2022 [21]. Despite two years of access to the vaccine, a large discrepancy between vaccinated children and adults remains. As of June 2024, only 8% of children aged 0–4 have received at least one dose of the vaccine, compared to 81% of all Canadians [22]. Patients under 6 months old remain ineligible for vaccination.

5. Conclusions

The pediatric oncology and BMT populations are vulnerable to diseases not only in the event of a future pandemic but also rely on immunity against routine diseases. Focusing on the risk of illness and the importance of disease prevention is paramount in such a vulnerable patient population. Since vaccine hesitancy varies depending on the disease and vaccine type, factors related to hesitancy should be openly explored both in general and for each vaccine type.

Author Contributions: Conceptualization, S.A.O., C.C. and T.H.T.; methodology, S.A.O., C.C. and T.H.T.; data analysis, S.A.O.; data collection, S.A.O., S.T. and T.H.T.; writing—original draft preparation, S.A.O. and T.H.T.; writing—review and editing, S.A.O., S.T., C.C. and T.H.T.; funding acquisition, S.A.O. and T.H.T. All authors have read and agreed to the published version of the manuscript.

Funding: This research was funded by the Barb Ibbotson Chair in Pediatric Hematology, Alberta Children's Hospital Research Foundation.

Institutional Review Board Statement: The study was conducted in accordance with the Declaration of Helsinki and approved by the Health Research Ethics Board of Alberta: Cancer Committee. (Ethics ID HREBA.CC-22-0342_REN1. Date of approval: 9 December 2022) for studies involving humans.

Informed Consent Statement: Informed consent was obtained from all subjects involved in the study.

Data Availability Statement: Data for the study are available by contacting the corresponding author.

Conflicts of Interest: S.O. and A.T. have no conflicts to declare. C.C. has received an honorarium from GSK. T.T. has received an honorarium from Servier, Jazz and Vertex. The funders had no role in the design of the study, in the collection, analyses, or interpretation of data, in the writing of the manuscript, or in the decision to publish the results.

References

1. MacDonald, N.E. Vaccine hesitancy: Definition, scope and determinants. *Vaccine* **2015**, *33*, 4161–4164. [CrossRef] [PubMed]
2. Top, K.A.; Pham-Huy, A.; Price, V.; Sung, L.; Tran, D.; Vaudry, W.; Halperin, S.A.; De Serres, G. Immunization practices in acute lymphocytic leukemia and post-hematopoietic stem cell transplant in Canadian Pediatric Hematology/Oncology centers. *Hum. Vaccin. Immunother.* **2016**, *12*, 931–936. [CrossRef] [PubMed]
3. Guilcher, G.M.T.; Rivard, L.; Huang, J.T.; Wright, N.A.M.; Anderson, L.; Eissa, H.; Pelletier, W.; Ramachandran, S.; Schechter, T.; Shah, A.J.; et al. Immune function in childhood cancer survivors: A Children's Oncology Group review. *Lancet Child Adolsc. Health* **2022**, *5*, 284–294. [CrossRef] [PubMed]
4. Cesaro, S.; Giacchino, M.; Fioredda, F.; Barone, A.; Battisti, L.; Bezzio, S.; Frenos, S.; De Santis, R.; Livadiotti, S.; Marinello, S.; et al. Guidelines on vaccinations in paediatric haematology and oncology patients. *BioMed Res. Int.* **2014**, *2014*, 707691. [CrossRef] [PubMed]

5. Charla, Y.; Kalra, M.; Chopra, N.; Choudhury, S. COVID-19 vaccination in pediatric cancer patients: A high priority. *Pediatr. Blood Cancer* **2021**, *68*, e29397. [CrossRef] [PubMed]
6. Children's Oncology Group. COVID-19 and Your Child, Teen, or Young Adult with Cancer. 2021. Retrieved from the Children's Oncology Group Website. Available online: https://childrensoncologygroup.org/downloads/COVID-19_and_Your_Child_with_Cancer_English.pdf (accessed on 2 December 2024).
7. Public Health Agency of Canada. Summary of NACI Statement of 3 May 2024: Guidance on the Use of COVID-19 Vaccines During the Fall of 2024. 2024. Retrieved from the Government of Canada Website. Available online: https://www.canada.ca/en/public-health/services/publications/vaccines-immunization/national-advisory-committee-immunization-summary-guidance-covid-19-vaccines-fall-2024.html (accessed on 2 December 2024).
8. Temsah, M.-H.; Alhuzaimi, A.N.; Aljamaan, F.; Bahkali, F.; Al-Eyadhy, A.; Alrabiaah, A.; Alhaboob, A.; Bashiri, F.A.; Alshaer, A.; Temsah, O.; et al. Parental Attitudes and Hesitancy About COVID-19 vs. Routine Childhood Vaccinations: A National Survey. *Front. Public Health* **2021**, *9*, 752323. [CrossRef] [PubMed]
9. Wimberly, C.E.; Towry, L.; Davis, E.; Johnston, E.E.; Walsh, K.M. SARS-CoV-2 vaccine acceptability among caregivers of childhood cancer survivors. *Pediatr. Blood Cancer* **2021**, *69*, e29443. [CrossRef] [PubMed]
10. Ilic, A.; Haardoerfer, R.; Michel, G.; Escoffery, C.; Mertens, A.C.; Marchak, J.G. Understanding caregivers' decision to vaccinate childhood cancer survivors against COVID-19. *Cancer Med.* **2023**, *12*, 21354–21363. [CrossRef] [PubMed]
11. Skeens, M.A.; Hill, K.; Olsavsky, A.; Buff, K.; Stevens, J.; Akard, T.F.; Shah, N.; Gerhardt, C.A. Factors affecting COVID-19 vaccine hesitancy in parents of children with cancer. *Pediatr. Blood Cancer* **2022**, *69*, e29707. [CrossRef] [PubMed]
12. Wigle, J.; Hodwitz, K.; Juando-Prats, C.; Allan, K.; Li, X.; Howard, L.; Fallon, B.; Birken, C.S.; Maguire, J.L.; Parsons, J.A. Parents' perspectives on SARS-CoV-2 vaccinations for children: A qualitative analysis. *CMAJ* **2023**, *195*, E259–E266. [CrossRef] [PubMed]
13. MacDonald, S.E.; Paudel, Y.R.; Kiely, M.; Rafferty, E.; Sadarangani, M.; Robinson, J.L.; Driedger, S.M.; Svenson, L.W. Impact of the COVID-19 pandemic on vaccine coverage for early childhood vaccines in Alberta, Canada: A population-based retrospective cohort study. *BMJ Open* **2022**, *12*, e055968. [CrossRef] [PubMed]
14. Ji, C.; Piché-Renaud, P.-P.; Apajee, J.; Stephenson, E.; Forte, M.; Friedman, J.N.; Science, M.; Zlotkin, S.; Morris, S.K.; Tu, K. Impact of the COVID-19 pandemic on routine immunization coverage in children under 2 years old in Ontario, Canada: A retrospective cohort study. *Vaccine* **2022**, *40*, 1790–1798. [CrossRef] [PubMed]
15. Opel, D.J.; Taylor, J.A.; Mangione-Smith, R.; Solomon, C.; Zhao, C.; Catz, S.; Martin, D. Validity and reliability of a survey to identify vaccine-hesitant parents. *Vaccine* **2011**, *29*, 6598–6605. [CrossRef] [PubMed]
16. Barrière, J.; Gal, J.; Hoch, B.; Cassuto, O.; Leysalle, A.; Chamorey, E.; Borchiellini, D. Acceptance of SARS-CoV-2 vaccination among French patients with cancer: A cross-sectional survey. *Ann. Oncol.* **2021**, *32*, 673–674. [CrossRef] [PubMed]
17. Prabani, K.I.P.; Weerasekara, I.; Damayanthi, H.D.W.T. COVID-19 vaccine acceptance and hesitancy among patients with cancer: A systematic review and meta-analysis. *Public Health* **2022**, *212*, 66–75. [CrossRef] [PubMed]
18. Villarreal-Garza, C.; Vaca-Cartagena, B.F.; Becerril-Gaitan, A.; Ferrigno, A.S.; Mesa-Chavez, F.; Platas, A.; Platas, A. Attitudes and factors associated with COVID-19 vaccine hesitancy among patients with breast cancer. *JAMA Oncol.* **2021**, *7*, 1242–1244. [CrossRef] [PubMed]
19. Waters, A.R.; Kepka, D.; Ramsay, J.M.; Mann, K.; Lopez, P.L.V.; Anderson, J.S.; Ou, J.Y.; Kaddas, H.K.; Palmer, A.; Ray, N.; et al. COVID-19 vaccine hesitancy among adolescent and young adult cancer survivors. *JNCI Cancer Spectrum* **2021**, *5*, pkab049. [CrossRef] [PubMed]
20. Public Health Agency of Canada. *Vaccine Hesitancy in Canadian Parents*; Public Health Agency of Canada: Ottawa, ON, Canada, 2022. Available online: https://www.canada.ca/content/dam/phac-aspc/documents/services/publications/healthy-living/vaccine-hesitancy-canadian-parents/vaccine-hesitancy-canadian-parents.pdf (accessed on 2 December 2024).
21. Moore, D. COVID-19 Vaccine for Children and Adolescents: Technical Report. Canadian Paediatric Society. 2023. Available online: https://cps.ca/en/documents/position/covid-19-vaccine-for-children-and-adolescents-technical-report (accessed on 2 December 2024).
22. Public Health Agency of Canada. Canadian COVID-19 Vaccination Coverage Report. 2024. Retrieved from the Government of Canada Website. Available online: https://health-infobase.canada.ca/covid-19/vaccination-coverage/ (accessed on 2 December 2024).

vaccines

MDPI

Article

Addressing Barriers Newcomer Families Face When Obtaining Routine Childhood Vaccines in Alberta, Canada

Siobhan M. Wong King Yuen [1,*], Emily J. Doucette [1], Caitlin Ford [2], Madison M. Fullerton [2,3], Ginamaria Vetro [2,4], Amanda Koyama [4], Jia Hu [2,5] and Cora Constantinescu [5,6]

1 Department of Pediatrics, Cumming School of Medicine, University of Calgary, Calgary, AB T2N 1N4, Canada
2 19 to Zero Inc., Rocky Mountain House, AB T4T 1B1, Canada; gina.vetro@19tozero.ca (G.V.)
3 Cumming School of Medicine, University of Calgary, Calgary, AB T2N 1N4, Canada
4 Calgary Catholic Immigration Society, Calgary, AB T2R 0G5, Canada
5 Department of Community Health Sciences, Cumming School of Medicine, University of Calgary, Calgary, AB T2N 1N4, Canada
6 Pediatric Infectious Diseases, Department of Pediatrics, Cumming School of Medicine, University of Calgary, Calgary, AB T2N 1N4, Canada
* Correspondence: siobhan.wongkingyuen@albertahealthservices.ca

Abstract: Background/Objectives: As the newcomer population in Canada continues to grow, we aimed to collaborate with newcomer families arriving in an urban center in Alberta, Canada to identify strategies to overcome identified barriers newcomers face in obtaining routine childhood vaccines (RCVs). **Methods**: We recruited newcomers living in Calgary, Alberta to participate in a workshop utilizing the Nominal Group Technique (NGT) to develop solutions addressing barriers to obtaining RCVs. Ranking exercises helped identify the top-proposed interventions based on perceived impact and feasibility for implementation. Based on the identified need for translated vaccine resources, infographics on school-based vaccines were developed. The infographics were pilot-tested in a first-language focus group before the final product was translated into 10 different languages. **Results**: Consensus from 15 NGT workshop participants identified five key solutions to facilitate obtaining routine childhood immunizations: (1) Increasing access to reliable vaccine information; (2) Ensuring vaccine information and healthcare services are available in different languages; (3) Increasing vaccine appointment availability and optimizing the booking system for ease of navigation; (4) Increasing the role of family doctors in vaccine counseling and administration; (5) Streamlining vaccine record tracking. We developed infographics on the vaccines children in Alberta can receive through school-based vaccine programs and these were pilot-tested with 16 participants in a first-language (Arabic) focus group. **Conclusions**: The collaborative and iterative process of solution development with newcomers provided a platform for knowledge translation through the development of educational resources on school-based vaccines, addressing the information barrier that newcomers identified when accessing RCVs.

Keywords: routine childhood vaccines; newcomer; immunizations; access; equity; qualitative methods

1. Introduction

The benefits of childhood vaccines have been well established. Immunizations have significantly reduced morbidity, disability, and mortality against severe infectious diseases at both individual and population levels [1–3]. Despite these benefits, childhood immunization rates in Canada remain suboptimal [2] and recent polling has demonstrated that parental opposition to vaccinating their children is on the rise, particularly in Alberta, Canada [4].

Newcomers, including immigrants, refugees, and temporary foreign workers, face unique challenges in obtaining routine childhood vaccines, which contributes to lower vaccination rates amongst newcomer families [5,6]. Charania et al. completed a scoping review of published literature assessing immunization coverage among migrants worldwide [7]. Their review suggests that newcomer populations, including both immigrant and refugee groups, generally experience a higher burden of vaccine-preventable disease and lower immunizations rates post-migration compared to the general population of their host country [5]. Language barriers, cultural competency, and difficulties accessing and utilizing healthcare were a few of the complex factors which decreased vaccination rates and increased the burden of vaccine-preventable diseases within newcomer populations [5]. In Canada, newcomers represent approximately a quarter (23%) of the population [8] with the projected plan from Immigration, Refugees and Citizenship Canada (IRCC) to welcome between ~365,000 and 390,000 new immigrants per year between 2024–2026 [9]. While newcomers to Canada have initially reported to be in better health compared to local-born counterparts, this "healthy immigrant effect" does not apply to selected health conditions such as infectious diseases [10]. Considering the vulnerability of this group, the decreasing rate of immunizations in Canada, and access issues faced by newcomers, it is imperative that we understand barriers and implement solutions for newcomer families to access routine childhood vaccines as part of their transition to life in Canada.

In a previous study conducted in 2022, our research team held several focus groups with 47 newcomer parents in one rural and two urban settings within Alberta, Canada [11]. Although the majority of individuals acknowledged the benefit of routine childhood vaccines, the participants identified five key barriers that newcomer families face in getting their children vaccinated, including: (1) a lack of reputable resources for routine childhood vaccines, (2) language barriers when looking for information and asking questions about routine childhood vaccines, (3) difficulty accessing a family physician, (4) lack of affordable and convenient transportation options to attend vaccine appointments, and (5) lack of available vaccine appointments [11]. It should be noted that within Alberta—unlike other Canadian provinces—family physicians do not administer routine childhood vaccines; instead, they are administered by separate appointments at public health clinics, through school-based vaccine programs, and some vaccines are available via pharmacies.

The purpose of this study was to collaborate with newcomer families arriving in an urban center in Alberta (Calgary) to identify strategies to overcome the identified barriers newcomer families face in obtaining routine childhood vaccines. Based on the 2021 census, Calgary had the third highest proportion of immigrants among Canada's 41 largest urban centers with foreign-born individuals making up 31.5% of Calgary's population and 1.9% being non-permanent residents [12] and in 2023, Calgary welcomed the most migrants per capita than any other Canadian city [13]. We used the Nominal Group Technique (NGT) as a structured method of idea generation, providing a platform for discussion and debate, and gauging participant consensus to generate ideas. An advantage of the NGT is that this methodology equally considers the views of all participants, avoiding one individual dominating the group, and has demonstrated validity [14,15]. An added benefit of the NGT method is its time efficiency, cost-effectiveness, and adaptability. Using the information gathered from the NGT, we then sought to provide knowledge translation through the development of educational resources on school-based vaccines. Ultimately, this project lays the foundation of a larger project goal, which is to increase newcomer acceptance, knowledge, and confidence in Canada's routine vaccine program.

2. Materials and Methods

Our study involved several different steps, including Nominal Group Technique (NGT) workshops for newcomer families, qualitative analysis, iterative development of vaccine infographics, and distribution of the resources to various community partners. Each step is described below and summarized in Figure 1.

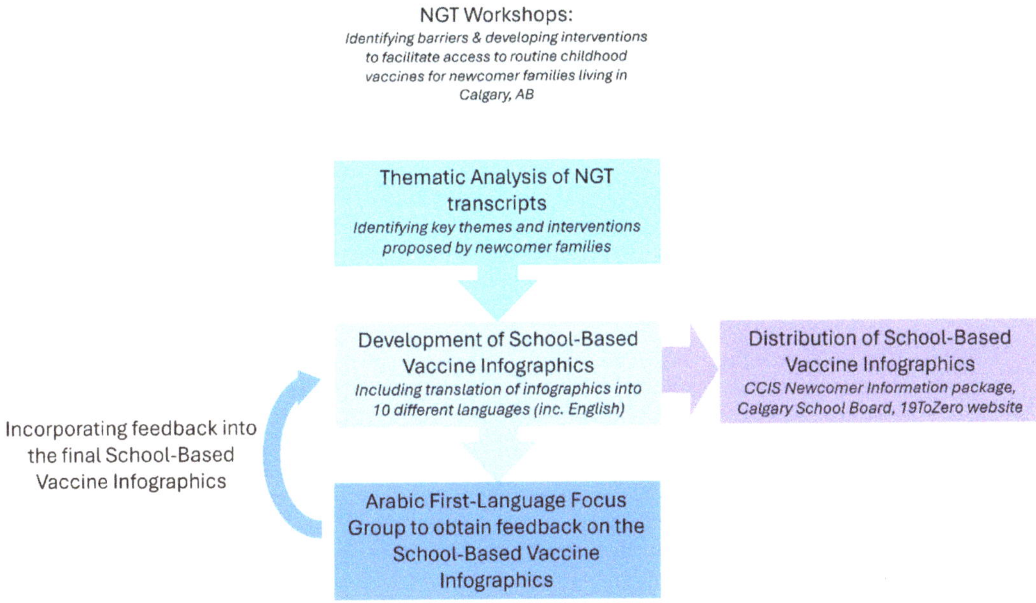

Figure 1. Overview of study methods.

2.1. Nominal Group Technique (NGT)

Our NGT sessions were adapted from the original NGT methodology [16] which consists of four steps: (1) Silent generations of ideas in writing, (2) Round-robin feedback from group members to record each idea, (3) Discussion of each recorded idea for clarification and evaluation, and (4) Individual voting on priority ideas (Figure 2). At the start of our workshop, facilitators gave a brief presentation to review the previously identified barriers that newcomer parents face in obtaining routine childhood vaccines as well as our project objectives. Next, participants were given 15 min to individually write down as many ideas to answer the following question: "What are potential solutions to the barriers newcomer parents face when accessing routine childhood vaccines?". Following individual generation of ideas, 45 min were dedicated to Round-robin feedback and discussion of each idea. The last part of our workshop consisted of participants ranking the solutions into the five most impactful and the five most realistic to implement solutions. The workshop time frame was two separate 1.5-h sessions (3 h total), completed over 2 days. Following the NGT workshops, the facilitators debriefed and shared field notes.

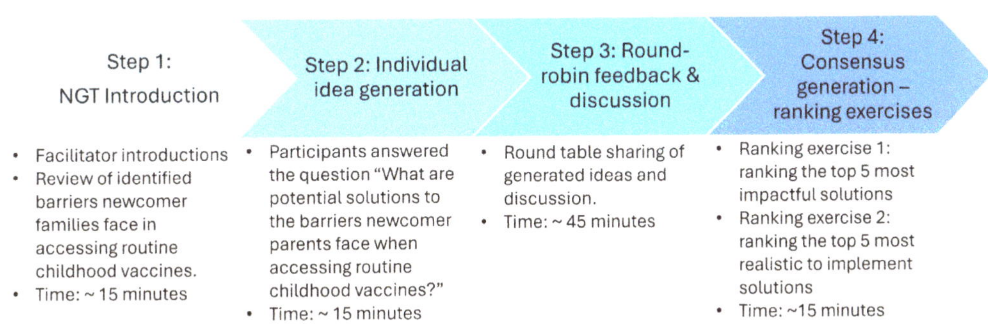

Figure 2. NGT workshop outline.

2.2. Nominal Group Theory Participant Recruitment

Two workshops utilizing NGT methodology were held on October 2nd and 4th, 2023 with a total of 15 newcomer individuals in Calgary, Alberta, Canada. Participants were recruited through the Calgary Catholic Immigration Society (CCIS) [17], a non-profit organization providing both settlement and integration services to newcomers in Southern Alberta. Participants were asked to attend an in-person workshop to develop solutions to ease the identified barriers accessing routine childhood vaccines in Calgary. To be eligible to participate, participants needed to be newcomers to Canada (including refugees, immigrants, and migrant workers) who migrated to Canada within the last five years, had at least one child 18 years old or younger, and needed to be able to communicate in English. Participants received a $50 honorarium each for their participation.

2.3. Qualitative Analysis

The NGT workshops were audio recorded and recordings were transcribed verbatim to support thematic analysis. Two qualitative researchers conducted in-depth iterative thematic analysis following Braun and Clark's 6-step framework [18]. NVivo Qualitative Data Analysis Software (QSR International, Version 14), a qualitative data analysis software, was used to organize data and facilitate analysis. Coding and thematic analysis were also supported by reviewing field notes recorded during each workshop. Regular communication between the data analysts ensured that final themes were agreed upon. In the discussion of themes, quotations from participants were provided along with their participant number, gender, and country of origin (Supplemental Data, Tables S1 and S2).

2.4. Ranking Exercises

Following the NGT discussion, participants were asked to rank the proposed interventions into the top five interventions that would provide the greatest impact in facilitating access to routine childhood vaccines for newcomer families and the top five interventions that were the most feasible to implement. Thirteen out of fifteen participant responses could be analyzed for the top five most impactful interventions while ten out of fifteen participant responses could be included in the analysis for the top five most feasible interventions. Excluded responses were those who were unable to complete the exercises correctly (e.g., no response to this exercise).

2.5. Development of School-Based Vaccines Infographics

Our group of researchers (including a pediatric resident at the Alberta Children's Hospital, researchers at 19 to Zero [19], and members of the CCIS team developed infographics on the vaccines children in Alberta can receive through school-based vaccine programs. In Grade 6, children receive the hepatitis B and human papillomavirus (HPV) vaccines and in Grade 9, diphtheria, tetanus, acellular pertussis (dTap) and meningococcal (Groups A, C, Y, W-135) conjugate vaccines. Vaccine information was obtained from resources available from Alberta Health Services [20] and our research team used an iterative process to distill information to the key elements for our infographics. The infographics were then translated into nine different languages (Arabic, French, Mandarin, Punjabi, Spanish, Tagalog, Tigrinya, Ukrainian, and Vietnamese), based on the demographic information of the most populous minority groups served at CCIS. Additionally, stakeholders with the Calgary Board of Education provided logistical advice for how to distribute the infographics to newcomer families within the Calgary school system.

2.6. School-Based Vaccine Infographic Focus Group

Following the development of the infographics, a one-hour first-language (Arabic) focus group was chosen as a case study with 16 participants recruited from CCIS to pilot-test the school-based infographics and gain feedback. Arabic is the fifth most spoken non-official language in Alberta [21] and given the large proportion of Arabic-speaking clientele served by CCIS, conducting a focus group in Arabic was the most feasible to complete in the time constraints of this study. The focus group started with a brief overview of the school-based vaccine program in Alberta. Most of the focus group was spent obtaining feedback on the clarity, design, relevance, and persuasion of the developed infographics, which was then used to improve the design and content of the infographics. CCIS interpreters were present during the focus group and were instrumental in helping our research team analyze feedback from the focus group. A final iteration of adjustments to the infographics was made based on feedback received during the newcomer first-language focus group.

3. Results

Two 1.5-h NGT workshops were held with 15 participants, representing 10 countries of origin (countries that participants had migrated to Canada from) (Table 1). Overall, the participants included ten females and five males, who had been in Canada between 6 months to 5 years and had between 1–3 children aged from >1 year to <18 years old per family. The age of participants was between 28–45 years.

Table 1. Participant demographics.

Age, mean (SD), range in years	34.6 (4.6), 28–45
Gender: n (%)	
Female	10 (67%)
Male	5 (33%)
Average number of children	1.6
Average age of children (years)	3
Average number of years in Canada	1.5
Country of origin, n (%)	
Algeria	1 (6.7%)
Brazil	1 (6.7%)
Eritrea	1 (6.7%)
Hungary	1 (6.7%)
India	6 (40%)
Lebanon	1 (6.7%)
Nigeria	1 (6.7%)
Pakistan	1 (6.7%)
Sudan	1 (6.7%)
Ukraine	1 (6.7%)

3.1. Identified Barriers Newcomer Families Experience in Obtaining Their Children's Routine Childhood Vaccines in Calgary, Alberta, Canada

During our workshops, five key barriers were identified by newcomer families when accessing routine childhood vaccines: (1) Difficulty navigating the appointment book system and lack of flexibility in appointment availability; (2) Lack of reliable and easy-to-access transport to attend vaccine appointments; (3) Language barriers during vaccine appointments and a lack of vaccine information in home language; (4) Rise in anti-vaccine rhetoric and vaccine conspiracy theories, including a lack of trustable vaccine information to help parents make vaccine decisions; (5) Difficulty accessing a family doctor for vaccine information and obtaining vaccines (Table S1).

3.2. Key Solutions Newcomer Families Identified to Facilitate Obtaining Their Children's Routine Childhood Vaccines

Parents identified five key areas, that if addressed, would facilitate routine vaccinations for their children: (1) Increasing access to reliable vaccine information; (2) Ensuring that vaccine information and healthcare service are available in different languages; (3) Increasing vaccine appointment availability, including utilization of community outreach programs, and optimizing the booking system for ease of navigation; (4) Championing family doctors to play a pivotal role in vaccine counseling and administration; (5) Streamlining vaccine record tracking.

3.3. Interventions

3.3.1. Interventions 1 & 2: Increasing Access to Reliable Vaccine Information and Ensuring Resources Are Available in Different Languages

Parents expressed difficulties finding information about vaccines as a barrier to obtaining their children's vaccines. Pertinent information that parents requested about vaccines included vaccine names, what disease(s) the vaccine protects against, ingredients contained within the vaccine, possible vaccine side effects, the vaccine schedule followed within Alberta, and the process for scheduling vaccines. Given that the Government of Alberta has the MyHealth Alberta website with the vaccine schedule and information [20], the focus of this intervention should be to educate newcomer families about this resource. Ensuring that families know how to access this website can be facilitated through their first medical appointment in Canada and public health can also direct families to this online resource.

Parents identified the need for healthcare services to be accessible in different languages. Parents discussed the difficulty and hesitancy they had around booking immunizations via phone with public health clinics given that translation services were not readily available. Thus, ensuring that interpreters are available during the vaccine booking process and during vaccine appointments will give newcomer families the confidence to participate in their children's immunizations. Additionally, ensuring that vaccine-related resources are available in different languages was also identified as a key factor in ensuring parents are well-informed about their children's vaccines.

Families thought distributing vaccine information at daycares and schools, at family doctors' offices and hospitals, at community and religious centers, and as part of newcomer orientation packages would be a helpful start to easing this barrier and empowering families with vaccine knowledge. Newcomer parents who had children born in Canada also identified that distributing vaccine information as part of the newborn information package would be beneficial as well, especially since most routine childhood vaccines are scheduled for infants and toddlers.

Vaccine information sessions were seen as a further step to help bridge the information gap about routine childhood vaccines and facilitate the process of obtaining vaccines. Parents were open to information sessions held at schools/daycares and community organizations, and even coordinated with IRCC pre-immigration workshops as helpful tools to facilitate immunizations once families have arrived in Canada. These information sessions were seen as an important link that families could establish with the Canadian healthcare system.

Families identified that the responsibility for knowing when their child was due for immunization was largely on them. Thus, developing an automated vaccine reminder system (via email/online) would help reduce the onus on families and prevent delays in their children receiving their scheduled vaccines. Following vaccine appointments, parents also would like a physical document to remind them when their child's next vaccine is due.

Additionally, families expressed hesitation when making decisions about seasonal vaccines (e.g., the annual influenza vaccine and COVID-19 vaccine) and thought having more information would guide their decision-making process.

3.3.2. Intervention 3: Improving Availability and Access to Vaccine Appointments

Parents voiced challenges attending vaccine appointments during working hours as it often meant that they needed to take time off work to attend these appointments. Although several public health clinics around the city of Calgary offer 1–2 evenings per week with extended clinic hours, parents strongly advocated for more extended evening clinic hours as well as weekend clinic appointments to reduce the burden of having to take time off regular commitments to attend their children's immunization appointments.

Families who do not have easy access to a personal vehicle noted transportation difficulties in attending the public health clinics. Transportation challenges were amplified when traveling with young children, in a new environment, and during winter conditions. In response to this need, many parents also identified that increasing the number of public health clinics around the city would facilitate access to immunizations.

Families were in favor of utilizing daycares, schools, local places of worship, and community organizations (such as cultural centers or newcomer centers) as places to obtain vaccine information as well as administer vaccines. Newcomer families described that their local community centers or religious centers were one of the first organizations that they affiliated with upon immigrating to Canada. Thus, hosting vaccine drives at these local organizations was seen as a means to facilitate vaccine access to newcomer families. Given that children attend daycare and school daily, parents also thought these settings would be ideal for vaccine drives for their children's routine immunizations.

Families identified challenges in booking their children for vaccines, thus developing a strategy to facilitate the vaccine booking process was a key intervention identified. Parents thought that a web-based booking system or a phone app would be helpful and the most accessible. Ensuring that these resources can be accessed in different languages would be key as well. If the booking system could be combined with vaccine information that would be the most ideal.

A key challenge that parents identified was needing to remember when their children were next due for immunization. A solution that was proposed by workshop participants was having "fixed open dates" for immunizations, set days where families can get their immunizations either at public health clinics without an appointment or vaccine drives at community organizations.

Families acknowledged that there is a general shortage of healthcare providers which places a strain on the healthcare sector and thus may limit extending public health appointments into the evening and over weekends. A solution that was proposed was utilizing foreign-trained healthcare workers to help staff immunization clinics. Although participants were cognizant of regulations healthcare professionals need to undergo to be able to practice within Canada, they thought immunizations were routine procedures whose practice variability from country to country was minimal and thus foreign-trained practitioners would be able to administer vaccines.

3.3.3. Intervention 4: Championing Family Doctors to Play a Pivotal Role in Vaccine Counseling and Administration

Parents compared the role that family doctors play in managing children's routine immunizations from their home country to the current practice that they have witnessed since they immigrated to Canada. Several parents recounted that family doctors played a much larger role in vaccine counseling and administering vaccines in their home country and reflected that they would like to see a similar role of family doctors in the immunization process in Calgary. Families reflected that family doctors were well positioned to provide counseling on their children's vaccine schedule, provide reminders for when vaccines were next due, and provide counseling on which vaccines are considered seasonal.

Families also voiced that family doctor clinics and walk-in clinics were more numerous throughout the city and thus easier to access compared to the sparser public health clinics. Thus, if family doctors could administer vaccines, parents thought this would ease transportation challenges and would increase flexibility to be able to obtain their children's routine immunizations.

3.3.4. Intervention 5: Streamlining Vaccine Record Tracking

Several families shared their impression that their children had received multiple duplicate vaccines upon immigration to Canada given that there was a lack of vaccine record sharing between different countries/health agencies. Parents expressed frustration that vaccine names differed between countries and felt strongly about the development of a vaccine equivalency table to facilitate record keeping and ensuring that their children get the right dosing of vaccines needed for immunization, regardless of the country in which they had received their vaccines. Families thought that a vaccine equivalency table would also be beneficial to healthcare agencies to determine which vaccines individuals had received despite different vaccine brand names.

Parents also advocated for access to an electronic vaccine passport or electronic certificates to facilitate vaccine record keeping, especially given that parents felt the burden of remembering when their children were due for vaccines was largely their responsibility. Although the infrastructure is in place for electronic vaccine passports in Alberta, more resources should be invested in helping families navigate these vaccine passports.

3.4. Ranking Exercise

To conclude our focus groups, participants were asked to rank the top five solutions proposed based on how impactful the intervention would be in facilitating newcomer family access to routine childhood immunizations (Table 2). Increasing access to vaccine resources, including increasing access to vaccine information via physical paper information or web-based platforms, and having vaccine information available in multiple resources was seen as the top solution to facilitate vaccination among newcomer families. The next most impactful strategy proposed was the development of global vaccine equivalency tables which would facilitate vaccine record keeping between different countries. Increasing immunization appointment availability was the third most impactful solution ranked by participants. Participants wished to see extended hours of vaccine appointments (late evening and weekend appointments), as well as increased public health clinics around the city of Calgary. Increasing the role of family doctors in administering vaccines and providing vaccine counseling was ranked as the fourth most prioritized solution for participants, including utilizing walk-in clinics for vaccine administration. Increasing parental access to vaccine records (via physical paper copies of immunizations and via electronic records) was the fifth most highly ranked intervention proposed to facilitate vaccine access to newcomer families.

Table 2. Top five most impactful interventions to increase the accessibility of routine childhood vaccines to newcomer families in Calgary, AB.

Ranking	Proposed Intervention
1.	Increasing access to reliable vaccine information
2.	Development of vaccine equivalency tables to facilitate vaccine record-keeping between different countries
3.	Increasing vaccine appointment availability and facilitating easier booking, including utilization of community outreach programs
4.	Championing the role of family doctors in vaccine counseling and administration
5.	Streamlining vaccine record tracking

In terms of the most feasible to implement interventions, most participants thought that increasing access to vaccine resources was the most realistic method of increasing access to vaccines for newcomer families. Creating a global vaccine equivalency table was ranked as the second most feasible intervention, followed by increasing public health clinic availability as the third most feasible intervention. Facilitating vaccine record-keeping for parents and increasing the role of family doctors were rated as the fourth and fifth most realistic interventions to increase newcomers' access to vaccines, respectively.

3.5. Developing School-Based Vaccine Infographics

Given that families identified a lack of vaccine information as a barrier to getting their children immunized, this was a tangible starting point to facilitate vaccine decision-making for newcomer parents. Parents identified uncertainty with regard to the age when their children should be receiving their routine childhood vaccines, a lack of clarity regarding the diseases that the vaccines prevented and possible vaccine side effects. To fill this knowledge gap, our research group developed infographics targeting school-based vaccines (Figure 3). School-aged children receive the Hepatitis B (HBV) and HPV-9 (human papillomavirus) vaccines in Grade 6 and the MenC-ACYW (meningococcal) and the dTAP (diphtheria, tetanus, and pertussis) vaccines in Grade 9. The infographic sheets were translated into nine different languages, including Arabic, French, Mandarin, Punjabi, Spanish, Tagalog, Tigrinya, Ukrainian, and Vietnamese. Including English, these were the top 10 languages spoken by newcomer families within Calgary as identified by CCIS. Based on the Arabic first-language focus group feedback, participants conveyed that maximizing visual presentation with bullet-point information was the preferred manner of relaying information and this was highlighted in our final product.

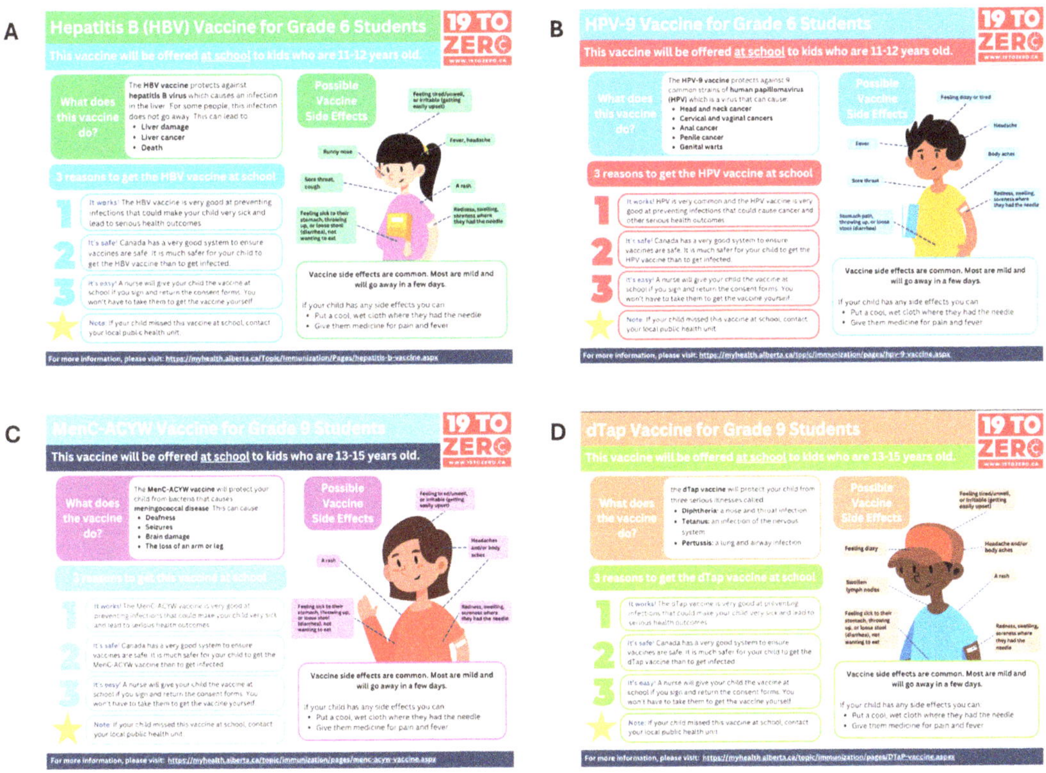

Figure 3. School-based vaccine infographics: (**A**) Hepatitis B (HBV) vaccine; (**B**) HPV-6 (human papillomavirus) (**C**) MenC-ACYW meningococcal; (**D**) dTAP (diphtheria, tetanus, pertussis) vaccine information sheets.

4. Discussion

In this study, we used the NGT to conduct workshops with newcomer families to identify barriers they face when accessing routine childhood vaccines, generate potential solutions to the barriers, and use the findings to inform the development of school-based vaccine infographics alongside researchers, healthcare workers, and community partners. The vaccine infographics were then pilot-tested during a first-language focus group with a small group of newcomer parents who provided feedback that was incorporated into the final version of the resources.

From the NGT workshops, we identified five barriers that newcomer families face in regard to immunization services in Alberta, including difficulty navigating the appointment booking system, lack of reliable access to transport to attend appointments, language barriers during appointments and lack of vaccine information in the home language, a rise in anti-vaccine rhetoric and vaccine conspiracy theories, and difficulty accessing a family doctor for vaccine information and obtaining vaccines. These findings are similar to those previously identified through focus groups conducted with newcomer families in Alberta, Canada by our research team [11], and have been identified in other communities worldwide [5].

Similar to our findings, a systematic review found that most immunization barriers can be separated into access-related barriers and acceptance-related barriers (including knowledge and information barriers) [5]. As newcomers are more likely to immunize themselves and their children when vaccine access barriers are removed when compared with non-newcomer populations [22], awareness of these information barriers provides a key opportunity to improve vaccine uptake. Our research emphasizes the identified need for reliable vaccine information when families are deciding about immunizations for their children.

The goal of our study was to ensure our research outcomes would effectively address the barriers newcomer families face in obtaining routine childhood vaccines and it was imperative that newcomer families were involved in the process of generating potential solutions. The strength of this study includes the extensive engagement with the target population, the iterative process of solution-development with a strong pragmatic, and action-oriented component via the focus groups and ranking exercises. The solution with the greatest potential impact and the most feasible solution based on participants' ranking was to increase access to reliable vaccine information. It has been shown that newcomers are more likely to trust health information received from healthcare providers and official sources such as community organizations and newcomer groups [23–25]. Given this information and the results of the focus groups and ranking exercise, we designed several one-page resources to provide key information on four routine childhood vaccines which children receive as part of the school-based immunization program within Alberta, and these resources were translated into nine different languages. The goal of creating these resources was to have them accessible online through government and health services websites, available in family physician offices, provided to newcomers in welcome packages from community groups, and distributed to parents via the Calgary school board.

The key strengths of this project include the co-development of vaccine resources based directly on the identified needs and solutions of newcomers who participated in the NGT workshops and collaboration with a multidisciplinary group of researchers, healthcare workers, and community partners. Further, the iterative process of resource development allowed for additional feedback from newcomers to be incorporated prior to dissemination. By conducting a first-language focus group, we have aimed to make our research more accessible and inclusive to members of society who may not traditionally participate in research activities due to language barriers. The infographics are also available in nine different languages, making them more likely to be used by newcomers than previous resources available in English only. This is also very timely work, as migration has steadily increased over the last few years worldwide and this helps in healthcare preparedness for host countries such as Canada.

The small number of NGT workshops conducted and recruitment from a single community organization may present a limitation to the overall generalizability of our findings. However, 2–3 workshops have been shown to successfully identify up to 80% of themes [26]. Given the narrow target population (newcomers to a Canadian urban center), the workshops were likely able to identify the most prominent themes as thematic saturation was met following analysis. Additionally, the NGT workshops were conducted in English only, which may have led to the exclusion of additional barriers faced by newcomers who do not speak English. The first-language focus group was conducted in

Arabic with only one cultural group meaning they required translators and interpreters for analysis. This resulted in methodological challenges for the English-speaking research team, including the inability to use direct quotes. Given the time constraints of the study, only one first-language focus group was conducted to confirm the resources adequately addressed the concerns of the population prior to dissemination. Further research will be needed to confirm our findings and more thoroughly evaluate the effectiveness of the infographics in English and the nine additional languages the infographics were translated into.

5. Conclusions and Future Directions

To date, the infographics have been shared with several partners across Canada in healthcare, education, and community service sectors to support meaningful engagement with newcomers around immunizations. While it is too early to evaluate the reach and impact of the resources on newcomer immunization rates, it can be expected that the resources will contribute to newcomer families feeling more knowledgeable about school-based vaccines, and more confident in making informed decisions for their children.

By creating tailored educational resources that have been disseminated through pre-existing information pathways with our community partners, we have started to address one of the several barriers experienced by newcomers when accessing information about immunizations in Canada through the school-based immunization programs. It is important to note that other access-related barriers, including a lack of transportation to clinics and inaccessible vaccine booking systems, that were identified are not addressed in this study. Table 3 assesses each of the interventions proposed by newcomer families and provides suggestions for how these can be implemented into practice. Further health systems research should be conducted to address these additional barriers, which can be aided by involving newcomers and community partners in the development of future resources.

Table 3. Suggestions for implementing proposed interventions into practice.

Proposed Intervention	Suggestions for Implementation
Increasing access to reliable vaccine information	• Expansion of the vaccine infographics for all routine childhood vaccines, which can similarly be included in newcomer orientation manuals • Distribution of vaccine resources to the offices of family doctors • Directing families to online vaccine material via their community centers (places of worship, cultural centers, schools, and daycares).
Ensuring that vaccine information and healthcare services are available in different languages	• Translating vaccine information and school immunization consents to the top 10 spoken languages within Calgary • Ensuring access to translators during the vaccine phone booking process • Ensuring access to translators during vaccine appointments with public health
Increasing vaccine appointment availability, including utilization of community outreach programs	• Engaging with vaccination centers to extend public health services into the evening and weekends and offer drop-in appointments • Utilizing physician trainees to host vaccine drives at community organizations • Utilizing community pharmacists to administer routine childhood vaccines
Championing family doctors to play a pivotal role in vaccine counseling and administration	• Distributing vaccine resources in the offices of family physicians • Expanding the role of allied health professionals (e.g., nurses, nurse practitioners) within the family physician offices in providing vaccine counselling and administration
Streamlining vaccine record tracking	• Development of an electronic passport to help track a child's immunization record

Supplementary Materials: The following supporting information can be downloaded at: https://www.mdpi.com/article/10.3390/vaccines12121380/s1, Table S1: Barriers identified by Calgary newcomer families when accessing routine childhood vaccines; Table S2: Interventions identified by Calgary newcomer families to facilitate access to routine childhood vaccines.

Author Contributions: Conceptualization, S.M.W.K.Y., C.F., M.M.F., J.H. and C.C.; methodology, S.M.W.K.Y., and E.J.D.; software, S.M.W.K.Y. and E.J.D.; validation, S.M.W.K.Y. and E.J.D.; formal analysis, S.M.W.K.Y. and E.J.D.; investigation, S.M.W.K.Y., E.J.D., M.M.F., G.V. and A.K.; resources, S.M.W.K.Y., E.J.D., C.F., M.M.F., G.V. and A.K.; data curation, S.M.W.K.Y. and E.J.D.; writing—original draft preparation, S.M.W.K.Y. and E.J.D.; writing—review and editing, S.M.W.K.Y., E.J.D., C.F., M.M.F., G.V., A.K., J.H. and C.C.; supervision, C.C. and J.H.; project administration, S.M.W.K.Y., E.J.D., C.F., M.M.F., G.V., and A.K.; funding acquisition, M.M.F., C.F., J.H. and C.C. All authors have read and agreed to the published version of the manuscript.

Funding: This research was funded by the Canadian Institutes of Health Research (Grant# 179904).

Institutional Review Board Statement: This study was conducted in accordance with the Declaration of Helsinki, and approved by the University of Calgary Conjoint Health Research Ethics Board (REB22 0277). Ethics approval was received on 13 June 2022.

Informed Consent Statement: Informed oral consent was obtained from all subjects involved in the study.

Data Availability Statement: The deidentified data presented in this study are available upon reasonable request from the corresponding author.

Acknowledgments: The authors wish to acknowledge Chelsea D'Silva for her advice in planning the NGT workshops.

Conflicts of Interest: C.C. has received honoraria from CCRN, FMWC and GSK. Authors C.F., M.M.F., G.V. and J.H. were employed by the company 19 to Zero Inc. The other authors declare no conflicts of interest. The funders had no role in the design of the study; in the collection, analyses, or interpretation of data; in the writing of the manuscript; or in the decision to publish the results.

References

1. MacDonald, N.E.; Harmon, S.; Dube, E.; Steenbeek, A.; Crowcroft, N.; Opel, D.J.; Faour, D.; Leask, J.; Butler, R. Mandatory infant & childhood immunization: Rationales, issues and knowledge gaps. *Vaccine* **2018**, *36*, 5811–5818.
2. Robinson, J.L. Potential strategies to improve childhood immunization rates in Canada. *Paediatr. Child Health* **2018**, *23*, 353–356. [CrossRef] [PubMed]
3. Public Health Agency of Canada. Benefits of immunization: Canadian Immunization Guide Canada: Government of Canada. 2016. Available online: https://www.canada.ca/en/public-health/services/publications/healthy-living/canadian-immunization-guide-part-1-key-immunization-information/page-3-benefits-immunization.html#p1c2a2 (accessed on 12 May 2024).
4. Angus Reid Institute. Parental Opposition to Childhood Vaccination Grows as Canadians Worry About Harms of Anti-Vax Movement [Updated 28 February 2024]. Available online: https://angusreid.org/canada-vaccines-childhood-vaccinations-anti-vax-mandates-covid-19-flu-mmr-side-effects/#gsc.tab=0 (accessed on 12 May 2024).
5. Kaufman, J.; Tuckerman, J.; Bonner, C.; Durrheim, D.N.; Costa, D.; Trevena, L.; Thomas, S.; Danchin, M. Parent-level barriers to uptake of childhood vaccination: A global overview of systematic reviews. *BMJ Glob. Health* **2021**, *6*, e006860. [CrossRef] [PubMed]
6. Wilson, L.; Rubens-Augustson, T.; Murphy, M.; Jardine, C.; Crowcroft, N.; Hui, C.; Wilson, K. Barriers to immunization among newcomers: A systematic review. *Vaccine* **2018**, *36*, 1055–1062. [CrossRef] [PubMed]
7. Charania, N.A.; Gaze, N.; Kung, J.Y.; Brooks, S. Vaccine-preventable diseases and immunisation coverage among migrants and non-migrants worldwide: A scoping review of published literature, 2006 to 2016. *Vaccine* **2019**, *37*, 2661–2669. [CrossRef] [PubMed]
8. Statistics Canada. Immigrants Make Up the Largest Share of the Population in over 150 Years and Continue to Shape Who We Are as Canadians Canada. 2022. Available online: https://www150.statcan.gc.ca/n1/daily-quotidien/221026/dq221026a-eng.htm (accessed on 16 May 2024).
9. Immigration, Refugees and Citizenship Canada. Government of Canada Reduces Immigration: Government of Canada. 2024. Available online: https://www.canada.ca/en/immigration-refugees-citizenship/news/2024/10/government-of-canada-reduces-immigration.html (accessed on 30 October 2024).
10. Ng, E.; Sanmartin, C.; Elien-Massenat, D.; Manuel, D.G. Vaccine-preventable disease-related hospitalization among immigrants and refugees to Canada: Study of linked population-based databases. *Vaccine* **2016**, *34*, 4437–4442. [CrossRef] [PubMed]
11. Fullerton, M.M.; Pateman, M.; Hasan, H.; Doucette, E.J.; Cantarutti, S.; Koyama, A.; Weightman, A.M.; Tang, T.; Coakley, A.; Currie, G.R.; et al. Barriers experienced by families new to Alberta, Canada when accessing routine-childhood vaccinations. *BMC Public Health* **2023**, *23*, 1333. [CrossRef] [PubMed]
12. Statistics Canada. Focus on Geography Series, 2021 Census of Population—Calgary, Census Metropolitan Area. Canada. 2022. Available online: https://www12.statcan.gc.ca/census-recensement/2021/as-sa/fogs-spg/Page.cfm?lang=E&topic=9&dguid=2021S0503825 (accessed on 16 August 2024).

13. Calgary Economic Development. Calgary Demographics Canada. 2024. Available online: https://www.calgaryeconomicdevelopment.com/insights/demographics/ (accessed on 30 October 2024).
14. Humphrey-Murto, S.; Varpio, L.; Wood, T.J.; Gonsalves, C.; Ufholz, L.A.; Mascioli, K.; Wang, C.; Foth, T. The Use of the Delphi and Other Consensus Group Methods in Medical Education Research: A Review. *Acad. Med.* **2017**, *92*, 1491–1498. [CrossRef] [PubMed]
15. Rankin, N.M.; McGregor, D.; Butow, P.N.; White, K.; Phillips, J.L.; Young, J.M.; Pearson, S.A.; York, S.; Shaw, T. Adapting the nominal group technique for priority setting of evidence-practice gaps in implementation science. *BMC Med. Res. Methodol.* **2016**, *16*, 110. [CrossRef] [PubMed]
16. Atherton, C.R. Group Techniques for Program Planning: A Guide to Nominal Group and Delphi Processes. By André L. Delbecq, Andrew H. Van de Ven, and David H. Gustafson. Glenview, Ill.: Scott, Foresman & Co., 1975. 174 pp. $4.75 paper and Interpersonal Conflict Resolution. By Alan C. Filley. *Soc. Work.* **1976**, *21*, 338.
17. Calgary Catholic Immigration Society. CCIS Alberta—Immigration Help | Resettlement & Training. Available online: https://ccisab.ca/ (accessed on 16 May 2024).
18. Braun, V.; Clarke, V. Using thematic analysis in psychology. *Qual. Res. Psychol.* **2006**, *3*, 77–101. [CrossRef]
19. 19 to Zero. 19 to Zero—Building a Healthier Future. Available online: https://www.19tozero.ca/ (accessed on 18 May 2024).
20. Alberta Health Services. Immunization and Vaccines. Alberta Health Services. 2024. Available online: https://myhealth.alberta.ca/topic/Immunization/Pages/default.aspx (accessed on 14 May 2024).
21. Business Council of Alberta. 2021 Census Population Trends: Linguistic Diversity Canada 2022. Available online: https://businesscouncilab.com/insights-category/analysis/2021-census-population-trends-linguistic-diveristy/ (accessed on 30 October 2024).
22. Quach, S.; Hamid, J.S.; Pereira, J.A.; Heidebrecht, C.L.; Deeks, S.L.; Crowcroft, N.S.; Quan, S.D.; Brien, S.; Kwong, J.C. Influenza vaccination coverage across ethnic groups in Canada. *Can. Med. Assoc. J. (CMAJ)* **2012**, *184*, 1673–1681. [CrossRef] [PubMed]
23. Kowal, S.P.; Jardine, C.G.; Bubela, T.M. "If they tell me to get it, I'll get it. If they don't....": Immunization decision-making processes of immigrant mothers. *Can. J. Public Health* **2015**, *106*, e230–e235. [CrossRef] [PubMed]
24. Brooks, S.P.; Sidhu, K.; Cooper, E.; Michelle Driedger, S.; Gisenya, L.; Kaur, G.; Kniseley, M.; Jardine, C.G. The influence of health service interactions and local policies on vaccination decision-making in immigrant women: A multi-site Canadian qualitative study. *Vaccine* **2024**, *42*, 2793–2800. [CrossRef] [PubMed]
25. Aghajafari, F.; Wall, L.; Weightman, A.; Ness, A.; Lake, D.; Anupindi, K.; Moorthi, G.; Kuk, B.; Santana, M.; Santana, A. COVID-19 Vaccinations, Trust, and Vaccination Decisions within the Refugee Community of Calgary, Canada. *Vaccines* **2024**, *12*, 177. [CrossRef] [PubMed]
26. Guest, G.; Namey, E.; McKenna, K. How Many Focus Groups Are Enough? Building an Evidence Base for Nonprobability Sample Sizes. *Field Methods* **2016**, *29*, 3–22. [CrossRef]

vaccines

MDPI

Article

Spectrum and Incidence of Adverse Reactions Post Immunization in the Taiwanese Population (2014–2019): An Analysis Using the National Vaccine Injury Compensation Program

Wan-Chun Lai [1], Chin-Hui Yang [2], Yhu-Chering Huang [1,3], Nan-Cheng Chiu [4] and Chih-Jung Chen [1,3,5,*]

[1] Division of Pediatric Infectious Diseases, Departments of Pediatrics, Chang Gung Memorial Hospital, Taoyuan 333, Taiwan; debbie61640@gmail.com (W.-C.L.); ychuang@cgmh.org.tw (Y.-C.H.)
[2] Taiwan Centers for Disease Control, Ministry of Health and Welfare, Taipei 100, Taiwan; inf@cdc.gov.tw
[3] School of Medicine, College of Medicine, Chang Gung University, Taoyuan 333, Taiwan
[4] Department of Pediatrics, MacKay Children's Hospital, Taipei 104, Taiwan; ncc88@mmh.org.tw
[5] Molecular Infectious Diseases Research Center, Chang Gung Memorial Hospital, Taoyuan 333, Taiwan
* Correspondence: james.ped@gmail.com; Tel.: +886-3-321200 (ext. 8228)

Abstract: Background: Post-marketing surveillance is crucial for gathering data on vaccine reactogenicity, enhancing public trust in immunization, and promoting vaccine uptake. This study aims to characterize adverse events following immunization (AEFIs) and estimate the incidence rates of adverse reactions (ARs) associated with vaccines included in Taiwan's Expanded Program on Immunization (EPI). This study utilizes data from Taiwan's Vaccine Injury Compensation Program (VICP). **Methods**: Vaccine injury claims submitted to the VICP between 2014 and 2019 were analyzed. ARs were defined as AEFIs adjudicated as "related" or "indeterminate" by the VICP committee. Data on the annual number of vaccine doses administered were obtained from the Taiwan CDC, which helped calculate the AR incidence rates. **Results**: A total of 491 AEFI claims were reviewed, with 327 (66.6%) categorized as ARs. The AEFIs were mainly associated with the Bacillus Calmette–Guérin (BCG) vaccine (43.4%) and the seasonal influenza vaccine (22.0%). Most EPI vaccines demonstrated low AR incidence rates, ranging from 1.68 to 13.6 per million doses, with the exception of BCG, which exhibited 162.5 ARs per million doses. Shifting BCG immunization from below 5 months to at least 5 months reduced osteomyelitis incidence significantly, from 41.4 to 7.9 ($p = 0.0014$), but increased abscess and lymphadenitis cases. **Conclusions**: EPI vaccines in Taiwan are highly safe, with minimal AR incidences in the general population. The BCG vaccine remains an exception, occasionally causing severe ARs like osteomyelitis. Adjusting the immunization schedule to an older age may mitigate some of these adverse effects.

Keywords: vaccine reactogenicity; adverse reactions; adverse events following immunization; vaccine injury compensation program

1. Introduction

The development and widespread use of effective vaccines play a fundamental role in controlling numerous serious and potentially lethal contagious diseases worldwide. The impact of vaccines is significant, with estimates suggesting that global immunization programs save four to five million lives annually [1]. Despite their high safety profiles, adverse events following immunization (AEFIs) are frequently encountered, although most are mild and resolved spontaneously within a short period. Serious adverse events (SAEs), while rare, can be associated with severe morbidity, long-term sequelae, or even death. Establishing a causal relationship between SAEs and vaccination on an individual case basis can be challenging, leading to legal conflicts between affected individuals, vaccine manufacturers, healthcare institutions, and governments. Moreover, safety concerns and misinformation about vaccines have emerged as critical issues contributing to vaccine hesitancy, suboptimal vaccine coverage, and the resurgence of vaccine-preventable diseases [2]. Data concerning the types and incidence of AEFIs, with their causality linked to vaccines (hereafter referred to as adverse reactions or ARs), are crucial for building public trust in vaccines and promoting vaccine uptake. However, such information is lacking in many countries.

In Taiwan, several systems are available for reporting AEFIs. These include the adverse drug reaction (ADR) reporting system operated by the Taiwan Drug Relief Foundation and the Taiwan National ADR Reporting Center, which is affiliated with the Taiwan Food and Drug Administration [3]. Additionally, the Vaccine Adverse Event Reporting System (VAERS) is managed by the Taiwan Centers for Disease Control (CDC), and there is also the National Vaccine Injury Compensation Program (VICP) [4]. All of these systems utilize passive reporting from individuals, healthcare providers, or pharmacists.

The VICP is considered a potential resource for the post-marketing surveillance of vaccine ARs. The Federal Republic of Germany established the first vaccine injury compensation system in 1961 [2]. In the United States, the surge in litigation related to vaccination in the 1970s led to vaccine shortages and a decline in the national vaccination rates as manufacturers withdrew production [5]. Concerns about a resurgence of vaccine-preventable diseases prompted the establishment of the national VICP between 1986 and 1988 as a public health safeguard in the United States [5,6]. In Taiwan, the VICP was introduced in 1988 following a serious adverse event where a boy developed polio-like symptoms after receiving the oral polio vaccine [7]. The program aims to raise awareness of vaccine safety, encourage immunization, and maintain a high vaccination coverage. It operates under a "no-fault" compensation scheme, compensating injured patients or their families through government funding once a causal link between an adverse event and immunization is established [8–10].

The Vaccine Adverse Event Reporting System (VAERS) is another channel for reporting AEFIs in Taiwan. However, the national VICP offers several advantages over the VAERS database for analyzing vaccine ARs in Taiwan. Firstly, the VICP was established in 1988, predating the VAERS. Secondly, due to public debates over high-profile AEFI cases adjudicated as "unrelated" by the VICP during the 2009 influenza A H1N1 pandemic, the VICP is more familiar to the Taiwanese public. Thirdly, while VAERS reporting is restricted to healthcare providers, the VICP is open to the public, allowing any Taiwanese citizen to file a claim of vaccine injury [11]. Such claims are encouraged by the Taiwanese government and can be easily submitted via an online application form (https://www.cdc.gov.tw/Vicp/Fill; accessed on 1 October 2024). Finally, after registration, a series of processes ensue, including local health bureaus collecting adverse event-related medical records and an expert committee determining causality. The causal relationship between AEFIs and vaccination is not determined in the VAERS. Thus, the VICP represents the most comprehensive database for the post-marketing surveillance of vaccine ARs in Taiwan. In this study, we aim to analyze the incidence and types of ARs associated with various vaccines using the VICP database from 2014 to 2019, before the COVID-19 pandemic.

2. Materials and Methods

2.1. Ethical Approval

This study was approved by the Research and Ethics Committee of Chang Gung Memorial Hospital (IRB: 202002607B1).

2.2. Claims to the Vaccine Injury Compensation Program (VICP)

The National Vaccine Injury Compensation Program (VICP) in Taiwan was established under Article 30 of the Communicable Disease Control Act. This program encompasses all officially approved vaccines used for disease prevention, irrespective of whether they are publicly funded or self-paid. In cases of suspected vaccine-related injury, claims may be filed within two years of becoming aware of the adverse event following immunization

(AEFI) or within five years from the first appearance of any AEFI symptoms. Claims can be submitted by the injured individuals themselves, guardians of individuals under 20 years old, or heirs of deceased individuals.

The local health bureau manages the claim process and is responsible for gathering all pertinent medical records related to the adverse event. These include clinical manifestations, laboratory data, examination reports, medical history, disease progression, treatment outcomes, and details about the vaccines involved. At least two medical experts from the VICP working group independently review these records and the relevant literature to assess the causality of the AEFI. If there is disagreement between the two experts, a third expert is consulted. The final decision on causality is reached collectively during a review conference attended by all members of the VICP working group, which comprises clinical physicians, pharmacists, pathologists, legal professionals, and impartial community members [7,12].

AEFI causality is classified as "related", "indeterminate", or "unrelated" to vaccination. Financial compensation is provided for cases adjudicated as "related" or with "indeterminate" causality. Compensation is also available for unrelated cases involving deceased individuals who underwent autopsy, those who had medical procedures to determine causality, and pregnant women who experienced stillbirth or miscarriage [13]. On average, the resolution process from claim filing to adjudication takes approximately six months, with claimants having the right to appeal within 30 days if dissatisfied with the outcome.

Following Wang's publication of updates to Taiwan's VICP in 2014 [7], this study collected data from claims adjudicated between 2014 and 2019. The VICP database records include claimants' age, sex, and residence, types of vaccines involved, dates of immunization, reported symptoms, clinical diagnoses, duration from vaccination to symptom onset, adjudication results, and compensation amounts. The data were collected from the VICP database. For this study, AEFIs adjudicated as "related" or "indeterminate" were classified as ARs to the vaccines. Adjudication outcomes are periodically published online by the Taiwan Centers for Disease Control [14]. Claims adjudicated from 2014 to 2019 were reviewed and analyzed in this study.

2.3. Definitions

Data on the total administered doses of each vaccine during the study period, as provided by the Taiwan CDC (Supplementary Table S1), were used to estimate the AR incidence for each vaccine. The immunization schedule in Taiwan is listed in Supplementary Table S2. If multiple vaccine types were administered simultaneously and the specific offending vaccine could not be precisely identified, the AEFI was attributed to all administered vaccines. The interval from vaccination to AEFI onset was calculated in days, with symptoms occurring on the day of vaccination counted as 0.5 days.

2.4. Statistics

Statistical analysis was performed using GraphPad Prism 9.0.0 and Microsoft Excel © 2022 Microsoft Corporation. Medians were compared using the Mann–Whitney U test, while categorical variables were compared using the Chi-square test and Fisher's exact test. A p-value of < 0.05 was considered statistically significant.

3. Results

From 2014 to 2019, the Vaccine Injury Compensation Program (VICP) of Taiwan received and adjudicated a total of 491 claims, with an annual range of 42 to 122 claims (mean 81.8 claims). Of these, 327 claims (66.6%) were adjudicated as either "related" (231 claims, 47.0%) or "indeterminate" (96 claims, 19.6%), while the remaining 164 claims (33.4%) were adjudicated as "unrelated" (Table 1). The total compensation disbursed for all claims amounted to approximately 30 million New Taiwan Dollars (~1 million USD) during the 2014–2019 period. The Bacillus Calmette–Guerin (BCG) vaccine was the most frequently identified offending vaccine, with 213 claims, followed by the influenza vaccine, with 108 claims (Figure 1a and Table 1). The incidence of adverse reactions (ARs) was generally low (Figure 1b,c), averaging 6.0 ARs per million vaccine doses, except for the BCG vaccine, which showed an incidence of 162.5 ARs per million doses.

Table 1. Claims of vaccine injury and adjudication results in the Taiwan vaccine injury compensation program from 2014 to 2019.

Vaccine Type	No. of Events (%)			
	Adverse Reactions			Unrelated Events
	Related	Indeterminate	Total	
BCG vaccine (n = 213)	188 (88.3)	18 (8.5)	206 (96.7)	7 (3.3)
Influenza vaccine (n = 108)	4 (3.7)	35 (32.4)	39 (36.1)	69 (63.9)
PCV13 (n = 41)	14 (34.1)	9 (22.0)	23 (56.1)	18 (43.9)
DTaP-Hib-IPV/DTaP-IPV-Hib-HepB vaccine (n = 36)	12 (33.3)	5 (13.9)	17 (47.2)	19 (52.8)
MMR vaccine (n = 24)	1 (4.2)	15 (62.5)	16 (66.7)	8 (33.3)
JE vaccine (n = 22)	5 (22.7)	5 (22.7)	10 (45.5)	12 (54.5)
PPV23 (n = 14)	7 (50.0)	0 (0)	7 (50.0)	7 (50.0)
Rotavirus vaccine (n = 12)	0 (0)	3 [a] (25.0)	3 (25.0)	9 (75.0)
Hepatitis A or B vaccine (n = 9)	0 (0)	2 (22.2)	2 (22.2)	7 (77.8)
Varicella vaccine (n = 7)	0 (0)	3 (42.9)	3 (42.9)	4 (57.1)
HPV vaccine (n = 5)	0 (0)	1 (20.0)	1 (20.0)	4 (80.0)
Total claims (n = 491)	231 (47.0)	96 (19.6)	327 (66.6)	164 (33.4)

[a] All three ARs involved intussusception. Abbreviations: BCG, Bacillus Calmette–Guérin; PCV13, 13-valent pneumococcal conjugate vaccine; PPV23, 23-valent polysaccharide pneumococcal vaccine; JE, Japanese encephalitis vaccine; DTaP-Hib-IPV, diphtheria, tetanus, acellular pertussis, *Hemophilus influenzae* type b, and inactivated poliovirus vaccine; DTaP-IPV-Hib-HepB, diphtheria, tetanus, acellular pertussis, *Hemophilus influenzae* type b, inactivated poliovirus, and hepatitis B; MMR, measles–mumps–rubella; and HPV, human papillomavirus.

(a)

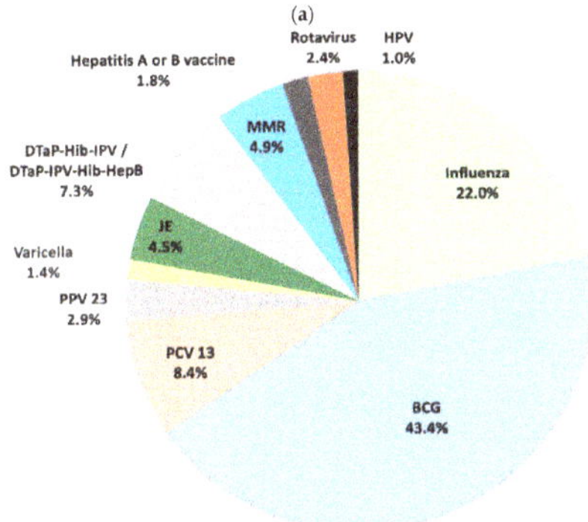

(b)

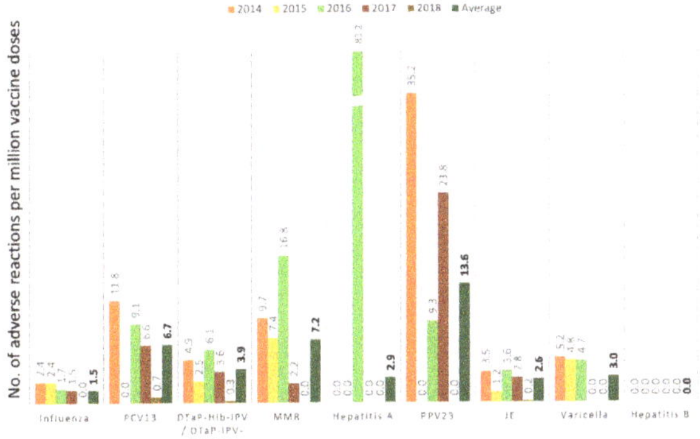

Figure 1. *Cont.*

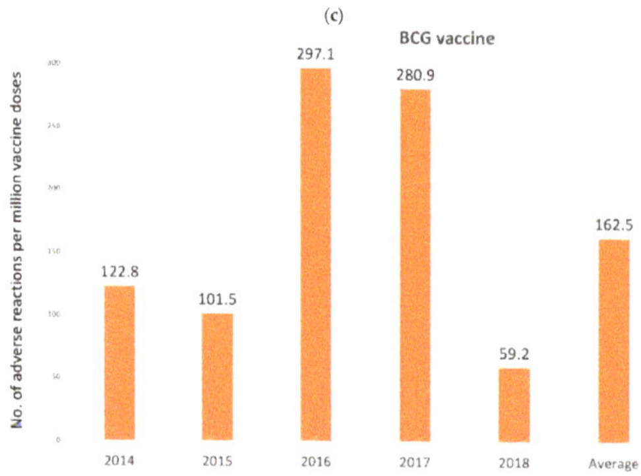

Figure 1. (**a**) Distribution of alleged vaccines in the claims received by the national vaccine injury compensation program in Taiwan during 2014 and 2019. Abbreviations: BCG, Bacillus Calmette–Guérin; PCV13, 13-valent pneumococcal conjugate vaccine; PPV23, 23-valent polysaccharide pneumococcal vaccine; JE, Japanese encephalitis vaccine; DTaP-Hib-IPV, diphtheria, tetanus, acellular pertussis, Hemophilus influenzae type b, and inactivated poliovirus vaccine; DTaP-IPV-Hib-HepB, diphtheria, tetanus, acellular pertussis, Hemophilus influenzae type b, inactivated poliovirus, and hepatitis B; MMR, measles–mumps–rubella vaccine; and HPV, human papillomavirus vaccine. (**b**,**c**) The incidence of the adverse reactions per million doses of vaccines. The average incidence is indicated on the right column with bold letters.

3.1. BCG Vaccine

Detailed AR data for the BCG vaccine can be found in Table 2 and Figure 2a. Abscess and lymphadenitis were the two most common ARs, typically observed at the vaccination site (left arm) and left axillary region but, occasionally, also at more distant sites such as the chest wall and supra- or infra-clavicular areas. Osteomyelitis was also notable, with an incidence of 22.9 episodes per million vaccine doses, accounting for 26.7% (55 out of 206) of all BCG-related ARs. BCG osteomyelitis mainly developed between 6 and 24 months post immunization, with an average onset interval of 15.9 ± 6.0 months (Figure 2b, Table 2). Lower-limb long bones were the most affected, followed by the sternum/ribs and the foot, ankle, or knee. Only one case of BCG spondylitis was identified.

Table 2. Post-immunization incidence and duration of various adverse reactions (ARs) of the BCG vaccine at different immunization ages, in 2014–2018.

Adverse Reactions/ Anatomic Sites	No. of AR (Incidence per Million Doses)				Months between Immunization and AR Onset, Median (Range)			
	Overall n = 917,030 Vaccine Doses	Age of Immunization			Overall n = 917,030 Vaccine Doses	Age of Immunization		
		<5 Months n = 410,621	≥5 Months n = 506,409	p		<5 Months n = 410,621	≥5 Months n = 506,409	p
Abscess	67 (73.1)	7 (17.1)	60 (118.5)	<0.0001	2.0 (0.6–14.9)	4.9 (0.6–10.2)	2.0 (0.6–14.9)	0.0195
Left arm	64	6	58		2.1 (0.6–14.9)			
Chest wall	1	1	0		7.2			
Left axillary	2	0	2		1.3 (1.1–1.5)			
Lymphadenitis	45 (49.1)	14 (34.1)	31 (61.2)	0.0724	1.8 (0.9–14.6)	4.7 (1.4–14.6)	1.6 (0.9–4.8)	<0.0001
Left axillary	34	11	23		2.0 (0.9–14.6)			
Not specified	8	2	6		1.5 (1.0–3.3)			
Clavicles	3	1	2		1.5 (1.4–1.7)			

Table 2. *Cont.*

Adverse Reactions/ Anatomic Sites	No. of AR (Incidence per Million Doses)				Months between Immunization and AR Onset, Median (Range)			
	Overall n = 917,030 Vaccine Doses	Age of Immunization			Overall n = 917,030 Vaccine Doses	Age of Immunization		
		<5 Months n = 410,621	≥5 Months n = 506,409	p		<5 Months n = 410,621	≥5 Months n = 506,409	p
Osteomyelitis	21 (22.9)	17 (41.4)	4 (7.9)	0.0014	14.5 (9.0–33.8)	14.5 (9.0–33.8)	14.3 (9.6–15.4)	0.4705
Lower limbs Long bone	10	6	4		15.4 (9.6–22.1)			
Sternum/rib	4	4	0		11.5 (9.6–13.7)			
Lower limb Foot, ankle, knee	3	3	0		12.1 (9.0–33.8)			
Unknown	2	2	0		18.4 (14.5–22.2)			
Upper limb Long bone	2	2	0		22.4 (22.0–22.9)			
Lumps	8 (8.7)	7 (17.0)	1 (2.0)	0.0262	10.4 (1.2–19.2)	14.1 (1.2–19.2)	2.5 (2.0–3.1)	...
Chest wall	7	6	1		14.1 (3.1–19.2)			
Four limbs	1	1	0		1.2			
Arthritis	3 (3.3)	1 (2.4)	2 (3.9)	>0.9999	14.0 (5.6–25.0)	14.0	15.3 (5.6–25.0)	...
Others [a]	5 (5.5)	1 (2.4)	4 (7.9)	0.3886	0.9 (<1d–14.9)	0.46	0.7 (<1d–1.5)	...

[a] Others: dermatitis (1), granuloma (1), urticaria (1), lupus vulgaris (1), and immunization stress-related response (1).

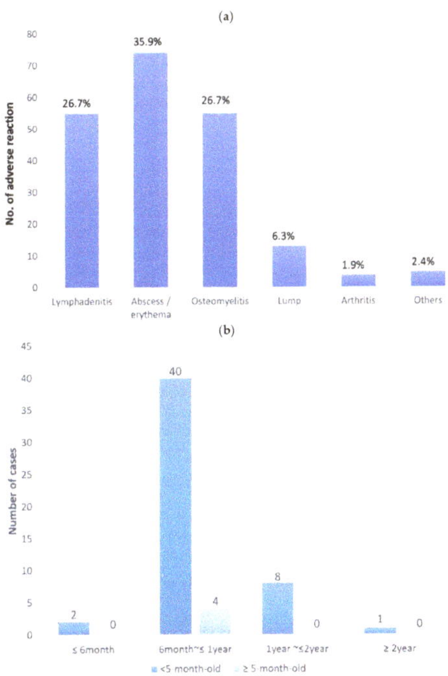

Figure 2. (**a**) The adverse reactions of the BCG vaccine. The percentages are the proportions of the indicated adverse reactions among all BCG-related adverse reactions. (**b**) The distributions of the intervals between the onset of the symptoms of osteomyelitis and BCG immunization stratified by the age of immunization.

In response to the relatively high incidence of BCG osteomyelitis, the vaccination schedule for infants was officially changed in January 2016 from within 24 h after birth to between 5 and 8 months of age. This schedule change resulted in a significant decline in the incidence of BCG osteomyelitis from 41.4 to 7.9 events per million doses between the 2014–2015 and 2016–2018 periods ($p = 0.0014$, Table 2). However, administering the vaccine in older infants led to a substantial increase in incidences of abscesses (from 17.1 to 118.5 events per million doses, $p < 0.0001$) and lymphadenitis (from 34.1 to 61.2 events per million doses, $p = 0.0724$). Lymphadenitis tended to occur sooner post immunization in infants vaccinated at 5–8 months compared to those vaccinated within 24 h of birth ($p < 0.0001$, Table 2).

3.2. *Influenza Vaccine*

The most common ARs for influenza vaccines were neurological disorders (28.2%), allergies (28.2%), and rheumatological disorders (17.9%) (Table 3 and Figure 3). The time interval from vaccination to disease onset varied greatly among these ARs. Most allergic reactions occurred within one day of vaccination (median < 1 day, range < 1 day to 60 days, Table 3), whereas neurological disorders had a significantly longer onset interval, with a mean and median duration of 39.9 and 6.0 days, respectively (Table 3).

Table 3. Incidences and demographics of various adverse reactions (ARs) of the influenza vaccine and intervals between immunization and the onset of the AR.

Categories of Adverse Reactions/Adverse Reactions	No. of ARs (Incidence per Million Doses)	Male (%)	Ages of Immunization in Years, Mean ± Standard Deviation	Days between Immunization and AR Onset, Mean ± Standard Deviation (Median, Range)
Neurology	11 (0.47)	6 (54.5)	47.9 ± 25.6	39.9 ± 108.0 (6.0, 1–365)
Guillain–Barré syndrome	6 (0.26)	4 (66.7)	52.2 ± 24.9	6.8 ± 5.6 (6.5, 1–14)
Transverse myelitis	2 (0.09)	1 (50.0)	41.5 ± 19.1	12.0 ± 14.1 (12, 2–22)
Acute myelitis	1 (0.04)	0 (0.0)	72.0	365.0
Acute disseminated encephalomyelitis	1 (0.04)	0 (0.0)	1.0	1.0
Tolosa–Hunt syndrome	1 (0.04)	1 (100.0)	58.0	6.0
Allergic reaction	11 (0.47)	4 (36.4)	26.2 ± 22.6	6.2 ± 17.9 (<1, <1–60)
Urticaria	10 (0.43)	4 (40.0)	28.5 ± 22.4	6.8 ± 18.7 (<1, <1–60)
Anaphylactic shock	1 (0.04)	0 (0.0)	3.0	<1.0
Rheumatology	7 (0.30)	3 (42.9)	26.7 ± 29.2	5.2 ± 5.4 (4.0, 0.5–17)
Idiopathic thrombocytopenic purpura	6 (0.26)	3 (50.0)	23.8 ± 28.6	6.0 ± 5.4 (4, 3–17)
Vasculitis	1 (0.04)	0 (0.0)	52.0	<1.0
Local reaction	3 (0.13)	2 (66.7)	4.3 ± 0.6	<1.0 (0.5, 0.5)
Respiratory	2 (0.09)	1 (50.0)	39.0 ± 11.3	<1.0 (0.5, 0.5)
Infectious	2 (0.09)	1 (50.0)	61.5 ± 10.6	1.5 ± 0.7 (1.5, 1–2)
Others [a]	3 (0.13)	2 (66.7)	14.3 ± 5.5	1.7 ± 2.0 (0.5, 0.5–4)
Total	39 (1.68)	19 (48.7)	32.3 ± 25.9	32.9 ± 97.7 (2, 0.5–365)

[a] Others: lipoatrophy (1), oral ulcer (1), and limb and chest pain (1).

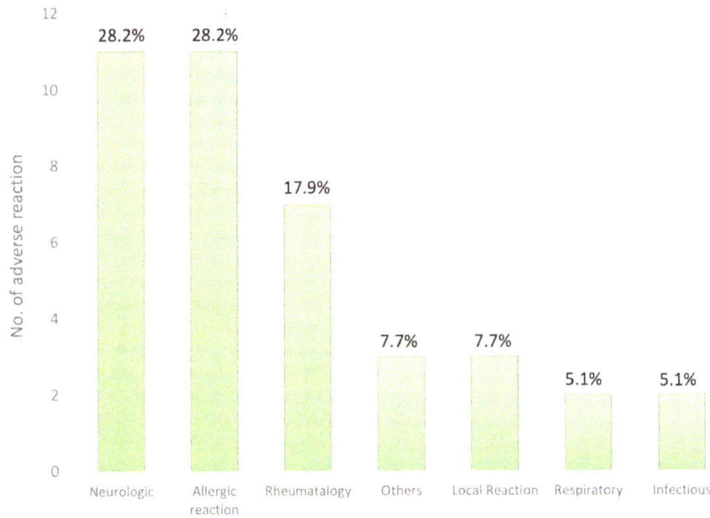

Figure 3. The adverse reactions of the influenza vaccine. The percentages indicate the proportion of adverse reactions.

Guillain–Barré syndrome (GBS) was the most frequently observed neurological AR (6 events, 54.5%), with an incidence of 0.26 events per million influenza vaccine doses. GBS predominantly affected adult vaccinees over 40 years of age and typically presented within two weeks post vaccination. Idiopathic thrombocytopenic purpura (ITP) occurred in both pediatric and adult vaccinees. Urticaria generally developed within one day of vaccination. Notably, one pediatric vaccinee experienced anaphylactic shock on the day of vaccination. There was one case of mortality linked to GBS, adjudicated as "indeterminate".

3.3. *Pneumococcal Vaccine*

Taiwan routinely administers two pneumococcal vaccines: the 13-valent pneumococcal conjugate vaccine (PCV13) for young children and the 23-valent pneumococcal polysaccharide vaccine (PPV23) for the elderly and individuals with underlying conditions [15]. The most common AR for both PCV13 (14 events, 60.9%) and PPV23 (6 events, 85.7%) was a severe local reaction, which typically occurred rapidly, with most reactions happening within one day post vaccination (69.6% for PCV13 and 85.7% for PPV23). Other less frequent ARs for PCV13 included urticaria (three events, 13.0%) and idiopathic thrombocytopenic purpura (ITP) (three events, 13.0%). Notably, severe local reactions presenting as extensive limb swelling were identified in two cases (28.6%) involving the PPV23 vaccine.

3.4. *Japanese Encephalitis (JE) Vaccine*

Since May 2017, Taiwan has replaced the mouse brain-derived JE vaccine with the live attenuated chimeric virus JE vaccine (Imojev®, Sanofi Pasteur, Lyon, France) and the inactivated Vero cell culture-derived JE vaccine (Jeval®, Adimmune, Taichung, Taiwan). These newer vaccines were associated with one adverse reaction case involving a skin rash after using the attenuated chimeric virus vaccine. In contrast, among the users of the older mouse brain-derived JE vaccine, four cases exhibited urticaria or skin rash, and there was one anaphylactic shock incident. A significant case involved a 5-year-old girl who experienced loss of consciousness within five minutes of receiving both the mouse brain-derived JE vaccine and the MMR vaccine. She was adjudicated as an "indeterminate" case, possibly due to anaphylactic shock or an immunization stress-related response.

3.5. Other EPI Vaccines

Table 4 outlines the incidences and characteristics of ARs related to other EPI vaccines. Notable ARs included the development of varicella, herpes zoster, and urticaria in a varicella vaccinee. For the DTaP-Hib-IPV or DTaP-IPV-Hib-HepB combination vaccines, the predominant ARs were severe local reactions (52.9%), cellulitis (17.6%), and ITP (17.6%). ITP was also the leading AR for the MMR vaccine, occurring in 9 out of 16 cases (56.3%), with a symptom onset interval ranging from 6 to 24 days post vaccination (mean of 14.2 days). One case involved optic neuritis in an HPV vaccinee, deemed "indeterminate" in relation to the HPV vaccine. A noteworthy incident involved a one-month-old boy who suffered from thrombocytopenia and accompanying intracranial hemorrhage nine days after HBV immunization, adjudicated as "indeterminate". Another case of the simultaneous administration of the hepatitis A vaccine (HAV) and the influenza vaccine led to anaphylactic shock, adjudicated as "indeterminate".

Table 4. Incidence and demographics of various adverse reactions and intervals between immunization and onset of ARs of selected EPI vaccines.

Vaccine Types	Adverse Reactions	No. of ARs (Incidence per Million Doses)	Gender Male (%)	Ages of Immunization in Years, Mean (Range)	Days between Immunization and AR Onset, Mean ± Standard Deviation (Median, Range)
PCV13 (*n* = 23)	Severe local reaction	14 (4.3)	7 (50.0)	15.5 (0.3–70.0)	1.4 ± 1.6 (1, 0.5–5)
	Urticaria	3 (0.9)	3 (100.0)	0.8 (0.3–1.0)	1.3 ± 1.4 (0.5, 0.5–3)
	ITP	3 (0.9)	1 (33.3)	21.8 (0.2–65.0)	17.7 ± 11.9 (23, 4–26)
	Cellulitis	2 (0.6)	0 (0.0)	31.0 (1.0–61)	<1.0 (0.5, 0.5–0.5)
	Intussusception	1 (0.3)	1 (100.0)	0.3	3.0
DtaP-Hib-IPV/DtaP-IPV-Hib-HepB (*n* = 17)	Severe local reaction	9 (2.3)	7 (77.8)	1.4 (0.3–2.0)	0.9 ± 0.5 (1.0, 0.5–2.0)
	ITP	3 (0.8)	1 (33.0)	1.5 (0.2–1.0)	19.0 ± 15.7 (26, 1–30)
	Cellulitis	3 (0.8)	2 (66.7)	2.0	1.2 ± 0.8 (1.0, 0.5–2.0)
	Seizure	1 (0.2)	0 (0.0)	0.2	<1.0
	Urticaria	1 (0.2)	1 (100.0)	0.3	<1.0
MMR (*n* = 16)	ITP	9 (4.3)	6 (66.7)	1.6 (1.0–6.0)	14.2 ± 6.9 (14.0, 6.0–24.0)
	Urticaria	4 (1.9)	2 (50.0)	3.3 (1.0–5.0)	1.1 ± 1.3 (0.5, 0.5–3.0)
	Cellulitis	1 (0.5)	0 (0.0)	1.0	3.0
	Anaphylactic shock	1 (0.5)	0 (0.0)	5.0	<1.0
	Erythema multiforme	1 (0.5)	1 (100.0)	1.0	4.0
JE (*n* = 10)	Urticaria	5 (1.3)	4 (80.0)	1.2 (1.0–2.0)	1.7 ± 1.9 (1.0, 0.5–5.0)
	Severe local reaction	3 (0.5)	2 (66.7)	2.0 (2.0–2.0)	0.8 ± 0.3 (1.0, 0.5–1.0)
	Anaphylactic shock	1 (0.3)	0 (0.0)	5.0	<1.0
	Cellulitis	1 (0.3)	1 (100.0)	2.0	2.0

Table 4. *Cont.*

Vaccine Types	Adverse Reactions	No. of ARs (Incidence per Million Doses)	Gender Male (%)	Ages of Immunization in Years, Mean (Range)	Days between Immunization and AR Onset, Mean ± Standard Deviation (Median, Range)
PPV23 (n = 7)	Severe local reaction	6 (11.6)	1 (14.2)	68.5 (62.0–75.0)	5.7 ± 11.9 (1, 0.5–30)
	Abscess	1 (1.9)	1 (100.0)	76.0	<1.0
VZV (n = 3)	Varicella and herpes zoster	1 (1.0)	1 (100.0)	1.0	60.0
	Varicella	1 (1.0)	1 (100.0)	1.0	6.0
	Urticaria	1 (1.0)	1 (100.0)	1.0	3.0
Hepatitis A or B (n = 2)	Anaphylactic shock	1 (2.9)	1 (100.0)	0.1	9.0
	ITP	1a	0 (0.0)	3.0	<1.0
HPV vaccine (n = 1)	Optic neuritis	1b	0 (0.0)	39.0	30.0

3.6. *Claims of Anaphylactic Shock and Mortality*

Anaphylactic shock was reported in three cases: one associated with the influenza vaccine, the other involving the simultaneous administration of the influenza and HAV vaccines, and a third in conjunction with the JE and MMR vaccines. In the latter two cases, immunization stress-related responses were also considered possible diagnoses. All these individuals survived, although data on their long-term follow-up were unavailable.

During the study period, there were 24 claims related to deaths (10 involving influenza, 3 rotavirus, 3 DTaP-Hib-IPV/DTaP-IPV-Hib-HepB, and 2 HepB) and 4 claims for life-threatening events (BCG and HepB, 2 each). Except for 1 fatality related to influenza vaccine-associated GBS, the remaining 23 death claims were adjudicated as "unrelated" to the vaccines. Notably, there were no claims involving congenital anomalies or birth defects.

4. Discussion

The BCG vaccine has been extensively used in regions where tuberculosis is prevalent and has shown optimal protection against severe manifestations such as meningitis and disseminated disease [16]. This study found that, among the EPI vaccines, BCG was associated with the highest incidence of ARs. In 2007, active surveillance by the Taiwan CDC led to a marked increase in the reported BCG-related AEFIs, particularly osteitis and osteomyelitis, with incidence rates rising approximately tenfold from 3.68 to 30.1 per million doses between the 2002–2006 and 2008–2012 periods [17,18]. Osteomyelitis symptoms typically emerged 6 to 12 months post vaccination, with diagnosis taking an average of 16.4 months [19]. Fortunately, BCG osteomyelitis generally has a good prognosis, with long-term sequelae being rare following adequate anti-tuberculosis therapy [19–21].

The relatively high incidence of BCG osteomyelitis in Taiwan prompted a change in the national immunization policy in 2016, delaying BCG administration from 24 h after birth to 5 to 8 months of age. Huang et al. observed a decrease in the incidence of BCG-related osteitis/osteomyelitis and an increasing rate of regional lymphadenitis and injection site reactions in the birth cohort from 2012 to 2017 following this policy change [22]. A more mature and robust immune response against BCG strains may account for this observation. Our study supports these findings, noting approximately a fivefold reduction in BCG-related osteitis and osteomyelitis while the timing after vaccination and the affected skeletal regions remained consistent. In Japan, the recommended age of BCG vaccination was less than 6 months after 2005 but subsequently changed to 5–8 months (latest amendment, <1 year) in 2013. National surveillance from 2013 to 2017 demonstrated that the incidence of developing BCG-associated osteitis/osteomyelitis and disseminated BCG was higher among those who received the BCG vaccine at <6 months of age than among those who were 6 months or older [23]. These data suggest that delaying BCG vaccination could reduce the incidence of these serious bone infections. However, potential disadvantages include the uncertainty of increased severe tuberculosis cases during the vaccination delay window, warranting further surveillance in infants under 5 months. Also, abscesses and lymphadenitis became more frequent with an older vaccination age, developing sooner post vaccination, causing prolonged and troublesome symptoms for caregivers. In response, the Taiwan CDC issued guidelines to better manage these ARs [24].

Along with the policy change in the vaccination age for BCG, the manufacturer of the BCG vaccines temporarily changed from the National Health Research Institutes (NHRI) in Taiwan to the Japan BCG Laboratory© between July 2016 and August 2020 due to the shortage in stockpile. However, both vaccines contained the same Tokyo-172 strains, fulfilling the WHO requirements. The intradermal route of administration did not change either. The manufacturer was changed back to the NHRI after August 2020. Continuing observation of the incidences of BCG abscess and osteomyelitis will be mandatory to clarify the role of different vaccine manufacturers in the occurrence of ARs of the BCG vaccine. Like the finding in this study, BCG was also the vaccine most frequently compensated for ARs in many other countries [25,26]. However, the estimated incidences of AEs following BCG vaccination varied greatly in different countries and ranged from 3.4 to 1540 per million vaccine doses [27–29]. Of note, an investigation into the AEs following BCG immunization from 2013 to 2018 in Korea indicated that the incidence was as high as 260 per million vaccine doses [30]. Consistent with our findings, abscesses and lymphadenitis were the major disease entities caused by BCG in Australia, Korea, Poland, and Oman [26,28,30].

Although the influenza vaccine was the second most frequent in AR-related claims, its overall AR incidence was extremely low. Severe ARs like neurological disorders, anaphylactic shock, and ITP were observed at rates below one per million doses, underscoring the influenza vaccine's excellent safety profile in post-marketing surveillance. Given its widespread use across global populations, injury claims remain common across regions and demographics [25,31], with a notable spike in 2010 due to extensive social media coverage during the 2009 H1N1 pandemic [7]. The low AR incidence data from this study are crucial for bolstering public trust and encouraging influenza vaccine uptake.

Guillain–Barré syndrome (GBS) is historically considered a significant AR of influenza vaccines, linked notably to the 1976 swine-origin influenza vaccine [32–34]. There remain public concerns regarding GBS and its association with influenza vaccination, notably during the 2009 H1N1 pandemic [35,36], although recent meta-analyses have not identified such associations [37]. Influenza vaccine-associated GBS is viewed as an immune-mediated condition, generally manifesting within six weeks post vaccination [38]. This study observed GBS occurrence within two weeks post immunization, reinforcing the notion that the benefits of influenza vaccination considerably outweigh potential AR risks.

Based on the findings of this study, it is recommended that Taiwan's health authorities consider further refining the immunization schedule and public education regarding vaccine safety. Specifically, the change in the BCG vaccination age from immediately after birth to 5–8 months has resulted in a significant reduction in cases of osteomyelitis, suggesting that the postponement of the BCG vaccine may be beneficial in mitigating severe adverse reactions. However, this policy change has been associated with an increase in reported abscesses and lymphadenitis, indicating the need for healthcare professionals to be vigilant in monitoring and managing these conditions. It is also imperative to maintain and enhance educational campaigns that reiterate the overall safety and importance of vaccines, as the low incidence of serious adverse reactions further supports the continued use of vaccines such as the influenza vaccine, which demonstrated excellent safety despite its common use. These educational efforts could help alleviate vaccine hesitancy by ensuring that the public is well-informed about the benefits of vaccination versus the low risks of adverse effects. Additionally, continued enhancement of the VICP to ensure transparency and accessibility may further boost public confidence in the nation's immunization activities.

5. Limitations

This study was based on a statistical analysis of the VICP database. There were some limitations regarding the system. First, identifying the specific vaccine responsible for systemic adverse reactions was challenging, particularly when multiple vaccines were administered simultaneously or in combination. Second, there was significant variability in the reported adverse event entities, which lacked a consistent form of reporting and a standardized terminology, potentially leading to misclassification. For example, severe local reactions with extensive limb swelling were often reported as cellulitis, which might not accurately reflect the nature of the reaction. Third, while adjudications were largely based on the available scientific evidence, there were no established quality criteria for the evidence used by the expert committee. In complex cases, this could result in subjective adjudications or reliance on evidence of a lower quality. Fourth, because the VICP operates as a passive reporting system, which is not mandatory, there was a potential for the underreporting of adverse reactions, particularly mild ones. However, the Taiwanese government encourages reporting through the VICP, supported by the possibility of financial compensation, so adverse reactions of significant severity and clinical importance were likely captured. Lastly, the time limitations for claim submission—either within two years of awareness of an adverse event or within five years of symptom onset—make it challenging to accurately estimate incidences of adverse events with long intervals post immunization, such as BCG osteomyelitis. Moreover, as VICP cases are closed once the final causality is determined and the financial compensation is made, information on long-term sequelae, in terms of both the physical and psychosocial aspects, is lacking.

6. Conclusions

Our study provides a comprehensive analysis of the adverse reactions associated with vaccines included in Taiwan's EPI using data from the VICP from 2014 to 2019. The findings confirm the overall safety of these vaccines, with most adverse events occurring at low incidence rates. Notably, the BCG vaccine, despite its effectiveness in preventing severe forms of tuberculosis, showed the highest incidence of adverse reactions, predominantly due to subacute or chronic infections by BCG strains, such as osteomyelitis. This underscores the need for carefully evaluating the risk–benefit ratio in regions with low tuberculosis prevalence, where routine BCG vaccination may require re-assessment of its necessity versus potential adverse effects.

While the influenza vaccine was the second vaccine most frequently associated with adverse claims, it maintained an excellent safety profile with very low incidences of severe adverse reactions such as Guillain–Barré syndrome. This reinforces its continued use and importance in public health efforts to prevent influenza outbreaks.

Our analysis highlights the critical role of continuous post-marketing surveillance and compensation programs like the VICP in ensuring vaccine safety and maintaining public trust. These programs are invaluable for identifying rare adverse events and facilitating data-driven adjustments in immunization schedules, such as the adjusted timing of the BCG vaccine, which significantly reduced the incidence of severe reactions. Future research and policies should focus on optimizing vaccination strategies, potentially incorporating more personalized approaches to mitigate risks while maximizing the benefits of immunization across diverse populations.

Supplementary Materials: The following supporting information can be downloaded at https://www.mdpi.com/article/10.3390/vaccines12101133/s1: Table S1: Total administered doses of various vaccines included in the extended program of immunization in Taiwan from 2010 to 2019; and Table S2: Immunization Schedule in Taiwan.

Author Contributions: W.-C.L. and C.-J.C. conceived this study. C.-J.C. designed this study and produced the protocol. Y.-C.H. and N.-C.C. assisted in the analysis of this study. C.-H.Y. collected the data on the total administered doses. W.-C.L. and C.-J.C. wrote the first draft of manuscript. All the authors read and approved the manuscript. All authors have read and agreed to the published version of the manuscript.

Funding: This research was funded by grants from Chang Gung Memorial Hospital [grant number CORPG3L0171, CORPG3L0172].

Institutional Review Board Statement: This study was approved by the Research and Ethics Committee of Chang Gung Memorial Hospital (IRB: 202002607B1).

Informed Consent Statement: Patient consent was waived due to the retrospective analysis of the de-identified VICP database, which contains no personally identifiable information, thereby protecting the privacy and confidentiality of all the individuals involved. Due to the de-identified nature of the data, this research was conducted in accordance with ethical guidelines that allow for the use of such information without the need for obtaining individual informed consent. This approach enabled this study to contribute valuable insights while maintaining strict adherence to privacy standards.

Data Availability Statement: The raw data of this study can be obtained by contacting the corresponding author.

Acknowledgments: We thanked the committee of the Vaccine Injury Compensation Program (VICP) in Taiwan for providing the electronic records of the adjudication results. We also thank the Centers for Disease Control in Taiwan for providing the statistics of annual administered doses of EPI vaccines.

Conflicts of Interest: The authors declare that they have no known competing financial interests or personal relationships that could have appeared to influence the work reported in this paper.

References

1. Carter, A.; Msemburi, W.; Sim, S.Y.; Gaythorpe, K.A.M.; Lambach, P.; Lindstrand, A.; Hutubessy, R. Modeling the Impact of Vaccination for the Immunization Agenda 2030: Deaths Averted Due to Vaccination against 14 Pathogens in 194 Countries from 2021 to 2030. *Vaccine* **2024**, *42*, S28–S37. [CrossRef] [PubMed]
2. Evans, G. Vaccine Injury Compensation Programs Worldwide. *Vaccine* **1999**, *17*, S25–S35. [CrossRef] [PubMed]
3. Taiwan National Adverse Drug Reactions Reporting System. Available online: https://adr.fda.gov.tw/logon (accessed on 20 September 2024).
4. Taiwan Centers for Disease Control. Vaccine Adverse Events Reporting System (VAERS). Available online: https://vaers.cdc.gov.tw/ (accessed on 20 September 2024).
5. Meissner, H.C.; Nair, N.; Plotkin, S.A. The National Vaccine Injury Compensation Program: Striking a Balance Between Individual Rights and Community Benefit. *JAMA* **2019**, *321*, 343. [CrossRef]
6. Cook, K.M.; Evans, G. The National Vaccine Injury Compensation Program. *Pediatrics* **2011**, *127*, S74–S77. [CrossRef]
7. Wang, P.C. Updates on Vaccine Injury Compensation Program in Taiwan and Program Evaluation. *Taiwan Epidemiol. Bull.* **2015**, *31*, 149–158.
8. Halabi, S.F.; Omer, S.B. A Global Vaccine Injury Compensation System. *JAMA* **2017**, *317*, 471. [CrossRef]
9. Looker, C.; Kelly, H. No-Fault Compensation Following Adverse Events Attributed to Vaccination: A Review of International Programmes. *Bull. World Health Organ.* **2011**, *89*, 371–378. [CrossRef]
10. Ridgway, D. No-Fault Vaccine Insurance: Lessons from the National Vaccine Injury Compensation Program. *J. Health Politics Polic. Law* **1999**, *24*, 59–90. [CrossRef] [PubMed]
11. Tsai, S.-Y.; Yeh, T.-Y.; Chiu, N.-C.; Huang, C.-T. National Safety Surveillance of Quadrivalent Recombinant Influenza Vaccine in Taiwan during NH 20/21. *Vaccine* **2022**, *40*, 3701–3704. [CrossRef]
12. Taiwan Centers for Disease Control. The Manual of the Vaccine Injury Compensation Program by Taiwan CDC. Available online: https://www.cdc.gov.tw/vicp (accessed on 20 September 2024).
13. Regulations Governing Collection and Review of Relief Fund for Victims of Immunization. 2004. Available online: https://law.moj.gov.tw/ENG/LawClass/LawAll.aspx?pcode=L0050021 (accessed on 20 September 2024).
14. Taiwan Centers for Disease Control. Annual Statistics on Compensation Services for Adverse Reactions to Vaccinations. Available online: https://www.cdc.gov.tw/Category/Page/OM4QgMRlmzYg5UDLHlnXRw (accessed on 20 September 2024).
15. Hsu, C.-Y.; Wang, E.-T.; Chou, Y.-M.; Yen, J.-J. Epidemiology of Invasive Pneumococcal Disease in Taiwan, 2008–2013. *Epidemiol. Bull.* **2014**, *30*, 180.
16. Colditz, G.A.; Berkey, C.S.; Mosteller, F.; Brewer, T.F.; Wilson, M.E.; Burdick, E.; Fineberg, H.V. The Efficacy of Bacillus Calmette-Guérin Vaccination of Newborns and Infants in the Prevention of Tuberculosis: Meta-Analyses of the Published Literature. *Pediatrics* **1995**, *96*, 29–35. [CrossRef] [PubMed]
17. Chan, P.-C.; Huang, W.-L.; Wang, K.-F.; Ma, C.-Y.; Lu, B.-Y.; Lin, F.-T.; Jou, R.; Yang, C.-H. The Active Surveillance of BCG-Related Adverse Events. *Taiwan Epidemiol. Bull.* **2012**, *28*, 13–22.

18. Chiu, N.-C.; Lin, M.-C.; Lin, W.-L.; Wang, S.-Y.; Chi, H.; Huang, L.-M.; Tang, R.-B.; Huang, Y.-C.; Liu, C.-C.; Huang, F.-Y.; et al. Mycobacterium Bovis BCG–Associated Osteomyelitis/Osteitis, Taiwan. *Emerg. Infect. Dis.* **2015**, *21*, 539–540. [CrossRef] [PubMed]
19. Yang, T.-L.; Lee, C.-M.; Lee, K.-L.; Yen, T.-Y.; Lu, C.-Y.; Lee, P.-I.; Chen, C.-M.; Huang, L.-M.; Chang, L.-Y. Clinical Features of Tuberculosis and Bacillus Calmette-Guérin (BCG) -Associated Adverse Effects in Children: A 12-Year Study. *J. Formos. Méd. Assoc.* **2021**, *120*, 443–451. [CrossRef]
20. Huang, C.-Y.; Chiu, N.-C.; Chi, H.; Huang, F.-Y.; Chang, P.-H. Clinical Manifestations, Management, and Outcomes of Osteitis/Osteomyelitis Caused by Mycobacterium Bovis Bacillus Calmette-Guérin in Children: Comparison by Site(s) of Affected Bones. *J. Pediatr.* **2019**, *207*, 97–102. [CrossRef]
21. Tsai, Y.-L.; Chen, Y.-J.; Lai, Y.-C. Long-Term Follow-up of Osteomyelitis Caused by Bacille Calmette-Guérin Vaccination in Immunocompetent Children. *Sci. Rep.* **2020**, *10*, 4072. [CrossRef]
22. Huang, W.; Chiu, N.-C.; Chi, H.; Huang, F.-Y.; Huang, C.-Y. Inoculation Age of Bacillus Calmette-Guérin Tokyo-172 Strain and Vaccine-Related Adverse Reactions in Taiwan Birth Cohort of 2012–2017. *Clin. Infect. Dis.* **2020**, *73*, e1554–e1559. [CrossRef]
23. Okuno, H.; Satoh, H.; Morino, S.; Arai, S.; Ochiai, M.; Fujita, K.; Naito, S.; Kato, A.; Ishii, K.; Oishi, K.; et al. Characteristics and Incidence of Vaccine Adverse Events after Bacille Calmette–Guérin Vaccination: A National Surveillance Study in Japan from 2013 to 2017. *Vaccine* **2022**, *40*, 4922–4928. [CrossRef]
24. Taiwan Centers for Disease Control. Information of the Management of BCG Abscess. Available online: https://www.cdc.gov.tw/Category/ListContent/4T8vDeSxOpmz0ILvF_D8Yw?uaid=QsqXMEzXYCw6Gp1n7YLSDA (accessed on 20 September 2024).
25. Kim, M.-K.; Lee, Y.K.; Kim, T.E.; Kong, I.; Yang, H.-J.; Suh, E.S. Surveillance and Compensation Claims for Adverse Events Following Immunization from 2011 to 2016 in the Republic of Korea. *Clin. Exp. Vaccine Res.* **2017**, *6*, 146–155. [CrossRef]
26. Patel, P.K.; Rawahi, B.A.; Jawari, A.A.; Abaidani, I.A.; Abri, S.A. Surveillance of Adverse Events Following Immunization in Oman, 2006–2015. *East. Mediterr. Health J.* **2018**, *24*, 119–126. [CrossRef]
27. Guo, B.; Page, A.; Wang, H.; Taylor, R.; McIntyre, P. Systematic Review of Reporting Rates of Adverse Events Following Immunization: An International Comparison of Post-Marketing Surveillance Programs with Reference to China. *Vaccine* **2013**, *31*, 603–617. [CrossRef] [PubMed]
28. Clothier, H.J.; Hosking, L.; Crawford, N.W.; Russell, M.; Easton, M.L.; Quinn, J.-A.; Buttery, J.P. Bacillus Calmette-Guérin (BCG) Vaccine Adverse Events in Victoria, Australia: Analysis of Reports to an Enhanced Passive Surveillance System. *Drug Saf.* **2014**, *38*, 79–86. [CrossRef] [PubMed]
29. Krysztopa-Grzybowska, K.; Paradowska-Stankiewicz, I.; Lutyńska, A. The Rate of Adverse Events Following BCG Vaccination in Poland. *Prz. Epidemiol.* **2012**, *66*, 465–469.
30. Roh, E.J.; Lee, Y.-K.; Lee, M.-H.; Kim, M.-K.; Kim, T.E.; Lee, S.G.; Chung, E.H. Investigation of Adverse Events Following Bacille Calmette-Guérin Immunization Using Immunization Safety Surveillance System in Korea Centers for Disease Control and Prevention. *Clin. Exp. Vaccine Res.* **2020**, *9*, 133–145. [CrossRef] [PubMed]
31. Thompson, K.M.; Orenstein, W.A.; Hinman, A.R. Performance of the United States Vaccine Injury Compensation Program (VICP): 1988–2019. *Vaccine* **2020**, *38*, 2136–2143. [CrossRef]
32. Schonberger, L.B.; Bregman, D.J.; Sullivan-Bolyai, J.Z.; Keenlyside, R.A.; Ziegler, D.W.; Retailliau, H.F.; Eddins, D.L.; Bryan, J.A. Guillain-Barre Syndrome Following Vaccination in the National Influenza Immunization Program, United States, 1976–1977. *Am. J. Epidemiol.* **1979**, *110*, 105–123. [CrossRef]
33. Langmuir, A.D.; Bregman, D.J.; Kurland, L.T.; Nathanson, N.; Victor, M. An epidemiologic and clinical evaluation of Guillain-Barré syndrome reported in association with the administration of swine influenza vaccines. *Am. J. Epidemiol.* **1984**, *119*, 841–879. [CrossRef]
34. Marks, J.S.; Halpin, T.J. Guillain-Barré Syndrome in Recipients of A/New Jersey Influenza Vaccine. *JAMA* **1980**, *243*, 2490–2494. [CrossRef]
35. Arias, L.H.M.; Sanz, R.; Sáinz, M.; Treceño, C.; Carvajal, A. Guillain-Barré Syndrome and Influenza Vaccines: A Meta-Analysis. *Vaccine* **2015**, *33*, 3773–3778. [CrossRef]
36. Salmon, D.A.; Proschan, M.; Forshee, R.; Gargiullo, P.; Bleser, W.; Burwen, D.R.; Cunningham, F.; Garman, P.; Greene, S.K.; Lee, G.M.; et al. Association between Guillain-Barré Syndrome and Influenza A (H1N1) 2009 Monovalent Inactivated Vaccines in the USA: A Meta-Analysis. *Lancet* **2013**, *381*, 1461–1468. [CrossRef]
37. Petráš, M.; Lesná, I.K.; Dáňová, J.; Čelko, A.M. Is an Increased Risk of Developing Guillain–Barré Syndrome Associated with Seasonal Influenza Vaccination? A Systematic Review and Meta-Analysis. *Vaccines* **2020**, *8*, 150. [CrossRef] [PubMed]
38. Vellozzi, C.; Iqbal, S.; Broder, K. Guillain-Barre Syndrome, Influenza, and Influenza Vaccination: The Epidemiologic Evidence. *Clin. Infect. Dis.* **2014**, *58*, 1149–1155. [CrossRef] [PubMed]

vaccines

MDPI

Article

COVID-19 Vaccine Hesitancy and Associated Oral Cholera Vaccine Hesitancy in a Cholera-Endemic Country: A Community-Based Cross-Sectional Study in the Democratic Republic of Congo

Arsene Daniel Nyalundja [1,2,†], Patrick Musole Bugeme [1,3,†], Alain Balola Ntaboba [2], Victoire Urbain Hatu'm [2], Guillaume Shamamba Ashuza [2], Jacques Lukenze Tamuzi [4], Duduzile Ndwandwe [5], Chinwe Iwu-Jaja [5], Charles Shey Wiysonge [5,6] and Patrick D. M. C. Katoto [1,4,5,7,*]

1 Center for Tropical Diseases and Global Health (CTDGH), Catholic University of Bukavu (UCB), Bukavu 285, Democratic Republic of the Congo; nyalu_arse.adn@outlook.com (A.D.N.); musolebugeme@gmail.com (P.M.B.)
2 Faculty of Medicine, Catholic University of Bukavu (UCB), Bukavu 285, Democratic Republic of the Congo; balola.ntaboball@gmail.com (A.B.N.); victoirehat@gmail.com (V.U.H.); shamambaguillaume@gmail.com (G.S.A.)
3 Department of Epidemiology, Johns Hopkins Bloomberg School of Public Health, Johns Hopkins University, Baltimore, MD 21205, USA
4 Department of Global Health, Faculty of Medicine and Health Sciences, Stellenbosch University, Cape Town 7505, South Africa; drjacques.tamuzi@gmail.com
5 Cochrane South Africa, South African Medical Research Council, Cape Town 7501, South Africa; duduzile.ndwandwe@mrc.ac.za (D.N.); chinwelolo@gmail.com (C.I.-J.); sheyc@who.int (C.S.W.)
6 Vaccine-Preventable Diseases Programme, World Health Organization Regional Office for Africa, Brazzaville P.O. Box 06, Congo
7 Centre for General Medicine and Global Health, Department of Medicine, University of Cape Town, Cape Town 7505, South Africa
* Correspondence: katoto.chimusa@ucbukavu.ac.cd
† These authors contributed equally to this work.

Abstract: COVID-19 vaccine hesitancy and its enablers shape community uptake of non-covid vaccines such as the oral cholera vaccine (OCV) in the post-COVID-19 era. This study assessed the impact of COVID-19 vaccine hesitancy and its drivers on OCV hesitancy in a cholera-endemic region of the Democratic Republic of Congo. We conducted a community-based survey in Bukavu. The survey included demographics, intention to take OCV and COVID-19 vaccines, reasons for COVID-19 hesitancy, and thoughts and feelings about COVID-19 vaccines. Poisson regression analyses were performed. Of the 1708 respondents, 84.66% and 77.57% were hesitant to OCV alone and to both OCV and COVID-19, respectively. Hesitancy to COVID-19 vaccines rose OCV hesitancy by 12% (crude prevalence ratio, [cPR] = 1.12, 95%CI [1.03–1.21]). Independent predictors of OCV hesitancy were living in a semi-urban area (adjusted prevalence ratio [aPR] = 1.10, 95%CI [1.03–1.12]), religious refusal of vaccines (aPR = 1.06, 95%CI [1.02–1.12]), concerns about vaccine safety (aPR = 1.05, 95%CI [1.01–1.11]) and adverse effects (aPR = 1.06, 95%CI [1.01–1.12]), as well as poor vaccine literacy (aPR = 1.07, 95%CI [1.01–1.14]). Interestingly, the belief in COVID-19 vaccine effectiveness reduced OCV hesitancy by 24% (aPR = 0.76, 95%CI [0.62–0.93]). COVID-19 vaccine hesitancy and its drivers exhibited a significant domino effect on OCV uptake. Addressing vaccine hesitancy through community-based health literacy and trust-building interventions would likely improve the introduction of novel non-COVID-19 vaccines in the post-COVID-19 era.

Keywords: non-COVID-19 vaccine; *Vibrio cholerae*; South Kivu; immunization; vaccine misinformation

1. Introduction

Cholera is a significant global health concern that threatens public health systems in low-resource settings, especially where the disease is commonly endemic [1]. The estimated burden of cholera accounts for 2.86 million (uncertainty range: 1.3–4.0 million) cases with 95,000 deaths (uncertainty range: 21,000–143,000) [2] and 1.9% of case fatality ratios (CFRs) [3]. While recent data suggest a decrease in cholera-related mortality globally between 1990 and 2019, significantly increasing mortality trends were observed in African regions [4]. In addition, Africa experiences the highest estimated CFR record of the decade at three times (2.9%) the agreed threshold (<1%) [5]. Global, multifaceted efforts have been undertaken to contain and control cholera, particularly in response to outbreaks, yet they remain insufficient to reduce the burden of disease related to cholera due to a combination of factors, including a lack of reliable data. Other challenges are not limited to complex humanitarian crises, political instability and protracted conflicts, health system fragility, climate change, limited and overstretched cholera workforce, multiple ongoing health emergencies, medical commodities supply chain, access to and availability of oral cholera vaccine (OCV), and more [1].

In the Democratic Republic of Congo (DRC), cholera is endemic in the eastern provinces, following an increasing seasonal trend during the rainy season [1,6,7]. The first cases of the disease were reported in 1973 during the seventh cholera pandemic, which began in Indonesia in 1961 [8]. Since the first cholera outbreak in 2021, the DRC reported 517,529 cases of cholera and 13,109 cholera-related deaths, ranking as the third and first country with the highest number of cholera cases and cholera-related deaths worldwide, respectively [9]. Sociopolitical instabilities and armed conflicts leading to massive internal and external displacement have been key factors in the cholera outbreak. For example, the most deadly and largest outbreak the country (more than 50,000 deaths) was observed in 1994 after the conflict in Rwanda [10]. Other factors, such as climate change and poor access to clean water, have been driving cholera across the country. In 2022, for example, a total of 18,403 suspected cases of cholera with a CFR of 1.6% were identified in 19 out of 26 provinces [6]. To control and eliminate cholera, the country implemented a nationwide strategy in 2007, "the Multisectoral Strategic Plan for Cholera Elimination" [11]. However, vaccination programs face enormous challenges including vaccine hesitancy [12], which is associated with vaccine safety and effectiveness concerns [13–15], trust in governments and scientists [16], complacency [15], knowledge gaps, poor health literacy, the infodemic and more. The government has received over 4 million doses targeting 2 million people. So far, over 1.4 million people have been vaccinated [17]. Although there are limited published studies on OCV uptake in the DRC, an OCV hesitancy rate of up to 67% has been recorded in a setting similar to the DRC [18]. However, mass vaccination against cholera provides herd immunity when more than 50% of the community receives two doses of a specific oral cholera vaccine [19].

Vaccine hesitancy, a highly variable and complex phenomenon, is patterned by specific contexts, time, and type of vaccines [20] and is classified by the World Health Organization (WHO) among the top ten threats to global health [21]. The COVID-19 pandemic further highlights this threat to global public health, especially in low-and-middle-income countries (LMICs), including the DRC, where vaccine-preventable diseases are the major contributors to the global burden of disease and where the COVID-19 vaccine uptake remained very low despite the availability of free vaccines. The DRC has one of the world's lowest rates of COVID-19 vaccine coverage, with only 19% of the population receiving at least one dose by November 2023 [22]. This is likely due to high COVID-19 vaccine hesitancy.

The multifaceted drivers that have shaped the reluctance of LMIC communities to receive COVID-19 vaccines may play an important role in the willingness to receive novel non-COVID-19 vaccines in the COVID-19 endemic era. In this work, we hypothesized that COVID-19 vaccine hesitancy would increase the likelihood of the community in the DRC hesitating to use other novel vaccines, such as the OCV. In addition, community reasons for COVID-19 vaccine hesitancy and thoughts and feelings about COVID-19 and its vaccines would be associated with cholera vaccine hesitancy. These data might guide the expanded Programme on Immunization (EPI) to implement effective interventions accordingly.

2. Materials and Methods

2.1. Study Design Setting and Population

We conducted a household-based survey from 1 to 31 March 2022 in three sites in Bukavu, South Kivu. Bukavu is the capital city of the South Kivu province in the eastern DRC, and administratively, it has three municipalities: Ibanda (urban), Kadutu (peri-urban), and Bagira (peri-urban). The city is located southwest of Lake Kivu, and west of Cyagungu, Rwanda, from which it is separated by the Rizizi River. In 2022, it has an estimated 1,190,000 urban population [23]. All adults (aged 18 and above) in Bukavu formed the target population. In this study, the inclusion criteria required a respondent per household to be 18 years or older at the time of the survey and who had lived in the region for at least 12 months.

2.2. Sampling and Sample Size

A deliberate minimum interval of 15 households was established to facilitate the random selection of subsequent households. In every municipality, the selection of the respondents at the household level was based on convenience, adhering to the criteria of choosing one respondent from each household. For each study site, a minimum estimated sample size of 350 respondents was determined as per the WHO's behavioral and social drivers of vaccines (BeSD) guidance [24].

2.3. Questionnaire

The survey contained closed-ended and Likert Scale questions adapted from the WHO's BeSD. After it was piloted, the structured questionnaire was used in both the official language, French, as well as in the local language, Swahili. The structured questionnaire included three sections:

1. Sociodemographic characteristics (7): age, gender, location, religion, religious acceptance of vaccination, educational level, profession, and monthly income;
2. Cholera vaccine (3): respondents were asked if they have been vaccinated against cholera, if they were ready to receive this vaccine as soon as it became available, and if they were willing to have their children vaccinated against cholera;
3. COVID-19 vaccine (4): vaccination against COVID-19, willingness to uptake COVID-19 vaccines if available, reasons for vaccination delayed or hesitancy, and perceptions about the COVID-19 vaccines.

Before administering the survey form, written informed consent was obtained for each respondent. Data were captured on tablets during the interview using KoboCollect (https://www.kobotoolbox.org/, accessed on 24 March 2023), an open-source Android application developed by KoboToolBox [24]. The survey was conducted by trained sixth-year medical students under the supervision of researchers affiliated with the Centre for Tropical Diseases and Global Health of the Catholic University of Bukavu.

2.4. Variables

The dependent variable was the willingness to uptake the cholera vaccine when available. The answers included "yes", "no", and "I do not know". For this type of question, hesitancy toward the cholera vaccine was defined as "no" or "I do not know", while "yes" was used to define vaccine acceptance. Independent variables were age, gender, location, religion, religious acceptance of vaccination, educational level, profession, monthly income, vaccination against COVID-19, willingness to uptake COVID-19 vaccines if available, reasons for delayed vaccination or hesitancy, and perceptions about the COVID-19 vaccines. Seven perceptions about the COVID-19 vaccines were identified, and each perception was designed as a 5-level Likert Scale question. The answers included "Strongly agree", "Slightly agree", "I am not sure/I have no opinion", "Slightly disagree", and

"Strongly disagree". To have binary variables, we merged "strongly agree" and "slightly agree" to become "yes" and the remainder to become "no".

2.5. Data Analysis

We used R (The R Foundation for Statistical Computing, Vienna, Austria) version 4.2.2 for data cleaning and analysis. Data were summarized as counts and percentages for categorical variables and medians with an interquartile range (percentile 25 and percentile 75) for quantitative variables. Chi-square and Wilcoxon rank-sum tests were used as appropriate for group comparisons. We used modified Poisson regression to determine the incidence rate ratio (IRR), analogous to the prevalence ratio (PR). We then used the generalized linear model (glm) function in R to create four unique models to uncover factors independently related to respondents' unwillingness to receive the cholera vaccine. Initially, the first model was adjusted to account for sociodemographic variables. Given the association between COVID-19 vaccine hesitancy and cholera vaccine hesitancy, the second and third models incorporated adjustments for variables related to the COVID-19 vaccine. The final model exclusively featured predictors that were significantly associated with vaccine hesitancy across the first three models, further adjusting for age as continuous variables and sex as binary variables, irrespective of their significance level. The results were presented as the PR with their 95% confidence interval (95%CI). All p-values were two-sided, and <0.05 indicated statistically significant results.

2.6. Ethics

This study was conducted in strict adherence to ethical principles. Access to the data was restricted solely to members of the research team, and any information that could potentially identify participants was meticulously removed or anonymized. Moreover, all participants provided informed consent for the publication of anonymized data. After a thorough explanation of any potential privacy risks, participants voluntarily agreed to the dissemination of findings in academic or professional forums. These measures were meticulously implemented to safeguard the privacy and confidentiality of all participants involved in the study.

3. Results

3.1. Sociodemographic Characteristics and Distribution of Cholera Vaccine Hesitancy among Respondents

A total of 1708 adults aged 38 years (median age, 95%CI 36–40 years) were surveyed in Bukavu, eastern DRC. Most of the respondents were males (54.34%), Christians (97.19%), aged between 25 and 39 years (33.14%), living in urban areas (54.75%), highly educated (62.59%), and employed (80.97%) but with a monthly income between USD 50 and USD 200 (40.20%). Overall, 84.66% of respondents were hesitant to receive OCV and were older than those who were willing to receive it when available (median age in years, 40 vs. 30, $p < 0.001$) (Table 1).

Table 1. Sociodemographic characteristics and predictors (Model 1) of OCV hesitancy among respondents.

Variables		Cholera Vaccine Hesitancy						*p*	cPR	95% CI		*p*	aPR	95% CI		*p*
		Yes		No		Total				Lower	Upper			Lower	Upper	
		n	%	n	%	n	%									
	Median$^{\$}$	40 (27–55)		30 (24–49)		38 (26–54)		**<0.001** *	1.02	1.01	1.03	**0.02**				
Age	>65	104	6.09	12	0.7	116	6.79	**<0.001**	Reference				Reference			
	18–24	234	13.70	76	4.45	310	18.15		0.84	0.77	0.92	**<0.01**	0.91	0.82	1.02	0.14
	25–39	474	27.75	92	5.39	566	33.14		0.93	0.86	1.01	0.11	0.98	0.89	1.07	0.68
	40–54	372	21.78	55	3.22	427	25.00		0.97	0.90	1.04	0.46	0.99	0.92	1.09	0.92
	55–65	262	15.34	27	1.58	289	16.92		1.01	0.94	1.09	0.75	1.03	0.94	1.12	0.46
Gender	Female	666	38.99	114	6.67	780	45.66	0.49	Reference				Reference			
	Male	780	45.67	148	8.67	928	54.34		1.02	0.98	1.06	0.45	0.99	0.95	1.03	0.69
Religion	Christian	1409	82.49	251	14.7	1660	97.19	0.20	Reference				-			
	Non-Christian	37	2.17	11	0.64	48	2.81		0.91	0.78	1.06	0.14				
Religious acceptance of vaccines	Yes	738	43.21	178	10.42	916	53.63	**<0.001**	Reference				Reference			
	No	708	41.45	84	4.92	792	46.37		1.11	1.07	1.15	**<0.01**	1.06	1.02	1.12	**<0.01**
Location	Urban	617	36.12	156	9.13	773	45.25	**<0.001**	Reference				Reference			
	Semi-rural	829	48.54	106	6.21	935	54.75		1.11	1.06	1.16	**<0.01**	1.10	1.03	1.19	**<0.01**
Education status	High	887	51.93	182	10.66	1069	62.59	**0.01**	Reference				Reference			
	Low	42	2.46	2	0.12	44	2.58		1.15	1.07	1.24	**0.04**	1.09	0.99	1.20	0.16
	Medium	527	30.27	78	4.57	605	34.84		1.04	1.01	1.09	**0.03**	1.01	0.98	1.06	0.32
Employment	Yes	1197	70.08	186	10.89	1383	80.97	**<0.001**	Reference				Reference			
	No	249	14.58	249	4.45	498	19.03		0.89	0.83	0.94	**<0.01**	0.96	0.91	1.03	0.18
Monthly income	>200	198	16.51	40	3.34	238	19.85	**<0.001**	Reference				Reference			
	<50	438	36.53	41	3.42	479	39.95		1.09	1.03	1.17	**<0.01**	1.09	0.98	1.21	0.06
	50–200	400	33.36	82	6.84	482	40.20		0.99	0.93	1.06	0.94	0.97	0.88	1.07	0.60

Median$^{\$}$ with interquartile range Q1–Q3: interquartile range; * Mann–Whitney U test; cPR: crude prevalence ratio; aPR: adjusted prevalence ratio. The bold for the number denotes a statistically significant *p*-value indicating notable significance within the data analysis.

3.2. Socio-Demographic Factors Associated with Cholera Vaccine Hesitancy

The first modified Poisson regression model was built to assess the association between sociodemographic characteristics and hesitancy to receive OCV once it was available (Table 1). After adjusting for different variables in the models, we found that hesitancy toward receiving OCV was 6% and 10% higher among respondents whose religion does not accept vaccination (aPR = 1.06, 95%CI [1.02–1.12]) and those who lived in a semi-rural area (aPR = 1.10, 95%CI [1.03–1.19]), respectively.

3.3. Effect of COVID-19 Vaccine Hesitancy on Willingness to Vaccine for Cholera

In our initial analysis, we investigated the association between COVID-19 vaccination attitudes and willingness to be vaccinated against cholera. We noted that individuals hesitant to receive the COVID-19 vaccine were approximately 12% more likely to express hesitancy towards the cholera vaccine (cPR = 1.12, 95%CI [1.03–1.21]) (Table 2). Following this, through two separate Poisson regression models, we evaluated how specific reasons and perceptions related to COVID-19 vaccine hesitancy influenced the prevalence of hesitancy to receive the cholera vaccine. Importantly, respondents who perceived that the COVID-19 vaccine could contain other viruses, such as Ebola (adjusted PR (aPR) = 1.05, 95% CI [1.01–1.11]), or could have other harmful health effects (aPR = 1.06, 95% CI [1.01–1.12]), or those who indicated having a lack of information about the vaccine (aPR = 1.07, 95% CI [1.01–1.14]) were found to have a higher prevalence of hesitancy towards the cholera vaccine (Table 3). In contrast, those who recognized that COVID-19 could be prevented by vaccination showed a 5% reduction in the prevalence of vaccine hesitancy (aPR = 0.95, 95% CI [0.91–0.99]) (Table 4).

Table 2. Association between cholera vaccine hesitancy and COVID-19 vaccine hesitancy.

Variables		Cholera Vaccine Hesitancy						*p*	PR	95% CI		*p*
		Yes		No		Total				Lower	Upper	
		n	%	n	%	n	%					
COVID-19 vaccine hesitancy	No	133	8.70	37	2.42	150	9.94	**<0.01**	Reference			
	Yes	1186	77.57	173	11.31	1359	90.06		1.12	1.03	1.21	**<0.01**

The bold for the number denotes a statistically significant *p*-value indicating notable significance within the data analysis.

Additionally, in a comprehensive model that accounted for statistically significant factors from the earlier models and controlled for age and gender, we identified that age, geographic location, and specific concerns about the COVID-19 vaccine (for instance, the fear it might contain viruses like Ebola) independently contributed to a higher prevalence of delaying or refusing the cholera vaccine. Notably, the understanding that COVID-19 is preventable through vaccination remained a significant factor; individuals with this knowledge exhibited a notably lower prevalence of hesitancy towards receiving the OCV when available (aPR = 0.76, 95%CI [0.62–0.93]).

Table 3. Association between reasons for COVID-19 vaccine hesitancy and OCV hesitancy (Model 2).

Reasons for COVID-19 Vaccine Hesitancy		Cholera Vaccine Hesitancy						p	cPR	95% CI		p	aPR	95% CI		p
		Yes		No		Total				Lower	Upper			Lower	Upper	
		n	%	n	%	n	%									
Vaccines could contain other virus such as Ebola, or more	No	948	62.95	162	10.76	1110	73.71	**0.03**		Reference				Reference		
	Yes	356	23.64	40	2.66	396	26.30		1.05	1.01	1.10	**0.01**	1.05	1.01	1.11	**0.04**
Fear of vaccine side effects	No	822	54.15	137	9.03	959	63.18	0.43		Reference				Reference		
	Yes	488	32.15	71	4.68	559	36.83		0.98	0.94	1.02	0.38	0.99	0.94	1.05	0.08
Inefficacity of the vaccine	No	1051	69.24	178	11.73	1229	80.97	0.08		Reference				Reference		
	Yes	259	17.06	30	1.98	289	19.04		1.04	1.01	1.10	0.04	1.03	0.98	1.10	0.29
Vaccine could have other harmful effects	No	1011	66.6	178	11.73	1189	78.33	**0.01**		Reference				Reference		
	Yes	299	19.70	30	1.98	329	21.68		1.07	1.02	1.11	**<0.001**	1.06	1.01	1.12	**0.03**
Do not know where to get this vaccine	No	1228	81.06	195	12.87	1423	93.93	0.80		Reference				Reference		
	Yes	78	5.15	14	0.92	92	6.07		0.97	0.89	1.07	0.59	0.98	0.88	1.09	0.79
Poor knowledge about the vaccine	No	118	73.65	189	12.45	307	86.10	**0.04**		Reference				Reference		
	Yes	192	12.65	19	1.25	211	13.90		2.36	2.04	2.744	**<0.001**	1.07	1.01	1.14	**0.03**

The bold for the number denotes a statistically significant *p*-value indicating notable significance within the data analysis.

Table 4. Association between COVID-19 vaccine perception and OCV hesitancy (Model 3).

Perceptions toward COVID Vaccine		Cholera Vaccine Hesitancy						p	cPR	95% CI		p	aPR	95% CI		p
		Yes		No		Total				Lower	Upper			Lower	Upper	
		n	%	n	%	n	%									
COVID-19 is a serious threat	No	576	33.72	59	3.45	635	37.17	**<0.01**		Reference				Reference		
	Yes	870	50.94	203	11.89	1073	62.83		0.89	0.86	0.92	**<0.001**	0.96	0.91	1.01	0.11
COVID-19 can be prevented by vaccination	No	942	55.15	105	6.15	1047	61.30	**<0.01**		Reference				Reference		
	Yes	504	29.51	157	9.19	661	38.70		0.84	0.81	0.88	**<0.001**	0.95	0.91	0.99	**0.01**

Table 4. *Cont.*

Perceptions toward COVID Vaccine		Cholera Vaccine Hesitancy						p	cPR	95% CI		p	aPR	95% CI		p
		Yes		No		Total				Lower	Upper			Lower	Upper	
		n	%	n	%	n	%									
The risks of COVID-19 disease are greater than the risks associated with its vaccine	No	843	49.36	106	6.21	949	55.57	**<0.01**		Reference				Reference		
	Yes	603	35.3	156	9.13	759	44.43		0.89	0.85	0.93	**<0.001**	0.99	0.97	1.02	0.81
The COVID-19 vaccines I have access to are safe	No	1136	66.51	152	8.9	1288	75.41	**<0.01**		Reference				Reference		
	Yes	310	18.15	110	6.44	420	24.59		0.84	0.79	0.89	**<0.001**	0.97	0.93	1.01	0.10
I believe that my government is capable of delivering the COVID-19 vaccine everywhere in my country, to everyone and equally	No	1055	61.77	148	8.67	1203	70.44	**<0.01**		Reference				Reference		
	Yes	391	22.89	114	6.67	505	29.56		0.88	0.83	0.93	**<0.001**	0.98	0.95	1.01	0.17
I trust the science behind the COVID-19 vaccine.	No	1054	61.71	135	7.90	1189	69.61	**<0.01**		Reference				Reference		
	Yes	392	22.95	127	7.44	519	30.39		0.85	0.81	0.89	**<0.001**	0.97	0.94	1.01	0.10
Trust in the government	No	1149	67.27	187	10.95	1336	78.22	**0.01**		Reference				Reference		
	Yes	297	11.39	75	4.39	372	15.78		0.92	0.88	0.98	**<0.001**	0.98	0.95	1.01	0.30

The bold for the number denotes a statistically significant p-value indicating notable significance within the data analysis.

4. Discussion

In this household-based cross-sectional study conducted in Bukavu, eastern DRC, we investigated the interplay between sociodemographic characteristics, perceptions towards the COVID-19 vaccine, and the overarching willingness to engage in cholera vaccination initiatives. Overall, a pronounced hesitancy toward OCV was discerned, with a notable inclination among the older demographic. Specifically, the analysis highlighted a significant association between COVID-19 vaccine hesitancy and hesitancy towards OCV, particularly attributed to fears of vaccine contamination with viruses like Ebola, concerns about adverse health effects, and insufficient vaccine-related information. Further, an incremental hesitancy associated with religious opposition to vaccination and residence in semi-rural areas was observed. Strikingly, the perception that vaccines are effective in preventing COVID-19 corresponded with a lower hesitancy towards receiving OCV.

The associations observed between vaccine hesitancy and various factors in this study are likely reflective of broader trends beyond the DRC. For example, misinformation surrounding vaccine safety and efficacy has been a longstanding challenge across various vaccination campaigns, contributing to hesitancy. This study's insights into the domino effect of COVID-19 vaccine hesitancy on OCV hesitancy highlight the long-term benefit of addressing misinformation and improving health literacy [25]. Importantly, while religious acceptance of vaccines did not significantly influence OCV hesitancy in our final model, it was linked to a notable rise in hesitancy in preliminary adjustments for sociodemographic characteristics. Additionally, previous studies conducted in similar settings indicated that OCV hesitancy was driven by religious reasons or tradition, along with community rumors regarding vaccine safety and confidence [26–30]. This highlights the influential role of community and religious leaders in vaccine uptake, corroborating literature that stresses their effectiveness in building trust and promoting health interventions over political or medical authorities [29,31].

Hence, the study further aligns with existing literature on the detrimental effects of public distrust in health institutions and government on vaccine hesitancy, exacerbated during the COVID-19 pandemic by the rapid spread of misinformation and conspiracy theories [32–36]. The emergence of an 'infodemic'—an overload of both accurate and false information—has been identified as a significant barrier to trust in health services, potentially explaining the observed association between vaccine hesitancy and religious acceptance of vaccination [37–40]. Yet, notably, our data suggest that those recognizing the preventive efficacy of vaccines against COVID-19 exhibited less hesitancy towards OCV, emphasizing the importance of health education in dispelling myths and promoting vaccine acceptance [40].

The importance of this study is further highlighted by the ongoing health challenges in Africa, particularly the persistent and widespread cholera outbreak and the high mortality rates due to diseases such as malaria, which continues to be a leading cause of death among children under five. The introduction of new life-saving vaccines against malaria, along with vaccines for HPV to prevent cervical cancer, marks a critical juncture in the continent's public health efforts. These vaccines represent a beacon of hope for reducing the disease burden and improving health outcomes. However, the effectiveness of these vaccination programs is significantly compromised by vaccine hesitancy, which will also constitute a barrier to achieving widespread vaccine coverage and the realization of their potential benefits. This study's findings, while focused on oral cholera vaccine hesitancy, shed light on broader vaccine hesitancy issues that could impact the uptake of other new vaccines.

From a policy perspective, leveraging the lessons learned from the COVID-19 pandemic's global and national response offers a strategic pathway for enhancing the Expanded Programme on Immunization (EPI) and overcoming challenges posed by vaccine hesitancy. The pandemic has emphasized the importance of building trust in health systems, fostering clear and effective communication, and engaging communities directly to encourage vaccine acceptance. These strategies are not only pivotal for COVID-19 vaccine uptake but are equally applicable to the rollout of new vaccines for malaria, which remains a leading cause of mortality among children under five in Africa, and HPV. Adapting strategies that have successfully increased COVID-19 vaccine acceptance in the context of EPI programs can provide a robust framework for addressing vaccine hesitancy. This approach, coupled with efforts to strengthen health systems and enhance health literacy, holds the promise of significantly improving vaccine coverage for malaria, HPV, and other vaccine-preventable diseases, paving the way for better health outcomes and a reduction in child mortality across the continent. The EPI in the DRC should capitalize on these insights to develop comprehensive guidelines targeting vaccine hesitancy. These guidelines should adopt a multifaceted approach, including community engagement and education, tailored messaging, equitable vaccine access, healthcare worker training, and robust surveillance systems. By integrating these components, the EPI can effectively promote vaccine acceptance and enhance immunization rates.

One of the primary weaknesses of this study is its reliance on self-reported data, which may introduce bias due to respondents' potential reluctance to disclose true vaccine hesitancy attitudes or misunderstandings about the vaccines in question. Furthermore, the cross-sectional design limits our ability to establish causal relationships between the identified factors and vaccine hesitancy. Additionally, while the study provides valuable insights into vaccine hesitancy within the context of the DRC, the findings might not be fully generalizable to other settings or populations due to cultural, socioeconomic, and health system differences. Despite these limitations, the study's strengths lie in its substantial sample size and the use of robust statistical methods to assess the factors associated with vaccine hesitancy. This approach has allowed for a nuanced understanding of the interplay between various determinants of hesitancy, offering critical insights that can inform targeted interventions to enhance vaccine uptake in similar contexts.

5. Conclusions

We found that addressing COVID-19 vaccination hesitancy and its drivers related to vaccine content, safety, and misinformation is critical to improving the uptake of new vaccines in the post-COVID era. This observation creates an opportunity for immunization programs that can leverage collaboration between academic and research institutions, civil societies, health system agencies, and government bodies to improve thinking and feeling about vaccines and vaccine-preventable diseases through community-related health literacy interventions.

Author Contributions: Conceptualization, A.D.N., P.M.B., P.D.M.C.K. and C.S.W.; methodology, A.D.N., P.M.B., P.D.M.C.K., J.L.T., D.N., C.I.-J. and C.S.W.; software, A.D.N.; validation, A.D.N., P.M.B., G.S.A., A.B.N., V.U.H., P.D.M.C.K., J.L.T., D.N., C.I.-J. and C.S.W.; formal analysis, A.D.N.; resources, P.D.M.C.K. and C.S.W.; data curation, G.S.A., A.B.N. and V.U.H.; writing—original draft preparation, A.D.N.; writing—review and editing, A.D.N., P.M.B., G.S.A., A.B.N., V.U.H., P.D.M.C.K., J.L.T., D.N., C.I.-J. and C.S.W.; visualization, A.D.N., P.M.B. and P.D.M.C.K.; supervision, J.L.T., D.N., C.I.-J., P.D.M.C.K. and C.S.W.; project administration, P.D.M.C.K. and P.M.B.; funding acquisition, P.D.M.C.K. All authors have read and agreed to the published version of the manuscript.

Funding: This work was supported by internal funding from the Center for Tropical Diseases and Global Health (CTDGH) at the Catholic University of Bukavu (UCB), awarded on 1 February 2022.

Institutional Review Board Statement: This study was approved by the Institutional Review Board of the Catholic University of Bukavu (UCB) (N/Ref: UCB/CIES/NC/002/2022) on 12 February 2022.

Informed Consent Statement: The survey was anonymous and voluntary. The aim, objectives, and scope of the study were clearly explained to the respondents verbally. Respondents who provided informed consent were surveyed after being informed of their right to withdraw or not respond at any point in the survey. Individuals who did not consent were not surveyed.

Data Availability Statement: The data and analytical code on which this article is based are available on request from the corresponding author (P.D.M.C.K.) or the first author (A.D.N.). To approve a request, it must be justified from a methodological point of view and receive the consent of all authors. All requests can be made after publication of this manuscript with no end date.

Acknowledgments: We wish to thank all the members of the Center for Tropical Diseases and Global Health (CTDGH) at the Catholic University of Bukavu (UCB) for their contribution to this study. Also, we wish to thank Cochrane South Africa at the South African Medical Research Council for supporting the article processing charge (APC) of this manuscript.

Conflicts of Interest: We declare no conflicts of interest. The views and opinions expressed in this article are those of the authors only and do not necessarily represent those of their affiliated institutions.

References

1. Cholera—Global Situation. Available online: https://www.who.int/emergencies/disease-outbreak-news/item/2022-DON426 (accessed on 24 March 2023).
2. Ali, M.; Nelson, A.R.; Lopez, A.L.; Sack, D.A. Updated Global Burden of Cholera in Endemic Countries. *PLoS Negl. Trop. Dis.* **2015**, *9*, e0003832. [CrossRef] [PubMed]
3. Cholera—Global Situation. Available online: https://www.who.int/emergencies/disease-outbreak-news/item/2023-DON437 (accessed on 24 March 2023).
4. Ilic, I.; Ilic, M. Global Patterns of Trends in Cholera Mortality. *Trop. Med. Infect. Dis.* **2023**, *8*, 169. [CrossRef] [PubMed]
5. Mavhunga, C. Cholera: World Health Organization warns of rising cases in Africa. *BMJ* **2023**, *380*, 488. [CrossRef]
6. Cholera—Democratic Republic of the Congo. Available online: https://www.who.int/emergencies/disease-outbreak-news/item/2023-DON441 (accessed on 24 March 2023).
7. Nkoko, D.; Giraudoux, P.; Plisnier, P.-D.; Tinda, A.; Piarroux, M.; Sudre, B.; Horion, S.; Tamfum, J.-J.; Ilunga, B.; Piarroux, R. Dynamics of cholera outbreaks in Great Lakes region of Africa, 1978–2008. *Emerg. Infect. Dis.* **2011**, *17*, 2026–2034. [CrossRef] [PubMed]
8. Weill, F.-X.; Domman, D.; Bercion, R.; Luquero, F.J.; Ngandjio, A.; Dosso, M.; Monakhova, E.; Garin, B.; Bouchier, C.; Pazzani, C.; et al. Genomic history of the seventh pandemic of cholera in Africa. *Science* **2017**, *358*, 785–789. [CrossRef] [PubMed]
9. Cholera Most Affected Countries. Available online: https://worldhealthorg.shinyapps.io/page8cholera_most_affected_countries/ (accessed on 24 March 2023).
10. Goma Epidemiology Group. Public health impact of Rwandan refugee crisis: What happened in Goma, Zaire, in July, 1994? *Lancet Lond. Engl.* **1995**, *345*, 339–344. [CrossRef]
11. Plan Stratégique Multisectoriel d'Elimination du Choléra en République Démocratique du Congo 2013–2017—Democratic Republic of the Congo | ReliefWeb. Published 13 March 2015. Available online: https://reliefweb.int/report/democratic-republic-congo/plan-strat-gique-multisectoriel-d-elimination-du-chol-ra-en-r (accessed on 24 March 2023).
12. de Figueiredo, A.; Simas, C.; Karafillakis, E.; Paterson, P.; Larson, H.J. Mapping global trends in vaccine confidence and investigating barriers to vaccine uptake: A large-scale retrospective temporal modelling study. *Lancet* **2020**, *396*, 898–908. [CrossRef] [PubMed]
13. Groenewald, C. To Vaccinate or Not? Decision-Making in the Time of COVID-19 Vaccines. *Cult. Stud. Crit. Methodol.* **2022**, *22*, 89–95. [CrossRef]
14. Baumgaertner, B.; Ridenhour, B.J.; Justwan, F.; Carlisle, J.E.; Miller, C.R. Risk of disease and willingness to vaccinate in the United States: A population-based survey. *PLoS Med.* **2020**, *17*, e1003354. [CrossRef]
15. Katoto, P.D.M.C.; Parker, S.; Coulson, N.; Pillay, N.; Cooper, S.; Jaca, A.; Mavundza, E.; Houston, G.; Groenewald, C.; Essack, Z.; et al. Predictors of COVID-19 Vaccine Hesitancy in South African Local Communities: The VaxScenes Study. *Vaccines* **2022**, *10*, 353. [CrossRef]
16. Simas, C.; Larson, H.J. Overcoming vaccine hesitancy in low-income and middle-income regions. *Nat. Rev. Dis. Primer.* **2021**, *7*, 41. [CrossRef]
17. RDC: 2 Millions de Personnes Ciblées par une Campagne de Vaccination Contre le Choléra (OMS) | ONU Info. Published 28 December 2021. Available online: https://news.un.org/fr/story/2021/12/1111362 (accessed on 24 March 2023).
18. Amani, A.; Bama, S.N.; Dia, M.; Lekelem, S.N.; Linjouom, A.; Makembe, H.M.; Njoh, A.A.; Lekeumo, F.Z.C.; Eyebe, S.; Nguefack-Tsague, G.; et al. Challenges, best practices, and lessons learned from oral cholera mass vaccination campaign in urban Cameroon during the COVID-19 era. *Vaccine* **2022**, *40*, 6873–6879. [CrossRef] [PubMed]
19. Deen, J.; Clemens, J.D. Licensed and Recommended Inactivated Oral CholeraVaccines: From Development to Innovative Deployment. *Trop. Med. Infect. Dis.* **2021**, *6*, 32. [CrossRef] [PubMed]
20. MacDonald, N.E.; Eskola, J.; Liang, X.; Chaudhuri, M.; Dube, E.; Gellin, B.; Goldstein, S.; Larson, H.; Manzo, M.L.; Reingold, A.; et al. Vaccine hesitancy: Definition, scope and determinants. *Vaccine* **2015**, *33*, 4161–4164. [CrossRef] [PubMed]
21. Ten Health Issues WHO Will Tackle This Year. Available online: https://www.who.int/news-room/spotlight/ten-threats-to-global-health-in-2019 (accessed on 24 March 2023).
22. COVID-19 Vaccines | WHO COVID-19 Dashboard. Datadot. Available online: http://data.who.int/dashboards/covid19/vaccines (accessed on 2 April 2024).
23. Bukavu, Democratic Republic of the Congo Population (2023)—Population Stat. Available online: https://populationstat.com/democratic-republic-of-the-congo/bukavu (accessed on 26 March 2023).

24. WHO. Understanding the Behavioural and Social Drivers of Vaccine Uptake WHO Position Paper—May 2022. *Wkly. Epidemiol. Rec.* **2022**, *97*, 209–224.
25. Data Collection on KoboCollect App (Older Version)—KoboToolbox Documentation. Available online: https://support.kobotoolbox.org/kobocollect-android.html (accessed on 24 March 2023).
26. Massing, L.A.; Aboubakar, S.; Blake, A.; Page, A.-L.; Cohuet, S.; Ngandwe, A.; Sompwe, E.M.; Ramazani, R.; Allheimen, M.; Levaillant, P.; et al. Highly targeted cholera vaccination campaigns in urban setting are feasible: The experience in Kalemie, Democratic Republic of Congo. *PLoS Negl. Trop. Dis.* **2018**, *12*, e0006369. [CrossRef] [PubMed]
27. Peprah, D.; Palmer, J.J.; Rubin, G.J.; Abubakar, A.; Costa, A.; Martin, S.; Perea, W.; Larson, H.J. Perceptions of oral cholera vaccine and reasons for full, partial and non-acceptance during a humanitarian crisis in South Sudan. *Vaccine* **2016**, *34*, 3823–3827. [CrossRef] [PubMed]
28. Schaetti, C.; Ali, S.M.; Chaignat, C.L.; Khatib, A.M.; Hutubessy, R.; Weiss, M.G. Improving Community Coverage of Oral Cholera Mass Vaccination Campaigns: Lessons Learned in Zanzibar. *PLoS ONE* **2012**, *7*, e41527. [CrossRef]
29. Heyerdahl, L.W.; Ngwira, B.; Demolis, R.; Nyirenda, G.; Mwesawina, M.; Rafael, F.; Cavailler, P.; Le Gargasson, J.B.; Mengel, M.A.; Gessner, B.D.; et al. Innovative vaccine delivery strategies in response to a cholera outbreak in the challenging context of Lake Chilwa. A rapid qualitative assessment. *Vaccine* **2018**, *36*, 6491–6496. [CrossRef]
30. Démolis, R.; Botão, C.; Heyerdahl, L.W.; Gessner, B.D.; Cavailler, P.; Sinai, C.; Magaço, A.; Le Gargasson, J.-B.; Mengel, M.; Guillermet, E. A rapid qualitative assessment of oral cholera vaccine anticipated acceptability in a context of resistance towards cholera intervention in Nampula, Mozambique. *Vaccine* **2018**, *36*, 6497–6505. [CrossRef] [PubMed]
31. Viskupič, F.; Wiltse, D.L. The Messenger Matters: Religious Leaders and Overcoming COVID-19 Vaccine Hesitancy. *PS Polit. Sci. Polit.* **2022**, *55*, 504–509. [CrossRef]
32. Choi, Y.; Fox, A.M. Mistrust in public health institutions is a stronger predictor of vaccine hesitancy and uptake than Trust in Trump. *Soc. Sci. Med.* **2022**, *314*, 115440. [CrossRef] [PubMed]
33. Trent, M.; Seale, H.; Chughtai, A.A.; Salmon, D.; MacIntyre, C.R. Trust in government, intention to vaccinate and COVID-19 vaccine hesitancy: A comparative survey of five large cities in the United States, United Kingdom, and Australia. *Vaccine* **2022**, *40*, 2498–2505. [CrossRef] [PubMed]
34. Tram, K.H.; Saeed, S.; Bradley, C.; Fox, B.; Eshun-Wilson, I.; Mody, A.; Geng, E. Deliberation, Dissent, and Distrust: Understanding Distinct Drivers of Coronavirus Disease 2019 Vaccine Hesitancy in the United States. *Clin. Infect. Dis. Off. Publ. Infect. Dis. Soc. Am.* **2022**, *74*, 1429–1441. [CrossRef] [PubMed]
35. Infodemic Management of WHO Information Net Work for Epidemics. Available online: https://www.who.int/teams/epi-win/infodemic-management (accessed on 24 March 2023).
36. Dash, S.; Parray, A.A.; De Freitas, L.; Mithu, I.H.; Rahman, M.; Ramasamy, A.; Pandya, A.K. Combating the COVID-19 infodemic: A three-level approach for low and middle-income countries. *BMJ Glob. Health* **2021**, *6*, e004671. [CrossRef]
37. Dodd, R.H.; Pickles, K.; Cvejic, E.; Cornell, S.; Isautier, J.M.; Copp, T.; Nickel, B.; Bonner, C.; Batcup, C.; Muscat, D.M.; et al. Perceived public health threat a key factor for willingness to get the COVID-19 vaccine in Australia. *Vaccine* **2022**, *40*, 2484–2490. [CrossRef] [PubMed]
38. Zhang, H.; Li, Y.; Peng, S.; Jiang, Y.; Jin, H.; Zhang, F. The effect of health literacy on COVID-19 vaccine hesitancy among community population in China: The moderating role of stress. *Vaccine* **2022**, *40*, 4473–4478. [CrossRef] [PubMed]
39. Bajos, N.; Spire, A.; Silberzan, L.; Sireyjol, A.; Jusot, F.; Meyer, L.; Franck, J.-E.; Warszawski, J.; The EpiCov Study Group. When Lack of Trust in the Government and in Scientists Reinforces Social Inequalities in Vaccination Against COVID-19. *Front. Public Health* **2022**, *10*, 908152. Available online: https://www.frontiersin.org/articles/10.3389/fpubh.2022.908152 (accessed on 24 March 2023). [CrossRef]
40. Sato, R. COVID-19 Vaccine Hesitancy and Trust in Government in Nigeria. *Vaccines* **2022**, *10*, 1008. [CrossRef]

vaccines

MDPI

Article

The Costs and Cost-Effectiveness of a Two-Dose Oral Cholera Vaccination Campaign: A Case Study in a Refugee Camp Setting in Thailand

Aaron S. Wallace [1,*], Kashmira Date [1], Sarah W. Pallas [1], Nuttapong Wongjindanon [2], Christina R. Phares [3] and Taiwo Abimbola [1]

1 Global Immunization Division, US Centers for Disease Control and Prevention, 1600 Clifton Rd NE, Mailstop H24-2, Atlanta, GA 30329, USA
2 Thailand Ministry of Public Health, U.S. Centers for Disease Control and Prevention Collaboration, Ministry of Public Health, Tiwanon Road, Nonthaburi 11000, Thailand
3 Division of Global Migration Health, Centers for Disease Control and Prevention, 1600 Clifton Rd NE, Mailstop H16-4, Atlanta, GA 30329, USA
* Correspondence: ccu7@cdc.gov

Abstract: Oral cholera vaccination (OCV) campaigns are increasingly used to prevent cholera outbreaks; however, little is known about their cost-effectiveness in refugee camps. We conducted a cost-effectiveness analysis of a pre-emptive OCV campaign in the Maela refugee camp in Thailand, where outbreaks occurred with an annual incidence rate (IR) of up to 10.7 cases per 1000. Data were collected via health sector records and interviews and household interviews. In the base-case scenario comparing the OCV campaign with no campaign, we estimated the campaign effect on the cholera IR and case fatality rate (CFR: 0.09%) from a static cohort model and calculated incremental cost-effectiveness ratios for the outcomes of death, disability-adjusted life-years (DALYs), and cases averted. In sensitivity analyses, we varied the CFR and IR. The household economic cost of illness was USD 21, and the health sector economic cost of illness was USD 51 per case. The OCV campaign economic cost was USD 289,561, 42% attributable to vaccine costs and 58% to service delivery costs. In our base case, the incremental cost was USD 1.9 million per death averted, USD 1745 per case averted, and USD 69,892 per DALY averted. Sensitivity analyses that increased the CFR to 0.35% or the IR to 10.4 cases per 1000 resulted in a cost per DALY of USD 15,666. The low multi-year average CFR and incidence of the cholera outbreaks in the Maela camp were key factors associated with the high cost per DALY averted. However, the sensitivity analyses indicated higher cost-effectiveness in a setting with a higher CFR or cholera incidence, indicating when to consider campaign use to reduce the outbreak risk.

Keywords: cholera; oral cholera vaccine; vaccination campaign; cost; cost-effectiveness

1. Introduction

In 2017, there were an estimated 21 million refugees globally, with approximately one-third living in camps and nearly one-half under the age of 14 [1]. Refugee camps can be particularly vulnerable to outbreaks of cholera disease due to crowding, poor sanitation, and poor housing infrastructure [2]. Bacteria that cause cholera infections are generally spread by contaminated water and food. Once contracted, cholera can cause severe diarrhea, leading to dehydration and death [3]. In cholera epidemics within refugee camp settings, case fatality rates (CFRs) can vary between 1% to over 50%, with this wide variation being due to treatment resource availability and sanitation-related behavioral factors to effectively manage these outbreaks [4–6]. Overcrowding and precarious conditions, such as those in refugee settings, may create an environment conducive to its rapid spread.

Increasingly, mass cholera vaccination campaigns are used to help reduce the incidence of or eliminate cholera in high-risk or outbreak settings [4]. In a 2017 position statement, the WHO recommended OCV use in endemic settings [3]. Prior experiences with OCV use (mainly Dukoral®, manufactured by Valvena Sweden AB, Solna, Sweden) in stable refugee settings have suggested the feasibility and utility of cholera vaccination in these situations, indicating that there may be real gains in cholera prevention and control with OCV use in such settings. As of 2024, the World Health Organization has pre-qualified three oral cholera vaccines: Dukoral®, Shanchol™ (manufactured by Sanofi Healthcare India Private Limited, Mumbai, India), and Euvichol-Plus® (manufactured by EuBiologics Co. Ltd., Seoul, Republic of Korea) [3]. Dukoral® is administered with a buffer solution and requires two doses for two years of protection for individuals over 5 years of age and three doses for children aged 2–5 years. Shanchol™ and Euvichol-Plus® do not require a buffer solution and can be safely given to individuals over 1 year of age, with two doses providing 3 years of protection. All three vaccines have a good safety profile based on results from multiple clinical trials [3].

Studies to document the impact, costs, and cost-effectiveness of OCV campaigns have been conducted in Tanzania, Bangladesh, and Indonesia [7–10]. Additional studies in Ethiopia, Haiti, and Malawi have examined OCV campaign costs only [11,12]; however, there are no published studies on the costs and cost-effectiveness of an OCV campaign within a refugee camp setting, in which the costs and cost-effectiveness may differ. In this study, we estimated the costs of the 2013 OCV campaign, the cost of cholera illness, and the cost-effectiveness of the vaccination campaign in a refugee camp setting [13]. Our findings aim to broadly inform the value of OCV vaccination for specialized populations, such as the Maela refugee camp in Thailand. In particular, the Thailand Ministry of Population and Health viewed the implementation of this OCV campaign as an effort to gain experience and develop strategies for OCV delivery in cholera-prone provinces and populations in the future; thus, conducting a cost-effectiveness analysis was a component of their analytical strategy.

2. Method

2.1. Study Setting and Population

The Maela camp is home to approximately 50,000 people who fled from Burma during the 1980s after a military regime came into power in Burma; it has been run by the United Nations High Commissioner for Refugees since 1984. The camp is located in a valley with a single road linking the camp to the nearest Thai city of Mae Sot, which is about one hour away by car. In 2005, the non-governmental organization (NGO) Premiere Urgence-Aide Medicale Internationale (PU-AMI) took over healthcare, water, and sanitation services for Maela and two other refugee camps.

The Maela camp has suffered multiple cholera outbreaks over the past 20 years, with the last confirmed cholera case occurring in 2010. In 2013, officials conducted a two-dose oral cholera vaccine (OCV) campaign for all 46,000 refugees in the camp to preemptively protect the population against a cholera outbreak. The 2013 OCV campaign used the Shanchol™ vaccine, which shares similar vaccine characteristics to the Dukoral vaccine in that both do not require a buffer solution for administration, and both can be given to all individuals over one year of age. Additional campaign details are documented elsewhere [13].

Lab-confirmed or presumed cases of cholera occurred in the camp in 2005, 2007, 2008, and 2010 [7]. These four outbreaks lasted between 17 and 26 weeks, with a total of 691 lab-confirmed cases and 1540 suspected cases during the 8-year period (2005–2012) leading up to the OCV campaign. The vast majority of reported cholera cases in Thailand were based in the Maela camp. Before 2008, some patients presenting with acute watery diarrhea (AWD) during lab-confirmed outbreaks were presumptively diagnosed with cholera, whereas after 2008, all patients seeking care for AWD during a confirmed outbreak were tested for cholera. During 2005–2012, the reported annual IR for confirmed or presumed cases ranged between 0.0 and 10.7 cases per 1000 refugees, with an annual average of 3.0 cases per 1000 individuals [13].

2.2. *Cost Analysis*

The cost analysis of the 2013 OCV campaign was conducted from the health sector and household perspectives. Cost data for the campaign were collected via reviews of financial records and interviews with involved organizations, and the costs of cholera illness were collected using household and health worker interviews. We calculated the costs separately by the health sector cost of illness (COI) per case, household COI per case, and OCV campaign cost. All costs were adjusted for inflation from 2013 to 2021 using the Thailand consumer price index and then converted to 2021 USD using the 2021 exchange rate of THB 33.98 to USD 1 [14,15]. The data analysis was conducted using Microsoft Excel 2013.

2.2.1. Health Sector Cost of Illness

We conducted semi-structured interviews of PU-AMI staff to ascertain the time spent treating cases of AWD and abstracted data from PU-AMI budgets of cholera treatment centers (CTCs) that were set up in previous cholera outbreaks. In the Maela camp, a CTC is only set up once a cholera case is confirmed; otherwise, the routine health sector in the camp is used for treating AWD cases and detecting and treating the first few suspected cholera cases in an outbreak. The health sector COI fixed costs comprised items and resources required to set up a cholera care and treatment center, such as tables, medical devices, chairs, water basins, and mats. The health sector COI variable costs included non-reusable items used in cholera care and treatment centers, such as cups, gloves, linens, and plastic bags, as well as variable costs of healthcare provider work hours per treated cholera case. The financial records contained information on CTC set-up expenses, medical supplies, patient material costs, and medicine costs. We calculated the health sector mean variable COI per case across the sample of cases, using the number of confirmed cases that occurred in the last Maela cholera outbreak of 2010 (N = 392).

2.2.2. Household Cost of Illness

As no cases of cholera had occurred in the camp since 2010, we used the cost of AWD illness as a proxy for the household COI for cholera. The illnesses generally have similar effects with regard to the length of illness and likely impact on days of work lost. In 2013, after the campaign, 40 primary cases of AWD were prospectively identified during discharge from health facilities and interviewed using a standardized questionnaire. For the purpose of this evaluation, we defined a case of AWD as any person aged 2 years or older who had three or more loose stools over 24 h, with or without concurrent vomiting. If the case had a caregiver, we interviewed the caregiver to ascertain workdays lost for the caregiver. We collected data on age, gender, monthly income, work details, travel time to/from the health facility, any incurred travel costs, length of diarrheal illness in days, length of time spent at the health facility, related healthcare costs (medicine, food, and treatment service payments), and number of days of missed work. We aimed to enroll 40 cases (based on the expected monthly volume of cases coming to facilities and the planned length of the data collection period) and conducted all interviews within one week of facility discharge. For cases of 2–17 years of age, the caregivers were interviewed about expenses incurred related to the case patient's illness as younger individuals may be unable to directly recall this information; for case patients of >17 years of age, the case patient was interviewed about their expenses related to the illness. Verbal consent was obtained from all interviewees. We calculated the mean household COI (at one week post-discharge) as the sum of the mean direct cost (i.e., the medical and non-medical costs incurred by households to treat or prevent illness) and the mean indirect cost (i.e., the monetary value of average daily wages lost by case patients and caregivers during the illness period) per case.

2.2.3. OCV Campaign Costs

PU-AMI, the Thailand Ministry of Public Health (MOPH), and the US Centers for Disease Control and Prevention (CDC) sponsored and implemented the two-dose OCV campaign in 2013. Two eight-day vaccination rounds occurred for all eligible individuals (over 1 year of age and not pregnant), with a two-day third round for those who had only received one OCV dose. The rounds were two weeks apart. In the two main vaccination rounds, 43,485 individuals were targeted. The first dose coverage was 81%, and the second dose coverage was 64%. Of the 90,000 OCV doses ordered, 63,085 OCV doses were administered, and 993 doses were wasted [13]. The 25,950 unused doses were repurposed for other OCV campaigns in Thailand, so only the 64,078 used doses were incorporated into the campaign cost estimates. The involved organizations provided cost data for the vaccine and service delivery from the health sector perspective. Detailed information about the campaign preparation and implementation is published elsewhere [13]. In short, PU-AMI conducted community-level informational meetings, circulated newsletters leading up to the campaign, and then set up vaccination campaign posts throughout the community during the campaign. Each post was staffed by 20–25 workers who screened individuals for eligibility (over 1 year of age and not pregnant) and issued vaccination cards. Costs from the household perspective to receive vaccination (i.e., costs and time spent on transport to and from the vaccination site) were calculated based on information provided through the survey of the 40 AWD cases regarding the duration of time traveling to/from a health facility, the proportion of those cases that reported paying for transport to/from the health facility, the proportion of cases who reported working, and their reported monthly salary.

We calculated the direct, indirect, and total OCV campaign costs and the cost per individual targeted and per fully vaccinated individual (FVI) from a societal (health sector and household) perspective. Direct OCV campaign costs included household costs of transport to the campaign session site, and indirect OCV campaign costs encompassed productivity losses due to time spent traveling to/from and receiving the vaccination at the vaccination post.

2.2.4. Cost-Effectiveness Analysis

To calculate the incremental cost-effectiveness, we compared a scenario where an OCV campaign occurred with a scenario where no OCV campaign occurred. In each scenario, we calculated the cost of treatment, OCV campaign, number of estimated cases, deaths, and DALYs and then calculated the differences between each scenario to arrive at an incremental value for each output (Table 1). Our analytic horizon was the three-year period after the campaign occurred, based on the estimated length of protection after OCV vaccination [3].

Table 1. External inputs for burden of cholera disease and oral cholera vaccine (OCV) campaign effectiveness conducted in Maela camp, Thailand, in 2013 for calculating cost-effectiveness.

Component	Description	Data Source	Base Case Value (Sensitivity Analysis Value)
Observed average cholera incidence	Historical cholera incidence observed in camp (2005–2013)	Government disease surveillance system	3.0 (10.0)
Cholera case fatality rate	Historical cholera case fatality rate observed in camp (2005–2013)	Government disease surveillance system	0.09% (0.35%)
Cholera illness duration	Average duration of cholera illness in days	[9]	4 days
Life expectancy	Average life expectancy	Government surveillance system data and World Bank [14]	51 years
OCV effectiveness	Vaccine effectiveness for two doses of Shanchol™ vaccine	[9]	65%
OCV duration of protection	Duration of vaccination protection for Shanchol™ vaccine	[9]	3 years

Table 1. *Cont.*

Component	Description	Data Source	Base Case Value (Sensitivity Analysis Value)
OCV campaign coverage	2013 OCV campaign 2-dose coverage	[13]	64% (100%)
GDP per capita	2017 Thailand GDP per capita	[14]	USD 6593
DALY weight	DALY weight for cholera illness	[16]	0.202

COI: cost of illness; OCV: oral cholera vaccination; VE: vaccine effectiveness; GDP: gross domestic product; DALY: disability-adjusted life years. Monetary values given in 2017 USD unless otherwise stated.

2.3. *Incremental Effectiveness of OCV Campaign*

We calculated the incremental effect of the campaign by calculating the difference in disease outcomes (deaths, cases, and DALYs) between each scenario (campaign versus no campaign) using a static cohort model. We used 2005–2013 data on the annual cholera incidence rate (IR) and annual cholera deaths derived from the disease surveillance system managed by PU-AMI and MOPH in the camp for the non-campaign scenario.

We then estimated the effect of the OCV campaign on cholera incidence, incorporating both the surveillance system data and other information on life expectancy after infection, disability weights, and duration of immunity as outlined in the approaches by Jeuland and Troeger [8,9] that are based on approaches outlined in the Disease Control Priorities Project [17].

The majority of data used in the scenario calculations were derived from our primary data collection efforts in the Maela camp and from the PU-AMI-managed disease surveillance system data, including the 2005–2013 observed CFR of 0.09%. The external data used were for vaccine efficacy (65% for two doses), disability weight for cholera (0.202), length of OCV protection (three years), and life expectancy at the age of infection (51 years) [8,9,18–20] (Table 1).

2.4. *Incremental Net Cost of OCV Campaign Versus No OCV Campaign*

We calculated the incremental cost of the campaign by calculating the difference in cost between each scenario (campaign versus no campaign). We used the following formula to calculate this difference:

Incremental cost of OCV campaign = [(Household COI + health sector COI) × (number of cases with OCV campaign) + (OCV campaign cost)] − [(Household COI + health sector COI) × (number of cases without OCV campaign)]

2.5. *Incremental Cost-Effectiveness Ratio Calculation*

We calculated the incremental cost-effectiveness ratios (ICER) for deaths, cases, and DALYs averted by the campaign by dividing the incremental cost of the campaign by the incremental effects of the campaign over the three-year period of assumed constant vaccine protection of 65%. To calculate the difference in DALYs between the campaign and non-campaign scenario (i.e., DALYs averted), we used the following formulas, assuming no age weighting:

Years of life lost to disability (YLD) averted_t = [((1 − CFR) × (vaccine efficacy_i) × (OCV campaign coverage) × (Population size) × (disease incidence)) × (duration of illness) × (disability weight)]

Years of life lost (YLL) averted = [(CFR × (vaccine efficacy) × (population size) × (OCV campaign coverage) × (disease incidence))/0.03] × [1 − exp(−0.03 × (life expectancy)]

DALYs averted_t = YLD_t averted + YLL_t averted

$$\text{Total DALYs averted} = \sum_{t=0}^{2} (\text{DALYs averted}_t)/(1+0.03)^t$$

where *t* is the year of the estimate (t = 0 is the first year after the vaccination campaign, and t = 2 is the third year after the vaccination campaign), and CFR is the observed case fatality rate for 2005–2013 (0.09%). We also conducted sensitivity analyses by varying the IR, CFR, campaign coverage, and COI to determine how much these indicators influenced the cost-effectiveness of the intervention. Lastly, we used the current guidance provided by the Thailand Health Intervention and Technology Assessment Program (HITAP) within the Ministry of Health to assess the health intervention cost-effectiveness as a proxy reference for a cost-effectiveness threshold for our analysis [21,22]. Based on research completed in the Thai healthcare setting on willingness to pay for a quality-adjusted life year (QALY), the current cost-effectiveness threshold, set in 2013, is THB 160,000, equivalent to USD 4708 in 2021 USD. This latter threshold was considered a proxy in this study, as we calculated an ICER in cost per DALYs. Previous studies have indicated the relevance of using QALYs and DALYs interchangeably [23].

3. Results

3.1. Household and Health Sector Cost of Illness

From the household perspective, the average direct and indirect COI per case were USD 3 and USD 18, respectively, summing up to a household economic COI of USD 21 per case or 30% of the mean monthly household income (USD 72) among surveyed households (Table 2). The direct medical costs were USD 1 per case, and the direct non-medical costs were USD 2, including transport costs (USD 0.20 per case) and food costs (USD 2). The indirect costs encompassed productivity losses due to time spent on treatment at the facility (USD 5 per case), time spent on travel (USD 2 per case), and time spent with illness at home (USD 13 per case). At the health sector level, the fixed and variable COI per case were USD 26 (52%) and USD 25 (48%), respectively (Table 2), summing up to a health sector economic COI of USD 51. The combined household and health sector economic COI was USD 72 per case, of which 72% was health sector costs, while 28% was household costs.

Table 2. Direct and indirect costs per case of cholera illness by perspective (household or health sector) in Maela camp in Thailand in 2013 in 2021 USD.

Household Cost of Illness	Mean Cost per Case (Standard Deviation)	% Total Cost
Direct medical		
Medicine and treatment services	USD 1.19 (USD 0.31)	6%
Direct non-medical		
Food	USD 1.85 (USD 0.44)	9%
Transport	USD 0.20 (USD 0.03)	1%
Indirect		
Lost income for case	USD 6.76 (USD 1.42)	32%
Lost income for caregiver	USD 11.03 (USD 2.36)	53%
Total household COI	USD 21.03 (USD 3.91)	100%
Health sector cost of illness		
Fixed cost	USD 26.43 (USD 4.14)	52%
Variable cost	USD 24.60 (USD 4.01)	48%
Total health sector COI	USD 51.03 (USD 7.93)	100%
Total COI (household + health sector)	USD 72.06 (USD 9.48)	

3.2. OCV Campaign Cost

The total cost of the OCV campaign was USD 289,561, consisting of USD 239,537 (80%) in health sector costs and USD 57,589 (20%) in household costs (Table 3). The total campaign costs per fully vaccinated individual (FVI) and per targeted individual were USD 10.47 and USD 6.67, respectively. The health sector direct costs included USD 122,977 for the vaccine used in this campaign (42% of total campaign costs, with USD 4.45 per FVI). The purchase price for two doses of the vaccine (a full course for a single individual) was USD 3.82. For vaccination delivery activities in the two campaign rounds, the health sector cost was USD 108,993 (38% of the total campaign costs, with USD 3.94 per FVI and USD 2.51 per targeted individual). From the health sector perspective, the vaccination delivery direct costs included USD 48,910 for cold chain equipment and fuel, USD 24,488 for vaccination materials (health cards, cups, and water), USD 14,985 for campaign staff remuneration, USD 13,984 for community mobilization materials, and USD 7115 for the transport of vaccines and materials. From the household perspective, the vaccine delivery direct costs consisted of USD 12,611 for transport costs (USD 0.46 per FVI), and the indirect costs consisted of USD 44,978 (USD 0.81 per FVI) in lost wages due to the household time spent attending the campaign. Based on a total of 63,057 doses administered (including first and second doses), the total cost per dose delivered was USD 4.59, the health sector cost per dose delivered was USD 3.68, and the household cost per dose delivered was USD 0.91.

Table 3. Total costs per targeted and fully vaccinated individual (FVI) associated with 2013 oral cholera vaccine (OCV) campaign in Maela camp in Thailand in 2021 USD.

	Total [1]	Per Targeted Individual [2]	Per FVI [3]	Per Dose
	Health sector cost			
Vaccine	USD 122,977 [1]	USD 2.83	USD 4.45	USD 1.95
Service delivery	USD 108,993	USD 2.51	USD 3.94	USD 1.73
	Household direct cost			
Transport	USD 12,611	USD 0.29	USD 0.46	USD 0.21
Household indirect cost				
Lost wages	USD 44,978	USD 1.04	USD 0.81	USD 0.70
Total cost	USD 289,561	USD 6.67	USD 10.47	USD 4.59

[1]. Total costs for two OCV rounds with target population of 43,485 individuals per round, with 81% coverage in first round and 64% coverage in second round. [2]. Cost per targeted individual based on target population of 43,485 individuals. [3]. Cost per fully vaccinated individual (FVI), where 64% of targets received two OCV doses (fully vaccinated).

3.3. Cost-Effectiveness

In the base case scenario, the OCV campaign was estimated to have averted 161 cases, 0.15 deaths, and 4.03 DALYs over the course of the 3-year duration of vaccine protection at an incremental cost of USD 281,336 (Table 4). The ICER for each outcome was USD 1,939,424 per death averted, USD 1745 per case averted, and USD 69,892 per DALY averted.

Table 4. Cost-effectiveness of 2013 oral cholera vaccine (OCV) campaign in base case scenario in Maela camp in Thailand in 2021 USD.

	Vaccination	No Vaccination	Difference (Vaccination Minus No Vaccination)
Effects			
Number of cases	226	387	−161
Number of deaths	0.20	0.35	−0.15
DALY averted over 3-year period of vaccination protection [1]	5.77	9.80	−4.03
Costs, 2021 USD			
Cost of vaccination program	USD 289,561	USD 0	USD 289,561
Health sector cost of illness	USD 11,547	USD 19,772	−USD 8225
Cost of treatment and vaccination program (incremental cost)	USD 301,108	USD 19,772	−USD 281,336
Cost-effectiveness ratios, 2021 USD			
ICER (case): incremental costs/case averted			USD 1745
ICER (death): incremental costs/death averted			USD 1,939,424
ICER (DALY): incremental costs/DALY (over duration of vaccination protection [1]) averted			USD 69,892

[1]: duration of vaccine protection against cholera estimated at 3 years, using a 3% discount rate.

In the sensitivity analysis scenarios, the ICER per DALY averted decreased to USD 15,666, with an annual incidence rate of 10.4 cases per 1000 individuals, and to USD 15,603 or a CFR of 0.35%, roughly three times the Thai cost-effectiveness threshold. If the OCV campaign had achieved 100% two-dose coverage, the ICER per DALY averted would have decreased to USD 57,621. If both the household and health sector COI were to be included at USD 72 per case, the ICER per DALY averted would decrease to USD 56,638.

If we assume the campaign to be the reason for the lack of any reported cholera cases during the three-year time horizon after the campaign, the cost per death and DALY averted would decrease to USD 559,416 and USD 52,811, respectively.

4. Discussion

In our study, the first to examine the cost-effectiveness of an OCV campaign in a refugee camp setting, we estimated that the incremental cost of the OCV campaign was USD 281,336 in our base case scenario, while the ICERs per death averted, per DALY averted, and per cholera case averted were USD 1.9 million, USD 69,892 and USD 1745, respectively. The aim of our study was not to inform a particular government decision in Thailand, and our findings suggest that this campaign would not be cost-effective using the willingness to pay thresholds (WTPs), such as the World Health Organization's three times gross domestic product per capita or the Health Intervention and Technology Assessment Program (HITAP) [24]. There is no conventional WTP threshold recommendation for refugee settings; however, it is noteworthy that the campaign could be cost-effective using the WHO thresholds in the scenario of higher cholera incidence rates (>10.0 cases per 1000 individuals) or a higher cholera CFR (>0.35%). The historical average annual CFR in the Maela camp is extremely low compared with other country settings where cholera outbreaks have occurred, with CFRs reported between 0.5% and 3% [7–10]. The very low CFR in Maela might indicate the ability of the local NGO, PU-AMI, to respond quickly with treatment for cholera cases when outbreaks have occurred, thereby nearly eliminating the risk of cholera-related death over the past ten years. Considering the vulnerability of refugee camps to outbreaks of cholera disease due to crowding, poor sanitation, and poor housing infrastructure, global health decision-makers, including non-governmental organizations financially responsible for refugee health, could consider the value of cholera vaccination in settings of high cholera incidence and high CFRs.

We used a static cohort model to estimate the post-campaign effects on cholera incidence and death, with 65% efficacy with two doses of the Shankol^{TM} vaccine, and, thus, the continued occurrence of cholera cases; however, surveillance system data from 2012 to 2015 indicate no cholera cases detected since the campaign.

In recent studies from Tanzania and elsewhere [7–9], results about the cost-effectiveness of OCV campaigns are mixed, largely due to variations in the assumed disease incidence rates and CFRs or the GDP per capita upon which the thresholds for cost-effectiveness are based. Higher health sector COI values were observed in Maela compared with Indonesia, India, and Bangladesh but lower compared with Tanzania. The household COI in Maela was about half the reported household COI from Tanzania. Costs for vaccine administration and the vaccine (USD 6.67 per targeted individual) were well below those reported elsewhere, which may be largely due to the confined nature of the camp and the decreasing cost of the Shankol^{TM} vaccine. Due to the relatively lower costs of OCV in the Maela camp campaign, the cost ratio between vaccine and delivery was about 50:50; in comparison, the Tanzania study, as well as studies from Vietnam, reported a ratio of approximately 25:75.

A number of study limitations exist. We used a convenience sample of household members, which may not represent the costs of illness for all cases. These individuals only provided information about costs one week after illness, so costs of any long-term sequelae (e.g., coma or renal failure) were not included. We also used the cost of AWD illness as a substitute for the cost of cholera illness. To the extent that cholera-specific symptoms and sequelae may differ from those of other causes of AWD, our COI estimates may not accurately reflect the cholera-specific COI [9,10]. The data we used to estimate the effects of the OCV campaign were based on historical surveillance system data, which could underestimate the true number of cholera cases that occurred [23]; however, due to the small and confined geographical nature of the camp and the active engagement of PU-AMI in the area, the surveillance system is likely more sensitive than similar systems in other low- and middle-income countries, where data quality can be a concern [25]. These results can remain valuable for many years into the future; however, it would be important to make additional inflation-associated adjustments to compare with the current costs of care. Shanchol™, alongside Euvichol™, which is essentially the same vaccine, are the main vaccines used for mass vaccination campaigns; thus, this analysis of a Shanchol™-based 2013 campaign continues to remain relevant for decision-makers.

5. Conclusions

Our sensitivity analysis indicates the key drivers under which this campaign would be substantially more cost-effective and should be key considerations when deciding on the use of an OCV campaign in a refugee camp setting. The cholera incidence rates and CFRs at which the OCV campaign would have been substantially more cost-effective were observed in Maela in one previous year of our study time frame and were at levels that are likely to be observed in other refugee camp settings where the infrastructure and organizational management may be much weaker than those available in the Maela camp. Our findings provide evidence to support the continued consideration of OCV campaigns in settings likely to have high incidence and case fatality rates as a key strategy for reducing the risk of cholera outbreaks.

Author Contributions: Conceptualization, A.S.W., K.D., S.W.P., N.W, C.R.P. and T.A.; methodology, A.S.W., K.D., S.W.P. and T.A.; validation, S.W.P. and T.A.; formal analysis, A.S.W., K.D., S.W.P. and T.A.; investigation, A.S.W., K.D., S.W.P., N.W, C.R.P. and T.A.; resources, K.D., N.W. and C.R.P.; data curation, K.D., N.W. and C.R.P.; writing—original draft preparation, A.S.W. and K.D.; writing—review and editing, A.S.W., K.D., S.W.P., N.W., C.R.P. and T.A.; visualization, A.S.W.; supervision, K.D., S.W.P. and T.A.; project administration, A.S.W., K.D. and T.A. All authors have read and agreed to the published version of the manuscript.

Funding: This research received no external funding.

Institutional Review Board Statement: The Human Subject Office in the Center for Global Health at the US Centers for Disease Control and Prevention approved the assessment as a non-research public health activity.

Informed Consent Statement: Informed consent was obtained from all individuals who were interviewed during data collection activities for this cost-effectiveness analysis.

Data Availability Statement: The datasets used and/or analyzed during the current study are available from the corresponding author upon reasonable request.

Conflicts of Interest: The authors declare no conflicts of interest.

References

1. *Global Trends, Forced Displacement in 2020*; UNHCR, The UN Refugee Agency: Copenhagen, Denmark, 2021.
2. Toole, M.J.; Waldman, R.J. The public health aspects of complex emergencies and refugee situations 1. *Annu. Rev. Public Health* **1997**, *18*, 283–312. [CrossRef] [PubMed]
3. World Health Organization, Cholera vaccines: WHO position paper—Recommendations. *Vaccine* **2017**, *34*, 477–500.
4. Naficy, A.; Rao, M.R.; Paquet, C.; Antona, D.; Sorkin, A.; Clemens, J.D. Treatment and vaccination strategies to control cholera in sub-Saharan refugee settings: A cost-effectiveness analysis. *JAMA* **1998**, *279*, 521–525. [CrossRef] [PubMed]
5. Waldman, R.J. Cholera vaccination in refugee settings. *JAMA* **1998**, *279*, 552–553. [CrossRef] [PubMed]
6. Tauxe, R.V.; Blake, P.A. Epidemic cholera in Latin America. *JAMA* **1992**, *267*, 1388–1390. [CrossRef] [PubMed]
7. Schaetti, C.; Weiss, M.G.; Ali, S.M.; Chaignat, C.L.; Khatib, A.M.; Reyburn, R.; Tebbens, R.J.D.; Hutubessy, R. Costs of illness due to cholera, costs of immunization and cost-effectiveness of an oral cholera mass vaccination campaign in Zanzibar. *PLoS Neglected Trop. Dis.* **2012**, *6*, e1844. [CrossRef] [PubMed]
8. Troeger, C.; Sack, D.A.; Chao, D.L. Evaluation of targeted mass cholera vaccination strategies in Bangladesh: A demonstration of a new cost-effectiveness calculator. *Am. J. Trop. Med. Hyg.* **2014**, *91*, 1181–1189. [CrossRef] [PubMed]

9. Jeuland, M.; Cook, J.; Poulos, C.; Clemens, J.; Whittington, D. Cost-Effectiveness of New-Generation Oral Cholera Vaccines: A Multisite Analysis. *Value Health* **2009**, *12*, 899–908. [CrossRef] [PubMed]
10. Hsiao, A.; Hall, A.H.; Mogasale, V.; Quentin, W. The health economics of cholera: A systematic review. *Vaccine* **2018**, *36*, 4404–4424. [CrossRef] [PubMed]
11. Ilboudo, P.G.; Le Gargasson, J.-B. Delivery cost analysis of a reactive mass cholera vaccination campaign: A case study of Shanchol™ vaccine use in Lake Chilwa, Malawi. *BMC Infect. Dis.* **2017**, *17*, 779. [CrossRef] [PubMed]
12. Teshome, S.; Desai, S.; Kim, J.H.; Belay, D.; Mogasale, V. Feasibility and costs of a targeted cholera vaccination campaign in Ethiopia. *Hum. Vaccines Immunother.* **2018**, *14*, 2427–2433. [CrossRef] [PubMed]
13. Phares, C.R.; Date, K.; Travers, P.; Deglise, C.; Wongjindanon, N.; Ortega, L.; Bhuket, P.R. Mass vaccination with a two-dose oral cholera vaccine in a long-standing refugee camp, Thailand. *Vaccine* **2016**, *34*, 128–133. [CrossRef] [PubMed]
14. World Bank. World Development Indicators: Official Exchange Rates. Available online: http://databank.worldbank.org/data/reports.aspx?source=2&series=PA.NUS.FCRF&country= (accessed on 28 October 2024).
15. World Bank. Consumer Price Index. Available online: https://data.worldbank.org/indicator/FP.CPI.TOTL?end=2021&locations=TH&start=1960&view=chart (accessed on 28 October 2024).
16. Salomon, J.A.; Vos, T.; Hogan, D.R.; Gagnon, M.; Naghavi, M.; Mokdad, A.; Begum, N.; Shah, R.; Karyana, M.; Kosen, S.; et al. Common values in assessing health outcomes from disease and injury: Disability weights measurement study for the Global Burden of Disease Study 2010. *Lancet* **2013**, *380*, 2129–2143. [CrossRef] [PubMed]
17. Jamison, D.; TBreman, J.; Measham, A.; Alleyne, G.; Claeson, M.; Evans, D. Disease Control Priorities Project. In *Disease Control Priorities in Developing Countries*; Oxford University Press: New York, NY, USA, 2006.
18. Wang, H.; Naghavi, M.; Allen, C.; Barber, R.; Carter, A.; Casey, D.; Charlson, F.; Chen, A.; Coates, M.; Coggeshall, M. Global, regional, and national life expectancy, all-cause mortality, and cause-specific mortality for 249 causes of death, 1980–2015: A systematic analysis for the Global Burden of Disease Study 2015. *Lancet* **2016**, *388*, 1459–1544. [CrossRef] [PubMed]
19. Bhattacharya, S.K.; Sur, D.; Ali, M.; Kanungo, S.; You, Y.A.; Manna, B.; Sah, B.; Niyogi, S.K.; Park, J.K.; Sarkar, B. 5 year efficacy of a bivalent killed whole-cell oral cholera vaccine in Kolkata, India: A cluster-randomised, double-blind, placebo-controlled trial. *Lancet Infect. Dis.* **2013**, *13*, 1050–1056. [CrossRef]
20. Sinclair, D.; Abba, K.; Zaman, K.; Qadri, F.; Graves, P.M. *Oral Vaccines for Preventing Cholera*; The Cochrane Library: London, UK, 2011.
21. Thavorncharoensap, M.; Teerawattananon, Y.; Natanant, S.; Kulpeng, W.; Yothasamut, J.; Werayingyong, P. Estimating the willingness to pay for a quality-adjusted life year in Thailand: Does the context of healht gain matter? *Clin. Outomces Res.* **2013**, *5*, 29–36. [CrossRef] [PubMed]
22. Revill, P.; Ochalek, J.; Lomas, J.; Nakamura, R.; Woods, B.; Rollinger, A.; Suhrcke, M.; Sculpher, M.; Claxton, K. Cost-Effectiveness Thresholds: Guiding Health Care Spending for Population Health Improvement; Centre for Health Economics, University of York. November 2015. Available online: http://www.idsihealth.org/wp-content/uploads/2015/01/CE-Thresholds-iDSI-Working-Group-Final-Report.pdf (accessed on 28 October 2024).
23. Augustovski FColantonioa, L.D.; Galante, J.; Bardach, A.; Caporale, J.E.; Zarate, V.; Chuang, L.H.; Pichon-Riviere, A.; Kind, P. Measuring the benefits of healthcare: DALYs and QALYs—Does the choice of measure matter? A case study of two preventive interventions. *Int. J. Health Policy Manag.* **2018**, *7*, 120–136. [CrossRef] [PubMed]
24. World Health Organization. *Making Choices in Health: WHO Guide to Cost-Effectiveness Analysis*; World Health Organization: Geneva, Switzerland, 2003; p. 9.
25. Zuckerman, J.N.; Rombo, L.; Fisch, A. The true burden and risk of cholera: Implications for prevention and control. *Lancet Infect. Dis.* **2007**, *7*, 521–530. [CrossRef] [PubMed]

vaccines

MDPI

Article

Using Human-Centered Design to Bridge Zero-Dose Vaccine Gap: A Case Study of Ilala District in Tanzani

Simon Martin Nzilibili [1,*], Hellen Maziku [2], Awet Araya [3], Ruthbetha Kateule [2], Millenium Anthony Malamla [2], Suna Salum [2], Furaha Kyesi [4], Lotalis Gadau [4], Tumaini Menson Haonga [1], Florian Tinuga [4], Rashid Mfaume [5], Zaitun Hamza [6], Georgina Joachim [4], Alice Geofrey Mwiru [3], Alex Benson [7], Oscar Kapela [1], Ona Machangu [1], Norman Jonas [1] and Ntuli Kapologwe [8]

1 Health Promotion Section, Ministry of Health, Dodoma P.O. Box 743, Tanzania; tumeha@yahoo.com (T.M.H.); kaperaoscar20@gmail.com (O.K.); onamach@gmail.com (O.M.); normanjonasmd@gmail.com (N.J.)
2 Department of Computer Science and Engineering, College of ICT, University of Dar es Salaam, Dar es Salaam P.O. Box 35091, Tanzania; nahelna@gmail.com (H.M.); rnackyy@gmail.com (R.K.); milleniummalamla@gmail.com (M.A.M.); sunnasalum382@gmail.com (S.S.)
3 Social Behavior Change UNICEF, Tanzania Country Office, Dar es Salaam P.O. Box 4076, Tanzania; aaraya@unicef.org (A.A.); amwiru@unicef.org (A.G.M.)
4 Immunization and Vaccine Development Program, Ministry of Health, Dodoma P.O. Box 743, Tanzania; furahakyesi@hotmail.com (F.K.); lgadawu@gmail.com (L.G.); floriantinuga@yahoo.com (F.T.); joachimgeorgina@gmail.com (G.J.)
5 Directorate of Health, Social Welfare and Nutrition Services at the President's Office, Regional Administration and Local Government, Dodoma P.O. Box 1923, Tanzania; srashid302@gmail.com
6 Council Health Management Team, Dar es Salaam City Council, Dar es Salaam P.O. Box 77742, Tanzania; drzelha@gmail.com
7 School of Journalism and Mass Communication, University of Dar es Salaam, Dar es Salaam P.O. Box 35091, Tanzania; benzanda@gmail.com
8 Department of Preventive Services, Ministry of Health, Dodoma P.O. Box 743, Tanzania; nkapologwe2002@gmail.com
* Correspondence: nzilibili@gmail.com

Abstract: Background: Immunization plays a substantial role in reducing the under-five mortality rate. However, Tanzania still has a significant number of zero-dose and under-vaccinated children and was ranked among the top ten African countries with the highest numbers of zero-dose children in 2022. The human-centered design (HCD) approach is more ethical and effective at addressing public health challenges in complex sociocultural settings. This study aimed to use the HCD approach to aid in identifying, prioritizing, and implementing community-centric interventions in Tanzania, particularly in the Ilala District of Dar es Salaam, to increase vaccine demand and close the zero-dose gap by at least 50%. **Methods:** The study involved co-creation workshops with 483 participants to identify, design, and test solutions. The study followed the UNICEF Journey to Health and Immunization framework to identify barriers and enablers influencing stakeholders in adopting and sustaining health- and immunization-related actions. **Results:** The study identified the causes of under-five defaulting and the zero-dose gap, i.e., the inadequate support of local community leaders in under-five vaccination sensitization and surveillance; poor infrastructure to new settlement areas; hesitancy and unwillingness of parents/guardians; absence of house numbers; limited/time-constrained availability of resources to facilitate mobile immunization services, etc. The participants were able to come up with 309 ideas, which were refined through multiple iterations using the impact—effort matrix and skimmed down to three (3) solutions: (i) having health facilities to notify and alert local leaders about vaccination dates; (ii) using parents, kids, and grownups who got vaccinated to influence others; (iii) using local government leaders and house representatives for vaccine advocacy. Of these, the solution involving local government leaders and house representatives for vaccine advocacy was implemented. An advocacy strategy

 https://doi.org/10.3390/vaccines13010038

was used to enhance the collaboration of the District Commissioner, Council leaders, and community leaders. A home-to-home interpersonal sensitization approach accompanied by the household delivery of vaccination services was employed. The findings reveal that the HCD framework was impactful in increasing collaborations/cooperation with local government leaders and community ownership of the under-five vaccination initiative. As a result, 67,145 houses, equal to 104%, were reached, surpassing the initial target of 64,800 houses, and 131,088 families, equal to 83% of the targeted 156,995 households, were sensitized through a home-to-home campaign approach. This study demonstrates the effectiveness of the approach. Researchers and practitioners are encouraged to adopt the HCD approach when addressing public health challenges, especially in complex sociocultural settings.

Keywords: zero dose; under-five vaccination; human centered design; advocacy; community-centric intervention

1. Introduction

The global mortality rate among children under five years of age declined by 59%, from 93 deaths per 1000 live births in 1990 to 37 deaths per 1000 live births in 2022 [1]. This significant reduction has been primarily attributed to the provision of childhood vaccinations, contributing to achieving the fourth United Nations Millennium Development Goal, which aimed to promote healthy lives for children and eliminate preventable deaths among newborns and young children [2]. Although substantial progress has been made in improving child survival, the magnitude of under-five mortality remains a significant burden in sub-Saharan Africa and South Asia [1,3]. Hence, continued efforts to reduce child mortality further are imperative.

In addition to the apparent health benefits, vaccination of under-five children is highly considered the most cost-effective, reliable, and robust public health intervention for curbing morbidity and mortality associated with preventable diseases [2,4]. Globally, immunization coverage has vastly expanded to cover all countries with the services available and accessible to rural and urban citizens of every nation [5]. In recent years, more efforts have been directed toward strict adherence to the vaccination schedule to immunize the under-five with vaccines such as Diphtheria–Tetanus, Measles–Rubella, and Polio [6]. The World Health Organization, in collaboration with governments of other countries, has implemented different strategies to upscale vaccine uptake among children [2]. As a result, these strategies increased the delivery of vaccination services and raised citizens' awareness of the vaccination benefits to under-fives. Yet, millions of children in Africa are still deprived of life-saving vaccinations, accounting for nearly half of the world's unvaccinated and under-vaccinated children [7].

Sub-Saharan African countries, particularly Tanzania, have recorded remarkable successes in nationwide child immunization coverage, attributed to vaccine availability, effective vaccine delivery mechanisms, and community sensitization and vaccination promotions [8]. Despite these accomplishments, significant challenges remain, including high rates of under-five mortality [9] and a considerable number of zero-dose and under-vaccinated children due to vaccine hesitancy [10]. In Tanzania, one in four children are not fully vaccinated. Many regions fail to meet the 90% coverage target set by the Reaching Every District (RED) strategy [10], and according to the WHO (2023), Tanzania, Angola, and Cameroon ranked among the top ten African countries with the highest numbers of zero-dose children in 2022 [11].

Various factors contribute to vaccine hesitancy, including trust, occupational status, education, marital status, wealth, place of residence, media exposure, and access to antenatal care (ANC) and postnatal care (PNC) [12–14]. These factors are shaped by social, economic, and cultural dynamics influencing parental vaccine awareness. For instance, the lack of trust in vaccines and healthcare practitioners is often fueled by misinformation, cultural beliefs, and past negative experiences with vaccination [13,15]. This distrust is a key factor contributing to the lack of confidence in the efficacy and safety of vaccines. Both occupations and education influence the extent to which an individual is exposed to vaccine-related information. For example, healthcare workers are exposed to detailed vaccine information, which can lead to either high acceptance or hesitancy [12,14]. Parental marital status can also influence vaccination hesitancy, as making a decision about whether to vaccinate a child often requires agreement between both parents [12,16]. Individuals with stable and higher financial resources generally have better access to healthcare services and vaccine-related information, making them more likely to accept vaccines compared to those with limited financial resources and influenced by other beliefs [14,17]. There is a critical need for effective interventions to overcome these barriers and ensure that children from hesitant families receive vaccinations. According to the WHO, interventions targeting vaccine hesitancy should be specifically tailored to the concerns of the respective target population to maximize their effectiveness [18].

Human-centered design (HCD) is a more ethical and practical approach to addressing public health challenges in complex sociocultural settings [19]. As conceptualized by the IDEO (2015), HCD emphasizes creating interventions tailored to the target population's needs, preferences, and experiences [20]. This approach prioritizes collaboration with end-user communities, engaging deeply with the impacted individuals and groups. By fostering this co-creation process, HCD ensures that solutions are effective, culturally, and contextually relevant, making them more sustainable and likely to succeed [21]. Despite the substantial contributions of HCD in addressing complex problems in public health, there is a lack of empirical evidence describing the implementation of an entire HCD project [19]. Most studies are centered on one or two aspects of HCD, i.e., stakeholder engagement [22], ideation [23], or prototyping [24]. To address this gap, this study described the use of the HCD approach in identifying, prioritizing, and implementing community-centered interventions to increase vaccine demand and close the zero-dose gap in Tanzania, focusing on the Ilala District in Dar es Salaam. Ilala is the leading district in Dar es Salaam, with a high number of zero-dose and under-vaccinated children [25]. The intention was to reduce the number of children with zero doses of Diphtheria–Tetanus–Pertussis (DTP) and Measles–Rubella (MR) vaccines by at least 50%. Key stakeholders, mainly caregivers, community health workers, healthcare providers, parents, and religious and community leaders, were actively engaged throughout the HCD process, ensuring that solutions were developed collaboratively with the direct beneficiaries.

The rest of this paper is organized as follows: the materials and methods section outline the research design, including co-creation workshops, data collection, analysis, challenge definition, solution design, and implementation methods. The results section presents findings on barriers to routine immunization, key opportunities for generating innovative solutions to reduce the zero-dose gap in Ilala, interventions, prototyped solutions, and their implementation. The discussion interprets these findings about the research objectives and relevant literature. Finally, the conclusion summarizes key insights, offers suggestions for improving digital systems, and highlights directions for future research.

2. Materials and Methods

2.1. Study Approach and Methodology

The study employed a human-centered design (HCD) approach, where participants in community-based co-creation workshops identified, prioritized, and implemented community-centric interventions to increase vaccination demand and address the zero-dose gap among under-five children in Tanzania. This approach leverages creativity and empathy to design solutions that are not only tailored to the community's specific needs but also foster active engagement and collaboration among stakeholders at all levels [19]. The study used persona models with fictional characters to represent key actors' immunization needs, values, aspirations, abilities, and limitations. Initially, five personas were considered: caregivers, community health workers (CHWs), healthcare workers (HCWs), religious leaders, and community leaders. However, rapid inquiry in Ilala revealed that mothers are often the breadwinners, with grandmothers assuming caregiving roles.

Additionally, men and traditional healers were identified as key stakeholders in the decision-making process related to immunization. As a result, the caregiver persona was adapted to include both female caregivers (mothers) and grandmothers, and additional personas for men and traditional healers were created. We followed the UNICEF Journey to Health and Immunization framework (2020), which takes into account six stages in the health journey, helping us identify both barriers and enablers for key stakeholders (personas) in taking and sustaining health and immunization-related actions [26].

2.2. Study Population and Sampling

The study was conducted in Ilala District, Dar es Salaam, Tanzania, from March to December 2023. Ilala was selected due to its high number of zero-dose and under-vaccinated children [25]. Drawing on their extensive experience in health promotion and vaccine delivery, the Ministry of Health (MoH) played a significant role in identifying key stakeholders for participation in various phases of the HCD process, which engaged 483 diverse participants. The involvement of these stakeholders brought their unique perspectives and valuable experiences to the co-creation workshops and community engagements, which is essential for designing solutions tailored to the community's needs and preferences. Participant involvement varied across the study's stages based on individual expertise and availability. Given the dual objectives of developing community-centered interventions and building stakeholder capacity in HCD, 24 participants were consistently engaged throughout all HCD phases. This ensured they acquired the necessary skills to implement the co-created interventions and sustain vaccine uptake efforts using participatory approaches within their communities, workplaces, and healthcare settings. This approach aligns with UNICEF's recommendation to integrate HCD into sub-national immunization coverage assessments to yield more impactful and sustainable initiatives [27]. A key innovation of this study was conducting multiple rounds of testing of the co-created interventions to challenge assumptions, collect feedback from communities, and uncover more user needs [28].

2.3. Co-Creation Workshops

The Ministry of Health defined the background and scope of the challenge, focusing on increasing support for and uptake of routine vaccinations, with the specific goal of reducing the number of children with zero doses of DTP and MR vaccines by at least 50%. To address this, two one-week co-creation workshops were conducted, where immunization stakeholders in Ilala were brought together to understand the immunization challenge, conduct rapid inquiry research, analyze and synthesize research findings, generate ideas, build prototypes, and engage communities to test and prioritize the prototypes iteratively.

Over three months, three weeks were dedicated to planning and implementing one of the prototypes deemed most desirable by the community.

2.3.1. Data Collection

In the HCD process, data are collected throughout all phases: problem diagnosis, solution design, and implementation. This process offers opportunities to uncover additional user needs, gather diverse perspectives, and identify hidden challenges. The study employed various data collection methods and tools through the co-creation workshops, including persona models, journey maps, rapid inquiry, brainstorming, discussions, prototyping, feedback grids, and prototype testing interviews.

2.3.2. Challenge Definition and Diagnosis

In the first co-creation workshop, 45 immunization stakeholders in Ilala participated in the HCD training workshop to understand the challenge from the perspectives of the key actors through persona models and capture the multi-dimensional nature of the challenge through journey maps. Personas were developed using worksheets where participants detailed each persona's motivations, frustrations, perceptions, routines, and influences. Challenge definition aims to understand users' needs, identify assumptions and gaps in existing data, and facilitate diagnosis through rapid inquiry research.

Rapid inquiry employs interactive research methods to quickly explore the social, cultural, political, and economic influences and motivations behind people's behaviors within a community. Participants used a rapid inquiry plan to explore areas of inquiry and ensure the right questions were directed to the right persona groups. Using discussion guides, participants prepared a list of questions and activities to be used during rapid inquiry. A discussion guide includes reminders of background information to share, open-ended questions to ask, and activities to administer. Sample activity included a worksheet that documents the day in the life of a given interviewee. At each point of the day, pain points and opportunities were identified. Participants visited health facilities and the Ilala community to conduct rapid inquiries to healthcare workers, community health workers, community leaders, and caregivers. Participants unpacked findings from the rapid inquiry using a Miro board and an interview highlights worksheet, capturing notes, quotes, and surprising moments. This was followed by analysis and synthesis of the unstructured data using open discussions and a 5-whys worksheet to uncover barriers, root causes, and opportunities for designing solutions.

2.3.3. Solution Design

The design of interventions using HCD approaches is achieved through idea generation, prototyping, and iterative testing. During brainstorming sessions, participants leveraged identified opportunities to generate 309 ideas to address barriers to routine immunization. These ideas were then prioritized based on desirability, viability, and feasibility metrics, narrowing them down to 49 ideas suitable for prototyping.

In the second co-creation workshop, 31 participants participated in HCD training to further prioritize ideas, create prototypes, and iteratively test and refine these prototypes. Using a participatory approach and a live poll, the impact–effort matrix was used to score and rank 49 ideas based on impact and feasibility. The top six ranked ideas were carried forward into the prototyping phase. Participants then reviewed these ideas to identify patterns and themes by comparing them with the remaining ideas.

Prototyping is the process of making ideas tangible. Prototypes are an early, quick, and cheap mechanism to test key assumptions and assess if interventions meet user needs, providing room for feedback and improvements [29]. Participants used idea dashboards to describe each of the six ideas and state how they work by capturing critical functionalities.

This process was followed by creating six paper prototypes for each idea. Community members tested the prototypes in Ilala. Feedback was unpacked on feedback grids to capture the features that users liked or did not like about the prototype, the questions asked, and new ideas that were suggested and worth trying. Participants analyzed the feedback on the grids and used it to iterate the prototypes by rebuilding them to incorporate new recommendations and remove some features. After 3 iterations of prototyping and testing through community engagements, the three most liked and desirable prototypes by the community of Ilala were selected for implementation.

2.3.4. Theory of Change

The Theory of Change (ToC) framework [30] was applied to integrate the learnings from the HCD process, guide the implementation plan, and track the progress of interventions over time. The ToC mapped the system of stakeholders, activities, outputs, and outcomes that were anticipated to lead to the long-term goal of reducing the number of children with zero doses of Diphtheria–Tetanus–Pertussis (DTP) and Measles–Rubella (MR) vaccines by at least 50%. The ToC facilitated the development of a shared strategy for change and laid out a clear plan for monitoring and evaluating progress, allowing the study to test assumptions and track both intermediate and long-term outcomes against the goal of reducing zero-dose cases.

2.3.5. Solution Implementation

The contribution of this study lies in applying HCD to the implementation phase of one of the three prioritized ideas. Existing literature indicates that the use of HCD beyond the design phase is still in its early stages, with most HCD studies not covering the entire project cycle [31,32].

The MoH, in collaboration with key stakeholders and representatives of participants who had undergone HCD training until the design phase, collaboratively established the implementation plan for the vaccine advocacy idea. The vaccine advocacy idea lies in using Ilala district leaders to advocate for vaccine uptake to community leaders and members. The team reviewed Ilala immunization health facility data to establish a five-year trend analysis for DPT3 and MR2 to identify low-performing areas needing prioritization during implementation. Through planning meetings and consultations, the team designed implementation tools and activities. The team set daily implementation targets for implementers to achieve and established criteria to guide the implementation duration for each ward. Key elements established during implementation planning include the number of advocacy stages, monitoring process, control mechanism, and reporting mechanism. Due to community engagements and open discussions, the advocacy prototype underwent another iteration to incorporate additional user needs and views.

During implementation, the District Commissioner (DC) advocated to 430 people in 2 different phases. In phase 1, the DC gathered council leaders to advocate for the sustainable and impactful implementation of vaccine mobilization and sensitization in their areas in the Ilala district. In phase 2, the DC, with other district leaders, gathered community leaders, HCWs, and CHWs in two low-performing constituencies to advocate for vaccine uptake. The DC shared the implementation target, where 56.5% of families in Ilala were expected to be reached (259,200 families). The DC provided two lists of wards: one where house-to-house mobilization would be completed in one week and another where it would extend over two weeks. Community-level advocacy presented an opportunity to gather feedback directly from the community leaders on the following key issues: understanding of HCD, opinions and views on the advocacy idea, and additional inputs to strengthen the implementation of HCD ideas.

House-to-house mobilization and sensitization commenced four days after completing the advocacy at the community level. In total, 189 CHWs were engaged to reach families in 26 wards in Ilala. Each CHW was accompanied by an HCW responsible for administering the vaccine. The CHW and HCW pair filled in vaccination data using a reporting tool designed based on specific indicators. The data were verified by the Street chairperson and submitted to the ward level for aggregation. The Ward Health Officers supervised the vaccination exercise in their respective wards. Ward-level vaccination data were verified and aggregated at the council level.

3. Results

3.1. Demographic Information

As shown in Table 1, the research involved a diverse group of 483 participants, with 24 consistently engaged throughout all phases of the human-centered design (HCD) process. Table 2 presents a list of participants involved in testing ideas and prototypes. Such stakeholders were categorized into various groups: researchers from higher learning institutions (HLIs); national government officials, mainly from the Ministry of Health (MoH); regional and district government leaders such as the Regional Medical Officer (RMO), District Executive Director (DED), District Commissioner (DC), mayor, and the Council Health Management Team (CHMT); local government leaders such as ward executive officers (WEOs), Mtaa executive officers (MEOs), Mtaa chairpersons, environmental health officers, and members of local government councils; civil society organizations such as the Shivyawata–Tanzania Federation of Disabled People's Organizations, the TADIO network of community radio stations in Tanzania, the Chavita (association of people with hearing impairment), and BBC Media Action; community health workers (CHWs) and caregivers; and international organizations such as UNICEF, WHO, JHPIEGO, and AMREF.

Table 1. Human-centered design (HCD) workshops participants list.

Participant Group	Number of Participants		
	HCD Training	Prototyping and Iterative Testing	Idea Implementation
Researchers from Higher Learning Institutions (HLIs)	12	7	7
National Government Officials from The Ministry of Health (MoH)	5	4	7
Regional and District Government Leaders (Regional Medical Officer (RMO), District Executive Director (DED), District Commissioner (DC), Mayor and Council Health Management Team (CHMT))	2	7	30
Local Government Leaders (Ward Executive Officer (WEO), Mtaa Executive Officer (MEO)/Local Executive Officer, Mtaa Chairpersons (Local/Street Chairperson), Environmental Health Officers, Members of Local Government Councils)	1	1	137
Civil Society (Tanzania Association of the Deafblind (TADIO), Tanzania Federation of Disabled People's Organizations (Shivyawata), Tanzania Association of the Deaf (Chavita), Media)	16	3	23
Community Health Workers	2	2	178
Health Care Workers	3	1	46
International Organizations (United Nations International Children's Emergency Fund (UNICEF), World Health Organization (WHO), Johns Hopkins Program for International Education in Gynecology and Obstetrics (JHPIEGO), and African Medical and Research Foundation (AMREF))	4	6	3
TOTAL	**45**	**31**	**431**

Table 2. Human-centered design (HCD) iterative testing participants list.

Participant Group	Number of Testers		
	Idea Testing-Round 1	**Prototype Testing-Round 2**	**Prototype Testing-Round 3**
Caregivers	2	4	2
Regional and District Government Leaders (RMO, DED, DC, Mayor, and CHMTs)		6	2
Local Government Leaders (Community Leaders)	1	2	2
Community Health Workers	1	8	2
Health Care Workers	1	8	2
Religious Leaders	1	2	
TOTAL	**6**	**30**	**10**

3.2. Identified Barriers and Key Opportunities

Based on a rapid inquiry and observation, multiple barriers to routine immunization, as depicted in Table 3, were identified from various perspectives, including those of fathers, female caregivers, community health workers (CHWs), religious leaders, healthcare workers (HCWs), community leaders, and grandmothers. Each group faces unique challenges that impact the delivery and uptake of vaccinations.

Table 3. Identified barriers for different persona groups.

S/N	Persona	Barriers
1.	Father	- There is the normalization of gender roles. - Fathers have been left out of child health initiatives, primarily targeting mothers. - Limited sources of health information reaching fathers. - The community prefers messages to go to mothers and fathers rather than fathers alone. - They questioned whether the father could take care of the baby alone.
2.	Female Caregivers	- Low motivation to skip earning to take children to clinics accounting for distance, long - wait times, and vaccine stockouts. - Many caregivers have no time or access to technology or social media, limiting their access to health information. - Claims that vaccine treatment shifts based on who is in the system and who is not; a very different experience for those who are not connected. - Many feel that traditional medicines are cheaper, trusted, and more accessible to them and would rather wait and treat their child traditionally if they fall ill.
3.	Community Mobilizers (CHWs)	- There is conflicting information about the role of the mobilizers and what they are doing for the community vs. the government, which impacts their influence. - Erratic incentives for mobilizers undermine their reputation; society thinks they are being paid, but it is an unpaid position. - Many in society feel that community mobilizers are paid and care more about the money than the community's health. - CHWs must complete a heavy amount of data reporting, which takes time and makes it hard to do part-time work. - Health equipment (masks, protective equipment) makes the community think of an outbreak, not safety.
4.	Religious Leaders	- The leader sees and hears about wrong vaccination practices in the community but does not have the correct information to correct it. - Religious leaders dismiss parents who did not take their children to be vaccinated in their interactions, which can cause echo chambers. - While higher-level religious leaders have formal training for immunization, local religious leaders are teaching themselves.

Table 3. *Cont.*

S/N	Persona	Barriers
5.	Health Care Workers (HCWs)	- Data reporting and logbook requirements are very time-consuming. - Vaccination centers are crowded with congested corridors, and workers are tired of keeping up with the influx of patients. - Patient feedback is not part of the job description, along with no employee feedback system. - HCWs work as they are trained. Updates are given through guidebooks but not personal guidance. - HCWs work in poor working conditions without incentives or overtime pay: "She ignores what she sees so she can do her work." - Since COVID-19, there has been an increase in the question of the importance of routine vaccination.
6.	Community Leaders	- Some community leaders have their attention divided between their constituents and professional clients. They are constantly receiving phone calls and plugged into helping the community. - Community leaders are also caregivers for elderly parents or children, which reduces their office days and hours. - Community leaders focus on social issues that matter to the community. They do not see health issues as social issues and, therefore, do not see child vaccination and do not consider it to be a part of their responsibilities.
7.	Grandmothers	- Some grandmothers are breadwinners and work odd hours to earn money and take care of the home. - They feel cut off and outside of the conversation around vaccination and immunization. - Grandmothers know about health and use traditional medicine practices and healing. - They are proactive about vaccinations, but they hear rumors such as a person dying a day after the vaccine, and these stories become stuck in people's minds.

From these identified barriers, nine key opportunities emerged, as shown in Figure 1, that were leveraged to generate innovative solutions to reduce the zero-dose gap in Ilala. These opportunities provided a foundation for targeted interventions to address each stakeholder group's specific needs and concerns, ultimately increasing immunization coverage in the region.

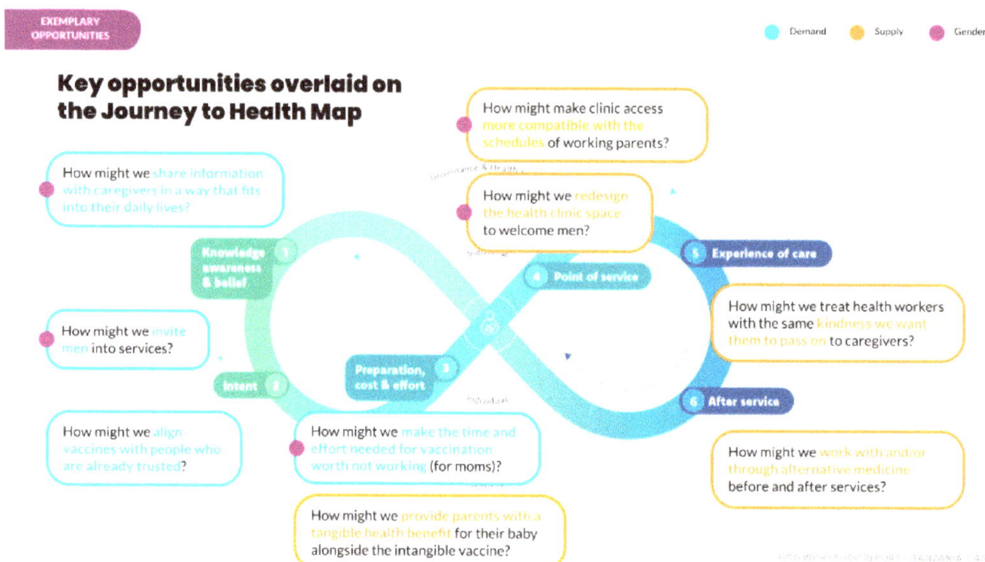
EXEMPLARY OPPORTUNITIES
Demand
Supply
Gender
Key opportunities overlaid on the Journey to Health Map
How might we share information with caregivers in a way that fits into their daily lives?
How might make clinic access more compatible with the schedules of working parents?
How might we redesign the health clinic space to welcome men?
Knowledge awareness & belief
1
4 Point of service
5 Experience of care
How might we invite men into services?
How might we treat health workers with the same kindness we want them to pass on to caregivers?
Intent
2
Preparation, cost & effort
3
6 After service
How might we align vaccines with people who are already trusted?
How might we make the time and effort needed for vaccination worth not working (for moms)?
How might we work with and/or through alternative medicine before and after services?
How might we provide parents with a tangible health benefit for their baby alongside the intangible vaccine?

Figure 1. Key opportunities mapped onto the journey to health map. Source: HCD Training Report in Ilala (2023).

3.3. Identified Interventions

From five opportunities, 309 ideas were generated through a collaborative brainstorming process involving diverse stakeholders, as summarized in Table 4.

Table 4. Number of ideas generated for each design challenge (opportunity).

S/N	Persona	Number of Generated Ideas	Design Challenge
1.	Traditional Healer	80 ideas	How might we work with/through alternative medicine?
2.	Religious and Community Leaders	80 Ideas	How might we align vaccines with people who are already trusted
3.	Health Care Workers	68 Ideas	How might we treat healthcare workers with the same kindness we want them to pass on to the caregivers?
4.	Caregivers (Mothers, Grandmothers)	60 Ideas	How might we make her get her child vaccinated worth not working?
5.	Men	21 Ideas	How might we invite men into services?

3.4. Prioritized Interventions

Of 309 ideas generated, 49 were prioritized after thorough discussion and broad thinking. The criteria used for prioritization were desirability, viability, and feasibility. These 49 ideas were then ranked through a participatory approach, with each idea being reviewed and discussed in detail. From this ranking process, the top six ideas listed in Table 5 were selected for further exploration.

Table 5. List of prioritized interventions.

S/N	Intervention
1.	Having health facilities notify and alert local leaders and Wajumbe (Local Government Representatives) about vaccination dates.
2.	Giving priority to fathers when they come to the hospital with kids.
3.	Improve CHWs' capacity to assist nurses and work with them.
4.	Use parents, kids, and grownups who got vaccinated to influence others.
5.	Use local government leaders and house representatives for vaccine advocacy.
6.	Put vaccination ads in religious places and centers.

During the discussions, participants highlighted key issues and questions, pointing out barriers and opportunities that could be explored further. One notable opportunity is the government's directive for health facilities to allocate resources through Health System Financing to enhance the capacity of CHWs. This initiative presents a valuable opportunity to strengthen CHW support. However, challenges remain, such as traditional healers' reluctance to partner with healthcare providers, suggesting that their views and needs should be incorporated into the design process. Additionally, there were concerns about the effectiveness of initiatives to invite fathers and make clinics more male-friendly, with participants questioning the value of such efforts if the vaccination environment remains unwelcoming. Finally, the current guidelines prioritize men who bring their children for vaccination, highlighting a potential area for further development and reinforcement.

3.5. Prototypes

Prototypes of the top six ideas were created in different forms, not limited to sketches or storyboards on rough papers or even role play scenarios. These prototyped ideas were iteratively tested (three iterations). Feedback from the community was collected after each iteration, allowing the ideas to be refined and improved. As a result, three (3) of the most desirable and impactful ideas emerged, shaped by the inputs and suggestions from the community. The three ideas that emerged are summarized in Table 6. It was also observed that community members preferred and emphasized the involvement of CHWs in all the ideas. Therefore, the idea of the capacitation of CHWs was merged into the three selected ideas, and new versions for each idea were created. Three rounds of iterative testing were conducted on the refined versions of the three chosen ideas, with feedback from each round used to further enhance the prototypes up to version 3.

Table 6. List of most desirable interventions.

S/N	Intervention
1.	Having health facilities notify and alert local leaders and Wajumbe (Local Government Representatives) about vaccination dates.
2.	Use parents, kids, and grownups who got vaccinated to influence others.
3.	Use local government leaders and house representatives for vaccine advocacy.

3.6. Prototype Implementation

The selected idea for implementation was advocacy through community leaders and community health workers (CHWs). Preparations for this implementation included creating a human-centered advocacy implementation plan involving collaboration with various stakeholders. The advocacy prototype was refined during this process based on feedback from the planning phase.

The refined prototype, as shown in Figure 2, underwent several modifications. Firstly, it broadened stakeholder inclusion by integrating previously omitted council leaders, such as the District Commissioner (DC), the Mayor, and the District Administrative Secretary (DAS). Secondly, the prototype streamlined the advocacy process by condensing the original four stages into two while still ensuring the participation of all relevant advocacy groups. The focus of the original prototype involved the DC advocating to ward-level leaders and Mtaa leaders (local/street leaders), who subsequently advocated to CHWs. However, since it was discovered during design research that CHWs maintain a closer relationship with the community, a more impactful approach would be for the DC to directly advocate for CHWs alongside ward leaders and Mtaa leaders (local/street leaders). Therefore, the advocacy flow was revised: the DC was now to advocate directly to council and community leaders. Community-level advocacy was restructured to incorporate the involvement of community health workers (CHWs), ward-level leaders, and street-level leaders.

During council-level and community-level advocacy, the DC championed vaccination to 430 participants, including government officials, regional leaders, district leaders, heads of departments, CHMTs, community leaders, CHWs, HCWs, media officers, and journalists.

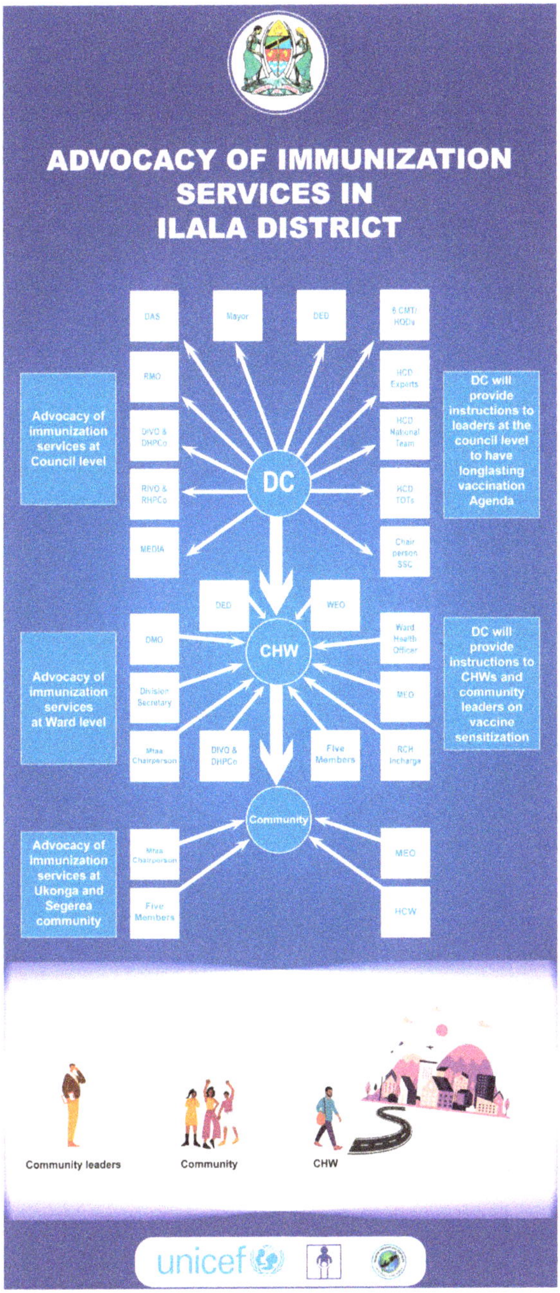

Figure 2. Refined prototype for the advocacy idea.

House-to-house mobilization and sensitization commenced immediately after the advocacy meetings in 26 wards in the Ukonga and Segerea Constituencies. Depending on the established criteria, the house-to-house mobilization process spanned five or ten days per ward. Each of the 189 CHWs paired with an HCW was assigned a daily house-to-house target of 40 households, assuming an average of 4 families per household and 160 families per day. Ward Health Officers supervised house-to-house mobilization exercises, verified daily vaccination data, and confirmed visits with photos of house numbers or postcodes. Special tools were created to gather and organize vaccination data at community, ward, and council levels. The tool was designed to record the number of families reached, zero-dose cases addressed, defaulter cases resolved, and the total count of children in each family and household. As a control measure, the Mtaa chairperson verified and stamped the daily data report for each CHW. CHWs were to document visited families.

The data collection tool used during the house-to-house vaccine mobilization exercise also included fields to capture challenges, achievements, and views from CHWs, HCWs, community leaders, and community members. The data collected were analyzed, and it was observed that the challenges, successes, and opinions were related to the following thematic areas: RCH Card, Infrastructure, Tools, Community Participation, Resources, Availability of Children, and Vaccine Education. Table 7 summarizes the key challenges frequently highlighted by the participants. Most of the feedback from community leaders and families was positive, highlighting that most families were cooperative and loved empowering CHWs to mobilize families alongside HCWs. A notable recommendation was that prior notifications should be provided through PAs, radios, and TV.

Table 7. List of challenges.

S/N	Challenge	Frequency
1.	Poor infrastructure (roads) due to rainy season	17
2.	Parents refusing having their children vaccinated	12
3.	The absence of tools such as gumboots, raincoats, and umbrellas	9
4.	Houses do not have house numbers	9
5.	Children born at home are not taken to health facilities	5

In the planning phase, it was initially estimated that, on average, four families resided in each house within the Ilala area. However, subsequent observations revealed a variance in the ratio of families to houses across different divisions. Specifically, in Ukonga, the ratio was two families per house, whereas in Segerea, the ratio was three families per house. Outliers may have influenced the estimated ratio of families per house, as some houses in Ilala were found to accommodate huge families, with numbers reaching up to 16 families per house. During the exercise, 67,145 houses were visited (104% of the goal) as summarized in Table 8 and shown in Figure 3. Within these visited houses, 156,995 families were recorded, of which 131,088 (83%) were offered vaccination services.

Table 2 shows the number of zero doses and 1753 defaulters. However, as depicted in Figure 3, fewer zero doses (387) were identified during the vaccination exercise, while a significantly higher number of defaulters (9899) were identified. While the results may be alarming, they align with the HCD problem diagnosis and research findings. These findings revealed that Ilala, the central urban hub in Dar es Salaam, attracts frequent family movements. Documenting children as defaulters may not accurately reflect their vaccination status, as there is a high likelihood that they moved and received vaccination services in HFs other than the ones they were born in. The frequent movements within and outside of Ilala highlight a pressing challenge: the need for a mechanism to track the vaccination process and synchronize vaccination records within Ilala.

Table 8. Household-level vaccine mobilization results.

S/N	Indicators	Ilala Community Vaccine Mobilization (Ukonga and Segerea)		
		Target	Actual	(%)
1.	Households reached	64,800	67,145	104
2.	Number of families present in the visited households	259,200	156,995	61
3.	Number of families reached	156,995	131,088	83
4.	Zero doses reached	2550	387	15
5.	Defaulters reached	1753	9899	565
6.	Total children vaccinated	4303	10,286	239
7.	Eligible children who were missed		2127	
8.	Total children in families that were reached		90,158	

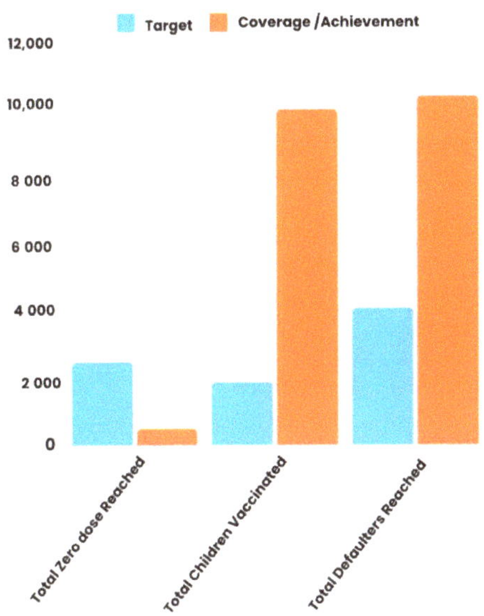

Figure 3. House-to-house sensitization and mobilization data.

3.7. Identified Theory of Change

The theory of change aims to map out the system of people and activities that are assumed to collectively bring about the desired change. It provides a framework for collaboratively monitoring progress over time, ensuring that each step taken contributes to long-term goals. By tracking intermediate outcomes along the way, the approach ensures that all stakeholders are aligned and working towards common objectives. Table 9 depicts the theory of change for each persona built from identified barriers and co-created ideas. For instance, to have increased vaccine coverage in Ilala by 50%, CHWs need to be empowered to take on responsibilities such as administering vaccines, keeping records, and weighing babies. As a result, the workload for HCWs is significantly reduced. This leads to improved work–life balance for HCWs, resulting in a more positive clinic environment and the potential to extend clinic hours. As a result, families are more likely to attend and support regular healthcare services, leading to increased trust and accessibility.

Table 9. Theory of change.

IMPACT	1. Increased Coverage by 50% in Ilala		
OUTCOME	**1.1 Families Support and Regularly Attend Services**		
Inputs	**Activities**	**Outputs**	**Intermediate Outcomes**
HCWs who are overworked + CHWs who are trusted by the community	Evolve CHWs' role to conduct routine vaccination activities like vaccination, record keeping, weighing babies	Less working hours for HCWs	Happier HCWs, better clinic experience, opportunity to open clinics for more hours
CHWs whose presence is critical to the community accepting services but who are believed to be motivated by money	Learned in prototyping: What helps CHWs gain trust and address misinformation? • Incentives like transport support • Tools like megaphones • Recognition from community • Recognition from health sector (including gov.)	CHWs have reliable, regular engagement with community (NOTE: sporadic engagement is causing rumors that they only work when paid)	Community trusts CHWs for advice and reminders
Caregivers who are not available when facilities are open + HCWs who do not have more time during the weekday	Offer services on Saturdays	More families receiving services	Women do not need to choose between making money and attending health services
OUTCOME	**1.2 Community ownership of vaccination and support of preventative medicine**		
Inputs	**Activities**	**Outputs**	**Intermediate Outcomes**
Grandmothers who have knowledge about vaccines + CHWs who are trusted by the community	Partner to provide outreach services to the community	Specific days where CHWs can reach out to grandmothers and provide vaccines	Vaccination is not only a mother's responsibility
Religious leaders who currently have informal training + Implementers in care who are not really trained	Receive formal training (beyond chairperson) that can be applied into their career	Links to information with their focus (religion)	Enhanced confidence during religious sermons
Community leaders who are involved in social issues in the community, but do not see health issues as social issues	Receive a health/vaccination induction after they come to office + Become involved in mobile clinics that are close to their community	More attendance at clinics	Social norm in community is to trust in vaccines

4. Discussion

The use of HCD as a framework of this study helped involve and engage local community leaders, health workers, community health workers, and local communities of the study area to identify community-specific impediments to vaccination of under-fives and determine the possible solutions to address the issue. This design emphasizes the need for vaccination interventions to involve the target population in the ideation, prototyping, and implementation stages. The study established the root causes of under-fives defaulting and the zero-dose gap. Among the challenges identified were the inadequate support from local community leaders in sensitizing and monitoring under-five vaccinations, poor infrastructure (especially roads) to newly settled areas during the rainy season, parental hesitancy and unwillingness, limited involvement of male spouses, the absence of house numbers, and the lack of an effective surveillance and notification system. These challenges align with findings from Vasudevan et al. [10], Shearer et al. [26], Hogan and Gupta [33] and Reñosa et al. [34].

Efforts to bridge the zero-dose gap among under-fives in Tanzania and the rest of the Sub-Saharan countries of Africa highly depend on the availability and proper record-keeping of vaccination data [25]. As evidenced by this study's findings, there needed to be more official data on unvaccinated children held by official designated authorities and those gathered in the study area. For example, the existing official vaccination data of the Ilala district showed that zero-dose vaccination is the most persistent vaccination challenge among the under-fives in the district, but this study found the opposite. As summarized in Figure 3, the study results suggest that vaccine defaulting among under-fives is the prevailing problem. According to the results, the district had a higher number of vaccine defaulters compared to the number of unvaccinated children. Consequently, the prevailing data discrepancies may lead to duplication of efforts and wrong demand-creation interventions.

The mismatch between existing official vaccination data and the field data collected in this study can be attributed to several factors. One major issue is the lack of an effective tracking and notification system for identifying vaccine defaulters, recording routine vaccination data, and sending reminders to parents and guardians. The current system relies on printed cards where healthcare workers manually record vaccination details, which are then kept by parents or guardians. This system poses challenges: cards can be lost, and parents may forget to check or remember vaccination dates. Additionally, some healthcare workers fail to record subsequent vaccination dates accurately. Consequently, this results in vaccine defaulting among under-fives. These findings align with existing research, which links parents' forgetfulness and inadequate knowledge of vaccination schedules to incomplete vaccinations [35–37]. Similarly, the lack of vaccination cards has been linked to non-adherence to immunization schedules [38].

Moreover, families migrating into the Ilala district and seeking better maternity services have led to incomplete vaccination records when they return to their regions of origin after the initial doses of vaccines such as DTP1 and BCG. This migration has contributed to a rise in vaccination rates for some vaccines, like DTP and BCG, while rates for others, such as MR2, have declined. Additionally, the rapid expansion of new settlements in the district, characterized by high population density, fertility rates, and limited access to health services, exacerbates vaccine defaulting. Due to transport challenges, mobile vaccination services, such as Huduma Mkoba, are infrequent in these areas.

The rapid urbanization and expansion of new settlements contribute to persistent vaccine defaulting and zero-dose cases among under-fives. These findings are consistent with Sambayuka et al. [25], who identified rapid urbanization in Dar es Salaam, particularly in the Ilala district, as a factor in persistent zero-dose and under-vaccination issues. The study also highlighted that the under-capacitation of healthcare workers impacts the delivery of vaccination counselling and contributes to vaccine hesitancy and defaulting.

Notably, the achievement of targets, as shown in Figure 3, confirms that face-to-face interpersonal communication through house-to-house vaccination advocacy effectively addresses the zero-dose gap and reaches vaccine defaulters. This approach facilitates the accurate capture of vaccination data and mitigates hesitancy and negative influences often associated with mass vaccination campaigns.

Generally, the HCD framework effectively captured the quantitative house-to-house vaccine mobilization data and qualitative data on the challenges and achievements. It guided the determination of community-specific solutions to bridge the zero-dose gap and persistent vaccination defaulting among the under-fives in the study area. This study observed that the majority of participants (council and local community leaders, health workers, community health workers, and grassroots communities) held positive views of the HCD framework for employing community-based solutions to address vaccination challenges among under-fives and bridge the zero-dose and vaccination defaulting gaps in the study area. This framework can be pre-tested in other districts of Tanzania to determine its efficacy in eradicating the country's zero-dose gap and under-vaccination of under-fives.

4.1. Lessons Learnt

The study demonstrated the transformative impact of engaging community members in every stage of the design and implementation process via co-creation workshops to address their challenges. Data-driven strategic advocacy and the involvement of trusted community members and leaders led to significant outcomes, including providing vaccination services to 131,088 families (83%). This effort reached 387 children with zero doses out of 2550 and identified many defaulters (9899 out of 1753). The success of this approach demonstrated the potential benefits of applying HCD innovation to public health issues, ensuring that the interventions were grounded in the realities and needs of the target population. The implementation team recommended extending this model to different regions and globally and integrating it with training institutions to ensure formalization and local sustainability.

4.2. Limitations of the Study

The study provides valuable insights into using an HCD approach to address vaccine hesitancy and increase uptake among under-five children. However, it was conducted in a single district. The Ilala district may not represent the entire country, limiting the generalizability of the findings to other regions with different cultural, economic, and healthcare dynamics. The insights and interventions developed in Ilala may not directly apply to rural or more socio-economically disadvantaged regions, which might face unique challenges in vaccination uptake. Additionally, the study focused primarily on stakeholders involved in child immunization, such as caregivers, CHWs, and HCWs. However, broader systemic challenges, such as supply chain issues, vaccine storage, and distribution, were not deeply examined. These factors could influence vaccine availability and accessibility, impacting the overall success of the interventions.

4.3. Recommendations

Future research should expand on these findings by conducting similar studies in diverse settings and incorporating broader factors influencing immunization coverage. The Ministry of Health and relevant stakeholders should institutionalize HCD as a core component of the immunization strategy. HCD should be used beyond immunization efforts. Scaling the use of HCD across regions will allow for identifying more nuanced community-specific challenges and co-creating tailored solutions to ensure formalization and local sustainability.

5. Conclusions

Reducing the zero-dose gap and the number of under-vaccinated children in Tanzania, a country with complex socioeconomic dynamics, requires an innovative, ethical, and practical approach like human-centered design (HCD). HCD helps overcome community hesitancy and misconceptions about vaccination by addressing the unique needs of each community and co-designing relevant, tailored interventions. The house-to-house campaigns implemented as part of the proposed community centric interventions raised awareness, increased vaccine uptake, and strengthened the community's role in health advocacy. This demonstrates that applying HCD principles in public health interventions can effectively tackle challenges like zero-dose vaccination while fostering community engagement and sustainable change.

Author Contributions: Conceptualization, S.M.N. and F.K.; Methodology, S.M.N., H.M. and R.K.; Software, H.M., R.K., M.A.M. and S.S.; Validation, S.M.N., H.M., A.A. and T.M.H.; Formal analysis, S.M.N., H.M., L.G., A.B. and O.K.; Investigation, S.M.N., F.K., L.G., A.G.M., A.B. and O.K.; Resources, F.T., R.M., Z.H. and A.G.M.; Data curation, H.M. and Z.H.; Writing—original draft, R.K., M.A.M., S.S., A.B. and O.K.; Writing—review & editing, S.M.N., H.M., A.A., R.K., M.A.M., S.S., F.K., L.G., T.M.H., F.T., R.M., Z.H., G.J., A.G.M., A.B., O.K., O.M., N.J. and N.K.; Visualization, H.M., R.K., M.A.M. and S.S.; Supervision, S.M.N., A.A., F.K., L.G., F.T., Z.H., G.J., O.M., N.J. and N.K.; Project administration, S.M.N., T.M.H., F.T., R.M., G.J., O.M., N.J. and N.K.; Funding acquisition, A.A. All authors have read and agreed to the published version of the manuscript.

Funding: This research was funded by UNICEF through the HCD approach and the Tanzanian Ministry of Health.

Institutional Review Board Statement: Not applicable.

Informed Consent Statement: This study and the findings generated were part of a routine implementation conducted to facilitate sensitization of vaccine uptake. The observed results and newness motivated the implementers to share the results with other implementers from different parts of the world so we can influence or help others with the same challenges.

Data Availability Statement: The original contributions presented in the study are included in the article, further inquiries can be directed to the corresponding author.

Conflicts of Interest: The authors declare no conflicts of interest.

Abbreviations

AMREF	African Medical and Research Foundation
CHAVITA	Tanzania Association of the Deaf
CHMT	Council Health Management Team
CHW	Community Health Worker
DC	District Commissioner
DED	District Executive Director
HCD	Human-Centered Design
HCWs	Healthcare workers
HLIs	Higher Learning Institutions
JHPIEGO	Johns Hopkins Program for International Education in Gynecology and Obstetrics
MEO	Mtaa Executive Officer
MoH	The Ministry of Health
RMO	Regional Medical Officer
SHIVYAWATA	Tanzania Federation of Disabled People's Organizations
TADIO	Tanzania Association of the Deafblind
UNICEF	United Nations International Children's Emergency Fund
WEO	Ward Executive Office
WHO	World Health Organization

References

1. World Health Organization (WHO). Child Mortality and Causes of Death. 2022. Available online: https://www.who.int/data/gho/data/themes/topics/topic-details/GHO/child-mortality-and-causes-of-death (accessed on 10 March 2023).
2. Oyo-Ita, A.; Oduwole, O.; Arikpo, D.; Effa, E.E.; Esu, E.B.; Balakrishna, Y.; Chibuzor, M.T.; Oringanje, C.M.; Nwachukwu, C.E.; Wiysonge, C.S.; et al. Interventions for improving coverage of childhood immunisation in low- and middle-income countries. *Cochrane Database Syst. Rev.* **2023**, *2023*, CD008145. [CrossRef] [PubMed]
3. Sharrow, D.; Hug, L.; You, D.; Alkema, L.; Black, R.; Cousens, S.; Croft, T.; Gaigbe-Togbe, V.; Gerland, P.; Guillot, M.; et al. Global, regional, and national trends in under-5 mortality between 1990 and 2019 with scenario-based projections until 2030: A systematic analysis by the UN Inter-agency Group for Child Mortality Estimation. *Lancet Glob. Health* **2022**, *10*, e195–e206. [CrossRef] [PubMed]
4. Enyew, E.B.; Tareke, A.A. Vaccination status and factors associated among children age 12–23 months in Ethiopia, based on 2016 EDHS: Logit based multinomial logistic regression analysis. *PLoS ONE* **2022**, *17*, e0264004. [CrossRef] [PubMed]
5. Liu, L.; Oza, S.; Hogan, D.; Chu, Y.; Perin, J.; Zhu, J.; Lawn, J.E.; Cousens, S.; Mathers, C.; Black, R.E. Global, regional, and national causes of under-5 mortality in 2000–15: An updated systematic analysis with implications for the Sustainable Development Goals. *Lancet* **2016**, *388*, 3027–3035. [CrossRef] [PubMed]
6. Talbird, S.; Carrico, J.; La, E.M.; Carias, C.; Marshall, G.S.; Roberts, C.S.; Chen, Y.; Nyaku, M. Impact of Routine Childhood Immunization in Reducing Vaccine-Preventable Diseases in the United States. *Pediatrics* **2022**, *150*, e2021056013. [CrossRef]
7. UNICEF and World Health Organization (WHO). *Progress and Challenges with Achieving Universal Immunization Coverage*; UNICEF and World Health Organization (WHO): Geneva, Switzerland, 2019. Available online: https://cdn.who.int/media/docs/default-source/immunization/coverage/who-immuniz.pdf?sfvrsn=72fd7237_2&download=true (accessed on 20 June 2023).
8. Galadima, A.N.; Zulkefli, N.A.M.; Said, S.M.; Ahmad, N. Factors influencing childhood immunisation uptake in Africa: A systematic review. *BMC Public Health* **2021**, *21*, 1475. [CrossRef]
9. Yaya, S.; Uthman, O.A.; Okonofua, F.; Bishwajit, G. Decomposing the rural-urban gap in the factors of under-five mortality in sub-Saharan Africa? Evidence from 35 countries. *BMC Public Health* **2019**, *19*, 616. [CrossRef]
10. Vasudevan, L.; Baumgartner, J.N.; Moses, S.; Ngadaya, E.; Mfinanga, S.G.; Ostermann, J. Parental concerns and uptake of childhood vaccines in rural Tanzania—A mixed methods study. *BMC Public Health* **2020**, *20*, 1573. [CrossRef]
11. World Health Organization (WHO). *Ending Disease in Africa: Status of Immunization Coverage in Africa as of the End of 2022*; WHO African Region: Brazzaville, Republic of Congo, 2023. Available online: https://www.afro.who.int/sites/default/files/2023-10/Status%20of%20immunization%20coverage_final-compressed_compressed.pdf (accessed on 15 July 2023).
12. Legesse, E.; Dechasa, W. An assessment of child immunization coverage and its determinants in Sinana District, Southeast Ethiopia. *BMC Pediatr.* **2015**, *15*, 31. [CrossRef]
13. Adedokun, S.; Uthman, O.; Adekanmbi, V.; Wiysonge, C. Incomplete childhood immunization in Nigeria: A multilevel analysis of individual and contextual factors. *BMC Public Health* **2017**, *17*, 236. [CrossRef]
14. Gebeyehu, N.A.; Asmare, A.G.; Dagnaw, T.K.; Birhan, A.B. Vaccination dropout among children in Sub-Saharan Africa: Systematic review and meta-analysis. *Hum. Vaccin. Immunother.* **2022**, *18*, 2145821. [CrossRef] [PubMed]
15. Cooper, S.; Schmidt, B.-M.; Sambala, E.Z.; Swartz, A.; Colvin, C.J.; Leon, N.; Wiysonge, C.S. Factors that influence parents' and informal caregivers' views and practices regarding routine childhood vaccination: A qualitative evidence synthesis. *Cochrane Database Syst. Rev.* **2021**, *10*, CD013265. [CrossRef] [PubMed]
16. Tu, P.; Smith, D.; Parker, T.; Pejavara, K.; Michener, J.L.; Lin, C. Parent-Child Vaccination Concordance and Its Relationship to Child Age, Parent Age and Education, and Perceived Social Norms. *Vaccines* **2023**, *11*, 1210. [CrossRef]
17. Bangura, J.B.; Xiao, S.; Qiu, D.; Ouyang, F.; Chen, L. Barriers to childhood immunization in sub-Saharan Africa: A systematic review. *BMC Public Health* **2020**, *20*, 1108. [CrossRef]
18. Dubé, E.; Leask, J.; Wolff, B.; Hickler, B.; Balaban, V.; Hosein, E.; Habersaat, K. The WHO tailoring immunization Programmes (TIP) approach: Review of implementation to date. *Vaccine* **2018**, *36*, 1509–1515. [CrossRef]
19. Bartlett, R.; Boyle, J.A.; Smith, J.S.; Khan, N.; Robinson, T.; Ramaswamy, R. Evaluating human-centred design for public health: A case study on developing a healthcare app with refugee communities. *Res. Involv. Engag.* **2021**, *7*, 32. [CrossRef] [PubMed]
20. IDEO.org. The Field Guide to Human-Centered Design, 1st ed. 2015. Available online: https://www.designkit.org/ (accessed on 5 April 2023).
21. Kindig, S. Solving Problems with Human-Centred Design: Gates Cambridge. 2015. Available online: https://www.huffingtonpost.co.uk/gates-cambridge-scholars/solving-problems-with-hum_b_8581626.html (accessed on 20 March 2023).
22. Hendricks, S.; Conrad, N.; Douglas, T.S.; Mutsvangwa, T. A modified stakeholder participation assessment framework for design thinking in health innovation. *Healthcare* **2018**, *6*, 191–196. [CrossRef]
23. Itad 2018. Evaluation of The Hewlett Foundation's Strategy to Apply Human-Centered Design to Improve Family Planning and Reproductive Health Services in Sub-Saharan Africa: Hewlett Foundation. Available online:

https://www.itad.com/knowledge-product/evaluation-of-the-hewlett-foundations-strategy-to-apply-human-centred-design-to-improve-family-planning-and-reproductive-health-in-sub-saharan-africa/ (accessed on 12 August 2023).
24. Mummah, S.A.; Robinson, T.N.; King, A.C.; Gardner, C.D.; Sutton, S. IDEAS (integrate, design, assess, and share): A framework and toolkit of strategies for the development of more effective digital interventions to change health behavior. *J. Med. Internet Res.* **2016**, *18*, e317. [CrossRef]
25. Sambayuka, B.; Mwendo, E.; Babyebonela, L.; Kisanga, J.A.; Marandu, S.; Tinuga, F.; Kinyunyi, P.; Kyesi, F.; Mfaume, R.; Guillot, A.; et al. Improving Urban Immunization and Reducing the Zero-dose Children: Results from Implementation Study in Dar es-Salaam, Tanzania. *Adv. Prev. Med. Health Care* **2023**, *6*, 1042. [CrossRef]
26. Shearer, J.C.; Nava, O.; Prosser, W.; Nawaz, S.; Mulongo, S.; Mambu, T.; Mafuta, E.; Munguambe, K.; Sigauque, B.; Cherima, Y.J.; et al. Uncovering the Drivers of Childhood Immunization Inequality with Caregivers, Community Members and Health System Stakeholders: Results from a Human-Centered Design Study in DRC, Mozambique and Nigeria. *Vaccines* **2023**, *11*, 689. [CrossRef]
27. UNICEF. *Embedding a Human Centered Design Approach into Sub-National Coverage and Equity Assessments (v3)*; UNICEF: New York, NY, USA, 2020.
28. Brown, T.; Wyatt, J. Design thinking for social innovation. *Stanford Soc. Innov. Rev.* **2010**, *8*, 30–35. [CrossRef]
29. Isa, S.S.; Liem, A. Exploring the role of physical prototypes during co-creation activities at LEGO company using case study validation. *CoDesign* **2020**, *17*, 330–354. [CrossRef]
30. Vogel, I. *Review of the Use of Theory of Change in International Development*; DFID: London, UK, 2012.
31. Bazzano, A.N.; Martin, J.; Hicks, E.; Faughnan, M.; Murphy, L. Human-centred design in global health: A scoping review of applications and contexts. *PLoS ONE* **2017**, *12*, e0186744. [CrossRef]
32. Göttgens, I.; Oertelt-Prigione, S. The application of human-centered design approaches in health research and innovation: A narrative review of current practices. *JMIR mHealth uHealth* **2021**, *9*, e28102. [CrossRef] [PubMed]
33. Hogan, D.; Gupta, A. Why Reaching Zero-Dose Children Holds the Key to Achieving the Sustainable Development Goals. *Vaccines* **2023**, *11*, 781. [CrossRef]
34. Reñosa, M.D.C.; Bärnighausen, K.; Wachinger, J.; Endoma, V.; Landicho, J.; Aligato, M.F.; Landicho-Guevarra, J.; Bravo, T.A.; Scott, K.; Bärnighausen, T.; et al. Messy but worth it: Human-centred design as applied within a successful vaccine-promotive campaign. *BMJ Glob. Health* **2024**, *9*, e014870. [CrossRef]
35. Ingle, E.A.; Shrestha, P.; Seth, A.; Lalika, M.S.; Azie, J.I.; Patel, R.C. Interventions to Vaccinate Zero-Dose Children: A Narrative Review and Synthesis. *Viruses* **2023**, *15*, 2092. [CrossRef]
36. Sigdel, B.; Jin, Y.; Dhakal, P.; Luitel, T.; Ghimire, P.K.; Wasti, S.P. Factors Affecting Compliance with Childhood Immunization in Ilam District of Nepal: A Case-Control Study. *Dialog Health* **2023**, *2*, 100140. [CrossRef] [PubMed]
37. Hamad, F.S.; Kalabamu, F.S. Missed Opportunities for Vaccination Among Children Under Five Years of Age: A Cross-Sectional Study at Mwananyamala Regional Hospital, Dar es Salaam, Tanzania. *Tanzan. Med. J.* **2021**, *32*, 126–136.
38. Muathe, E.C.; Kamau, M.; Rajula, E. Exploring Strategies to Improve Adherence to Immunization Schedule: A Study among Children Attending Maternal and Child Health Clinic at Kenyatta National Hospital, Nairobi, Kenya. *Int. J. Pediatr.* **2020**, *2020*, 4730205. [CrossRef]

vaccines

MDPI

Article

Impact of Measles, Mumps, and Rubella Vaccination on Hospitalizations and Human Capital: Evidence from Copenhagen School Health Records

Onur Altindag [1,2], Jane Greve [2,3] and Erdal Tekin [2,4,*]

1 Department of Economics, Bentley University, Waltham, MA 02452, USA; oaltindag@bentley.edu
2 Institute of Labor Economics (IZA) and National Bureau of Economic Research (NBER), 53113 Bonn, Germany; jagr@vive.dk
3 VIVE—The Danish Center for Social Science Research, 1052 Copenhagen, Denmark
4 School of Public Affairs, American University, Washington, DC 20016, USA
* Correspondence: tekin@american.edu

Abstract: Background: This paper investigates the long-term effects of the measles, mumps, and rubella (MMR) vaccine on healthcare, education, and economic outcomes using a novel dataset from the Copenhagen School Health Records Register. **Methods:** To address potential endogeneity, we use within-sibling variation in vaccination status induced by different periods of vaccine availability in Denmark. **Results:** Our findings reveal that, prior to the establishment of herd immunity, vaccinated cohorts experienced substantial protection against hospitalizations related to MMR. During the same period, we also observe modest improvements in educational outcomes and positive—though statistically insignificant—estimates for labor market outcomes among siblings with discordant vaccination status. We find no impact of vaccination on hospitalizations, education, or economic outcomes for cohorts born after herd immunity was established, a period when everyone benefited from herd protection regardless of individual vaccination status. **Conclusions:** MMR vaccination, before herd immunity, reduced hospitalization due to Measles, Mumps, and Rubella. The impact on later outcomes, such as education, income, and employment lacks statistical precision at conventional levels. Evidence suggest positive self-selection in vaccination among families with high socioeconomic status.

Keywords: measles, mumps, and rubella; MMR; vaccine; Denmark; school; vaccination; healthcare; education; economic outcomes

1. Introduction

The development of vaccines marks one of the most remarkable public health breakthroughs in human history, transforming global health by substantially reducing disease burdens through direct protection against infections and the establishment of herd immunity. A notable example of this achievement is the introduction of the measles vaccine in 1963 in the United States, followed by a combined measles, mumps, and rubella (MMR) vaccine in 1971. Before these vaccines, nearly everyone was infected with major outbreaks every two to three years, with approximately 30 million cases and 2.6 million annual deaths worldwide [1,2] (in the United States alone, it has been estimated that 3 to 4 million people were infected each year, leading to approximately 400 to 500 deaths, 48,000 hospitalizations, and 1000 cases of encephalitis [3]). The introduction of measles vaccine produced immediate and significant benefits, drastically reducing mortality and morbidity associated with the disease. For instance, by 1965, the number of measles cases in the U.S. began to plummet, with only about 22,000 cases reported in 1968—a drop of over 97 percent in just three years. Globally, the World Health Organization estimates that vaccination efforts have averted approximately 57 million deaths globally between 2000 and 2022 [4].

There is an extensive literature in economics suggesting that interventions that improve health early in life might contribute to improvements in human capital later [5–8]. However, it is proposed that the developmental advantages linked to vaccine-induced health improvements could be particularly strong with the measles vaccine. This suggestion stems from the widespread epidemiological evidence documenting reductions in infectious disease mortality in many parts of the world following measles vaccination, which cannot be solely attributed to preventing acute measles deaths [9–12]. One explanation for the stronger than expected benefits of the measles vaccine is the concept of "trained immunity", where vaccines, particularly live-attenuated ones like the measles vaccine, bolster the innate immune system's response to various pathogens through epigenetic and metabolic changes [13–15]. Alternatively, a series of studies hypothesize that it is the concept of "measles-induced immune amnesia", that leads to the loss of immune memory cells, resulting in excess non-measles morbidity and mortality, which may last up to five years after measles infection [11,16,17]. These discoveries imply that the total benefits of the measles vaccine, as inferred from the wider literature on vaccine impact, may be underestimated.

Recently, these findings have sparked interest in the social sciences literature aimed at understanding the impact of the measles vaccine on human capital and labor market outcomes. Specifically, studies have examined the impact of introducing the measles vaccine or implementing mass measles vaccination campaigns in several countries, including the United States [18,19], the United Kingdom [20], Mexico [21], and South Africa [22] (the vast majority of the literature on the effects of childhood vaccination focuses on mortality rather than other outcomes—we do not discuss this literature in the interest of space). Atwood [18] shows that the introduction of the measles vaccine in the United States caused increases in earnings and employment among cohorts after the licensing of the vaccine, where the increase in earnings was driven by greater productivity rather than an increase in hours worked. Barteska et al. [19] also explores the United States context, emphasizing the consequences of the mass vaccination campaign introduced four years after the licensing of the measles vaccine. Their paper considers educational attainment rather than solely focusing on labor market outcomes. Their results suggest that the mass vaccination campaign led to an increase of 0.1 years in education among the affected cohorts, albeit only among males. Atwood and Pearlman [21] investigated the impact of a nationwide measles vaccination program in Mexico on the human capital and labor market outcomes of men. They documented substantial increases in educational attainment, employment, and income due to the program with effect sizes two to ten times greater than those found in the U.S. In the context of the United Kingdom, van den Berg et al. [20] showed that exposure to vaccination in early childhood has no influence on years of education. They found a positive effect on adult height, but only among those possessing higher levels of genetic endowment for height, as identified by polygenic scores. Finally, Anekwe et al. [22] examined the impact of measles vaccination on education levels among children in a poor and rural South African community. We identified several studies examining the relationship between vaccination and cognitive and human capital outcomes in developing countries—using propensity score matching, Nandi et al. [23] found that children vaccinated against measles have improved child anthropometry, cognition, and schooling outcomes in Ethiopia, India, and Vietnam. Bloom et al. [24] showed that full vaccination against measles, polio, and tuberculosis is associated with improvements in cognitive test scores in the Philippines, also using propensity matching to control for selection into vaccination status. Lastly, Driessen et al. [25] examined the phased implementation of a vaccination campaign in Bangladesh and showed that vaccination led to increased school enrolment among boys. However, these studies may not fully account for the potential endogeneity stemming from measles exposure or the vaccination decision). This study differs from the others in that it employs a mother fixed-effects model to account for the characteristics that may influence the vaccination decision of parents such as risk attitudes and future aspirations. Using variation based on a sample of 607 children who shared the same mother, but differed in measles vaccination status, the study revealed that measles vaccination increases the average school grade attainment by 0.188 grades.

In this study, we examined a range of human capital and healthcare outcomes to evaluate the long-term impacts of MMR vaccination. Human capital is captured by various measures of education and labor market productivity derived from Danish administrative registries spanning 1977 to 2018. Specifically, educational measures include an indicator for not completing ten years of mandatory education by age 16, an indicator representing those whose highest level of education is ten years or less by age 21, and an indicator for being not in education, employment, or training (NEET) at age 21. Labor market outcomes include an indicator for employment status, annual labor market income, and an indicator for the receipt of social benefits, all measured at age 24. These outcomes collectively capture important aspects of human capital, reflecting both educational attainment and long-term economic engagement [26–29]. For healthcare, we assess hospitalization due to MMR by age 5 and between ages 2 and 12, obtained from administrative records from 1977 to 2006. These data are combined with a unique dataset from the Copenhagen School Health Records Register to evaluate the impact of MMR vaccination on health outcomes for birth cohorts born between 1977 and 1986. Employing a sibling fixed-effects approach, our research design relies on within-family variation in vaccination status driven by differences in vaccine availability over time. By focusing on periods before and after the establishment of herd immunity in Denmark, this design mitigates the selection bias and enables the causal estimation of the effects of MMR vaccination on hospitalizations, as well as educational and labor market outcomes. Overall, this study provides new insights into both the direct and indirect impacts of MMR vaccination. By examining cohorts exposed to varying levels of herd immunity, we contribute to understanding the broader implications of vaccination, including its influence on health, educational, and economic outcomes.

2. Materials and Methods

2.1. The Introduction of the Measles Vaccine in Denmark

The combined version of the measles, mumps, and rubella (MMR) vaccine was incorporated into the Danish Vaccination Program (DCVP) on 1 January 1987. Before 1987, 98 percent of the population had contracted measles in Denmark, but this proportion significantly decreased following the introduction of the MMR vaccine [30].

Denmark introduced the MMR vaccine relatively late compared to neighboring countries such as Sweden, Finland, and Norway, where it had been in use since the early 1980s [31]. The delayed adoption of the MMR vaccine in Denmark stemmed from various factors, including the perception of measles, mumps, and rubella as less urgent health threats compared to other diseases. Additionally, Denmark's reliance on rubella screening programs rather than vaccinations created a path dependency that hindered the integration of new vaccine-based strategies. Institutional inertia, along with political and economic factors further contributed to the delay. However, changes in international health policy during the 1980s, focusing on cost-effectiveness and broader public health benefits, eventually persuaded Danish politicians to include the MMR vaccine in the DCVP.

Prior to the introduction of the MMR vaccine, vaccines against diseases like diphtheria, tetanus, pertussis, and polio were already included in the program. The MMR vaccine had been available for several years before it was officially introduced into the national program, with parents often paying for it out of pocket. The measles vaccine was additionally recommended for high-risk children (EPI-NEWS, 11/1982), leading to ambiguity in the expected direction of self-selection. On one hand, the cost of the vaccine (as it was not free) likely encouraged positive self-selection, whereby healthier children from families with higher socioeconomic status were more likely to be vaccinated. On the other hand, the recommendation for high-risk groups may have resulted in children with poorer baseline health being more frequently vaccinated. Official statistics, which are consistent with our analysis, suggest that the effect of positive self-selection was more pronounced. For instance, in 1983, the Statens Serum Institute distributed 9416 doses of the measles vaccine, 3734 doses of the mumps vaccine, and 653 doses of the rubella vaccine. In the years leading up to 1987 between 15,000 and 25,000 children were vaccinated (EPI-NEWS, 48/1986). The majority of these doses were administered to healthy children at the request of their parents, rather than to those in high-risk groups [32].

Vaccines within the DCVP are provided free of charge and administered by general practitioners (GPs). According to the Danish Health Care Act (Sundhedsloven), all children residing in Denmark are offered seven preventive GP visits (known as Børneundersøgelser) before beginning school. These visits are scheduled at five weeks, five months, one year, two years, three years, four years, and five years of age. During the initial visit after birth, the GP informs parents about the immunizations included in the program. Since the first MMR vaccination is given at 15 months of age, parents must arrange an additional appointment with their primary care physician, beyond the seven preventive visits. Prior to 1987, parents were required to pay for the MMR vaccination, with the cost of one dose of MMR vaccine in 1985 being DKK 110 (including tax), equivalent to around DKK 225/USD 31 in 2020, excluding any GP fees (EPI-NEWS, 44/1985). The fees charged by GPs for administering vaccinations varied ranking from DKK 150 to 300 in 2020. Adjusting this cost to 1985 prices, the fee accounts for approximately half of the vaccine's price.

Upon the introduction of the MMR vaccination into the DCVP, there was a short transition period lasting approximately one year. During this phase, all children aged 2–12 who had not previously contracted measles or mumps were offered the vaccine, leading to a large-scale immunization effort [33]. From 1987 to 2016, the National Board of Health advised MMR immunizations at 15 months (MMR1) and 12 years (MMR2) (A booster dose (MMR2), administered at the age of 4, was introduced in 2008. The rationale for the change was to increase herd immunity by increasing the immunity of children aged under 12 years [34]).

2.2. Data

2.2.1. Copenhagen School Health Records Register

The Copenhagen School Health Records Register (CSHRR) contains comprehensive health data collected through school health examinations [35]. The data in the CSHRR were primarily collected during mandatory school health examinations conducted at the entry and exit points of school education in Copenhagen (the school health records only exist for Copenhagen—approximately 20% of the Danish population lives in Copenhagen). The Danish National Health Service Registry (DNHSR) started recording MMR vaccine data from 1990 onward. However, prior to 1996, procedural constraints prevented the direct linkage of services to children under 16 years old. Consequently, detailed information on the immunization status of individuals born before, during, and after the introduction of the MMR vaccine in Denmark in 1987 was previously unavailable. To improve data accessibility, we undertook a substantial effort to digitize individual vaccination records from the physical files of the Copenhagen School Health Record Register for cohorts born between 1977 and 1994 [32]. This process involved a detailed history taken from parents regarding their child's health and vaccination record. We digitized the physical files of these records, including detailed vaccine information, enhancing the accessibility and usability of the data for research purposes. As a result of these efforts, the CSHRR now includes data on the type of MMR vaccination administered (MMR1 or MMR2), along with the dates of these vaccinations. The data were described in detail, compared with vaccine information available from reimbursement records for later cohorts, and validated in Altindag et al. [32].

We use the vaccine information for cohorts from 1977 to 1994. The raw data include 68,239 children. Following the approach in Altindag et al. [32], we exclude children from our study who had missing information about all vaccines, as can be seen in Altindag et al. [32]. The children with missing information on any additional vaccines other than MMR mainly consist of children whose parents did not provide any vaccine information in their children's health card. Removing the children with no information on any vaccines does not introduce significant selection into the sample. This resulted in a total of 58,735 observations remaining in our sample. Furthermore, as a sizeable proportion of immigrants not born in Denmark have missing information on immunizations, we exclude these observations, focusing on 52,816 children born in Denmark in our main analysis. Although excluding children not born in Denmark makes the sample more comparable to the full Danish population, we acknowledge that it is not fully representative of the entire population in Denmark.

As we describe in the empirical strategy, our primary research design relies on within-sibling comparisons in the MMR vaccination status to mitigate the bias arising from the potential endogeneity of vaccination decisions. In our full sample of 52,816 children, 27,734 are siblings born to 12,452 unique mothers. Among sibling pairs born before 1987, 30% have discordant vaccination statuses. For sibling pairs that include siblings born both before and after 1987, 24% have discordant vaccination statuses. In sibling pairs born after 1987, 17% display differing vaccination statuses (see Table A1).

2.2.2. Healthcare, Education, and Labor Market Outcomes

We link our samples from the CSHRR to several administrative registers maintained by Statistics Denmark using a unique civil registration number, which facilitates connections between children and their parents and siblings. For the children, we include information on birth year, gender, birth order, and parental education, with parental information measured in the year before birth.

Using extensive records on hospital admissions and diagnoses from 1977 through 2006, we construct binary indicator variables for being hospitalized with MMR before age 5 and at ages between 2 and 12, respectively. The later age-restriction is motivated by the age-range where the children receive the MMR vaccination (age 15 months and 12 years).

Next, we construct the measures of educational and labor market outcomes for the children using administrative registries from 1977 through 2018. The educational outcomes include an indicator for not completing ten years of education with a final exam before age 16. In Denmark, it is mandatory to receive at least 10 years of education; however, approximately 10% do not complete the final exam after 10 years of education [36]. This indicator is a measure of the expected long run human capital outcome as these children have a high probability of not completing any further education [36]. As individuals with no formal education beyond basic education tend to perform less successfully in the labor market, the lack of formal education is widely regarded as a significant economic and social issue in most countries. Therefore, we constructed an indicator representing those whose highest completed education is ten years or less by the age of 21. Similarly, we created an indicator for whether individuals are employed or pursuing further education, meaning that they are not part of the group categorized as not in education, employment, or training (NEET) at the age of 21.

We consider three labor market outcomes measured at age 24. These include an indicator for being employed (where the main income during the year is from wage or self-employment), annual gross wage income (we use the inflation-adjusted annual gross wage, with the baseline year set as 2018), and an indicator for receiving social benefits, such as unemployment or social security benefits. While the first two outcomes serve as indicators of long-term economic well-being, we are limited by measuring these outcomes at the age of 24, the age at which labor market data are available for all cohorts (we have access to registry data up until 2018). At this age, some individuals may still be enrolled in education and therefore not yet employed or earning an income. The latter outcome, which measures the probability of receiving social benefits, reflects a relatively weak attachment to the labor market and offers an additional way to assess long-term economic consequences.

Table 1 presents the descriptive statistics for the child and mother characteristics and the outcome variables for both the full sample and the sibling sample included in the analysis. Both samples exhibit similar child characteristics and socioeconomic outcomes: 49% of the children are female, both have an identical dropout rate before grade 9 (12%), and the same proportion of youths active at the age of 21 (83%). The key differences lie in family structure due to the sibling sample only consisting of families with multiple children. The sibling sample has more children per family (2.36 vs. 1.71), and mothers who are more likely to be married (63% vs. 58%). While variables related to family composition and maternal characteristics show statistically significant differences, the two samples are largely comparable in terms of children's hospitalization, education, and labor market outcomes.

Table 1. Descriptive statistics.

	Full Sample		Sibling Sample		Mean Difference
	n	%	n	%	
Child characteristics					
Female	25,906	49.0%	13,958	49.0%	0.0
Birth year, mean (Std. dev.)	1986.1	(5.3)	1986.3	(4.9)	−0.2
Mother characteristics					
Number of children in family, mean (Std. dev.)	1.70	(0.84)	2.36	(0.69)	−0.64
One child	24,347	46.1%	0.00	0.00	46.1
Two children	20,466	38.7%	20,466	71.9%	33.1
Three children	5761	10.9%	5761	20.2%	−9.3
Four children	1624	3.1%	1624	5.7%	−2.6
Five or more children	2242	4.2%	2242	7.8%	−3.6
Married	30,152	57.6%	17,854	63.3%	−5.7
Basic education	22,590	43.1%	12,770	45.3%	−2.1
Vocational or high school	16,618	31.7%	8099	28.7%	3.0
Further education	13,146	25.1%	7334	26.0%	0.9
Age at birth, mean (Std. dev.)	28.32	(20.50)	28.29	(23.16)	0.03
Hospitalizations due to measles, mumps, and rubella (per 100,000 births)					
Ages 0–5, mean (Std. dev.)	6.97	(83.18)	6.24	(78.73)	0.73
Ages 2–12, mean (Std. dev.)	4.37	(65.99)	3.75	(61.12)	0.62
Human capital and labor market outcomes					
Dropping out before grade 9	6320	12.2%	3308	11.8%	0.4
Not advancing beyond grade 9	13,556	26.6%	7334	26.7%	−0.1
Active at age 21 (not NEET)	42,438	83.2%	22,905	83.3%	−0.1
Employed at age 24	22,843	45.4%	12,144	44.7%	0.6
Annual wage income at age 24, mean (Std. dev.)	160,710	(11,877)	159,824	(120,222)	885
Received social benefits at 24	15,541	29.4%	8449	29.7%	−0.3

Notes: Number of observations is 52,816 in the full sample and 27,734 in the sibling sample. NEET is an acronym used to define young people not in education, employment, or training. Annual real wage income is in DKK, adjusted for inflation using 2018 as the base year. Wage information only exists for those with positive values, with 41,945 observations for the full sample and 22,018 for the sibling sample. Comparing the means of the full and sibling samples, the following variables are significantly different at $p = 0.001$: birth year, number of children, mother's partner status, and education.

2.3. Empirical Strategy

We employ a within-sibling difference-in-differences approach to estimate the short- and long-run effects of MMR immunization among children in our sample. The distinct phases of vaccination in Denmark allow for a unique comparison of siblings with discordant vaccination statuses across two periods: 1977–1986 and 1987–1994.

The first period includes cohorts born in 1977 through 1986, during which the MMR vaccine was not part of the national immunization program. Although the vaccine was available on the market, uptake was low, and herd immunity had not been established. Consequently, all children born during this period were exposed to circulating measles, mumps, and rubella viruses, with only vaccinated children receiving individual protection.

The second period covers birth cohorts from 1987 to 1994. During this time, a large-scale immunization campaign was launched, and the MMR vaccine became freely available through the national immunization program. Due to high vaccination rates and the establishment of herd immunity, most children born after 1986 were not exposed to measles, mumps, or rubella viruses, regardless of their individual vaccination status. Therefore, only cohorts born between 1976 and 1986 are expected to exhibit any effects from the MMR vaccine, as they were exposed to circulating pathogens. Therefore, the post-1986 herd immunity period offered an opportunity to perform a placebo test, where any observed effects, including the primary health impacts of the MMR vaccine, should diminish or disappear.

Moreover, our approach relies on sibling fixed effects, which substantially mitigates any bias from self-selection into vaccine uptake. Since, most often, the same parents make the immunization decision for all siblings, the decision should primarily be influenced by time-varying conditions, likely due to supply-side factors, rather than by socio-economic and cultural characteristics that might be correlated with both vaccination status and later-life health and economic outcomes.

In this context, our regression model can be specified as follows:

$$y_{itm} = \alpha + \tau \text{MMR}_{it} + \delta(\text{MMR}_{it} \times \text{Post}_t) + \lambda_t + \mu_m + \gamma X_{imt} + \epsilon_{itm}, \quad (1)$$

where y_{itm} represents the short- and long-run outcomes for child i born in year t to mother m. The right-hand side variables include a constant α, an indicator for individual immunization status for MMR_{it} and its interaction with an indicator variable Post_t that equals one if the child is born on or after 1987. The regression also controls for birth year fixed effects λ_t, sibling fixed effects μ_m, a vector of controls X_{imt} including sibling-varying factors such as birth order fixed effects and gender. We denote the residual fluctuation around the outcome with ϵ_{itm}.

In Equation (1), τ shows the effect of the vaccine for a child born during the high-exposure period, while $\tau + \delta$ represents the vaccine effect for the no-exposure period. We expect any vaccine effects on child health and later life outcomes to be captured by τ and estimate null effects for the latter. To illustrate the extent of bias in naive estimates, we also present results without sibling fixed effects. Additionally, we provide estimates without X_{imt} to confirm that child-level characteristics do not significantly impact vaccine uptake. Standard errors are clustered at the sibling level to account for within-sibling correlation across our regression outcomes.

The causal interpretation of τ relies on the assumption that the factors driving discordance in MMR immunization status across siblings are not endogenous to health and later-life economic outcomes. In addition, the vaccine should have an impact on our outcomes if the vaccinated individual was born before 1987, with no effect expected for cohorts born after herd immunity was established by the 1986 massive immunization campaign.

3. Results

3.1. Immunization Campaign and Herd Immunity

We begin by analyzing the incidence rates of hospitalizations for the under-5 population in Copenhagen due to measles, mumps, and rubella (MMR) over the 75 months before and 75 months after the initiation of the nationwide vaccination campaign. This descriptive analysis helps us empirically establish the onset of widespread immunity in our sample. Figure 1 shows the monthly time trend of the annualized incidence rate of hospitalization in the under-5 population in our analysis sample from the Copenhagen School Health Records Register (CSHRR), which includes children born in Denmark between 1977 and 1994. The figure is centered around January 1987, the start of the nationwide vaccination campaign. The vertical line around 12 months after the introduction of the vaccine in the DCVP indicates the transition period during which all children aged 2–12 were offered the vaccine.

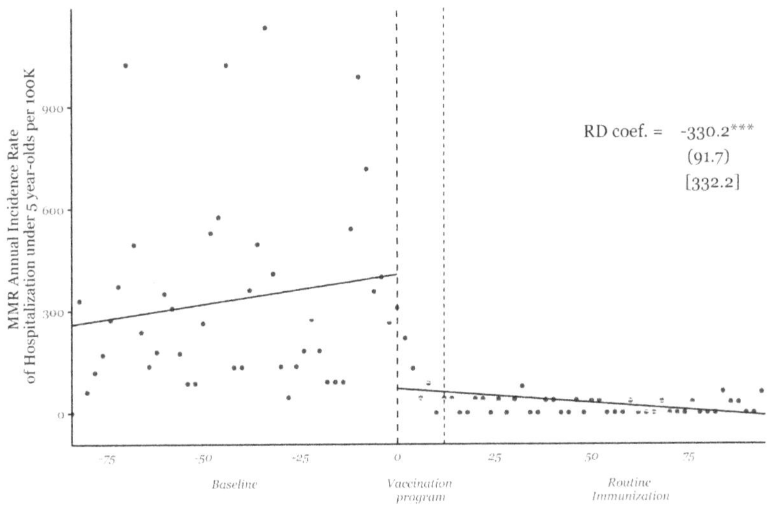

Figure 1. Annualized incidence rate of hospitalization in the under-5 population in Copenhagen and fitted linear trends: 75 months before and after the introduction of the nationwide vaccination campaign (vertical line at 0). The vertical line 12 months after the introduction indicates the transition period during which all children aged 2−12 were offered the vaccine. Regression discontinuity (RD) method estimate the drop in hospitalization incidence rate (see Equation (2)). *** $p < 0.01$.

We also fit linear trend lines for the 75 months before and after the vaccination campaign and provide a regression discontinuity estimate to quantify the sudden drop in hospitalization incidence due to the massive and successful immunization effort. Formally, we estimate the following regression:

$$HR_t = \alpha + \beta \text{Post}_t + f(S_t) + \epsilon_t \quad \text{for all} \quad S_t \in (c - h, c + h), \tag{2}$$

where HR_t denotes the incidence rate of hospitalization at time t, Post_t is a binary variable that equals 1 for the period following the nationwide vaccination campaign and 0 otherwise, and S_t represents the running variable calculated as the number of months relative to January 1987. We fit two continuous linear functions, $f(S_t)$, on either side of the regression sample, encompassing data from h months before and after the vaccination campaign. We use an ad hoc bandwidth of 75 months as this specification is primarily intended to distinguish between two distinct periods in terms of widespread herd immunity in Copenhagen. Given the birth cohort structure of the data, we calculated robust standard errors using the Newey–West estimator, which accounts for heteroskedasticity and autocorrelation up to lag 1.

In this model, β captures the abrupt drop in the hospitalization incidence rate attributable to the vaccination campaign in Denmark. Figure 1 clearly illustrates that the immunization campaign was highly successful, nearly eliminating MMR-related hospitalizations. The annualized monthly incidence rate of hospitalization was 332.2 cases per 100,000 children under 5 years old before the campaign, which virtually dropped to zero following the MMR campaign and subsequent routine immunizations, thanks to the establishment of widespread immunity. While these figures pertain to Copenhagen, similar trends and declines are observed in (a population-based version of) nationwide data. Figure 1 using data from Denmark is available upon request from the authors.

Given that measles is highly contagious, achieving and maintaining herd protection is challenging. Although there are still rare and sporadic cases of measles, the data clearly show that measles has been eliminated as a significant contagious disease in Denmark following the vaccination campaign.

These results highlight the two distinct periods that we analyze in our study. Before the vaccination campaign, only those who were individually vaccinated were protected against these viruses. However, after the campaign, the individual vaccination status became less critical due to the immediate establishment of widespread community protection.

3.2. Cohort Analysis of MMR-Related Hospitalizations

Next, we focus on our sibling sample to estimate the direct health effects of MMR immunization before and after the vaccination campaign among siblings with discordant vaccination status. The regression results presented in Table 2 illustrate the impact of MMR vaccination on the number of hospitalizations due to measles, mumps, and rubella per 10,000 births within 5 years after birth and between 2 and 12 years of age, across different specifications. Columns (1) and (4) show the baseline OLS estimates, where the model controls only for cohort fixed effects. The coefficient on the vaccine effect for the pre-1987 cohort is significant and negative in both columns, indicating a substantial reduction in hospitalizations during the high-exposure period. Specifically, the estimates suggest that vaccination reduced hospitalizations by 8.65 per 10,000 births within 5 years (column 1) and by 6.66 per 10,000 births within 12 years (column 4).

Table 2. Impact of MMR vaccination on hospitalizations due to measles, mumps, and rubella.

	Hospitalization Within 5 Years			Hospitalization Between Age 2–12		
	(1)	(2)	(3)	(4)	(5)	(6)
Pre-1987 cohort	−8.65 ***	−10.64 ***	−10.61 ***	−6.66 ***	−8.92 ***	−8.93 ***
	[−12.28, −5.02]	[−17.46, −3.83]	[−17.46, −3.76]	[−9.68, −3.63]	[−14.68, −3.16]	[−14.71, −3.15]
Post-1987 cohort	−0.32	1.25	1.23	−0.73	0.33	0.42
	[−1.33, 0.69]	[−2.63, 5.14]	[−2.61, 5.07]	[−1.71, 0.25]	[−2.80, 3.47]	[−2.70, 3.53]
Post–Pre difference	8.34 ***	11.90 ***	11.84 ***	5.93 ***	9.25 ***	9.35 ***
	[4.56, 12.11]	[3.88, 19.92]	[3.82, 19.86]	[2.75, 9.11]	[2.53, 15.98]	[2.62, 16.07]
N	52,816	27,734	27,734	52,816	27,734	27,734
Outcome mean	13.45	12.10	12.10	8.60	7.54	7.54
Clusters (mother)	37,534	12,452	12,452	37,534	12,452	12,452
R^2	0.01	0.47	0.47	0.01	0.48	0.48
Cohort FE	X	X	X	X	X	X
Sibling FE		X	X		X	X
Gender FE			X			X
Birth Order FE			X			X

Notes: *** $p < 0.01$ [95% CI]. Standard errors are clustered at the mother level. The outcome is the number of hospitalizations due to measles, mumps, and rubella per 10,000 births for children within the first 5 years of life and for children aged 2–12 years.

In columns (2) and (5), we add sibling fixed effects, which are the preferred specifications because they control for unobserved family-level characteristics that may influence both vaccine uptake and health outcomes. The results remain similar, with the vaccine effect for the pre-1987 cohort still significant and slightly larger in magnitude, reducing hospitalizations by 10.64 per 10,000 births for children within the first 5 years of life, and by 8.92 per 10,000 births for children aged 2–12 years.

Columns (3) and (6) further include controls for gender and birth order fixed effects, which show similar results. As in the previous analysis, the relative changes indicate herd immunity for cohorts born after 1987. Compared to the outcome mean, column (3) shows a decrease of approximately 87% (10.61/12.10) within 5 years, and column (6) shows a complete elimination of hospitalization cases within 12 years after birth for cohorts born before 1987.

The coefficients for the post-1987 cohort are not statistically different from zero across all columns, consistent with the expectation that the vaccine's direct impact would diminish due to the establishment of herd immunity during the no-exposure period. The difference between the pre- and post-1987 effects, captured by the post–pre difference, is significant in all specifications, reinforcing the idea that the vaccine had a substantial protective effect during the high-exposure period but not in the period after the vaccination campaign.

3.3. *Indirect Effect of MMR Vaccine on Later Life Economic Outcomes*

In addition to the documented health benefits of the MMR vaccine, we explore its potential longer-term non-targeted effects on education, labor market outcomes, and income. Table 3 presents the impact of MMR vaccination on educational outcomes for two cohorts: those born before the 1987 vaccination campaign, those born on or after it, and the difference between the two.

Table 3. The impact of vaccination on the probability of dropping out, not advancing, and being active before and after the introduction of the MMR vaccine.

	Dropping Out Before Grade 9			Not Advancing at Age 21			Active (Not NEET) at Age 21		
	(1)	(2)	(3)	(4)	(5)	(6)	(7)	(8)	(9)
Pre-1987 cohort	−2.81 *** [−3.69, −1.93]	−1.39 [−3.28, 0.50]	−0.97 [−2.86, 0.92]	−7.14 *** [−8.46, −5.82]	−2.75 ** [−5.19, −0.32]	−2.21 * [−4.64, 0.22]	4.96 *** [3.89, 6.04]	2.49 ** [0.23, 4.75]	2.20 * [−0.07, 4.46]
Post-1987 cohort	−3.99 *** [−5.36, −2.62]	−0.52 [−3.07, 2.03]	−0.30 [−2.84, 2.23]	−9.17 *** [−10.87, −7.47]	−1.55 [−4.61, 1.51]	−1.45 [−4.49, 1.60]	5.74 *** [4.22, 7.27]	−0.40 [−3.20, 2.40]	−0.45 [−3.25, 2.35]
Post-Pre difference	−1.18 [−2.80, 0.45]	0.87 [−2.21, 3.95]	0.67 [−2.40, 3.73]	−2.03 * [−4.17, 0.11]	1.20 [−2.64, 5.04]	0.76 [−3.06, 4.59]	0.78 [−1.08, 2.64]	−2.89 [−6.42, 0.65]	−2.65 [−6.18, 0.88]
N	51,687	27,108	27,108	50,998	26,465	26,465	50,998	26,465	26,465
Outcome Mean	10.03	9.99	9.99	28.41	28.06	28.06	84.47	84.75	84.75
Clusters (mother)	36,756	12,177	12,177	36,479	11,946	11,946	36,479	11,946	11,946
R^2	0.01	0.51	0.51	0.01	0.59	0.59	0.01	0.52	0.52
Cohort FE	X	X	X	X	X	X	X	X	X
Sibling FE		X	X		X	X		X	X
Gender FE			X			X			X
Birth order FE			X			X			X

Notes: *** $p < 0.01$, ** $p < 0.05$, * $p < 0.1$. [95% CI]. Standard errors are clustered at the mother level.

For the pre-1987 cohort, the results using sibling fixed effects indicate some improvement in educational outcomes. Specifically, we observe a statistically insignificant reduction of 0.97 to 1.39 percentage points in the likelihood of dropping out before Grade 9; a statistically significant decrease of 2.21 to 2.75 percentage points in the likelihood of not advancing beyond Grade 9 (an 8.2% to 9.8% improvement relative to the outcome mean of 28.06%); and a 2.2 to 2.49 percentage point increase in the likelihood of being active (either employed, in education, or in training), which represents a 2.6% to 2.9% improvement relative to the outcome mean of 84.75%.

For cohorts born after the herd immunity period, there are no significant differences between MMR-vaccinated children and their non-vaccinated siblings. Furthermore, we lack the statistical power to detect a significant difference-in-differences estimate across the outcomes in any of the specifications.

3.4. Economic Outcomes Associated with MMR Vaccination

We assess the association of the MMR vaccination with longer-term economic outcomes, including employment, annual wage income, and social benefits, as presented in Table 4. The OLS results without sibling fixed effects again suggest a positive self-selection, particularly for cohorts who were vaccinated when the MMR vaccine was not part of the nationwide immunization program. Estimates for net-of-sibling fixed effects are substantially muted and statistically insignificant for all outcomes and specifications. For older vaccinated cohorts, before 1987, discordant siblings suggest a 1.3 to 1.9 percentage point increase in employment compared to a mean of 49.6%, a 0.5 to 2% increase in real wage income measured at the age of 24, and a 1.6–1.8% decrease in the probability of receiving social benefits at the age of 24. For cohorts born on or after 1987, there is no such consistent pattern across point estimates and outcomes. The difference-in-differences estimates are accordingly unable to differentiate the vaccine effect in two distinct periods in Denmark.

Table 4. Impact of vaccination on wage income and the probability of being employed and receiving social benefits at age 24 before and after the introduction of the MMR vaccine.

	Employed at 24 (Wage or Self-Employed)			Wage Income at 24 (Annual Earnings > 0)			Social Benefits (Received at Age 24)		
	(1)	(2)	(3)	(4)	(5)	(6)	(7)	(8)	(9)
Pre-1987	1.28 *	1.30	1.88	1839	789	2896	−3.98 ***	−0.46	−0.53
	[−0.15, 2.71]	[−1.56, 4.17]	[−0.97, 4.73]	[−1685, 6023]	[−5954, 10,320]	[−3597, 12,448]	[−5.28, −2.67]	[−3.05, 2.13]	[−3.12, 2.07]
Post-1987	−0.34	0.66	0.81	−3476	−4504	−4226	−7.68 ***	1.07	1.03
	[−2.14, 1.46]	[−2.82, 4.15]	[−2.66, 4.28]	[−6724, 2887]	[−10,913, 8560]	[−10,474, 8932]	[−9.36, −6.00]	[−2.07, 4.20]	[−2.11, 4.17]
Pre-Post diff.	−1.62	−0.64	−1.07	−5314	−5294	−7122	−3.70 ***	1.53	1.56
	[−3.91, 0.67]	[−5.01, 3.74]	[−5.43, 3.29]	[−10,244, 2068]	[−15,786, 9067]	[−17,516, 7122]	[−5.83, −1.58]	[−2.44, 5.50]	[−2.41, 5.53]
N	50,368	25,888	25,888	41,945	19,069	19,069	52,816	27,734	27,734
Outcome Mean	50.6	49.6	49.6	147,545	147,659	147,659	30.3	29.6	29.6
Clusters	36,188	11,708	11,708	31,691	8815	8815	37,534	12,452	12,452
R-squared	0.01	0.55	0.56	0.00	0.57	0.58	0.01	0.55	0.55
Cohort FE	X	X	X	X	X	X	X	X	X
Sibling FE		X	X		X	X		X	X
Gender FE			X			X			X
Birth Order FE			X			X			X

Notes: *** $p < 0.01$, * $p < 0.1$. [95% CI]. Standard errors are clustered at the mother level.

4. Discussion

This study investigates the long-term impacts of the MMR vaccine on both health and economic outcomes. By using a unique dataset from the Copenhagen School Health Records Register, we use the variation in the vaccination statuses of siblings between two distinct phases of vaccination in Denmark to account for family-level heterogeneity that could confound the estimated effects of the MMR vaccine.

Our findings underscore the critical role of the MMR vaccine in reducing hospitalizations due to measles, mumps, and rubella among children in Denmark, particularly during the high-exposure period prior to the nationwide immunization campaign in 1987. The introduction of the vaccine not only diminished the immediate health risks associated with these diseases but also contributed to a near elimination of MMR-related hospitalizations post-vaccination, demonstrating the effectiveness of the vaccine in establishing herd immunity.

Beyond the direct health benefits, our study investigates the potential broader socioeconomic advantages provided by the MMR vaccine. Our empirical results suggest that MMR vaccination prior to herd immunity was associated with modest improvements in educational outcomes, including a reduction in the likelihood of not completing ten years of education with a final exam before age 16, a decrease in the likelihood of completing only ten years or less of education by the age of 21, and an increase in the likelihood of being employed or pursuing further education, thus avoiding classification as not in education, employment, or training at age 21. We also examine economic outcomes such as employment, real wage income, and reliance on social benefits, which show patterns consistent with the educational findings. However, these estimates lack statistical precision, limiting our ability to draw strong conclusions about the vaccine's effects on human capital.

Finally, for all human capital outcomes, the association between vaccination and human capital accumulation decreases substantially in magnitude across all outcomes and cohorts when we include sibling fixed effects, which suggests strong positive self-selection by parents of higher socioeconomic status in vaccinating their children.

These results contribute to the growing body of literature examining the effects of the measles vaccine on human capital and labor market outcomes. Using population-level administrative data from Denmark, our analysis offers new insights into the long-term impacts of measles vaccination within the context of a developed country with universal healthcare. Given the limited number of studies on these outcomes and the mixed findings in the existing literature, our investigation provides much-needed evidence to advance the field towards a consensus.

Our investigation differs from the concurrent measles literature in three aspects. First, all previous studies—with the exception ofAnekwe et al. [22]—rely on a research design that leverages variation in pre-vaccination measles infection rates across states or regions and cohort differences in vaccine exposure driven by year of birth in a difference-in-differences framework. In this paper, we use unique data on the actual measles vaccination status of individuals born between 1977 and 1994, which we recently digitized from the Copenhagen School Health Records Register. These data encompass comprehensive health information collected through school examinations. With actual information on the vaccination status linked to rich administrative data obtained from demographic and health registers, our primary strategy for identification is based on a sibling fixed-effects design, in which we compare the long-term outcomes of siblings with discordant vaccination status.

Second, the setting of our analysis differs substantially from those in the concurrent measles literature. Importantly, the measles vaccine was introduced in Denmark in 1987, much later than in most other countries. Unlike the United States, the United Kingdom, and Mexico—where the vaccine was introduced decades earlier in 1963, 1968, and 1973, respectively—Denmark's later adoption allows for a more contemporary analysis of the effect of the measles vaccine. Therefore, the evidence from the current analysis aligns with more recent changes in both educational systems and labor markets, offering insights that are relevant to the current context.

Third, existing studies exclusively focus on education and labor market outcomes. In contrast, we are equipped with a wide range of health information including hospitalizations from administrative data registers. We use these data to first demonstrate that the sharp declines in hospitalizations due to measles following the introduction of the vaccine as well as to investigate non-specific health effects within a unified framework.

Limitations

Despite the strengths of our sibling fixed-effects research design—which includes a long period of herd immunity providing a powerful placebo test—this study is not without limitations. One concern is the potential for residual confounding due to unobserved factors that change within families over time. For example, shifts in living conditions, parental preferences, economic fluctuations, differing sibling health conditions (including contraindications to vaccinate), or later social restrictions (e.g., kindergarten or school policies for unvaccinated children) could influence vaccination decisions and potentially bias the results if they are correlated with the outcomes.

For later-life human capital outcomes, such as education, income, and employment, our analysis lacks statistical precision at conventional levels. This is primarily because these outcomes are measured much later in life, making them inherently noisier due to the extended time lag between the cause (vaccination) and the effect. Over this time, various other factors contribute to human capital formation, potentially mitigating any negative effects associated with a lack of vaccination. As a result, isolating the specific impact of vaccination on these outcomes becomes more challenging, leading to less precise estimates. It is important to note that our sample may also be underpowered to capture later downstream outcomes since we only have data until the age of 24 and some individuals may still be enrolled in education, meaning we do not fully capture the long-term effects on economic and labor market outcomes.

Finally, the environment in which children grow up can greatly influence the effects of vaccines. Since our study was conducted in Denmark—a country with a comprehensive healthcare system and low levels of health stressors—it may not fully capture the potential benefits that vaccination programs could have in less-resourced settings. In environments where adequate nutrition is lacking, anemia rates are higher, and other health challenges are more prevalent, the benefits of vaccination may be significantly amplified.

5. Conclusions

This study examines the long-term impacts of the MMR vaccine on health, education, and labor market outcomes using a unique dataset and a sibling fixed-effects research design. Our findings confirm the significant role of MMR vaccination in reducing hospitalizations due to measles, mumps, and rubella prior to the establishment of herd immunity. Beyond health, we find that vaccination before herd immunity modestly improved educational outcomes, with positive but statistically imprecise estimates for labor market measures such as employment and labor market income. The evidence also suggests positive self-selection in vaccination, particularly among families with higher socioeconomic status, emphasizing the need to account for such factors when evaluating vaccine effects.

Author Contributions: Conceptualization, O.A., J.G. and E.T.; Methodology, O.A., J.G. and E.T.; Formal Analysis, O.A. and J.G.; Investigation, O.A., J.G. and E.T.; Resources, O.A., J.G. and E.T.; Data Curation, O.A. and J.G.; Writing—Review and Editing, O.A., J.G. and E.T.; Supervision, O.A., J.G. and E.T.; Project Administration, O.A., J.G. and E.T.; Funding Acquisition, O.A., J.G. and E.T. All authors have read and agreed to the published version of the manuscript.

Funding: The authors disclose the receipt of the following financial support for the research, authorship, and/or publication of this article: Data collection and research was funded by the Novo Nordisk Foundation (grant NFF180CO034296).

Institutional Review Board Statement: This project is not a clinical study and no institutional review board statement was required. We use secondary data (the Copenhagen School Health Record Registry) merged with other registry data.

Informed Consent Statement: The paper uses psydonomized registry data, implying that individual consent was not required.

Data Availability Statement: This paper uses confidential data from Danish administrative registry databases. Therefore, we are not able to make these data publicly available. However, researchers can apply for access to data from Statistics Denmark. Researchers based in institutions outside Denmark can access the data through an affiliation with a Danish authorized research institution. We agree to guiding interested researchers in pursuing these data. In replication files, we will provide all scripts/codes that perform the empirical analyses.

Acknowledgments: We thank Matvei Andersen for excellent research assistance. The CSHRR was initiated by Thorkild I. A. Sørensen and built by the Institute of Preventive Medicine, the Capital Region of Denmark. We thank Jennifer Lyn Baker for her support and work in the digitization of the vaccine information in the CSHRR. We also thank participants at the workshop Health Innovations, Vaccines, Individual Behaviors, and Inequalities in Health and Care, at the Danish Center for Social Science Research and Value of Vaccination Research Network (VoVRN) community and David Bloom for comments and suggestions.

Conflicts of Interest: The authors declared no potential conflicts of interest with respect to the research, authorship and/or publication of this article.

Abbreviations

The following abbreviations are used in this manuscript:

MMR	Measles, Mumps, and Rubella
CSHRR	Copenhagen School Health Records Register
DVP	Danish Vaccination Program
GP	General Practitioners

Appendix A

Table A1. Number of Discordant Siblings and Discordance Rate.

		Sibling 2		
Pre-campaign		No vaccine	Vaccine	Total
Sibling 1	No vaccine	686	803	1489
	Vaccine	793	3043	3836
	Total	1479	3846	5325
	Discordance rate			0.30
Pre- and post-campaign		No vaccine	Vaccine	Total
Sibling 1	No vaccine	316	719	1032
	Vaccine	777	4404	5181
	Total	1093	5123	6216
	Discordance rate			0.24
Post-campaign		No vaccine	Vaccine	Total
Sibling 1	No vaccine	264	487	751
	Vaccine	471	4411	4882
	Total	735	4898	5633
	Discordance rate			0.17
Full sibling sample		No vaccine	Vaccine	Total
Sibling 1	No vaccine	1142	1756	2898
	Vaccine	1798	10,586	12,384
	Total	2940	12,342	15,282
	Discordance rate			0.23

Note: The table shows the discordance in vaccine status among siblings with the same mother (within mother). The discordance rate is the number of discordant sibling pairs relative to the total number of sibling pairs.

References

1. Strebel, P.M.; Cochi, S.L.; Hoekstra, E.; Rota, P.A.; Featherstone, D.; Bellini, W.J.; Katz, S.L. A world without measles. *J. Infect. Dis.* **2011**, *204*, S1–S3. [CrossRef] [PubMed]
2. Wolfson, L.J.; Strebel, P.M.; Gacic-Dobo, M.; Hoekstra, E.J.; McFarland, J.W.; Hersh, B.S. Has the 2005 measles mortality reduction goal been achieved? A natural history modelling study. *Lancet* **2007**, *369*, 191–200. [CrossRef] [PubMed]
3. Centers for Disease Control and Prevention. History of Measles. 2024. Available online: https://www.cdc.gov/measles/about/history.html (accessed on 5 October 2024).
4. Minta, A.A. Progress toward measles elimination—Worldwide, 2000–2022. *MMWR Morb. Mortal. Wkly. Rep.* **2023**, *72*, 1262–1268. [CrossRef] [PubMed]

5. Almond, D.; Currie, J. Killing me softly: The fetal origins hypothesis. *J. Econ. Perspect.* **2011**, *25*, 153–172. [CrossRef]
6. Almond, D.; Currie, J.; Duque, V. Childhood circumstances and adult outcomes: Act II. *J. Econ. Lit.* **2018**, *56*, 1360–1446. [CrossRef]
7. Currie, J.; Almond, D. Human capital development before age five. In *Handbook of Labor Economics*; Elsevier: Amsterdam, The Netherlands, 2011; Volume 4, pp. 1315–1486.
8. Bharadwaj, P.; Løken, K.V.; Neilson, C. Early life health interventions and academic achievement. *Am. Econ. Rev.* **2013**, *103*, 1862–1891. [CrossRef]
9. Aaby, P.; Bukh, J.; Lisse, I.M.; Smits, A.J. Measles vaccination and reduction in child mortality: A community study from Guinea-Bissau. *J. Infect.* **1984**, *8*, 13–21. [CrossRef]
10. Aaby, P.; Samb, B.; Simondon, F.; Seck, A.M.C.; Knudsen, K.; Whittle, H. Non-specific beneficial effect of measles immunisation: Analysis of mortality studies from developing countries. *BMJ* **1995**, *311*, 481–485. [CrossRef]
11. Mina, M.J.; Metcalf, C.J.E.; De Swart, R.L.; Osterhaus, A.; Grenfell, B.T. Long-term measles-induced immunomodulation increases overall childhood infectious disease mortality. *Science* **2015**, *348*, 694–699. [CrossRef]
12. Mogensen, S.W.; Aaby, P.; Smedman, L.; Martins, C.L.; Rodrigues, A.; Benn, C.S.; Ravn, H. Introduction of standard measles vaccination in an urban African community in 1979 and overall child survival: A reanalysis of data from a cohort study. *BMJ Open* **2016**, *6*, e011317. [CrossRef]
13. De Bree, L.; Koeken, V.A.; Joosten, L.A.; Aaby, P.; Benn, C.S.; van Crevel, R.; Netea, M.G. Non-specific effects of vaccines: Current evidence and potential implications. In *Seminars in Immunology*; Elsevier: Amsterdam, The Netherlands, 2018; Volume 39, pp. 35–43.
14. Aaby, P.; Benn, C.S. Developing the concept of beneficial non-specific effect of live vaccines with epidemiological studies. *Clin. Microbiol. Infect.* **2019**, *25*, 1459–1467. [CrossRef]
15. Aaby, P.; Netea, M.G.; Benn, C.S. Beneficial non-specific effects of live vaccines against COVID-19 and other unrelated infections. *Lancet Infect. Dis.* **2023**, *23*, e34–e42. [CrossRef] [PubMed]
16. Frederick, E. How measles causes the body to 'forget'past infections. *Science* **2019**, *366*, 560–561. [CrossRef] [PubMed]
17. Laksono, B.M.; de Vries, R.D.; Verburgh, R.J.; Visser, E.G.; de Jong, A.; Fraaij, P.L.; Ruijs, W.L.; Nieuwenhuijse, D.F.; van den Ham, H.J.; Koopmans, M.P.; et al. Studies into the mechanism of measles-associated immune suppression during a measles outbreak in the Netherlands. *Nat. Commun.* **2018**, *9*, 1–10. [CrossRef] [PubMed]
18. Atwood, A. The long-term effects of measles vaccination on earnings and employment. *Am. Econ. J. Econ. Policy* **2022**, *14*, 34–60. [CrossRef]
19. Barteska, P.; Dobkowitz, S.; Olkkola, M.; Rieser, M. Mass vaccination and educational attainment: Evidence from the 1967–68 Measles Eradication Campaign. *J. Health Econ.* **2023**, *92*, 102828. [CrossRef]
20. van den Berg, G.J.; Scholder, S.v.H.K.; Vitt, N. *Early Life Exposure to Measles and Later-Life Outcomes: Evidence from the Introduction of a Vaccine*; School of Economics, University of Bristol: Bristol, UK, 2023.
21. Atwood, A.; Pearlman, S. The Long Term Benefits of Vaccination Campaigns: Evidence from Measles. *J. Health Econ.* **2025**, *101*, 102974. [CrossRef]
22. Anekwe, T.D.; Newell, M.L.; Tanser, F.; Pillay, D.; Bärnighausen, T. The causal effect of childhood measles vaccination on educational attainment: A mother fixed-effects study in rural South Africa. *Vaccine* **2015**, *33*, 5020–5026. [CrossRef]
23. Nandi, A.; Shet, A.; Behrman, J.R.; Black, M.M.; Bloom, D.E.; Laxminarayan, R. Anthropometric, cognitive, and schooling benefits of measles vaccination: Longitudinal cohort analysis in Ethiopia, India, and Vietnam. *Vaccine* **2019**, *37*, 4336–4343. [CrossRef]
24. Bloom, D.E.; Canning, D.; Shenoy, E.S. The effect of vaccination on children's physical and cognitive development in the Philippines. *Appl. Econ.* **2012**, *44*, 2777–2783. [CrossRef]
25. Driessen, J.; Razzaque, A.; Walker, D.; Canning, D. The effect of childhood measles vaccination on school enrolment in Matlab, Bangladesh. *Appl. Econ.* **2015**, *47*, 6019–6040. [CrossRef]
26. Card, D. The Causal Effect of Education on Earnings. In *Handbook of Labor Economics*; Elsevier: Amsterdam, The Netherlands, 1999.
27. Bynner, J.; Parsons, S. Social exclusion and the transition from school to work: The case of young people not in education, employment, or training (NEET). *J. Vocat. Behav.* **2002**, *60*, 289–309. [CrossRef]
28. Heckman, J.J.; Lochner, L.J.; Todd, P.E. Earnings functions, rates of return and treatment effects: The Mincer equation and beyond. *Handb. Econ. Educ.* **2006**, *1*, 307–458.
29. Oreopoulos, P. Do dropouts drop out too soon? Wealth, health and happiness from compulsory schooling. *J. Public Econ.* **2007**, *91*, 2213–2229. [CrossRef]
30. Kirkedal, A.B.K.; Møller, J.E.; Stensballe, L.G.; Zoffmann, V. Parents' and Health Professionals' Attitudes to Advancing Primary MMR Vaccine Administration from Fifteen to Six Months of Age—A Qualitative Thematic Analysis Embedded in a Randomized Trial. *Vaccines* **2022**, *11*, 67. [CrossRef]
31. Berg, A.H.; Blume, S.S. Reasonable Grounds? The Delayed Introduction of MMR Vaccine in Denmark and the Netherlands, 1977–87. *Med. Hist.* **2020**, *64*, 355–373. [CrossRef]

32. Altindag, O.; Andersen, M.; Baker, J.L.; Greve, J.; Tekin, E. Information on Measles, Mumps and Rubella Vaccine in the Copenhagen School Health Records Register. *Scand. J. Public Health* **2024**, 14034948241247882. [CrossRef]
33. Rønne, T.; Kaaber, K.; Petersen, I. Kendskab og holdninger samt tilslutning de første 2 år til de nye vaccinationer mod mæslinger, fåresyge og røde hunde. *Ugeskr Læger* **1989**, *151*, 2418–2422.
34. Rasmussen, L.D.; Fonager, J.; Knudsen, L.K.; Andersen, P.H.S.; Rønn, J.; Poulsen, M.W.; Franck, K.T.; Fischer, T.K. Phylogenetic and epidemiological analysis of measles outbreaks in Denmark, 2013 to 2014. *Eurosurveillance* **2015**, *20*, 30027. [CrossRef]
35. Baker, J.L.; Olsen, L.W.; Andersen, I.; Pearson, S.; Hansen, B.; Sørensen, T.I. Cohort profile: the Copenhagen school health records register. *Int. J. Epidemiol.* **2009**, *38*, 656–662. [CrossRef]
36. Danish Ministry of Children and Education. Elever der Ikke Aflægger alle Obligatoriske 9.-Klasseprøver. 2021. Available online: https://www.uvm.dk/-/media/filer/uvm/publikationer/2021/210112-elever-der-ikke-aflaegger-alle-obligatoriske-9-klasseproever-ua.pdf (accessed on 1 March 2025).

MDPI AG
Grosspeteranlage 5
4052 Basel
Switzerland
Tel.: +41 61 683 77 34

Vaccines Editorial Office
E-mail: vaccines@mdpi.com
www.mdpi.com/journal/vaccines

www.ingramcontent.com/pod-product-compliance
Lightning Source LLC
Chambersburg PA
CBHW041015270926
51850CB00024B/285
9783725846856